Learning
Electrocardiography
A Complete Course
Fourth Edition

Learning
Electrocardiography
A Complete Course
Fourth Edition

Jules Constant MD
State University of New York at Buffalo
Buffalo, NY

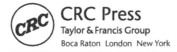

CRC Press
Taylor & Francis Group
Boca Raton London New York

CRC Press is an imprint of the
Taylor & Francis Group, an **informa** business

First published 2009 by Informa Healthcare USA, Inc.

Published 2019 by CRC Press
Taylor & Francis Group
6000 Broken Sound Parkway NW, Suite 300
Boca Raton, FL 33487-2742

© 2009 by Taylor & Francis Group, LLC (original copyright 2002 by The Parthenon Publishing Group, Ltd.)
CRC Press is an imprint of Taylor & Francis Group, an Informa business

First issued in paperback 2019

No claim to original U.S. Government works

ISBN 13: 978-0-367-44691-8 (pbk)
ISBN 13: 978-1-84214-206-6 (hbk)

Visit the Taylor & Francis Web site at
http://www.taylorandfrancis.com

and the CRC Press Web site at
http://www.crcpress.com

Contents

Causes of PVCs. Reentry Theory. Multiform Versus Multifocal PVCs. Ectopic Focus Theory. PVCs Versus Parasystole. Parasystole Defined. Parasystole and Coupling. Parasystolic Entrance and Exit Blocks. Parasystole and Fusion Beats. Parasystole Recognition. Reciprocal Beats. Ectopic Tachycardias. Atrial Fibrillation. Atrial and Ventricular Rates. Characteristics of f Waves. Causes of AF. AF and Digitalis. AF with Aberrant Conduction. Atrial Flutter. Atrial Flutter F Wave Characteristics. F Wave-QRS Relations. Causes of Atrial Flutter. Atrial Tachycardia. Reciprocal Beat Theory for ATs. AT in the WPW and Lown-Ganong-Levine Syndromes. AT with Block. Junctional Tachycardias. Wandering and Shifting Atrial Pacemakers. Multifocal or Chaotic AT. Isorhythmic Dissociation. Electrical Alternans. Ventricular Tachycardia. Mechanisms and Causes of VT. Chronic VT. Arrhythmogenic Right Ventricular Dyslplasia (ARVD). The Brugada Syndrome. Differentiation of VT from Supraventricular Tachycardias. AV Dissociation. Capture and Fusion Beats. Distinguishing VT from Its Commonest Mimic, a Regular Supraventricular Tachycardia with Aberrancy: Summary. Bidirectional Tachycardia. Ventricular Flutter and Fibrillation. Systematic Approach to Interpretation of an Arrhythmia

Preface

This book is designed for beginners and for fellows in cardiology. The two levels are separated by placing an asterisk in front of all material that is only for the fellow. The question and answer (Socratic) format is used because it focuses attention and also allows one to cover up the answer and use it as programmed learning on a second reading. Further, it requires the author to be brief and concise.

The book incorporates the author's experience of giving brief courses to physicians, medical students, and nurses several times a year for two decades. For example, the book concludes with a step-by-step method of reading an electrocardiogram (ECG). This is an invaluable aid for a student who is handed an ECG to read for the first time in an elective program in cardiology. Similarly, at the end of the discussion of arrhythmias is a step-by-step protocol for interpreting an arrhythmia. The hexaxial system in two planes is used to explain directional data, so the student becomes familiar with hexaxial system techniques by following the ECGs, most of which are mounted on a hexaxial system diagram. The method of drawing a spatial vector has been included for instructors who wish to show students how the electrical activity of the heart is represented on a chest wall.

In addition to the hundreds of new references, the fourth edition has many new diagrams and electrocardiograms. There are new explanations for such things as indeterminate axes, anterior QRS axes, R/S ratio progressions (normal and abnormal), the absence of initial force changes in some patients with divisional blocks, the T negativity in V1 in newborns, and the use of multifocal versus multiform PVCs.

Also to be found are new methods of ECG diagnosis of such phenomena as infarction in the presence of left bundle branch block, posterior infarction from T waves, right ventricular infarction, inferior infarction in the absence of a Q in lead 3 with anterior divisional block, pericarditis from ST/T ratios and P-R segments, apical hypertrophy, cachetic hearts, left pneumothorax, tricuspid regurgitation, right atrial overloads, and atrial infarction.

Many new uses for electrocardiography are introduced, including how an ECG can predict malignant hyperthermia, how to predict coronary events by treadmill testing, how to determine the cause of left ventricular enlargement, how to test for accessory AV pathway refractoriness, how to use simultaneous leads to diagnose divisional blocks in difficult cases, and how to use the new pacemaker codes.

Computer analysis of electrocardiograms is probably capable of correctly reading a perfectly normal ECG. When any abnormality is found, major disagreements may occur in about 25% of reviewed ECGs. Without review of the ECGs by a cardiologist, significant changes are missed.

1. Cardiac Anatomy and Physiology

A BRIEF NOTE FOR BEGINNING STUDENTS[1]

The heart consists of four chambers: two atria, mainly for receiving blood, and two ventricles, mainly for pumping blood.

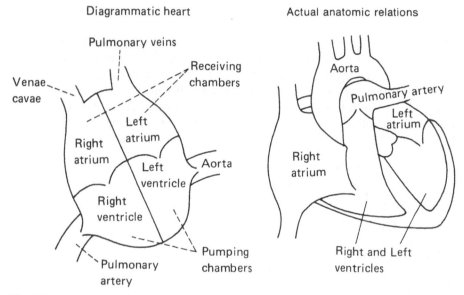

Diagrammatic heart   Actual anatomic relations

The right atrium is on the <u>anatomical right</u>, i.e., on the right from the point of view of a person standing facing you.

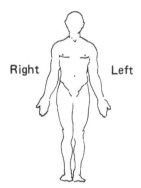

A man in the <u>anatomical position</u> is standing and facing you. <u>His</u> right is what is meant by <u>right</u> in anatomy and in electrocardiography.

[1] Physicians may find this section useful for giving their patients a brief background of knowledge that explains their cardiac problems more fully.

The electrical activity of the heart begins high in the right atrium in an area about 2.5 cm long called the sinoatrial (SA) node. This node is a collection of specialized muscle fibers with the ability to produce electrical impulses rhythmically. It is known as the normal 'pacemaker' of the heart.

After the electrical activity of the atria begins at the SA node, it spreads throughout both atria, producing the outline on an electrocardiogram (ECG) called the P wave.

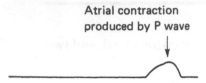

This P wave electrical activity reflects depolarization, i.e., cells coming out of their resting state. Once out of their resting state, the atria contract and push blood into the ventricles. The depolarizing impulse reaches the ventricles by way of a bridge of tissue where the atria meet the ventricles at the top of the interventricular septum (the thick muscular wall between the ventricles). This bridge, the atrioventricular (AV) node, consists of cells whose function is to slow conduction. It extends the slowed impulse to a bundle of conducting fibers known as the bundle of His.

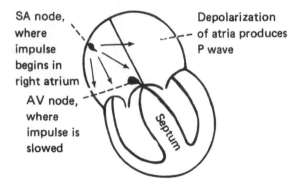

Once in the ventricular septum the bundle of His divides into two conduction fibers known as the right and left bundle branches. The terminal conduction fibers in the ventricular walls are called Purkinje fibers, after the anatomist who first described the fibers in 1845.

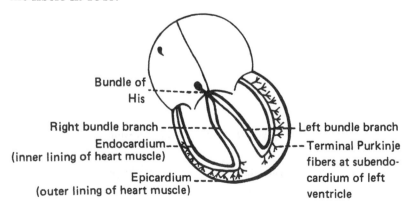

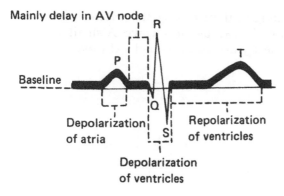

Conduction through the AV node, bundle of His, and bundle branches does not show on an ECG, so that only the baseline is drawn on ECG paper during their depolarization. This isoelectric interval that precedes the depolarization of the ventricle is called the P-R segment.

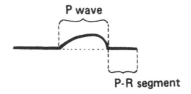

The bundle branches further subdivide the electrical current in the septum until the inner surface of the ventricles (subendocardium) is reached. Then the impulse spreads from the subendocardium to the epicardium (outer surface of the heart muscle). As both ventricles are depolarized in this way, from inner to outer surface, the electrical current produces a complex on ECG paper known as the QRS.

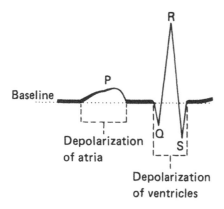

Finally, the ventricular cells repolarize, returning to their resting state. Return to the resting state causes the outline on ECG paper known as the T wave. A smaller ventricular repolarization wave often follows the T wave and is called a U wave.

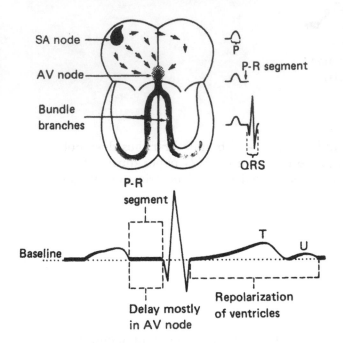

2. Electrical Activity of the Heart

1. Is there experimental proof that the heart actually produces electrical current?
   ANS.: Yes. When a frog leg is kept alive in an appropriate solution and the nerve is stimulated electrically, the muscle contracts. If the same nerve–muscle preparation is placed on the beating frog heart, the leg muscle contracts with each heartbeat.

2. What is meant by polarization of a cell?
   ANS.: It means that the resting cell has excess potassium inside and excess sodium outside and is thereby in a state of ionic imbalance. The selectively permeable cell membrane maintains the imbalance by allowing potassium and sodium to pass through it only at certain times when energy is available. The inside of the resting cell is always negative relative to the outside of the cell. (An easy way to remember this distinction is that both words *inside* and *negative* contain an *n*.)

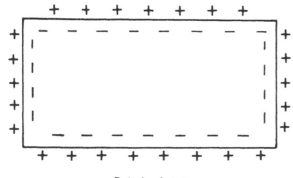

Polarized state

3. What is meant by depolarization of a cell?
   ANS.: It is the flow of ions (the electron carriers) across the cell membrane. When the membrane suddenly changes its permeability, sodium moves into the cell and potassium moves out. (In addition to the major flux of sodium and potassium, calcium flux also occurs.)

4. What is the relation between depolarization and contraction of heart muscle?
   ANS.: Depolarization initiates the process of contraction.

3. How an Electrocardiograph Works

FUNCTIONS OF AN ELECTROCARDIOGRAPH

1. What are the only two functions built into an electrocardiograph (ECG machine) by the electronic engineers?

    ANS.: The ECG machine is designed to show only the direction and magnitude of the electrical current produced by the heart. (It follows, then, that anyone who reads ECGs must be able to tell the direction of current at any point in the cardiac cycle.)

2. If current is flowing in all directions at once, how can an ECG writing arm follow all these directions in order to draw a single line?

    ANS.: The writing arm, or stylus, of an ECG machine can only swing up and down on a moving paper strip in response to resultant forces at each moment in time. (A resultant is the final force that is produced when forces with more than one direction and magnitude act on anything.)

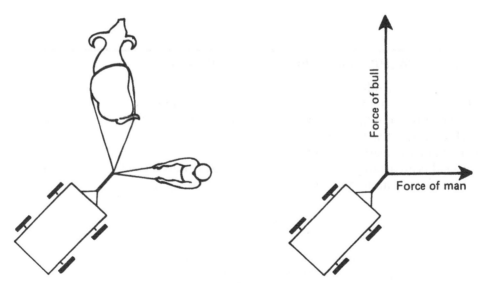

The direction in which the wagon travels is the resultant of the two forces pulling it.

3. How is a resultant calculated from two forces represented as arrows in the diagram?
   ANS.: By drawing a parallelogram using arrows whose direction represents the direction of the force and whose length represents the magnitude of the force. The resultant is a diagonal from the point of origin to the opposite angle.

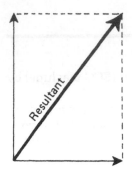

4. The ECG machine can draw the resultant of hundreds of forces occurring simultaneously in the heart. What term describes this function?
   ANS.: The term *resolving machine* may be used. The electrocardiograph resolves all the individual forces into their resultant and gives the direction and magnitude of the resultant force at each moment.

HOW THE ECG MACHINE MEASURES CURRENT DIRECTION

1. What is an ECG electrode?
   ANS.: It is a metal plate that can transmit electrical current from the body provided it has direct contact with the skin. A wire connects it to the ECG machine, which links it with one or more other electrodes.
2. What is meant by a 'lead', and how is it named?
   ANS.: A lead is an arrangement of two or more electrodes joined by wires that pass through the galvanometer of the electrocardiograph.

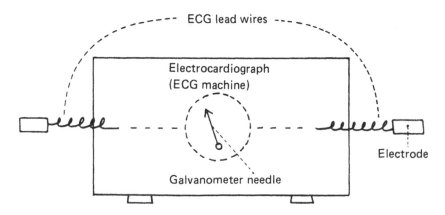

ECG lead = electrodes + lead wires + galvanometer.

The electrodes are placed at specific sites on the body, and the leads are named according to the body sites involved in the circuit. For example, leads with electrodes placed only on the limbs are called L1, L2, L3, aVR, aVL, and aVF. When electrodes are also placed on the chest, the leads are called precordial V leads and are numbered V1, V2, etc., depending on the chest site used.

3. What moves the writing arm, or stylus, of an ECG machine?

  ANS.: The galvanometer. It is a current meter that pivots a needle to and fro, depending on the direction of current passing through it. The galvanometer needle movement is directly responsible for the up-and-down motion of the stylus. The stylus is made to pivot upward if electrical current flows in one direction through the lead and downward if current flows in the opposite direction.

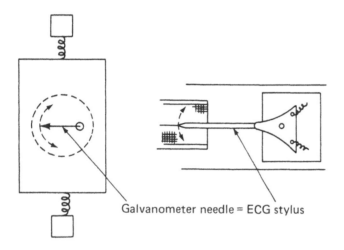

Galvanometer needle = ECG stylus

4. What is meant by a positive electrode?

  ANS.: It is a lead's electrode that engineers have arbitrarily designated positive. They have arranged it so that the movement of current toward this arbitrary electrode causes an upward deflection on ECG paper. *This concept is the most important in electrocardiography and must be memorized.* Put another way, if current through a lead makes the stylus of the ECG machine pivot upward, the current is flowing toward a positive electrode. We need only to learn the sites of the positive electrodes on the body in order to determine the direction of current that produces the ECG deflections.

4. Electrocardiographic Configuration and Nomenclature

ECG OF VENTRICULAR DEPOLARIZATION

1. What do we call the complex of waves that results from depolarization of the ventricles?
   ANS.: The QRS.
2. What is meant by the 'baseline' of an ECG?
   ANS.: The baseline is the horizontal line made by the stylus when electrical current is absent or too weak to disturb the galvanometer.
3. What is meant by a 'positive' or 'negative' deflection?
   ANS.: A positive deflection merely means a movement of the ECG stylus above the baseline, i.e., an upward deflection. A negative deflection means a movement below the baseline, or a downward deflection. It has no relation to positive or negative electricity but is merely customary usage for upward or downward movements.

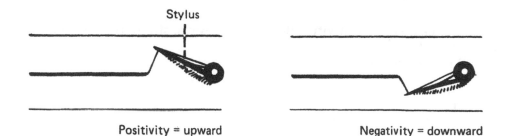

Positivity = upward   Negativity = downward

Note: The stylus is really an extension of the galvanometer needle, which is placed in the machine in such a way that it rotates up and down rather than from right to left.

4. What is a Q wave?
   ANS.: An initial *negative area* of the QRS. It is not the initial downward or negative deflection, as a wave cannot be made merely by one deflection.

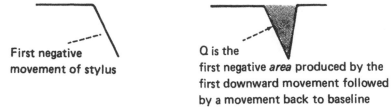

First negative movement of stylus

Q is the first negative *area* produced by the first downward movement followed by a movement back to baseline

A negative <u>area</u> can be produced only by a downward movement plus a movement <u>back to the baseline</u>.

5. What is an R wave?
   ANS.: The first positive area (above the baseline) produced by depolarization of the ventricles. An R wave may or may not be preceded by a Q wave.

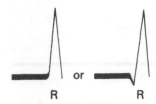

6. What is an S wave?
   ANS.: The first negative area that follows an R wave during depolarization of the ventricles.

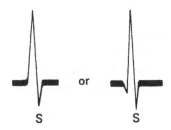

7. What do we call a second positivity following the S wave, still during depolarization of the ventricles?
   ANS.: An R prime written R′.

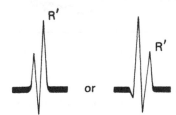

8. What do we call a negative area after an R′?
   ANS.: An S prime (S′), e.g.,

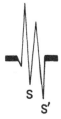

9. How does a deep notch on an R wave differ from an S wave?
   ANS.: The notch does not go below the baseline, e.g.,

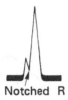

Notched R

10. What label do we give to a completely negative depolarization complex?
    ANS.: QS.

Q S

11. How can you symbolize the magnitude of the Q, R, or S deflection in writing?
    ANS.: By using lower-case letters for small amplitudes and capital letters for large amplitudes.

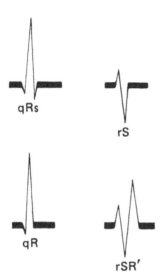

Note: Hereafter, we use the term QRS to denote the ventricular depolarization complex even with only a Qs, qR, rS, or R wave. This terminology is used simply to avoid having to repeat 'ventricular depolarization complex.'

ECG OF VENTRICULAR REPOLARIZATION

1. What are the ECG waves that result from ventricular repolarization?
   ANS.: The S-T, T, and U waves.
2. What is a T wave?
   ANS.: A T wave is the relatively long wave that follows a QRS and represents repolarization of the ventricle. The T wave may be low, high, negative, positive, or biphasic.

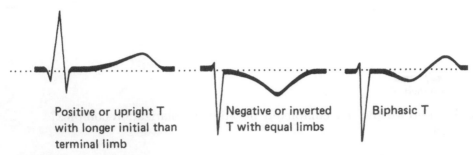

Positive or upright T
with longer initial than
terminal limb

Negative or inverted
T with equal limbs

Biphasic T

The normal T usually has a long initial limb and a shorter terminal limb, but it may also have equal limbs, as in the negative T above.

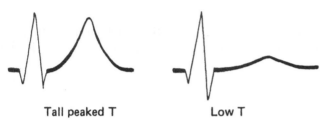

Tall peaked T   **Low T**

The tall peaked T and the low T are possible normal variants but may also be abnormal.

3. What is meant by an S-T segment?
   ANS.: It is the part of the T wave between the end of the QRS and the point at which the slope of the T wave appears to become steeper abruptly. The T is often simply called the S-T, T to show that the S-T is really just an arbitrary division of the repolarization wave. In many leads there is no obvious S-T segment because there is no point at which the slope changes abruptly.

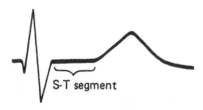

S-T segment

   Note: It is occasionally called the RS-T segment, especially in the older literature, probably because the QRS may end with either an R or an S.

4. What do we call the junction between the QRS and the S-T?
   ANS.: The J point. (J stands for 'junction.')

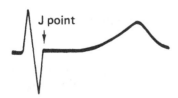

J point

5. What do we call an S-T that is
    a. Above the baseline?
    b. Below the baseline?
    ANS.: a. An elevated or positive S-T.
          b. A depressed or negative S-T.

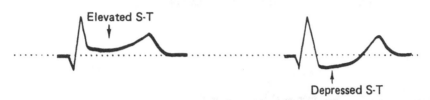

6. Is this 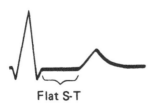 a terminal R′?

ANS.: No, it is only an S-T elevation because the QRS always finishes at or toward the baseline. An R′ must have an *area*; it cannot simply be a deflection above the baseline. The QRS ends at the baseline when there is S-T elevation.

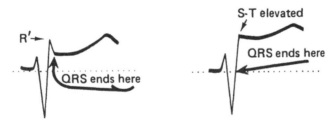

7. What do we call an S-T that is horizontal?
    ANS.: It is called flat or straight.

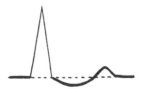

8. What is an S-T usually called when it is upward concave but *below the baseline*?
    ANS.: Sagging, e.g.,

9. What do we call an upright T that is decreased in amplitude?

    ANS.: A low T. Do not call a low T a 'flat' T. The term *flat* should be used only for S-T segments. An isoelectric T should be called a low T.

10. What is any wave between a T and the next P called?

    ANS.: A U wave. (See p. 326 for the cause of U waves.)

        Note: A small U wave is present in most ECGs.

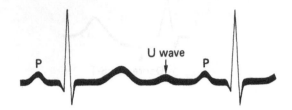

5. Electrocardiographic Language of Direction

1. How are the degrees of a circle named in electrocardiography so that no numbers over 180° are used?

   ANS.: The lower half of the circle is measured from 0° to 180° clockwise and given a *plus* sign. The upper half of the circle is measured from 0° to 180° upward, and the degrees are given a *minus* sign.

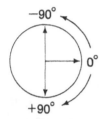

2. What is the electrocardiographic word for a radius with an arrow at the end?

   ANS.: A vector.

3. What is the mathematical meaning of the word *vector*?

   ANS.: It is a quantity with both magnitude and direction, represented by a straight line with an arrowhead.

4. What aspect of the meaning of vector do we stress in electrocardiography?

   ANS.: We are far more interested in the *direction* than in the magnitude of a vector. Thus we tend to use the word *vector* to describe merely a direction of current.

5. Describe approximately the direction in which current is traveling in the following diagrams.

   ANS.: A = + 60°, B = − 30°, C = + 150°, and D = − 60°.

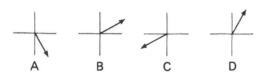

A   B   C   D

6. What is meant by 'right' and 'left' in ECG language?

ANS.: We mean the anatomical right and left, meaning the right and left from the point of view of a patient standing in front of you. Be sure you understand this principle, because, *from this chapter on, right and left are used in the anatomical sense; i.e., it means the patient's right and left.*

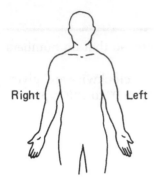

7. Why not use the system of counting all degrees clockwise from 0° to 360°?

Because small angles and numbers are easier to visualize and work with than large ones. For example, it is easier to visualize an angle of 60° above 0° (i.e. – 60°) than 300° down and around from 0° (i.e. + 300°).

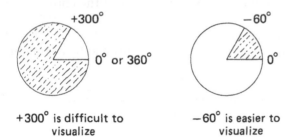

+300° is difficult to   −60° is easier to
    visualize   visualize

6. Bipolar Limb Leads

LEADS 1, 2, AND 3

1. What happens on ECG paper when current flows toward a positive electrode?
   ANS.: The current causes the stylus to produce an upward deflection on the ECG paper.
2. What is the importance of knowing that current flowing toward a positive electrode produces an upward deflection on ECG paper?
   ANS.: Because then it must also be true that current flowing toward a *negative* electrode produces a *downward* deflection on ECG paper. Therefore all we have to do is to learn the sites of the negative and positive electrodes of the various leads and we can then tell the direction of the current produced by the heart.
3. What is the purpose of an ECG lead?
   ANS.: It shows the extent to which a current is traveling in the direction of the line joining the electrodes.
4. What is meant by a bipolar limb lead?
   ANS.: A bipolar limb lead has a positive and a negative electrode placed on any two limbs, with the electrodes joined by wire connected to a galvanometer. The galvanometer needle moves in proportion to the difference in the number of electrons between the two limbs. The current deflecting the needle is due to the flow of electrons from the limb with more electrons to the limb with fewer electrons.
5. If there are 12 million electrons at a right arm electrode and 2 million at a left arm electrode, what is the difference as measured by a bipolar limb lead? What is this difference called?

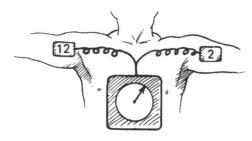

   ANS.: The difference is 10 million electrons, and it is known as a *potential difference*. Therefore a bipolar lead measures the potential difference between two electrodes.
6. What direction of current is measured by a lead with electrodes on the left and right arm?
   ANS.: A horizontal direction, i.e., the same as a line joining 0° and 180° on a circle. (It is known as the X axis in geometry.)

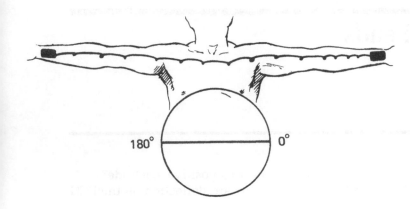

7. If the positive electrode is on the left arm and the negative electrode on the right arm, what is this lead called?
   ANS.: Lead 1 (L1).

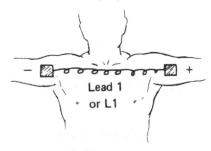

8. Where are the positive and negative electrodes for lead 2 (L2)?
   ANS.: The positive electrode is on the left leg, and the negative electrode is on the right arm.
9. What direction of current does L2 measure?
   ANS.: In terms of degrees on a circle, it measures the direction from the center of the circle to + 60° or, in the opposite direction, from the center of the circle to − 120°. The L2 axis is said to be from + 60° to − 120°

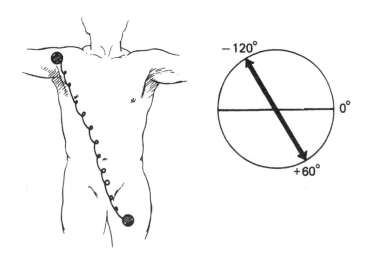

10. Where are the positive and negative electrodes for lead 3 (L3)?
    ANS.: The positive electrode is still on the left leg, but the negative electrode is on the left arm.
11. What direction of current is measured by L3?
    ANS.: Surprisingly, the direction measured by L3 is not straight down from the left arm to the left leg but at an angle of + 120° if measured from the center of the circle or an angle of − 60° if measured in the opposite direction. The L3 axis is said to be from + 120° to − 60°.

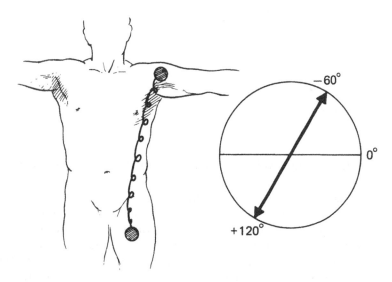

12. By what other name is the leg electrode called?
    ANS.: The foot electrode.
13. Is the foot electrode ever made the negative electrode of a bipolar lead?
    ANS.: No.
14. Which leg must be used as the foot electrode?
    ANS.: Either leg may be used; it should make no difference. By convention, however, the left leg is used. The right leg electrode is a ground electrode to eliminate electrical interference.
    Note: Originally, ECGs were taken without an electrode on the right leg, but at that time a different system of grounding was used.
15. What is the other term for the bipolar limb leads?
    ANS.: *Standard limb leads.* As this term was applicable only when there were no unipolar leads, there is no place for it in modern nomenclature.

TRIAXIAL SYSTEM AND EINTHOVEN'S TRIANGLE

1. If one makes an equilateral triangle from the three bipolar leads, what is it called?
   ANS.: Einthoven's triangle. In this concept, Einthoven, who invented the electrocardiograph in 1903, supposed that the three extremities formed the apexes of an equilateral triangle of which the heart, an electrical source, was assumed to be the center.

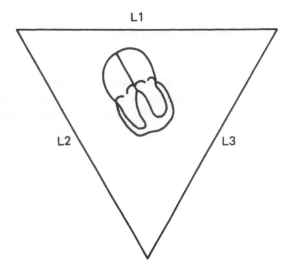

2. What is meant by saying that an electrode placed more than 12 cm from the heart is at electrical infinity?

    ANS.: If an electrode is placed less than 12 cm from the heart, the amplitudes of the deflections are influenced by the proximity to the heart. Thus the closer the electrode is to the heart, the greater is the amplitude. If, on the other hand, an electrode is placed further than 12 cm from the electrical center of the heart, no matter how much farther it is placed (even on the wrist or ankle), the *amplitude* of the deflection measured by that lead does not change significantly. This fact tells us that the limb leads are not affected by their distance from the heart. However, the precordial leads, which are placed on the chest wall, should be affected by their proximity to the electrical center of the heart.

3. How does the concept of electrical infinity from the heart help you to decide whether electrodes can be placed on a shoulder or amputated limb?

    ANS.: It should make no difference whether an extremity electrode is placed on a shoulder, a wrist, a thigh, or an ankle, all are at infinity from the heart. (The electrical center of the heart is at about the fourth or fifth rib level, near the center of the chest.)

*4. Was Einthoven correct in thinking that an equilateral triangle could represent the direction of the bipolar leads?

    ANS.: No. Even though the bipolar electrodes are at infinity from the electrical center of the heart, they may not necessarily be at points that are equidistant from each other and therefore may not fit the characteristics of an equilateral triangle. Einthoven's theory nevertheless works adequately in helping to determine the directions of current.

5. Why can the three sides of Einthoven's triangle be shifted so that they appear to radiate from the center of the heart?

* Material marked with an asterisk is included for reference and for advanced students in cardiology.

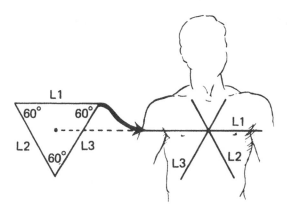

ANS.: The reason that one can do this shifting is that lead 1 measures not only current flowing between the right and left arm but also that flowing horizontally from side to side in the chest. This theory is based on the concept of the body as a volume conductor; i.e., the body acts like a tub of salt water, so that current flowing in any direction can be measured between any two points on the body.

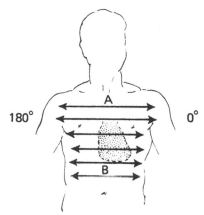

A lead at either A or B would measure side-to-side axes of current produced by a source (heart) in the center of the chest.

Similarly, L2 measures not only the current between the right arm and left leg but also all that which flows on the chest from + 60° to − 120°.

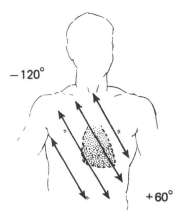

L3 measures all current traveling from + 120° to − 60° on the chest.

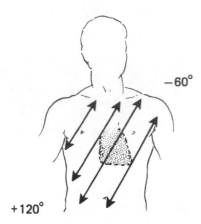

Therefore to make a convenient diagram of the three axes measured by the limb leads, one need merely shift the horizontal (X) axis to the electrical center of the chest (at about the fifth interspace level) and shift the L2 and L3 axes to run through this electrical center.

6. What is this diagram of directions radiating from the electrical center of the heart called?

ANS.: The triaxial system.

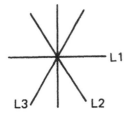

7. How to Draw a QRS Vector with the Triaxial System

QRS DURATION

1. What is the distance between the smallest vertical lines on ECG paper called?

   ANS.: It depends on paper speed because the vertical lines are time lines. At the usual paper speed of 25 mm per second, the smallest time lines are 40 msec (0.04 sec) apart. Pediatric cardiologists tend to run the paper at double speed, i.e., at 50 mm per second, so that their time lines are 20 msec (0.02 sec) apart.

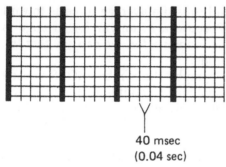

   40 msec
   (0.04 sec)

   At the usual paper speed of 25 mm per second, the small vertical divisions are time lines 40 msec (0.04 sec) apart.

2. What is the range of duration of the adult QRS?

   ANS.: 60 to 90 msec (0.06–0.09 sec). It tends to be shorter in women, children, and blacks. (In children or in cachectic adults, the QRS may be no more than 40 msec.)

3. What ECG artifact tends to make a normal QRS appear to be longer than 90 msec (0.09 sec)?

   ANS.: A slurring of the terminal forces common with direct writing machines may make it difficult to find the exact end of the QRS. The first change of slope at the end of a terminal R or S wave is best taken as the end of the QRS.

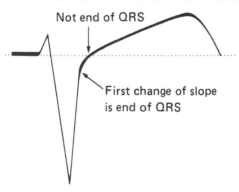

   Not end of QRS

   First change of slope is end of QRS

QRS DIRECTION RECOGNITION

1. Why is it important to be able to tell the direction of a QRS?

   ANS.: Almost all conduction abnormalities as well as ventricular overload problems are manifested as changes in the axis of the QRS; e.g., left ventricular hypertrophy tends to turn the QRS axis leftward or superiorly, and right ventricular hypertrophy turns it rightward or inferiorly.

2. What is meant by the direction of an entire QRS?

   ANS.: It refers to the direction in which current is traveling for most of the time that it is producing the QRS, i.e., the average direction. For example, in this 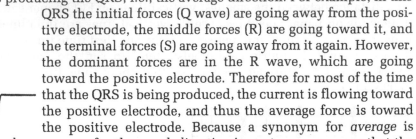 QRS the initial forces (Q wave) are going away from the positive electrode, the middle forces (R) are going toward it, and the terminal forces (S) are going away from it again. However, the dominant forces are in the R wave, which are going toward the positive electrode. Therefore for most of the time that the QRS is being produced, the current is flowing toward the positive electrode, and thus the average force is toward the positive electrode. Because a synonym for *average* is *mean*, and a synonym for the word *direction* is *vector*, we can say that the mean vector is toward the positive electrode.

   Note: In many textbooks of electrocardiography the symbol ÂQRS is used for *mean QRS vector*. However, this symbol may be confusing to beginners.

3. If during most of the 70 msec (0.07 sec) of a QRS current is traveling toward the positive electrode of L1, what would the QRS look like if the machine were switched to L1? Why?

   ANS.: The QRS would be predominantly upward because when current flows predominantly toward a positive electrode it produces an upward deflection in that lead's ECG tracing.

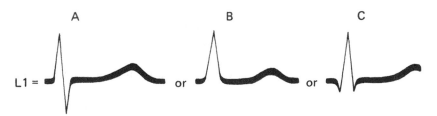

All the above are predominantly upright or positive because there is more area above than below the baseline. A and C are least parallel to the lead line of L1. B is most nearly parallel to the direction measured by L1.

4. What is another way of saying that the QRS is going predominantly toward a positive electrode?

   ANS.: The average, or mean, vector for the QRS is toward that positive electrode.

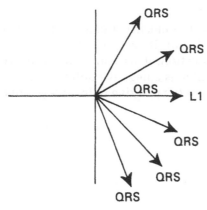

All these QRS vectors are going <u>predominantly toward</u> the positive electrode of L1. Note that they are all <u>less than 90°</u> from the lead line of L1.

5. How can we define the word *toward* in ECG language?
   ANS.: It means that the QRS is going in a direction that is less than the perpendicular to the positive lead line or positive arm of the lead.
   Note: The positive line or positive arm of L1 is from the electrical center to 0°.

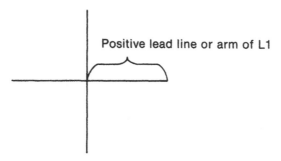

Therefore a force is going toward the positive electrode of L1 if it is going in a direction that is less than either − 90° or + 90°, giving a large arc of possibilities.

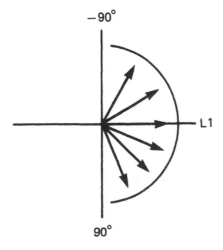

6. How is a positive electrode analogous to an eye?
    ANS.: It can be compared to an eye looking at the electrical center of the chest (from which all electrical impulses originate). It sees any current moving even slightly toward it as an upward deflection. It sees any current moving even slightly away from the electrical center as a negative deflection.
7. If the mean QRS is going predominantly away from the positive pole, or 'eye,' of L1, what does the QRS in L1 look like?
    ANS.: It looks predominantly negative, with most of the area of the QRS below the baseline.

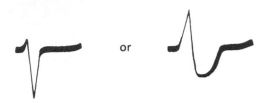

8. In what direction may the mean QRS travel in order to produce a predominantly positive QRS in L1?
    ANS.: In any direction in an arc that is less than 90° from the lead line measured by L1.

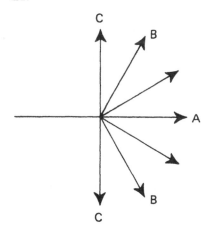

QRS vectors A to B in the above will produce a mean QRS that is predominantly positive in L1; i.e., the 'eye' of L1 will see predominantly upward deflections. Vector A, which is parallel to the leadline of L1, will show a QRS that is almost entirely positive.

Lead 1

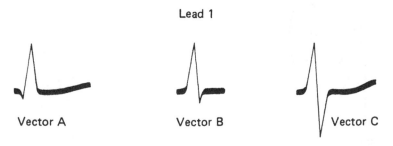

Vector A   Vector B   Vector C

Vector B, which is *nearly* perpendicular to the lead line of L1, will show a QRS in L1 that is nearly equal in positivity and negativity (almost as much above the baseline as below) but still predominantly above. Only if the mean QRS were *exactly* perpendicular to the lead line of L1 would the area above the baseline *equal* the area below (vector C in the foregoing diagram).

9. If, for half the duration of depolarization, current is traveling away from the positive electrode, or 'eye,' of L1, and for the other half it is traveling toward it, what will the QRS in L1 look like?

   ANS.: It will be equiphasic; i.e., one-half the QRS area will be above the baseline and one-half below it.

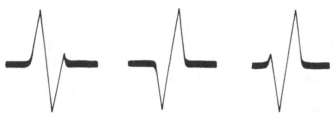

All the above are equiphasic; i.e., they have equal areas of negative and positive phases.

10. What is the mean direction of the QRS if it is equiphasic in L1?

    ANS.: Because it cannot be going toward or away from the positive electrode, it must be going exactly perpendicular to the lead line of L1; i.e., it must be going at either $-90°$ or $+90°$.

TELLING DIRECTION BY THE METHOD OF PERPENDICULARS

1. What is meant by a 'perpendicular' to a lead line?

   ANS.: A perpendicular is a line that lies at $\pm 90°$ or at right angles to a lead line. (This concept is very important.)

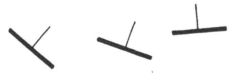

All the above thin lines are perpendicular to the thick ones and vice versa.

2. What do we call an ECG complex that has as much area above as below the baseline?

   ANS.: Equiphasic.

   Note: Isoelectric is a poor term to describe this complex because it implies no movement at all, either above or below the baseline; *biphasic* does not tell you that the amounts above or below the baseline are equal.

3. If a mean QRS vector is equiphasic in L1 (perpendicular to L1), in what direction is it going?

   ANS.: There are two possibilities: straight up at $-90°$ or straight down at $+90°$.

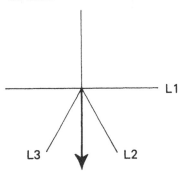

Note: This concept is a key one. Even if you forget why it is so, you must know that if you run an ECG on a given lead and find that the stylus records an equiphasic QRS, the average direction of that subject's QRS is in a direction perpendicular to that lead. This method is one used for determining the direction of all vectors at a glance. Simply by learning the directions measured by the routine leads and looking for the lead with the equiphasic complex, you can eliminate all but two possible directions.

Of course, if current is flowing perpendicular to a lead for the entire duration of the QRS, no QRS shows on the ECG paper. We know that when we see a QRS, however, we must be dealing with many directions of currents that can move the stylus above and below the baseline. It takes about 60 to 90 msec to produce the QRS. In that case, the average direction of the multidirectional forces during the 60 to 90 msec *can* be perpendicular to a lead line, and when it is perpendicular it manifests an equiphasic complex.

4. How can you tell whether such a mean vector is going toward − 90° or + 90°?

ANS.: By looking at lead 2 or lead 3. If they show predominant positivity—i.e., most of the QRS is above the baseline—the QRS vector must be traveling predominantly toward their positive electrodes. Only a + 90° vector could do this.

Only the inferior (+ 90°) QRS vector could produce an upright deflection in L2 and L3.

5. If the mean QRS is perpendicular to L2, what does the QRS look like in L2?

ANS.: It is equiphasic.

6. If L2 has an equiphasic QRS, in which direction does the mean QRS vector go?
    ANS.: − 30° or + 150°, i.e., perpendicular to L2. For example,

    If L2 = 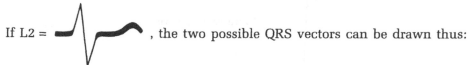 , the two possible QRS vectors can be drawn thus:

    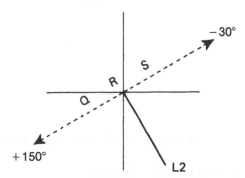

    Note that an equiphasic lead limits the vector direction to <u>only two possibilities</u>. This fact is the secret of the inspection method of finding vector directions.

7. How can you tell by rapid inspection of the ECG whether the direction of the QRS vector in the diagram is − 30° or + 150°?
    ANS.: Look at L1. If it is toward − 30°, it is going toward the positive electrode of L1 and gives a positive deflection in this lead. If it is toward + 150°, it shows as a negative deflection in L1.
8. Why is finding the equiphasic lead so helpful in plotting a vector?
    ANS.: The equiphasic lead eliminates all possibilities *except two*. Merely looking at one other lead tells you which of the two it is.

    e.g.,   L3 =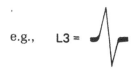

    If an ECG shows that L3 is equiphasic, as in the complex above, the mean QRS has only two possible directions, +30° or −150°.

    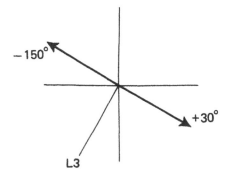

9. Is the following QRS complex predominantly positive or negative?

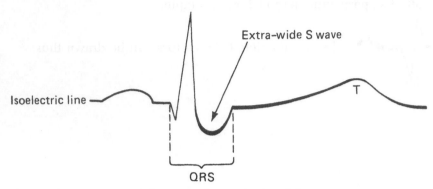

The QRS here is extra wide because of a conduction defect.

ANS.: Predominantly negative because the area below the isoelectric line is greater than that above.

Note: Use areas and not merely amplitudes to plot vectors.

10. What can you do to find the direction of a QRS if none of the bipolar leads is equiphasic?

ANS.: You can look for an equiphasic complex in the unipolar limb leads aVR, aVL, or aVF (see Chap. 8).

8. Unipolar Limb Leads

1. What was the original purpose of unipolar leads, as invented by Wilson et al. [2] in 1934?

   ANS.: They hoped to measure the absolute electrical force at the site of a positive electrode. That is, their purpose was to record, if it was present, an electrical force of, let us say, 10 electrons at the left arm and not merely to record the potential difference of forces between two limbs.

2. What is necessary to measure the absolute level of electrical force at the site of a positive electrode?

   ANS.: The nonpositive opposite pole of the lead must be at zero potential. This means that it must have no electrical force at all; i.e., it must be a zero electrode.

3. How can the negative effect of a bipolar lead be eliminated so that instead of having a negative and positive pole, it has a zero and positive pole?

   ANS.: By a mechanism built into the ECG machine that joins the negative electrodes of the three lead wire extremities so that their forces cancel each other out and make one common electrode. (Lead electrodes are placed on only three extremities; the right leg electrode is only a ground.)

4. What is this common zero electrode called?

   ANS.: The central terminal.

5. Where in relation to the heart is this central terminal effect located?

   ANS.: Approximately at the electrical center of the heart (at about the fourth or fifth interspace level of the mid-chest, theoretically near the middle of the left side of the ventricular septum, where ventricular activation begins).

6. What did Wilson call these leads that measure electricity from the electrical center of the heart to the limbs?

   ANS.: V leads. Thus the lead from the central terminal to the left arm was called VL, to the right arm VR, and to the foot VF, because it measured the absolute voltage in each limb.

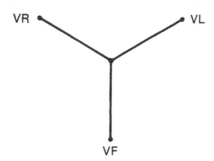

7. What new directions of current did VR, VL, and VF measure?
   ANS.:

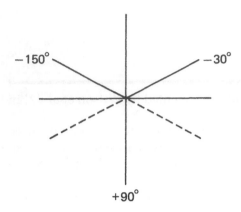

   VR measured − 150° (and + 30° in the opposite direction); VL measured − 30° (and + 150° in the opposite direction); and VF measured + 90° (and − 90°).

8. Why did these unipolar leads have to be augmented?
   ANS.: Because the ECG complexes recorded by Wilson's system were too small to be of much use. (The augmented leads are called aVR, aVL, and aVF.)

9. What, then, does the 'a' in aVL and aVF mean?
   ANS.: Augmented.

*10. How are the unipolar leads augmented?
   ANS.: Goldberger [1] changed the connection of the central terminal so that it is not attached to the positive electrode of the lead actually being taken. Therefore if aVL is being taken, aVL's negative wire is automatically disconnected by the ECG machine from the central terminal. (This maneuver augments the voltage by a factor of 1.5.)

11. What direction results from joining the negative electrodes of only two of the three limbs into a common negative electrode and using the third limb as a positive electrode?
   ANS.: It is the same as if the negative electrodes from two limbs were averaged to make a common negative electrode halfway between the two negative limbs. For example, if the left arm has the positive electrode, the negative right arm and leg electrodes are joined together to make a single negative electrode. (The common terminal so constructed is slightly negative, but this negativity is of no consequence. However, in reality it is actually a modified bipolar system.) By convention it is called a unipolar system.

* Material marked with an asterisk is included for reference and for advanced students in cardiology.

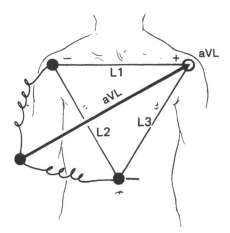

When the negative pole of the right arm and of the foot are joined together to make a common negative electrode, a new lead line is made that passes through the electrical center of the chest to the site of the positive electrode, here on the left arm. Note that the new lead line for this lead bisects the L2 side of Einthoven's triangle. Because the position of the positive (+) electrode is on the left arm, it is called aVL.

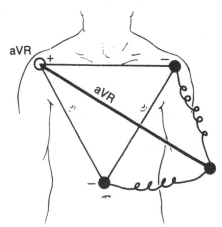

Another new lead is aVR, made by making the <u>right arm positive</u> and joining the left arm and leg to make a common negative electrode.

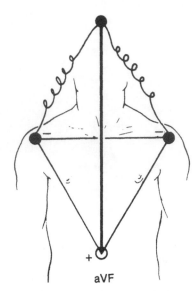

aVF

Another new lead is aVF, made by joining both arms to produce a common negative electrode and connecting them to a <u>positive leg electrode</u>.

12. What is the relative voltage of the augmented unipolar leads when compared with bipolar leads?
    ANS.: Augmented unipolar leads have only about four-fifths (actually 87 percent) the voltage of the bipolar leads. For example, if L1 equals aVL in height, aVL is actually one-fifth greater in voltage.
13. What is the advantage of the three augmented unipolar leads?
    ANS.: They provide us with three new vector directions.
14. What direction is measured by the lead joining the central terminal to the left arm electrode, i.e., aVL?
    ANS.: Upward at an angle of – 30° or downward in the opposite direction.

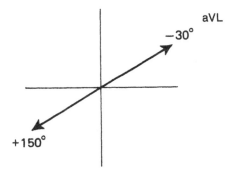

15. What direction is measured by the lead joining the central terminal to the right arm, i.e., aVR?
    ANS.: It measures only the current that goes upward at an angle of – 150°, or in the exactly opposite direction.

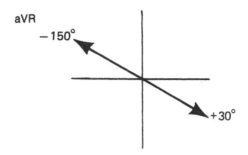

16. What direction is measured by the lead joining the central terminal to the foot electrode, i.e., aVF?

ANS.: Upward at − 90° or downward at + 90°, the Y axis of geometry.

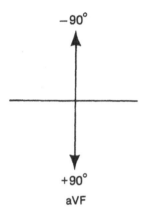

REFERENCES

1. Goldberger, E. A simple indifferent electrocardiographic electrode of zero potential and a technique of obtaining augmented unipolar extremity leads. *Am. Heart J.* 23:483, 1942.
2. Wilson, F. N., Macleod, A. G., and Barker, P. S. Electrocardiograms that represent the potential variations of a single electrode. *Am. Heart J.* 9:447, 1934.

9. Frontal Plane Hexaxial System

HOW TO DRAW A FRONTAL PLANE HEXAXIAL SYSTEM

1. What is meant by the frontal plane?

   ANS.: It is easiest to think of it as the plane of a wall against which the patient is standing while facing you, i.e., in the anatomical position. Even though routine ECGs are not taken in the upright position, we think of the directions of current as if they were occurring in a patient standing in the anatomical position.

2. How many axes of electricity can be measured by both the bipolar and unipolar leads in the frontal plane?

   ANS.: Six.

3. If all six directions are drawn like spokes radiating from the electrical center of the heart, what is this diagram called?

   ANS.: The hexaxial reference system.

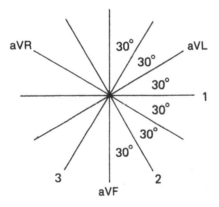

4. Is it necessary to memorize the hexaxial system?

   ANS.: Yes, because without it no vector can be quickly visualized or drawn merely by inspecting the ECG.

   Note: The next few questions and answers are designed to teach you an easy way to learn the frontal hexaxial system.

5. What is the first step in drawing the hexaxial system quickly?

   ANS.: Draw a horizontal and a vertical axis through the imaginary electrical center of the heart.

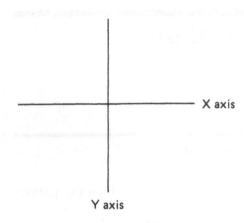

6. What lead axes does this drawing automatically give us?
   ANS.: L1 and aVF.

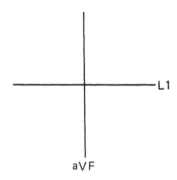

   Note: Leads L1, L2, etc. need be labeled only on the positive electrode side of the electrical center. This method helps you to memorize where the positive and negative electrodes are.

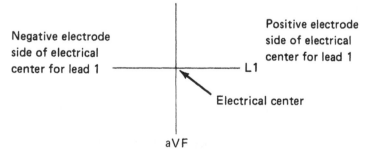

7. Does any single rule cover how to draw the other four axes easily after the horizontal and vertical axes are drawn?
   ANS.: Yes. The other four axes are at 30° angles from the horizontal or vertical axes; i.e., aVR and aVL are at 30° above the horizontal axis, and L2 and L3 are at 30° on each side of the vertical axis.

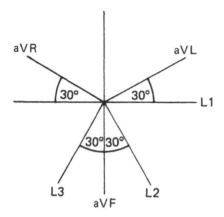

Note: When learning to make the hexaxial system it is not necessary at first to extend the axes to show their full length on each side of the electrical center. It is much easier at first to draw the axes as if they have only a positive arm going from the center of the heart to the positive electrodes, that is,

than to draw this.

Practice drawing this freehand, from memory. Put the lead names at the sites of the positive electrodes.

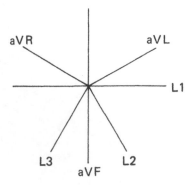

Note: After you have memorized the foregoing method of drawing the hexaxial system, the extensions to the negative electrodes should be put in as dotted lines; e.g.,

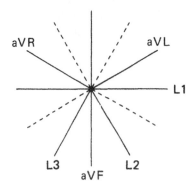

An entire lead on the hexaxial system stretches from the positive electrode through the electrical center to the negative electrode.

An easy way to remember how to draw the hexaxial system and the positive electrode sites is to first draw the X and Y axes, giving you L1 and aVF.

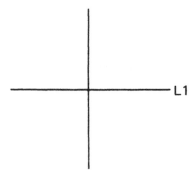

Then imagine a body superimposed on it with the arms slightly raised 30° and each leg 30° from the vertical.

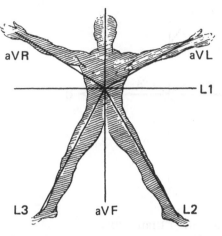

The hands and feet are the positive electrode sites.

No matter what method is used to memorize how to draw the hexaxial system, there is no point in going further without having it completely at your recall. Practice drawing it now. Do five from memory before going any further.

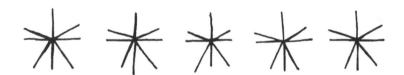

HOW TO PLOT VECTORS IN THE HEXAXIAL SYSTEM

1. If aVF has an equiphasic QRS, what is the mean vector?
   ANS.: Draw the hexaxial system and look for the perpendicular to aVF. You will find it at 0° or 180°; i.e., there are only two possible directions.

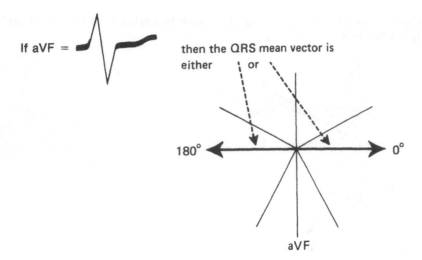

If aVF =   then the QRS mean vector is either   or

2. How can you tell if the QRS mean vector is 0° rather than 180°?

   ANS.: Look at any other lead, e.g., L1. If the QRS is directed toward 0°, it gives a predominantly positive complex in L1. On the other hand, if the QRS is pointing toward the negative electrode of L1 and 180°, it produces a negative complex in L1.

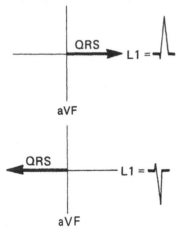

Both the above QRS vectors are perpendicular to the lead line of aVF, but one produces a positive QRS in L1, and the other produces a negative QRS in L1.

3. If L2 has a flat (or isoelectric) T wave, and aVL has a predominantly positive T wave, in which direction is the mean T vector?

   ANS.: − 30°; i.e., it is perpendicular to L2 and on the positive side of aVL.

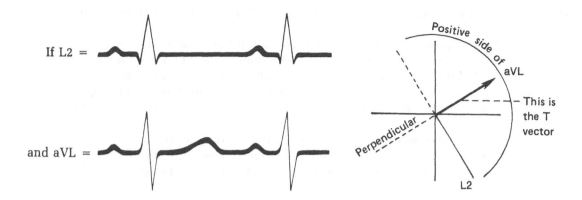

4. Why is it sometimes possible to use the word *isoelectric* for an equiphasic T wave?
   ANS.: Because T waves sometimes have such low voltage that an equiphasic lead may show no deflections above or below the baseline.
5. Can the S-T segment have a vector?
   ANS.: Yes, any point on the ECG that can be named has a vector.

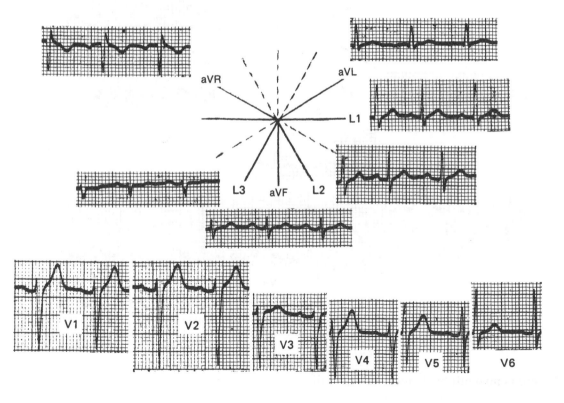

ECG 1. This normal ECG is from an asymptomatic 33-year-old man with a normal heart. Lead aVF has the equiphasic QRS. Therefore the QRS direction is perpendicular to the lead line of aVF, i.e., 0° or 180°. Because lead 1 is positive, the direction of the QRS is 0°.

6. What is the quickest way of visualizing a mean frontal vector if there is no equiphasic lead?

ANS.: Look for the most nearly equiphasic limb lead. If that lead were equiphasic, it limits the direction to only two possible ones. After choosing the one of the two that fits with what you see in any other lead, shift the vector a little to the proper direction in relation to that nearly equiphasic lead; i.e., if the nearly equiphasic lead is actually slightly negative, shift the vector to a little more than 90° from that lead line. For example, see ECG 2, where the QRS in L3 is the most nearly equiphasic. If it were equiphasic, the vector would be at + 30°. However, L3 is actually slightly positive (more area above than below the baseline). Therefore the vector is slightly less than the perpendicular to L3, or about + 45°.

Note: A low voltage lead that is equiphasic may change from slightly positive to slightly negative with respiration (see ECG 5A; p. 75).

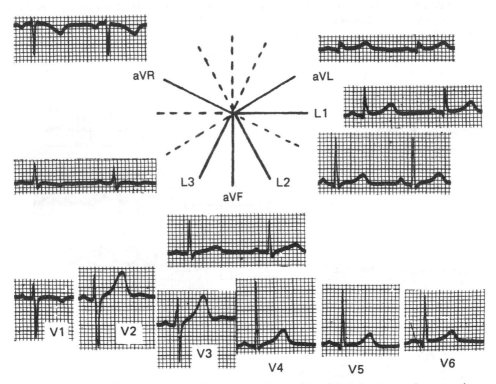

ECG 2. This ECG is from a 27-year-old woman with a mild pelvic infection and a normal heart. The T in lead 3 is almost equiphasic but is actually slightly negative. Thus the T vector is slightly beyond lead 3's perpendicular of + 30°; it lies at about + 20°.

7. If there is no equiphasic lead, can the tallest QRS be used to tell the direction of the QRS?

ANS.: In general, the QRS must be traveling parallel to the line with the tallest complex. However, because the unipolar leads have only about 85 percent of the amplitude of bipolar leads, a vector may be taller in L2 than in aVF, yet be going exactly between them (+ 75°). Therefore use only the bipolar leads for comparison of amplitude. For example, in ECG 2, the QRS in L2 is the tallest of the limb leads 1, 2, or 3. Therefore the vector is most parallel to the lead line of L2, or + 60°. However, because it is taller in L1 than in L3, the vector is pointing slightly more toward L1 and L3, or toward 45° to 50°. *Note:* The general rule for finding the direction of any vector is to decide which limb lead has recorded the conspicuously largest or smallest resultant deflection. The vector is parallel to the axis of the lead with the largest deflection or nearly perpendicular to the lead with the smallest deflection. If the smallest deflection is exactly equiphasic, the vector is exactly perpendicular to that lead. Use the *area* above and below the baseline, not the amplitude, to determine the resultant vector. You can determine the direction of a QRS and T vector within a 5° error by this method.

SEMICIRCLE METHOD OF PLOTTING FRONTAL VECTORS

*1. What probably was the greatest obstacle to the use of the vector approach for understanding the scalar ECG?

ANS.: The old method of plotting vectors by means of measuring units of amplitude along two axes and making a resultant made it impossible to tell the direction of an electrical force without pencil and paper. Usually leads 1 and 3 were used. In this example, if lead 1 has an amplitude of 6 units and lead 3 has an amplitude of 8 units, perpendiculars can be drawn with a resultant vector from the electrical center to the point at which the perpendiculars meet.

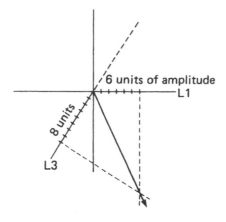

When this method of determining the direction of a vector was used, it was impossible to tell at a glance the direction of a P, QRS, or T. Thus the reading of ECGs was an occult art that was virtually unteachable. Also, it has been shown that if different combinations of leads are used to determine the axes by the preceding method, there can be as much as a 35° difference in axis [1].

---

* Material marked with an asterisk is included for reference and for advanced students in cardiology.

REFERENCE

1. Okamoto, N., Kaneko, K., Simonson, E., and Schmitt, O. H. Reliability of individual frontal plane axis determination. *Circulation* 44:213, 1971.

10. Normal Frontal Plane QRS, T, and P Vector Ranges and Patterns

NORMAL QRS RANGE

1. Why is it important to be able to draw an *average*, or *mean*, QRS, T, or P vector?
   ANS.: Because abnormalities of ventricular depolarization change the direction of the mean QRS vector; abnormalities of repolarization change the mean T direction; and abnormalities of pacemaker site or of atrial overload can change the direction of the P waves.
2. In which direction would you expect the QRS vector to point in the frontal plane? Why?
   ANS.: Inferior and to the left, because it is the direction of the main body of the left ventricle, which is inferior and to the left of where depolarization begins near the middle of the ventricular septum.

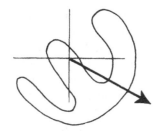

3. What is the normal range of direction of mean QRS vectors for the vast majority of adults?
   ANS.: The normal range is from 0° to + 90°, or the entire left lower quadrant of the frontal plane [2, 4, 7].

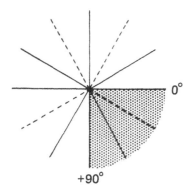

The normal range of adult mean QRS vectors is in the shaded area.

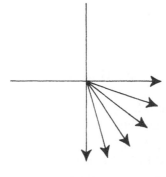

Any of these mean QRS vectors may be normal.

You can now derive patterns from vector observations to tell at a glance whether you are looking at a normal or an abnormal ECG.

Note: a.   Although an axis above 0° (left axis deviation) is occasionally normal, most subjects with an axis of even − 10° have either left ventricular hypertrophy or a conduction defect. The normal variant superior axis is discussed on page 118.

*b.   Up to age 1 month the normal axis may even be 180° to the right due to the right ventricular dominance in the newborn. Between 1 month and 1 year, it may still be rightward as much as 135°. From age 1 to puberty, it may be + 120°, but after puberty it is not expected to be more than + 100° [7].

*c.   For the first month of life the QRS is rarely more leftward than + 70° [6]. Therefore all infants in this age group should have a negative QRS in aVL.

4. Why is a predominantly negative QRS in the usual adult lead 1 rarely normal?
   ANS.: Because it means that the QRS would fall into an abnormal range of a semicircle

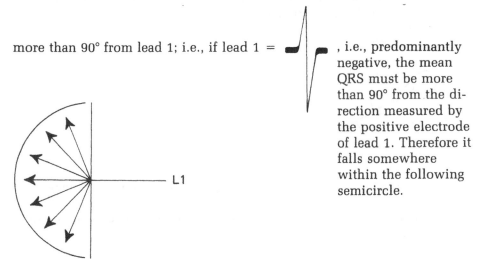

more than 90° from lead 1; i.e., if lead 1 = , i.e., predominantly negative, the mean QRS must be more than 90° from the direction measured by the positive electrode of lead 1. Therefore it falls somewhere within the following semicircle.

Any of these arrows could be the vector for a predominantly negative L1, and they are all outside the usual normal adult range. (See shaded area in question 3 diagram.)

5. When can a normal adult QRS be predominantly negative in lead 1?
   ANS.: In the very young or in some subjects under age 35 who have long, thin chests (see ECG 3).

6. How can raising the chest to a 60° angle change the ECG

   (a) QRS axis? (b) voltage?
   ANS.: a. It can shift it either leftward or rightward by as much as 20°.
          b. It can decrease voltage in the left precordial leads [1].

* Material marked with an asterisk is included for reference and for advanced students in cardiology.

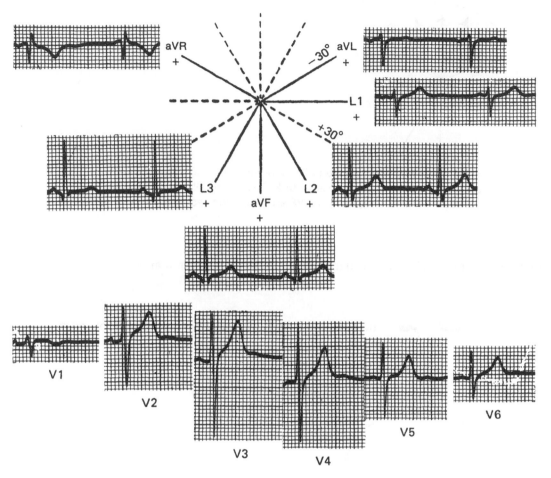

ECG 3. A right axis deviation of about 110° in a normal 30-year-old man with a long, thin chest. Right ventricular hypertrophy must always be considered in an adult with such a right axis.

7. Which leads other than lead 1 should not have a negative QRS in the normal adult ECG?

ANS.: As can be seen from the normal shaded area in the diagram in question 3, neither lead 1, lead 2, nor lead aVF can normally have a predominantly negative QRS;

i.e., if lead 2 = 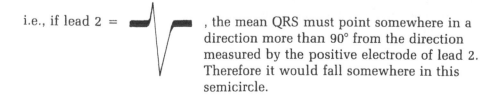 , the mean QRS must point somewhere in a direction more than 90° from the direction measured by the positive electrode of lead 2. Therefore it would fall somewhere in this semicircle.

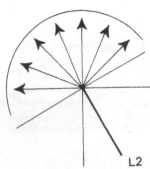

L2

Any one of these arrows could be the QRS vector for an L2 with a predominantly negative complex. Note that they are all outside the normal QRS range. The same reasoning would show that negativity in aVF also places the vector in an abnormal area.

8. Show how aVF negativity would place the vector in an abnormal area.
   ANS.:

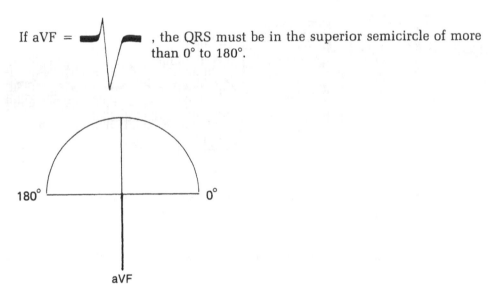

If aVF = ⟨waveform⟩ , the QRS must be in the superior semicircle of more than 0° to 180°.

180°   0°

aVF

Any QRS in the above semicircle area is outside the usual normal range of 0° to + 90°.

9. Prove that negativity in aVL could be normal.
   ANS.: Draw a perpendicular to aVL through the electrical center, and draw a vector just beyond it.

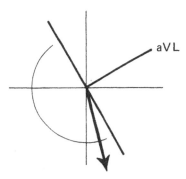

Note that a vector on the negative side of the perpendicular to aVL may still be in the normal range for the QRS (0° to + 90°).

10. Prove that a negative QRS in lead 3 may be normal.
    ANS.: Draw a perpendicular to the lead line of lead 3 on the hexaxial system through the electrical center, and draw a vector just beyond it.

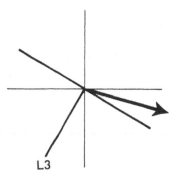

Note that this vector is still in the normal range for the QRS.

NORMAL T RANGE

1. What is the normal range for the frontal T wave vector?
   ANS.: In the adult, 0° to + 90°, exactly the same as for the QRS.
       Note: Up to 1 month of age, the T may be slightly more than + 90°. The rightward range reaches adult levels after 1 month of age. Up to the late teens, however, occasionally the T is slightly more leftward than 0°, especially in athletes [5].

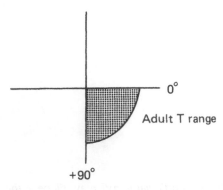

*2. Would you expect the T vector to have the same direction as the QRS?
    ANS.: Because the QRS represents depolarization and the T represents repolarization, you might expect them to have exactly opposite directions.
*3. In what direction would you expect depolarization and repolarization to occur through the thick wall of ventricular muscle?
    ANS.: Because bundle branches finally arborize as fine Purkinje fibers in the subendocardium, you would expect both depolarization and repolarization to proceed from endocardium to epicardium and so produce opposite QRS and T vectors.
*4. Why then are the QRS and T vectors in about the same direction?
    ANS.: Because repolarization does not occur from endocardium to epicardium but, instead, from the outer to the inner surface of the ventricle. (The reason this happens is discussed in Chap. 20.)

NORMAL P RANGE

1. What is the direction of depolarization of the atria in the frontal plane?
    ANS.: The usual concept is that depolarization spreads radially from the SA node in concentric waves similar to those made by a pebble thrown into a pond, toward the AV node, which is inferior and to the left.

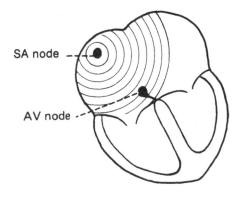

2. What then is the expected normal direction of the P vector?
    ANS.: Inferior and to the left.

3. What is wrong with the concentric wave 'pebble-in-a-pond' theory of atrial depolarization?

 ANS.: There are three specialized conduction pathways, each one as thick as a finger, between the SA and AV nodes, as well as one between the atria.

 Note: There has been much controversy over the existence of internodal pathways because their Purkinje-like conduction cells are interspersed with 'working,' or ordinary, atrial muscle. These ordinary atrial fibers may be the mode of lateral spread from the conduction fibers to the atrial muscle.

4. What is the normal range for the frontal P vector at all ages?

 ANS.: 0° to + 90°.

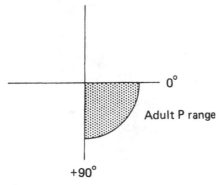

The shaded area is the normal P range.

Therefore the adult QRS, T, and P conveniently have the same normal range.

 Note: In adults the inferior P range is rarely over + 75°, so that a flat or equiphasic P in lead 1, i.e., + 90°, is probably pathological and means either an ectopic P or, more likely, chronic obstructive pulmonary disease.

PATTERN COROLLARY: *A negative QRS, T, or P in leads 1, 2, or aVF is probably abnormal in the adult ECG.*

On the basis of this law, leads 1, 2, and aVF may be called the 'critical leads' for absolute abnormalities of QRS, T, and P vectors. Because the aVR lead line bisects the angle between critical leads 1 and 2, it is also a critical lead and may therefore have no predominantly *positive* QRS, T, or P.

 Note: a. Always look with suspicion at the 'upper limits' type of vector. For example, a 0° QRS may be normal for a stocky adult but abnormal for a slender youth because age and body build affect the vector rotations.

 b. You should learn the general rule of the 'critical leads' for negativity now. Later you will learn the few exceptions to this rule, i.e., when it is normal for an adult to have a negative QRS not only in lead 1 but also in lead 2 and in aVF.

INDETERMINATE AXES

1. What kind of normal mean QRS vector cannot be plotted on a hexaxial system?

 ANS.: One in which the QRS is equiphasic in two or more limb leads.

2. When is the QRS equiphasic in two or more limb leads?
   ANS.: When the terminal half of the QRS is independent of the initial half (see ECG 4).
3. When are the initial and terminal halves of the QRS independent of one another?
   ANS.: When terminal conduction is along the outflow tract of the right ventricle. This subject is discussed under 'Right Bundle Branch Block Pattern' on page 115.

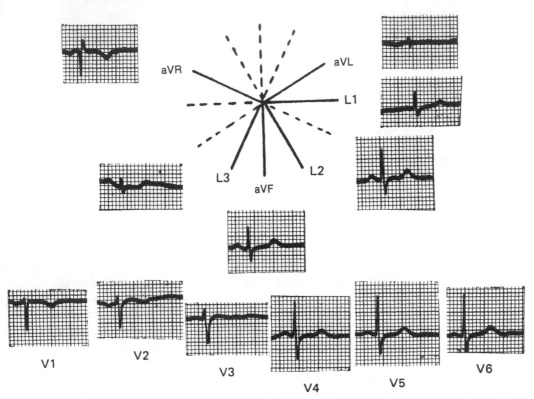

ECG 4. A 54-year-old woman with a normal heart. A routine ECG shows four limb leads to be nearly, and two exactly, equiphasic. This normal variant is caused by the terminal depolarization occurring up the outflow tract of the right ventricle. Because the outflow tract, or infundibulum, of the right ventricle is superior and to the right, the terminal part of the QRS is superior and to the right, causing an S wave in all limb leads except aVR.

4. When does terminal conduction normally proceed along the outflow tract of the right ventricle?
   ANS.: In young people. As people grow older, terminal conduction is more likely to occur in the high posterior part of the left ventricle. When the middle-aged or older patient has terminal conduction along the outflow tract of the right ventricle, suspect right ventricular hypertrophy.

EFFECT OF AGE AND CHEST SHAPE ON QRS AXES

1. How does the QRS axis change physiologically with chest shape?
   ANS.: The QRS is vertical or rightward in the long, thin chest and leftward or horizontal in the squat, relatively wide chest.

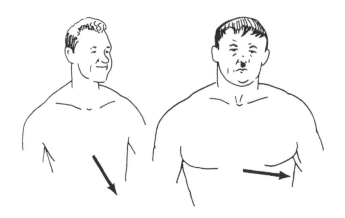

2. How does the QRS direction tend to change with age?
   ANS.: From rightward or inferior during childhood to leftward or horizontal during old age. It may rotate from 180° in an infant up to age 1 month to 0° in the adult [7].

   Note: a. The more leftward QRS seen with increasing age is not as likely due to an increase in blood pressure with age as it is to a conduction defect secondary to thickening of the coronary intima and the resultant ischemia and scarring that occurs with age [3, 4].

        b. The greater the relative body weight, the more leftward is the QRS axis in all age groups [4].

REFERENCES

1. Bergman, K. S., et al. Effect of body position on the electrocardiogram. *Am. Heart J.* 117:204, 1989.
2. Carter, E. P., and Greene, C. H. The ECG and ventricular preponderance. *Arch. Intern. Med.* 24:638, 1919.
3. Lober, P. H. Pathogenesis of coronary sclerosis. *Arch. Pathol.* 55:357, 1953.
4. Simonson, E. The effect of age on the electrocardiogram. *Am. J. Cardiol.* 29:64, 1972.
5. Van Ganse, W., et al. The electrocardiogram of athletes. Comparison with untrained subjects. *Br. Heart J.* 32:160, 1970.
6. Wenger, N. K. The electrocardiogram of the normal newborn infant. *J. Med. Assoc. Ga.* 54:58, 1965.
7. Ziegler, R. F. *Electrocardiographic Studies in Normal Infants and Children.* Springfield, Ill.: Thomas, 1951, P. 52.

11. Horizontal Plane Electrocardiogram

PLACING THE CHEST ELECTRODES

1. What are the synonyms used for chest leads?
   ANS.: V leads, or precordial leads.
2. Where are the electrodes for V1 and V2 placed?
   ANS.: In the *fourth* intercostal space at the right and left sternal edge, respectively.
   Note: The commonest error is to place the V1 and V2 in the *second* right and left interspaces.

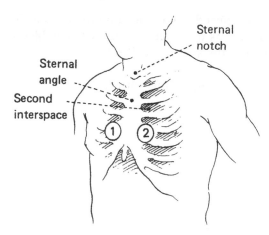

Technicians should note that the sternal angle is the slight protuberance or bump felt at the junction of the upper smaller and lower main portion of the breast bone, or sternum.

3. How is the fourth interspace found?
   ANS.: Feel the angle of Louis, or the sternal angle. It is the first protuberant part of the sternum down from the sternal notch. The second rib's cartilage is attached here. The interspace *below* this spot is the second interspace. Count below this interspace to find the fourth.
   Note: A common error is to try to find the fourth right interspace by counting down from below the collarbone or clavicle, believing it is the first interspace. This choice turns out to be correct only about 50 percent of the time.
4. Where is the electrode for V4 placed?
   ANS.: In the fifth left interspace in the mid-clavicular line. It is equivalent to the midpoint of the left half of the chest in the mid left thorax.

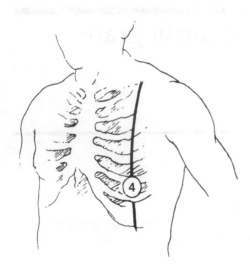

Note: This electrode was originally supposed to be placed on the apex beat, but the apex beat in the supine position is palpable in only a few subjects over age 30. ECGs are routinely taken in the supine position.

5. Where is the electrode for V3 placed?
    ANS.: Equidistant between V2 and V4 and in a straight line with them.

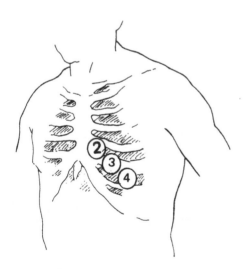

6. Where are the electrodes for V5 and V6 placed?
    ANS.: In the anterior and mid-axillary lines, respectively, at the same horizontal level as lead V4.

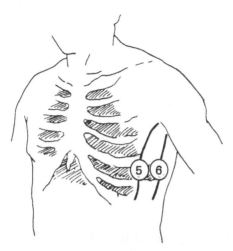

Because the left axilla means the left lateral side of the chest, the anterior axillary line is really an imaginary or arbitrary line that separates the front from the left lateral side.

With all the V lead electrodes placed on one diagram, the chest would look like this:

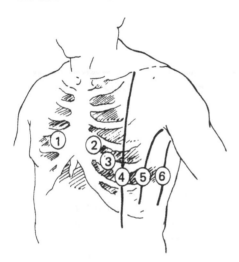

7. Why are not all the chest electrodes placed in a straight horizontal line at either the fourth or fifth interspace?

   ANS.: Originally, it was thought that potentials exactly underneath the exploring chest electrode were being picked up. Therefore to pick up left ventricular potentials, an electrode at the apex beat was thought necessary. Because the apex beat is always lower than the main body of the right ventricle, the apex was explored by electrodes one interspace lower. When the mid-clavicular line fifth interspace was substituted for the apex beat, the eccentric electrode placement was retained as a compromise.

8. In what plane are directions of current measured by precordial leads?

   ANS.: The horizontal plane. This plane includes all front-to-back and side-to-side directions. It is the same plane as the floor if the subject is standing.

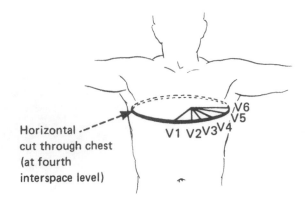

Horizontal
cut through chest
(at fourth
interspace level)

V1 V2V3V4
V5
V6

Note: The term *transverse plane*, which appears at first glance to be more accurate than *horizontal plane*, is not necessary. The term *transverse* was thought better because when a subject is recumbent a transverse cut through the chest is not the horizontal plane; i.e., it is not in the plane of the floor. However, in medicine all the terminology of anatomy is applied to patients as if they were in the 'anatomical position,' i.e., standing up and facing the examiner.

HOW TO PLOT VECTORS IN THE HORIZONTAL PLANE: HORIZONTAL PLANE HEXAXIAL SYSTEM

1. Are the horizontal plane leads a bipolar or unipolar system?
   ANS.: A unipolar system.
2. Are the horizontal plane leads an augmented unipolar system?
   ANS.: No. They are Wilson's original V leads.
3. Why can we use the original unaugmented central terminal of Wilson for the precordial leads when the voltage of such leads is too small for limb leads?
   ANS.: The positive precordial electrodes are so close to the heart that the amplitude is quite adequate for practical purposes. Remember that as soon as an electrode is less than 12 cm from the heart it becomes very sensitive to proximity effects, so that the closer electrodes get to the heart, the greater are the amplitudes of the deflections they record.
4. What does the central terminal or zero electrode represent anatomically?
   ANS.: The electrical center of the heart, where all the QRS and T vectors have their origin.
5. Where is this electrical center in the chest in the horizontal plane?
   ANS.: About halfway through the chest and, because the heart is slightly to the left of center, slightly to the left.

* Material marked with an asterisk is included for reference and for advanced students in cardiology.

6. Draw the horizontal plane hexaxial system.
   ANS.: *Step 1:* Draw a bird's-eye view of the horizontal plane.

Posterior

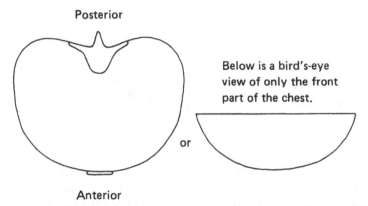

Below is a bird's-eye
view of only the front
part of the chest.

or

Anterior

You have a choice of drawing either the entire chest or just the front half.

Step 2: Place an imaginary electrical center in the figure. Because slightly more of the heart is on the left side of the chest, the electrical center should be placed eccentrically to the left, about halfway between the front and back of the chest.

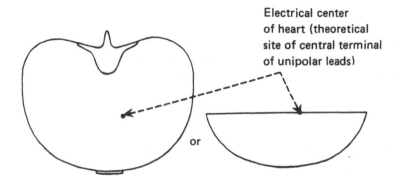

Electrical center
of heart (theoretical
site of central terminal
of unipolar leads)

or

Step 3: Place the positive chest electrodes in their position around the thorax.

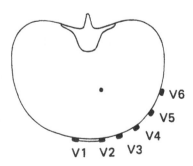

V6
V5
V4
V1 V2 V3

Step 4: Join the electrical center to each positive electrode.

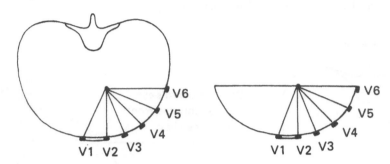

7. Which direction of current do the chest leads measure?

   ANS.: The direction shown by radii in the horizontal plane. Imagine that each positive electrode is like an eye looking at the electrical center of the heart. If current flows toward an eye in a direction that is less than the perpendicular to the positive lead line, the eye sees a positive or upright deflection.

   Note: Because the electrodes for V4, V5, and V6 are placed lower on the chest wall than those for V1 and V2, some vertical frontal vectors are also being recorded.

8. If the mean QRS is equiphasic in V3, what is the direction of this QRS vector on the horizontal plane diagram?

   ANS.:

   If V3 = , the QRS must be perpendicular to the 'eye' of V3. This means that there are only two possibilities for the direction of the QRS because there are only two directions perpendicular to V3.

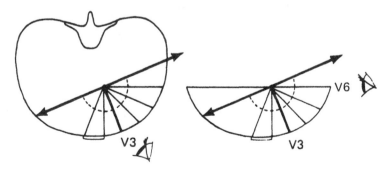

9. How can you tell whether the QRS vector is going anteriorly or posteriorly in this situation?

   ANS.: By seeing which chest leads have positive QRS complexes. For example, in the above diagram, if V6 = with a predominantly positive QRS, the V6 electrode 'eye' sees the QRS forces moving predominantly toward it. Therefore the vector must be going posteriorly.

HOW TO DRAW A SPATIAL VECTOR

*1. How did Grant [2] plot horizontal vectors?
    ANS.: By plotting both frontal and horizontal plane directions in the same diagram, so that he actually had a three-dimensional figure [2].

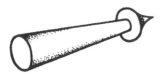

*2. On what discovery did Grant's method of plotting a three-dimensional vector depend?
    ANS.: He showed that if chest electrodes are placed like polka dots in every area of the chest, both front and back, the complexes are seen to form a pattern in which there are only negative QRS complexes on one-half of the chest and only positive complexes on the other half [2].
    If the chest wall is considered a cylinder, the anterior view can be drawn with positive and negative complexes on it. Here is one possible pattern:

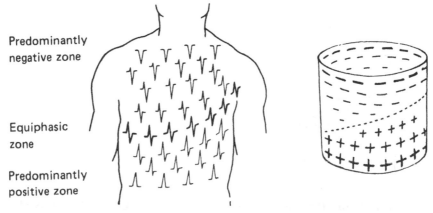

If a line is drawn through all the equiphasic complexes on the chest wall, it separates the positive from the negative side of the chest, and so divides the chest into two parts, as if by a belt.

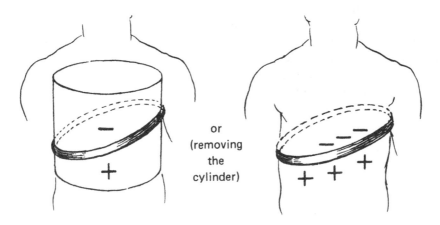

*3. What is the belt of equiphasic complexes called?
ANS.: The null zone. (It has occasionally been called the equatorial zone.)

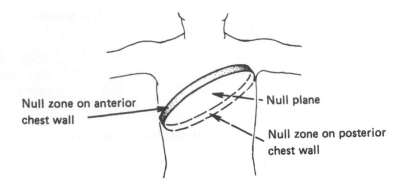

*4. Where is the electrical center of the heart on the chest wall in the frontal plane?
ANS.: Two sites have been proposed:
A—at the V2 position.
B—in the middle of the chest, about 1 to 2 cm below the V1 and V2 leads.

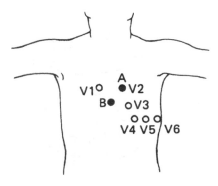

Note: In this book, the position of B, proposed by Grant [2], is used as a close approximation.

*5. What is the relation between a vector and its null plane?
ANS.: Because the null plane is everywhere perpendicular to its vector, the vector must be perpendicular to its null plane.

*6. What is the relation between a vector and the electrical center of the heart?
ANS.: All vectors are pictured as originating from the electrical center of the heart.

*7. How can you draw the relation between a vector and its null plane?
ANS.: The vector is like the axle of a wheel, the wheel being the null plane. The axle has a pointer at one end.

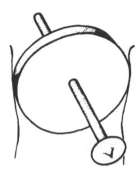

*8. What is this 'axle pointer' representation of a vector called?
    ANS.: A spatial vector because it is in three dimensions. It is symbolized as
    SÂQRS.
*9. What is meant by the frontal plane projection of a spatial vector, i.e., given this
    spatial vector and its null plane?
    ANS.:

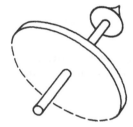

*10. What is its frontal plane projection in the hexaxial system?
     ANS.:

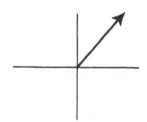

*11. How do we find the null plane tilt?
     ANS.: By finding the rim of the null plane on the chest wall, i.e., by finding the null
           zone. We have already found two points on the null zone by drawing one
           diameter of the null plane. To draw a null zone we must find a third point
           on the chest wall through which the null zone belt passes. You can draw a
           circle or ellipse through three points but not through two.
*12. How do we find the null zone from an ECG with a + 60° QRS in the frontal plane?
     ANS.: Draw the one null plane diameter that is perpendicular to the frontal plane
           vector. The two points where this diameter touches the chest wall are on the
           null zone because the null zone of every vector runs like a belt around the
           chest wall.

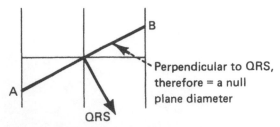

Draw diameter AB because that is the one that is perpendicular to the frontal plane vector. The null plane for this QRS vector touches the chest wall in two places, A and B. Threfore we now have two points on the null zone for this vector.

To find a third point on the null zone we use the precordial leads. For example, if the precordial leads look like this

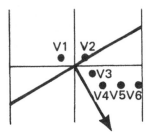

the V3 electrode is on the null zone because its QRS is equiphasic. Now we can draw our null zone through A, B, and V3 by drawing the chest leads into the cylinder that represents the chest.

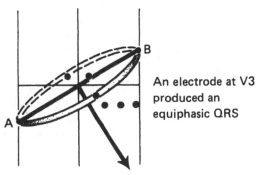

Note that the electrical center of the heart is arbitrairly placed roughly between and just below V1 and V2.

Now draw an arc connecting points A, V3, and B. This is the anterior half of the null zone on the anterior chest wall. Next draw a symmetrical arc to represent the posterior half of the null zone.

An electrode at V3 produced an equiphasic QRS

An electrode placed at either point A or B ought to give an equiphasic QRS.

Now we can draw the pointer or arrowhead showing the direction of an axle perpendicular to our null plane.

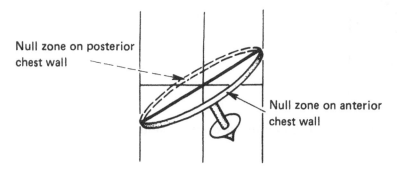

Null zone on posterior chest wall

Null zone on anterior chest wall

*13. What is the synonym in electrocardiography for a V lead that shows a QRS on the equiphasic area of the chest wall?
ANS.: Transition zone.

*Steps in Drawing a Spatial QRS Vector[1]

*1. Draw the frontal plane vector on the hexaxial system. Let us assume that in this ECG it is at 50°.

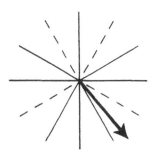

*2. Draw the sides of the chest wall on the hexaxial system.

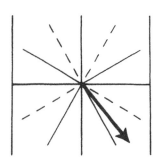

*3. Draw one diameter of the null plane. It is done by drawing a perpendicular to the frontal plane vector.

---

[1] It is not necessary to understand the previous section in order to draw a spatial vector. Memorize the steps described, and understanding will come with use.

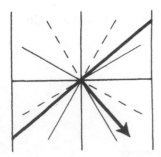

*4. Draw the chest electrode positions on the hexaxial system.

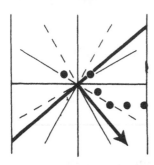

*5. Mark the chest lead with the equiphasic complex. Let us assume that V3 is equiphasic; i.e., the transition zone is at V3.

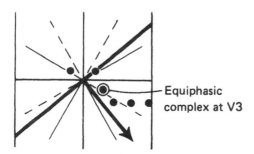

Equiphasic complex at V3

*6. Join all the equiphasic areas by an arc across the anterior and posterior chest, forming an ellipse.

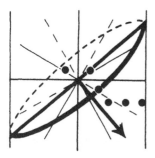

It takes three points to form the anterior part of the ellipse, two of which are the junction of the chest wall and the line perpendicular to the null plane. The third point is at the site of the electrode that produced the equiphasic complex. The posterior half of the ellipse is merely drawn as a mirror image of the anterior half.

*7. Make the anterior part of the ellipse heavy and the posterior part dotted. Now visualize the tilt of the null plane and draw an arrowhead of the vector with the same tilt. It is done by drawing an arrowhead with an ellipse exactly the same shape as the null plane ellipse. Then put the point on either the posterior or the anterior surface of the arrowhead, depending on its tilt.

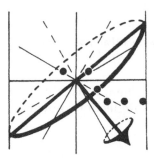

Note: If all the chest leads show an upright complex (common with T or P vectors), there is no equiphasic chest lead to tell you where to place the null zone. Draw the null zone anywhere above all the electrode sites so as to place them all on the positive side of the null plane.

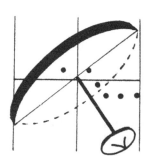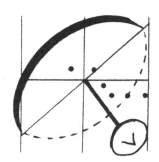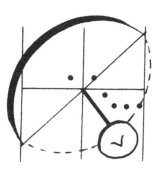

Note that all these null planes fit a frontal vector of 50° with all chest leads on the positive side of the null plane. You can tell that the vector is anterior but cannot say how anterior.

HORIZONTAL PLANE NORMAL VECTORS

Normal QRS Ranges and Patterns

1. What is the normal range of anteroposterior directions of the QRS?

ANS.: The QRS points toward the left ventricle, i.e., leftward and backward from 0° to − 60°. Note that directions in the horizontal plane are conveniently measured as radii of a circle, using a plus sign for all anterior directions and a minus sign for all posterior directions.

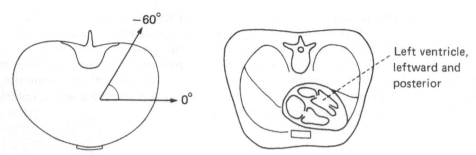

The LV is leftward and posterior, and the mean QRS range is also leftward and posterior.

2. How does this range of directions affect the appearance of V1?

ANS.: It makes the QRS in V1 appear predominantly negative. There is usually a small r and deep S or even no r at all and only a negative deflection known as a QS.

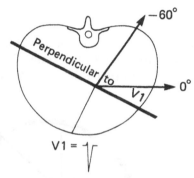

The range of directions 0° to − 60° make V1 appear predominantly negative because all the included vectors are beyond the perpendicular to V1.

Note: To derive the appearance of a chest lead, draw a perpendicular to the lead line through the electrical center. Any mean vectors that are in a

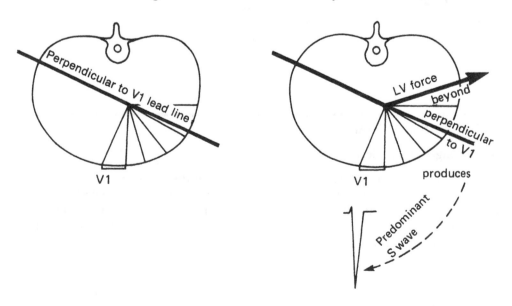

direction that is more than 90° from the lead line show up as a predominantly negative or downward complex.

3. How does the normal range of QRS directions in the horizontal plane affect the appearance of the QRS in the left precordial leads V5 and V6?
   ANS.: All vectors in the range of 0° to – 60° make V5 and V6 look predominantly positive.

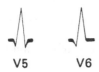

4. Which precordial leads are most like lead 1 in that their positive electrodes are almost directly to the left of the electrical center and primarily measure the X axis?
   ANS.: V5 and V6.

5. If leads V5 and V6 are somewhat like lead 1, should they normally show predominantly positive or negative deflections?
   ANS.: Because lead 1 normally shows positive QRS, T, and P waves, V5 and V6 also should (and normally do) show predominant positivity.

6. Because the positive electrodes of V1 and V6 are the most widely separated chest electrodes, which lead can be considered as most opposite to V6, looking at vectors from nearly the opposite side of the chest?
   ANS.: V1.

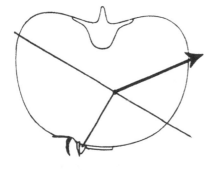

The eye of V1 sees

An electrode may be likened to an eye that is looking at the electrical center of the heart. Current flowing from the electrical center in any direction that is more than 90° from the line joining the eye to the electrical center is seen as a downward, or negative, deflection. Conversely, any current flowing toward the 'eye' is seen as un upright, or positive, deflection.

7. If V1 looks at the same vectors as V6 but from the opposite side of the chest, should V1 normally appear predominantly positive or negative?
   ANS.: In V1 the QRS is always normally predominantly negative (but the P and T may be either positive, negative, or biphasic).

PATTERN COROLLARY: *The chest or 'V' leads should show a progressive QRS change from an R/S ratio that has a predominantly negative QRS in V1 to a more positive QRS on the left precordium.*

8. What positivity does the V1 electrode 'see'?

    ANS.: The initial septal forces. The left ventricle begins depolarization about one-third of the way down the left side of the septum, which is then depolarized from left to right as well as anteriorly. These septal forces dominate during the first 10 to 30 msec of the QRS and produce a small positive wave, or r, in V1. This small r may be called the 'septal r'.

    Conversely, V5 and V6 see a small initial negative wave, or q, which may be called a 'septal q'.

*9. Why do leads V1, V2, and V3 usually show gradually higher R waves as the electrode site is moved from the right chest to the middle of the chest?

    ANS.: The R waves should increase in amplitude from V1 to V3 because the initial 0.03 sec (30 msec) forces are predominantly septal and become larger as they travel more and more obliquely through the septum. Because they are directed more and more anteriorly as well, they become more parallel to successive leads V1, V2, and V3.

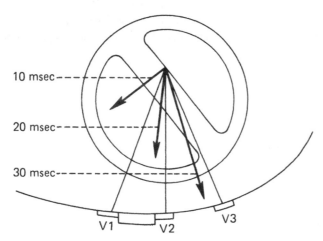

The septal forces (10-, 20-, and 30-msec vectors) shown here gradually increase in size. Each enlarging vector becomes successively more parallel to each lead as it records from right to mid-chest.

10. Why is it misleading to use the loss of progression of R height across the precordium to imply loss of anterior forces, i.e., anterior infarction or fibrosis?

    ANS.: R wave height depends partly on how close the positive electrode is to the heart. For example, V5 and V6 commonly have a lower R than does V4 even though the QRS is *relatively* more positive.

11. If not the R wave height, then what parts of the QRS do progress across the precordium?

    ANS.: The R/S ratio. The R gradually becomes greater than the S as one moves toward the V6. We should speak of a 'progression of the R/S ratio across the chest' (see ECG 5).

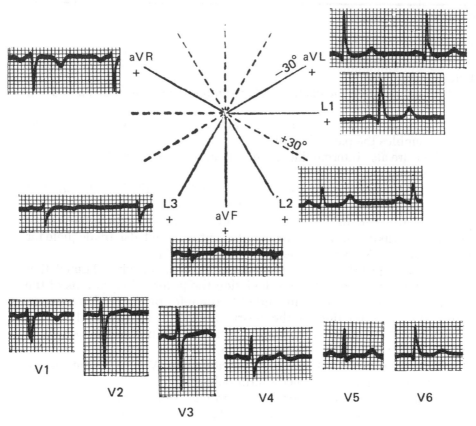

ECG 5. The R in V3 is taller than the R in V4, yet the R/S ratio is still progressing normally. This ECG is from an 82-year-old woman with labile hypertension and moderate anemia due to a bleeding peptic ulcer.

12. How does respiration affect the transition (equiphasic) lead?
    ANS.: Inspiration can shift it because inspiration can rotate the mean QRS vector. In the frontal plane, inspiration rotates the QRS inferiorly, presumably by a downward pull from the diaphragm. In the horizontal plane a deep inspiration can rotate the QRS anteriorly, and therefore the transition zone may shift toward V1.

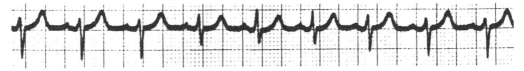

ECG 5A. Changes in R wave amplitude with respiration in a nearly equiphasic lead. The complexes gradually change from negative to positive over five beats. This change can happen in any lead that is nearly equiphasic, but it is especially common in leads 3 and aVF and the transitional lead of the precordium. If this were lead 3 or aVF, the QRS that is positive would represent the peak of inspiration because with inspiration the QRS turns inferiorly, i.e., toward the positive electrodes of leads 3 and aVF.

---

*Electrical Positions of the Heart

*1. What is meant by

a. Horizontal electrical position?
b. Vertical electrical position?

ANS.: a. Horizontal position means that aVL resembles the pattern of V5 and V6, and aVF resembles the pattern of V1.

b. Vertical position means that aVF resembles the pattern of V5 and V6, and aVL resembles the pattern of V1.

Note: There are also intermediate semivertical, semihorizontal, and indeterminate positions.

*2. What have electrical positions offered to the interpretation of ECGs that could not be done better by understanding the axes of vectors?

ANS.: Nothing. They seem to be a carryover from the days when the vector approach was unknown. They are not only confusing but also inadequate for describing all the axes seen in electrocardiography [3].

Note: Electrical positions were introduced by Wilson, who claimed that in normal subjects with right axis deviation the potential variations of the right ventricular surface are transmitted to the left arm. This phenomenon requires sufficient rotation of the heart around its longitudinal axis to allow aVL to 'see' more of the right ventricle than the left, which is an impossibility even with extreme rotation.

*3. What does it actually mean if V4, V5, and V6 resemble aVF; i.e., what does a 'vertical electrical position' mean in vector terminology?

ANS.: It means that V4, V5, and V6 positive electrodes are low enough below the electrical center of the patient's heart to be below the null plane.

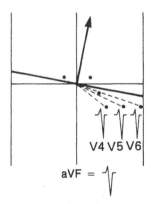

V4, V5, and V6 show Y axis forces and look somewhat like leads 2 and aVF because they are below the null plane and beyond 90° to the frontal plane vector.

*4. What does it imply about the chest electrodes if V5 and V6 look like lead 1 or aVL?

ANS.: It implies that V5 and V6 positive electrodes are placed relatively high on the patient's chest and are near the level of the electrical center.

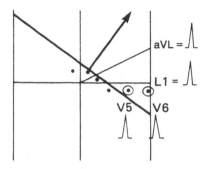

Note that V5 and V6 show X axis forces because they are above the level of the null plane and are less than 90° to the frontal QRS vector. (The electrical center is often over the V2 electrode, as in the above illustration.)

5. What is meant by clockwise and counterclockwise rotation of the heart?

    ANS.: It refers to anatomical rotation around its longitudinal axis as viewed from the apex. (See p. 385, question 6, Chap. 24 for further explanation.)

Normal T Ranges and Patterns (Horizontal Plane)

1. What is the normal range of direction of the T in the anteroposterior (horizontal) plane in the adult?

    ANS.: As in the frontal plane, where the T wave is never to the left of a leftward QRS, so in the horizontal plane it points anteriorly to the normally leftward and posterior QRS. The range is shifted about 45° anterior to the QRS range.

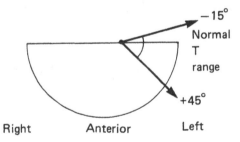

Note: Like the QRS, the T is also 10° more anterior in patients over age 30.

2. How does this direction of the T vectors control the appearance of the T in V1 compared with its appearance in V6?

    ANS.: If the T vector points at + 45°, which is the most anterior end of its normal range,

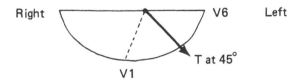

it gives an almost equally positive T in both V1 and V6. Usually, however, the T in V6 is taller than the T in V1. (See chest lead strips that follow.)

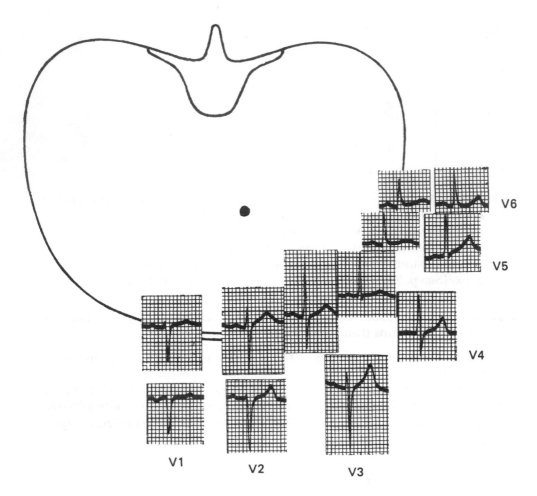

If, however, the T is at its most posterior position (− 15°), it produces a negative T in V1 and a positive T in V6.

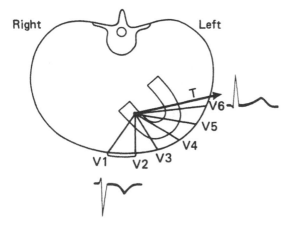

Note: The T is rarely negative from V1 to as far as V4 in the adult. A T as posterior as this is normally seen only in children and in some adults with a juvenile T pattern. (See Note for question 4.) Even by puberty only about 2 percent of children have T negativity as far as V4 [1].

3. How does the T look in V1 and V6 if it has turned anteriorly to an abnormal degree, as shown?

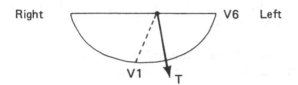

ANS.: It is higher in V1 than in V6 (probably even negative in V6). Also, because the chest electrodes for V1 to V3 may be very close to the heart, this proximity may give rise to very high T waves in these leads.

PATTERN COROLLARY FOR T: *The normal precordial T shows either equal positivity in all leads or a gradual increase in positivity from V1 (which may even have a negative T) to V6 (which normally never has a negative T).*

Note: Positivity does not refer to height but to whether the T is above or below the baseline, i.e., positivity is merely the reverse of negativity. A positive T wave in V1 normally becomes taller in V2 to V4 because the latter leads are closer to the heart. See illustrations for question 2.

4. Why is the T sometimes positive in V1 when the QRS is negative?

ANS.: Because the T vector is normally slightly anterior to the QRS. Remember that *positivity* in a chest lead means 'anteriorness'; i.e., the vector is moving *toward* the electrode on the chest wall.

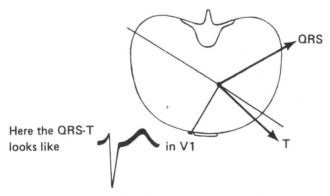

Although the QRS in the diagram is predominantly negative in V1, the T is positive because it is anterior to the QRS. This pattern is the normal relationship.

Note: If the T is posterior to the QRS, it tends to produce negative T waves across the right precordium. This phenomenon is normal in children. If it persists into adulthood, it is called the juvenile T pattern. In the adult it must be distinguished from the abnormal T of either myocardial ischemia or right ventricular overload. (This subject is discussed in Chaps. 21 and 25.)

Normal P Ranges and Patterns (Horizontal Plane)

1. Which atrium normally dominates the horizontal plane P vector?
   ANS.: The right atrium because it is the more anterior atrium and thus closer to the precordial electrodes.
2. The P vector is an average of anterior forces from the right atrium and posterior forces from the left atrium. (The left atrium is a midline posterior structure; see illustration below.) Where is the most anterior P vector expected to be if it is the resultant of anterior and posterior forces with the anterior forces dominant?
   ANS.: At about the same place as that of the T wave, i.e., about + 45°.

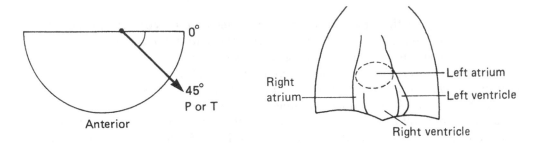

*3. Is the most posterior range of the P vector anterior or posterior to the most posterior T of − 15°?
   ANS.: The most posterior P is anterior to the most posterior T wave vector. The most posterior P vector is about 0°.

Posterior limits

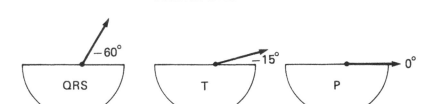

4. How is the P in V1 and V2 likely to appear if 0° is the most posterior normal direction?
   ANS.: V1 may have either a positive, negative, or biphasic P wave, but V2 is either positive or biphasic.

---

*PEDIATRIC, FRONTAL, AND HORIZONTAL P, QRS, AND T DIRECTIONS

*1. How does the P wave direction differ in infants and adults?
   ANS.: In infants it tends to be slightly more posterior; i.e., it is commonly biphasic or negative in both V1 and V2. (Remember that the farther over toward the left precordium a transition zone is for any vector, the more posterior it is.)

*2. Why does the newborn have a right axis deviation? How far to the right?

ANS.: Infants are born with right ventricular hypertrophy (RVH). The infant's right ventricular myocardium is as thick as or thicker than that of the left ventricle owing to the high pulmonary vascular resistance during fetal life. It takes several months for the infant's heart to undergo the normal involution that makes the myocardium of the right ventricle thinner than that of the left ventricle. The QRS axis can even be as far to the right as 180° on the first day, and usually it remains more than 100° for the first week.

*3. How does the RVH of infancy show itself during the first week of life other than by right axis deviation?

ANS.: By an anterior QRS; i.e., the R wave in V1 is larger than the V6 (opposite to that in the adult). Infants also have an R/S ratio exceeding 1 in all chest leads.

*4. How does the RVH of infancy show itself during the first month of life?

ANS.: There is commonly a reversal of the R/S ratio progression during the first month; i.e., the R/S gradually decreases from V1 to V6, so that V1 has an Rs and V6 has an rS [1].

*5. How does the T change in V1 with age?

ANS.: It is upright during the first 1 to 4 days. After this time, it is invariably negative. An upright T in V1 after the first few days usually signifies a right ventricular overload. (The T is negtive in V1 in premature newborns possibly because of a deficiency of beta stimulation.)

REFERENCES

1. Alimurung, M. M., et al. The unipolar precordial and extremity electrocardiogram in normal infants and children. *Circulation* 4:420, 1951.
2. Grant, R. P. Spatial vector electrocardiography. *Circulation* 1:878, 1950.
3. Urschel, D. L., and Abbey, D. C. Mean spatial vectorcardiography: The normal QRS and T vectors. *Am. Heart J.* 45:65, 1953.

12. Normal P, P-R, QRS, and T Height, Width, and Duration

1. What is the normal height and width of a P wave?

    ANS.: The upper limit of a P wave height and duration is '2.5 × 2.5' in the adult, meaning that it is 2.5 mm high and 2.5 small divisions wide, i.e., 100 msec (0.10 sec) in width.

    Note: in actual practice it is rare to find a normal adult P wave more than 2 mm high.

2. What is meant by a P-R interval?

    ANS.: It is the distance from the beginning of the P wave to the beginning of the QRS. It measures the time from the beginning of atrial depolarization to the beginning of ventricular depolarization. In some countries it is called the P-Q interval.

3. What is the normal P-R interval range?

    ANS.: It is 120 to 200 msec (0.12–0.20 sec), i.e., three to five small divisions. The faster the rate and the younger the person, the shorter should be the P-R interval.

4. What can cause periodic short and long P-R intervals?

    ANS.: Alternate use of slow and fast pathways through the *AV node*. It is postulated that increased vagal tone increases the refractory period of the fast pathways so that conduction is only over the slow pathway. A decrease in vagal tone shortens the effect of refractory period of the fast pathway and conduction through the AV node is improved [5].

5. What is the effect of gender on the QRS width?

    ANS.: It tends to be shorter in women [6].

6. When is the width of a QRS expected to be narrower than 60 msec (0.06 sec)?

    ANS.: a. In young children and in blacks it can be as short as 40 msec.

    b. In black subjects, the QRS tends to be not only narrower but also taller than in whites. The reason is unknown.

    c. In cachectic patients, such as those with cancer, the QRS may also be narrower than 80 msec [4].

7. What is the normal height of a T wave?

    ANS.: It should be at least 10 percent of a QRS, provided the QRS is predominantly positive with almost no S wave. (A complex with almost all R wave and very little S is known as a 'left ventricular complex.')

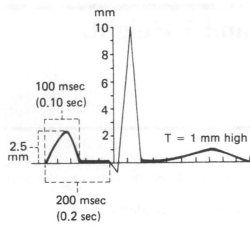

Upper normal limits for P wave (2.5 × 2.5) and P-R intervals (200 msec), and the lowest normal height for T waves (10% of a QRS that has almost no negativity).

You are now ready to read an ECG. Turn to the last pages in the book for a systematic approach to reading an ECG.

REFERENCES

1. Alimurung, M. M., et al. The unipolar precordial and extremity electrocardiogram in normal infants and children. *Circulation* 4:420, 1951.
2. Grant, R. P. Spatial vector electrocardiography. *Circulation* 1:878, 1950.
3. Urschel, D. L., and Abbey, D. C. Mean spatial vectorcardiography: The normal QRS and T vectors. *Am. Heart J.* 45:65, 1953.
4. Feldman, H., et al. Relationship between QRS width and neoplasm. *J. Electrocardiol.* 15:361, 1982.
5. Kinoshita, S., et al. Periodic variation in AV conduction time. *Am. J. Cardiol.* 53:1288, 1984.
6. Simonson, E., et al. Sex differences in the ECG. *Circulation* 22:598, 1960.

13.*Dipole Concept

*1. What is a dipole?
ANS.: A dipole is a potential force caused by a negative and a positive electrical charge in close proximity.

*2. How does a dipole relate to a vector?
ANS.: A dipole can produce a vector.

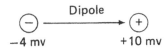

-4 mv   +10 mv

The potential difference between – 4 millivolts (mv) and + 10 mv is 14 mv. Shown here is a dipole with a right-to-left direction and a magnitude of 14 mv. Therefore it is a vector.

*3. How does the heart's current relate to the dipole concept?
ANS.: As each myocardial cell is depolarized, the heart produces dipoles. The production of current by the heart is really the production of a sequence of dipoles.

*4. How does a dipole relate to the entire human body?
ANS.: Each cardiac dipole turns the entire body into positive and negative zones.

*5. How is a dipole in the center of the chest capable of turning the whole body into positive and negative areas, with the same potential difference and vector directions as the tiny dipole itself?
ANS.: The body is a volume conductor; i.e., it acts like a tank full of electrolyte solution (e.g., normal saline) that can carry electrical current easily in all directions.
Note: When a single vector force is used to describe the resultant of all the dipoles produced simultaneously by depolarization of many cardiac cells that happen to depolarize simultaneously, it is known as an equivalent dipole. Because the dipole theory assumes that the chest is a perfect sphere that conducts equally well in all directions, an electrode anywhere on the body should theoretically pick up all dipoles equally well. Because this assumption is wrong, there are proximity effects. Some dipoles are picked up only by chest electrodes placed close to the heart and are not seen in the distant limb electrodes.

* Material marked with an asterisk is included for reference and for advanced students in cardiology.

3.*Dipole Concept

14. How to Produce a Good ECG Tracing

TERMINOLOGY

1. What is the ECG machine called?
   ANS.: An electrocardiograph.
2. What is the tracing called?
   ANS.: An electrocardiogram (ECG). (Compare *telegraph* with *telegram*.)
3. Why is the abbreviation ECG equivalent to EKG?
   ANS.: EKG is an abbreviation of the German word *Elektrokardiogram*; ECG is an abbreviation of the English word. (Some prefer EKG to avoid possible confusion with EEG [electroencephalogram].)

ELECTROCARDIOGRAPHS

1. The current evolved by the heart muscle is extremely small. How is it amplified?
   ANS.: Modern instruments use transistorized amplifiers that magnify the electrical forces before passing them through a galvanometer.
2. What is a galvanometer?
   ANS.: It is a current meter using a wire loop suspended between the poles of a permanent magnet. A pointer attached to the wire moves toward the positive or negative magnetic pole according to the direction and strength of current in the wire. This pointer can be made the writing arm, or stylus, of an ECG machine.

STANDARDIZATION

1. When the 1-millivolt (mv) button is pressed, how high should the stylus move?
   ANS.: 10 small divisions. This procedure is known as 'standardizing' the machine.

This chapter has been adapted to the needs of technicians and nurses as well as physicians.

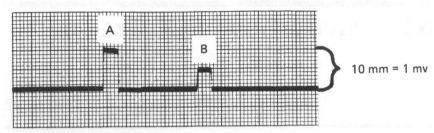

A = full or normal sensitivity or standardization. B = half-sensitivity or half-standardization. This expression is often shortened to ½S. It is used when the QRS complexes are too large to fit on the paper. Here 1 mv = 5 mm.

2. How many millimeters high is one small division?

ANS.: ECG paper has a standardized height, so that the small divisions are 0.1 ($^1/_{10}$) mv apart. In the past, 0.1 mv was always 1 mm high. However, with the smaller machines now available, one small division may be less than 1 mm high. Thus many ECG readers call each division 0.1 mv rather than 1 mm. However, it is easier to speak in terms of millimeters than tenths of millivolts. Therefore in this book the term millimeters is used for amplitude.

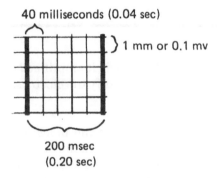

PAPER SPEED AND TIME MARKINGS

1. What is the usual paper speed?
   ANS.: 25 mm per second.
2. At 25 mm per second, how far apart in time are the
   a. Small divisions (thin lines)?
   b. Large divisions (thick lines)?
   ANS.: a. 0.04 sec (40 msec).
         b. 0.20 sec (200 msec).
3. What can change the paper speed without your realizing it?
   ANS.: Using a paper not manufactured for a particular model of machine can change the paper speed. A paper roll that is too heavy slows the paper advancement, and a roll that is too light speeds it up.
4. How can you check paper speed for accuracy without calling a serviceman?
   ANS.: Introduce alternating current (AC) into the baseline. Touch either an electrode or the machine with one hand, and touch a current-carrying accessory such as a lampstand with the other. If the line current is alternating at 60 Hz

and the paper is advancing at 50 mm per second, five large divisions (0.5 sec) should contain 30 deflections. Running the machine at both double speed (50 mm/second) and double sensitivity (1 mv = 20 mm) makes it easier to count the deflections. A difference of more than 2 percent between time markings and the actual paper speed is unsatisfactory.

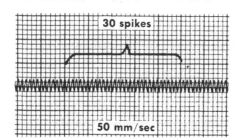

5. When is double speed (50 mm/second) used to take routine ECGs?
   ANS.: Usually in pediatric ECGs because the faster heart rates of infants and young children obscure details at 25 mm per second.
6. On many types of ECG paper, vertical lines appear at regular intervals on the margin. What do they signify?
   ANS.: Three-second intervals. (Some rare types use 2-second intervals.)

APPLYING ELECTRODES

1. Should small or large quantities of electrode paste be used?
   ANS.: Small amounts. Large quantities tend to produce wandering baselines by allowing slight movements of the electrodes on the slippery paste.
2. Does rubbing the skin reduce skin resistance?
   ANS.: Yes, but only if there is enough abrasion to damage surface cells, as by light scratches with fingernails or a rough towel. This rubbing can be done without undue discomfort to the subject. If the skin does not become reddened, abrasion has been too mild.
3. Why must skin resistance be equal at all electrode sites?
   ANS.: A difference in skin resistance can produce local currents that distort the ECG. Sometimes it can even produce AC interference.
   Note: Rubbing must be more vigorous on the legs because skin resistance is higher there than in the arms or chest.
4. Why should the ECG machine be turned on while the electrodes are being applied?
   ANS.: It allows the machine to warm up and so saves time.
5. How can you apply a suction cup to a hairy chest?
   ANS.: Use plenty of paste and then a rotary or twisting movement during firm application.
6. How can you judge the best pressure for a strap that holds an electrode to a limb?
   ANS.: Introduce your finger under the strap and secure the strap snugly over the finger. When the finger is removed, the strap will be neither too tight nor too loose.

Note: Too-tight rubber strap pressure, surprisingly, is the commonest cause of muscle tremor artifacts.

7. Where on the arms should the electrodes be placed?
   ANS.: On the upper arm, which is preferred because
      a. There is only fine hair on the upper arm.
      b. Finger movement does not cause muscle contraction artifacts in the upper arm. Contraction above the elbow joint is required to produce upper arm artifacts.
      c. If the forearm is used, technicians tend to put the electrodes on the thick, hairy posterior surface.

SPECIAL LEADS

1. Where are chest electrodes placed for V3R and V4R leads? When are they used?
   ANS.: They are right-sided chest leads that are the mirror image of regular electrodes V3 and V4, as shown.

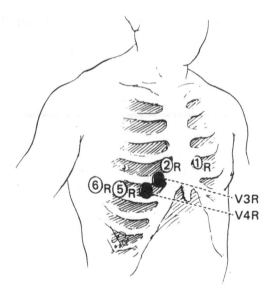

   They are used for:
      a. Diagnosing right ventricular hypertrophy and infarction.
      b. Establishing the diagnosis of dextrocardia.
*2. What is a VE lead? When is it used?
   ANS.: It is a lead produced by a chest electrode placed on the xiphoid, or ensiform, cartilage. It is used to explore for P waves in atrial ectopic rhythms.
*3. What is an esophageal lead?
   ANS.: An exploring chest lead with the positive electrode at the tip of an esophageal tube that is passed through the nose and swallowed, so that the electrode contacts the area of the esophagus that is against the left atrium. It is occasionally useful when it is necessary to magnify P waves that are

* Material marked with an asterisk is included for reference and for advanced students in cardiology.

difficult to see owing to rapid rates or ectopic foci. A 'Lewis lead' is often used for this purpose. In this type of lead you place the right arm electrode at the first right interspace and the left arm electrode at V1, then switch to L1. When you learn about CR leads in question 5, you will note that the Lewis lead is a modified CR1 lead.

Note: You can tell that you are at the atrial level with an esophageal electrode by noting that at the atrial level

a. The P waves are larger than the QRS.

b. The esophageal tube, measured in centimeters, has decended roughly 15 to 25 cm from the nares.

*4. When is the L3 on deep inspiration used?

ANS.: It has been said that a q in L3 that is due to an infarct remains on deep inspiration, whereas the normal q disappears. This 'rule' has so many exceptions that most centers have discarded the maneuver [5].

*5. What is a CR lead? What are its advantages?

ANS.: It is a bipolar lead with the negative electrode on the *right* arm and the positive electrode placed on the chest as an exploring electrode. It exaggerates voltage in the left precordium. Not only may notched T waves become deep and easily seen with a CR lead, but P waves can be exaggerated for the study of arrhythmias.

Note: You can make a CR lead by switching the ECG to lead 1 and using the left arm electrode as an exploring electrode in place of the usual precordial electrodes.

6. What is a CL lead?

ANS.: It is a bipolar lead with the negative electrode on the *left* arm and the positive electrode placed on the chest as an exploring electrode.

7. When is a CL lead used today?

ANS.: A modification known as the MCL 1 lead is often used in coronary care units with the positive electrode at the V1 position. The negative electrode is placed under the outer third of the left clavicle (instead of the left arm). The ground wire is placed under the outer third of the right clavicle. It allows

a. The mid-precordium and left precordium to be free for defibrillation or external compression.

b. An easily visible P wave to be seen for the monitoring of arrhythmias.

c. Easy recognition of right or left bundle branch block development.

PATIENT AND BED ASPECT

1. In what position should the patient be when the ECG is recorded? Why?

ANS.: Supine if possible. The criteria for normal ECGs are based on records of patients in the supine position. If the patient cannot lie flat, the record should be taken in the lowest chest elevation that is comfortable for the patient.

Note: If the patient's chest is raised to about 60°, the QRS axis may become more leftward to as high as − 30°, or more rightward by more than 20° [1].

2. How can patient nervousness or discomfort spoil an ECG?
   ANS.: By producing muscle tremor artifacts.
3. How can patient discomfort be minimized?
   ANS.: a. Assure the patient that the electrocardiograph is merely a device that measures the amount and direction of the small amount of electricity generated by the heart.
   b. Expose only the patient's chest and arms and keep his or her abdomen and thighs warm with adequate covering and a warm room.
   c. Use pillows to adjust the head for maximum comfort.
   d. Do not put rubber straps on tightly.
   e. Give infants a delayed feeding bottle and distract them with dangling lights, toys, or keys. A mother can restrain or comfort an infant or child, but she should wear rubber gloves.

ELIMINATION OF AC INTERFERENCE

Routine Methods

1. How can you recognize AC interference?
   ANS.: It is a rapid (often audible) vibration of the stylus that produces regular spikes of similar amplitude that widen the baseline and make it fuzzy. In the United States the frequency of the spikes is 60 per second.

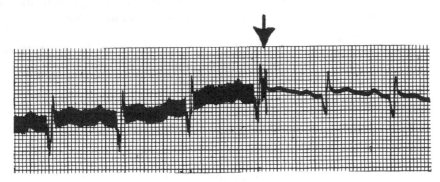

aVF

At the arrow, the technician's hand was removed from the left arm electrode, and the 60-cycle interference was abolished.

2. How can the patient and the bed be made less likely to produce AC interference?
   ANS.: a. By not allowing the patient's feet and hands to touch any part of the bed other than the mattress.
   b. By disconnecting the wall plug of any electrical apparatus near to or touching the bed.
   Note: Merely turning off an electrical appliance near the bed is not sufficient to eliminate interference. It must be unplugged from the wall.

3. Do hearing aids cause interference?
   ANS.: Not the modern transistorized ones.
4. Is it necessary to remove the patient's watch to prevent damage to it or to prevent interference?
   ANS.: No. See p. 99 for effects of a battery-operated watch.
5. How can bed position improve a record?
   ANS.: A power cable running parallel to the bed may create AC interference, which can be eliminated by rotating the bed 90°.
   Note: The power cable should never cross over the patient or bed, nor should it ever cross the cable that connects the patient's electrodes with the ECG machine.
6. If a patient is seated because of some problem that prevents his or her being placed in the supine position, how can you eliminate AC interference from the floor?
   ANS.: Place books or magazines under the patient's feet to insulate them from the floor.
7. What feature of some ECG machines is designed to help eliminate AC interference?
   ANS.: A special lever or button is provided to reverse the polarity of the wall plug from inside the machine. This switch can often eliminate AC interference.

Grounding

1. Must both leg electrodes be attached to the patient if only an L1 or L2 is desired?
   ANS.: The right leg is usually essential for grounding. However, in an emergency such as a cardiac arrest, a rhythm strip could be tried using just two limb electrodes, e.g., right arm and left leg (L2) or right and left arms (L1). Only if too much interference occurs need the right leg electrode be put on.
2. How should you ground a machine that shows AC interference despite correction of everything obviously wrong?
   ANS.: One grounding wire with a clip at each end is attached to the metal part of the ECG machine and to another metal object in the room such as a water pipe, a radiator, or the metal frame of the patient's bed.
   Note: A fractured lead wire can manifest as AC interference or as complete failure to record certain leads.
3. If this grounding wire does not work, what further techniques should be tried?
   ANS.: a. Make sure that there is no paint under either end of the ground wire clip.
   b. Connect two ground wires to the machine. Attach one to the bed and the other to a water pipe.
   c. Try touching different parts of the patient's skin. (Occasionally this maneuver works, contrary to expectation, especially if you touch the machine with the other hand.)
   Note: Always disengage the patient cable of a cardiac monitor if an ECG machine is about to be connected to the patient. The monitor and your ECG machine must go to a common ground. Otherwise a static charge might travel from one machine to the other with your patient the unwitting connector, and ventricular fibrillation may result.

Eliminating Persistent AC Interference

1. List the more subtle method of eliminating AC interference if all other grounding techniques fail.
   ANS.: a. Move the patient and machine to another part of the room, as far from the walls as possible.
   b. Make certain that all oil or metal particles are washed off the skin with alcohol.
   c. Be sure any unattached lead wire is on the bed and not touching the floor or bed frame. Have the chest electrode in the V1 position attached while taking limb leads.
   d. See if there is paste on the cable tip and check that the tip is tightly attached to the binding post.
   e. See that any electrical apparatus in adjoining rooms is disconnected.
2. How can you tell whether the AC interference is due to a fault in the machine itself?
   ANS.: If after all precautions have been taken AC interference is still present even when the patient cable is removed, a blown patient-circuit fuse is the most likely cause.
3. What materials used to clean electrodes can produce AC interference?
   ANS.: Abrasive materials because metallic compounds in the resulting scratches can cause artifacts and AC interference.

PROTECTING THE ECG MACHINE AGAINST DAMAGE

1. When during a surgical procedure does the stylus of an ECG machine need protection?
   ANS.: If diathermy cautery is used, the ECG machine should be disconnected from the wall to prevent damage to the stylus and to avoid blowing a fuse.
2. What other situation requires disconnecting the ECG machine from the wall to protect it?
   ANS.: When defibrillation or electroversion is being carried out. However, some machines have a special circuit to protect them in these situations. You must ask the manufacturer whether yours does.

ERRORS AND ARTIFACTS IN RECORDING

Lead Reversal and Lead Placement Artifacts

1. What should make you suspect immediately that you have reversed the right and left arm leads?
   ANS.: If all the components of the ECG in L1 are inverted; i.e., the P, QRS, and T are all negative (see ECG 6).

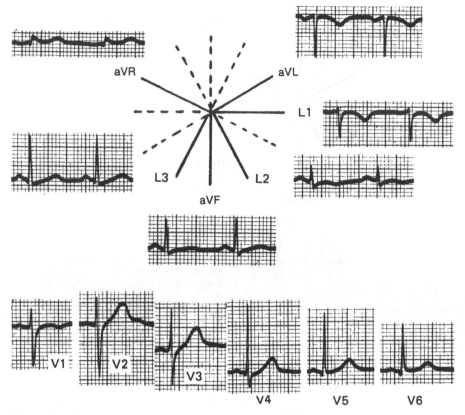

ECG 6. This ECG is from the same normal woman as ECG 2 (p. 46). However, note that now L1 has a negative P, QRS, and T, and aVR has a positive QRS and T, denoting right and left arm lead reversal. Note also that the chest leads are not affected.

2. What is the only other possible cause of negativity of all complexes in L1?
    ANS.: Uncomplicated mirror-image dextrocardia, in which the left ventricle, left atrium, aortic arch, and stomach are all on the right side. This situation is also known as situs inversus.

    Note: a. The ECG diagnosis of dextrocardia is made obvious by looking at the chest leads. The chest leads utilize a unipolar system and do not reflect lead reversal. That is, they look normal even if the limb leads are reversed (V1 is predominantly negative and V6 positive) (see ECG 6). In dextrocardia, V1 and V2 are negative, and V6 is also mostly negative (see ECG 7).

    *b. The triad of dextrocardia, bronchiectasis, and sinusitis is known as Kartagener's syndrome.

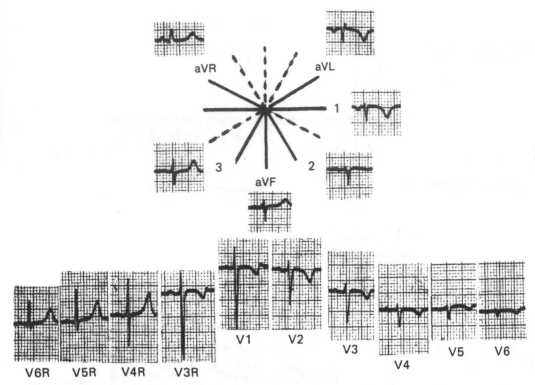

ECG 7. This ECG is from a 12-year-old child with mirror-image dextrocardia (situs inversus) and a normal heart. Right and left precordial leads show that it is not reversed limb leads that caused the negative P, QRS, and T in L1.

*3. When should you suspect that the right arm and left leg leads are reversed?
 ANS.: If the P is negative in leads 1, 2, and 3. (The P is *never* normally negative in leads 1 and 2.)

 4. What generally happens to the QRS in a normal young subject if the V1 lead is placed in the third rather than the fourth right interspace?
 ANS.: A terminal positivity (R′) is commonly seen.

 5. What happens if electrode paste is spread so that it runs into the site of two chest electrodes?
 ANS.: Confluence of paste between various chest electrodes causes a similarity of QRS configuration because the electrodes joined by paste then form a common electrode. Be certain that there is dry skin between electrode positions on the chest (see ECG 8).

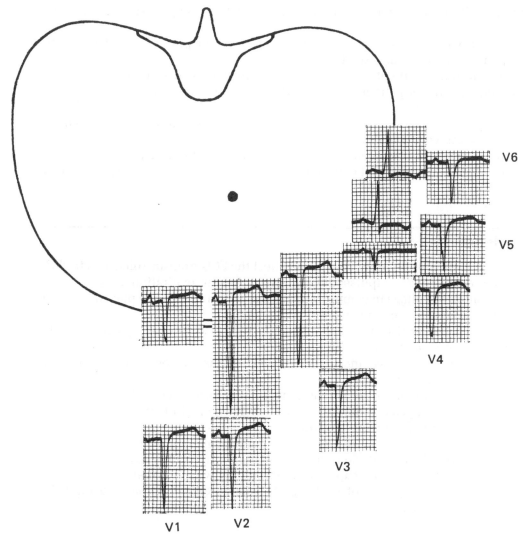

ECG 8. Chest leads from a 50-year-old man with an alcoholic cardiomyopathy and biventricular overload. The top row was taken with the electrode paste separated by dry areas. The bottom row was taken with paste smeared across the chest joining all electrode sites. Note the similarity of complexes that smearing produced.

Wandering or Jumping Baselines

1. What are the causes of a wandering baseline in addition to not waiting for the stylus to settle before turning the switch to run?

   ANS.: a. Patient movement due to tension, curiosity, or talking.

   b. Metal dust on the skin, or dirt in the paste.

   c. Dirty lead-wire tips.

   d. Too loose application of electrodes.

   e. In chest leads only: excessive respiratory movement.

2. If all these failings are corrected and the wandering baseline persists, what may be wrong?

   ANS.: There may be marked variations in voltage from the power line, with a faulty or inadequate voltage stabilizer.

3. What can cause intermittent or jumping irregularities of the baseline?

   ANS.: Slight jarring or patient movement if, in addition, there is

   a. Poor contact of one or more electrodes with the skin, especially in patients who work in atmospheres laden with metallic dust or who have excessively oily skin.

   b. Poor contact between the lead-wire tip and the binding post.

   c. A loose connection between the patient cable or power cable plug and its socket.

Amplitude Artifacts

1. How can a forceful cardiac apex movement affect the ECG from an apical electrode?

   ANS.: A greater apical impulse during inspiration or expiration may cause a variation of voltage in complexes recorded with an electrode placed over the apical impulse, i.e., in leads V4, V5, or V6.

2. How can a forceful cardiac apex movement affect the ECG from an apical electrode other than changing amplitude with respiration?

   ANS.: It can cause the appearance of small, irregular baseline oscillations that may resemble somatic tremor.

3. What can cause a sudden decrease in amplitude in a normal record?

   ANS.: Contaminated paste, a defective amplifier tube, or dirt between the binding post and cup of a suction electrode.

   Note: Some television sets can cause radiofrequency interference, which may lower the amplitude of an ECG complex if an ECG machine without special radiofrequency suppression circuits is within 2 meters of the television set. The policy of shutting off bedside television sets during ECG recording is suggested [4].

Somatic Tremor Artifacts

1. What is the commonest cause of somatic tremor artifacts?

   ANS.: Too-tight rubber straps on the limb electrodes.

2. What are some other causes of somatic tremor artifacts?

   ANS.: a. Anxiety or physical discomfort, especially if the room is chilly.

   b. Parkinsonism.

   c. Hyperthyroidism.

   Note: The muscle tremor of parkinsonism can produce either of the following:

   a. A regular sequence of undulations at the same rate as the clinical tremor. The undulations may resemble the F waves of atrial flutter at about five oscillations per second.

   b. Very fine irregular oscillations at a frequency of 30 to 150 Hz unrelated to the clinical tremor rate [6].

3. How can you sometimes decrease the effect of somatic tremor if loosening the rubber strap does not work?

ANS.: a. By placing the limb electrodes near or on the shoulders or thighs, where the tremor is less marked.

b. By covering the exposed chest with a towel or blanket.

*4. What artifact can nearby electrical equipment produce?

ANS.: a. A ringing phone can produce tiny 20-Hz spikes. Dialing a phone can produce tiny irregularities similar to those of somatic tremor.

b. A nasogastric suction pump can produce false atrial flutter waves [2].

c. A battery-operated watch may leak current and produce spikes similar to those produced by a runaway pacemaker [3].

REFERENCES

1. Bergman, K. S., Stevenson, W. G., Tillisch, J. H., Stevenson, L. W. Effect of body position on the diagnostic accuracy of the electrocardiogram. *Am. Heart J.* 117:204–206, 1999.

2. Crampton, R. S., and Hunter, F. P., Jr. False atrial flutter from nasogastric suction pump. *J.A.M.A.* 223:1160, 1973.

3. Lesch, M., and Greene, H. L. Electrocardiographic artifact due to malfunction of an electric watch. *J.A.M.A.* 228:26, 1974.

4. Lichstein, E., and Gupta, P. K. Television set distortion of electrocardiogram. *J.A.M.A.* 223: 1285, 1973.

5. Shettigar, U. R., et al. Diagnostic value of Q-waves in inferior myocardial infarction. *Am. Heart J.* 88:170, 1974.

6. Soderstrom, N. Some typical patterns of muscular tremor in routine electrocardiograms. *Acta Med. Scand.* 152:209, 1955.

15. Initial Activation and the Septal Vector

1. The bundle of His ends by bifurcating into a right and left bundle branch. How far from the beginning of the bundle of His does the bifurcation occur?
   ANS.: The bifurcation occurs after 1 cm of the His bundle, just as it emerges from the fibrous ring that joins atrium to ventricle (see the diagram of question 4).
2. How long is the main left bundle in humans before it breaks up into its branches, or divisions? What are these divisions?
   ANS.: The main left bundle is 1 to 2 cm long before it bifurcates into a proximal posterior, a distal anterior, and a smaller septal division.
3. Where in the septum does the bundle of His bifurcate into right and left bundle branches?
   ANS.: Very high, still in the region of the membranous septum, which is the thin translucent part of the ventricular septum just below the aortic valve.
4. Which is narrower, the left or right bundle branch?
   ANS.: The main right bundle, which is a slender strand 1 to 2 mm thick.

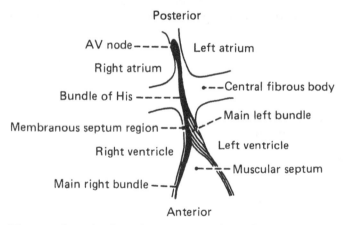

Diagram of proximal conduction system from above, i.e., a bird's-eye view.

5. How close to the endocardium of the right side of the septum does the main right bundle travel?
   ANS.: It is very close to the right ventricular cavity.
   Note: A catheter in the right ventricle that is pressed against the septum can cause various degrees of delayed conduction along the right bundle branch.
6. Where does the right bundle arborize, or divide, into small branches?
   ANS.: The right bundle passes down the right side of the septum as a slender bundle until it reaches the lowest part of the apex of the right ventricle. There it passes into a bridge of muscle between the septum and the anterior papillary muscle. (This bridge is the moderator band.) The right bundle does not arborize until it reaches the anterior papillary muscle of the right ventricle.

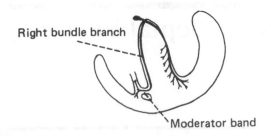

7. Where does the left bundle branch arborize, and which part of the heart would be expected to be depolarized first?
   ANS.: It arborizes on the left side of the septum, about one-third of the way down between base and apex. Therefore the left side of the septum should be depolarized first.
8. Which parts of the heart are actually activated first?
   ANS.: Three subendocardial areas are synchronously excited as if there were three divisions to the left bundle [3]:
   a. Middle of the left side of the septum (septal fascicle).
   b. A high anterior left ventricular subendocardial area near the septum (anterior fascicle).
   c. A low posterior left ventricular subendocardial area near the septum (posterior fascicle).
9. If the left side of the septum is activated first, what must be the direction of conduction through the septum; i.e., is the direction of septal activation from left to right or vice versa?
   ANS.: From left to right.

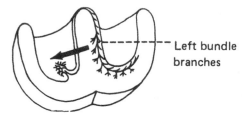

Note that the septal vector is from left to right.

Note: Studies in dogs and human subjects have shown that the septum is activated from right to left almost immediately after the initial left-to-right forces have begun; i.e., there is a double envelopment of the septum by the forces of early depolarization [1, 2]. Therefore the initial left-to-right vector seen in most normal subjects represents the *dominant* initial vector and not an absence of right-to-left forces. The dominance of left-to-right initial forces is probably due to the relatively small area involved on the right side of the septum in contrast to the large area on the left side that is depolarized early [1].

10. How long does it take to activate the septum?
    ANS.: About 35 msec (0.035 sec).

* Material marked with an asterisk is included for reference and for advanced students in cardiology.

Note: It actually takes about 65 msec (0.065 sec) for the current of depolarization to cross the septum when the current starts from only one side. However, the septum is bilaterally invaded from right to left as well as from left to right, so that despite some delay in the onset of right-to-left conduction depolarization is actually completed in about 35 msec.

11. What other parts of the left ventricle are activated during the first 35 msec?
    ANS.: The subendocardium of most of the free wall of the left ventricle (not the high posterior areas).

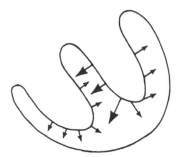

All these vectors actually make up the 'septal' vectors.

Note: Within 35 msec the epicardium has already been reached over the three areas that were activated earliest.

12. Why, then, is the initial vector of the QRS called a 'septal' vector?
    ANS.: Because the septal forces are thought to dominate the initial vectors (for unknown reasons). The resultant vector is from left to right.
        Note: In subjects without a septum, i.e., with a single ventricle, the initial vector may still be from left to right and produce a 'septal' vector with q waves in aVL and lead 1. (This situation occurs only if the infundibulum of the rudimentary right ventricle is situated on the right side of the single ventricle.)

13. What are the three major directions in which ventricular depolarization is divided?
    ANS.: *Vector 1:* The 'septal' vector (from left to right).
        Vector 2: Through the major muscle mass of the left ventricle (inferior, to the left, and posterior).
        Vector 3: Either through the posterior basal portion of the left ventricle or up the outflow tract of the right ventricle, i.e., either straight posterior or superior and to the right. There are thus two possible third vectors.

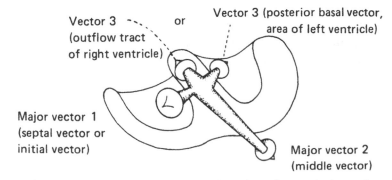

With increasing age, vector 3 changes from the right ventricular outflow tract to the posterior basal region of the left ventricle.

14. What is the major vector 1 (major initial QRS vector) usually called?
    ANS.: The 'septal' vector. Because septal forces usually dominate the initial vec-
    tors, it justifies use of the term *septal*, and we shall henceforth dispense with
    quotation marks on this term.
15. If the septal vector is normally from left to right, in which limb leads is a septal q
    (slight initial negativity) normally expected?
    ANS.: Any limb lead may normally have a q wave.

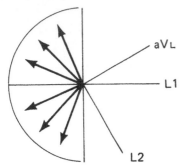

*All the vectors in this semicircle are from left to right and therefore could be septal
vectors.*

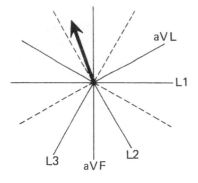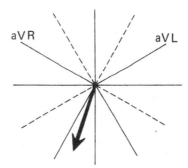

16. Where is a septal q expected in the horizontal plane or chest leads?
    ANS.: In the left precordium, i.e., around V6, because V6 also tends to measure
    current along the X axis, as does lead 1.
17. Where is a septal r expected in the horizontal plane?
    ANS.: In the right precordial leads, i.e., V1 or V2.

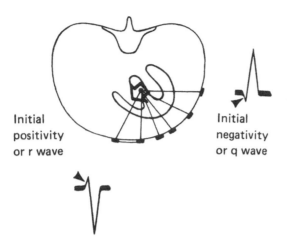

Initial
positivity
or r wave

Initial
negativity
or q wave

Note: The initial forces should reverse if the septum is reversed. This reversal occurs in corrected transposition (inversion of the ventricles). The initial vector is from right to left. This fact is especially useful to know when a ventricular septal defect is also known to be present. Because a ventricular septal defect generally causes a deep Q in the left precordium, and the absence of such a Q then suggests a corrected transposition as well.

REFERENCES

1. Amer, N. S., et al. Activation of the interventricular septal myocardium studied during cardiopulmonary bypass. *Am. Heart J.* 59:224, 1960.
2. Durrer, D. Electrical aspects of human cardiac activity. *Cardiovasc. Res.* 2:1, 1968.
3. Durrer, D., et al. Total excitation of the isolated human heart. *Circulation* 41:899, 1970.

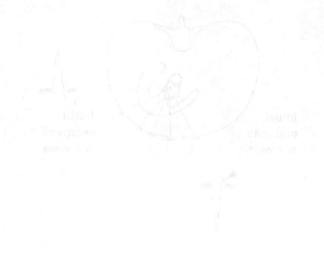

16. Bundle Branch Block

RIGHT BUNDLE BRANCH BLOCK (RBBB)

Initial QRS Vector in RBBB

1. What is meant by the 'initial QRS vector'?

   ANS.: It means any part of the first portion of the QRS that includes the initial forces. The term does not imply any exact duration so long as the very first forces are considered. If the beginning forces are in a direction different from the mean QRS vector, the *initial* vector refers to these beginning forces, e.g., vector 1 or the septal vector (see p. 103).

2. The right main bundle passes down close to the subendocardium of the right side of the septum and gives off few fibers as it extends to the apex of the right ventricle (RV), where it passes into the base of the anterior papillary muscle via the moderator band. The left bundle, on the other hand, breaks up near the upper third of the left side of the septum to send branches into the septum (see illustration on p. 102). If the right bundle branch is blocked, how is the direction of the septal activity affected?

   ANS.: It is not affected at all because the right bundle branch does not contribute significantly to septal activation. Septal depolarization is dominated by the left bundle, which breaks up high on the left side of the septum. The right bundle breaks up or arborizes low in the RV.

   RULE 1 for RBBB: *RBBB does not affect the direction of the initial QRS vector.*

Direction of the Terminal QRS Vector in RBBB

1. What is meant by the 'terminal QRS forces'?

   ANS.: Any portion of the last third of the QRS that inclues the final forces. If these final forces are in a direction different from the middle QRS vectors, it refers to these forces (vector 3) and may normally last 10 to 30 msec.

*2. Why is it unnecessary to go into detail about the middle or major vector 2 (the vector of the mass of the left ventricle) in RBBB?

   ANS.: The terminal vector in RBBB changes in the middle of the QRS, so that at least the second half of the middle vector is affected.

3. How does the RV manifest on the QRS of the normal ECG?

   ANS.: It does not show. Because the normal RV is only about one-half the thickness of the left ventricle (LV), it does not contribute significantly to the normal ECG.

* Material marked with an asterisk is included for reference and for advanced students in cardiology.

4. When *does* the RV contribute to the ECG?

    ANS.: a. When the RV hypertrophies. It then approaches the LV in thickness and competes for electrical control of the ECG.

        b. When depolarization of the RV is delayed, as in RBBB, so that it does not depolarize simultaneously with the LV. It then finishes depolarization after the LV has finished.

     *c. When the RV is depolarized early, as in some preexcitation syndromes and in left bundle branch block (LBBB).

5. What can delay depolarization of the RV?

    ANS.: A block in the right bundle branch. This block is not necessarily an anatomical block. It may be a physiological or functional slowing of conduction and thus be intermittent and varying in degree from time to time. RBBB is sometimes called 'RBB delay.' Whether the right bundle branch has delayed or slowed conduction or it is completely blocked, the LV still finishes its depolarization first, and so right ventricular depolarization occurs last. Therefore the words *block* and *delay* have similar effects and may be interchanged.

    Note: A QRS may be considered to be the final result of fusion between right and left bundle depolarization. Asynchrony of depolarization caused by any degree of slowing through either major pathway can result in a QRS configuration of varying degrees of RBBB or LBBB.

6. If conduction down the right bundle is blocked or slowed, which part of the QRS shows right ventricular forces?

    ANS.: Because right ventricular activation is delayed, the LV is depolarized first, and the *final* forces show the late right ventricular depolarization.

7. How is the RV placed anatomically in relation to the LV?

    ANS.: The RV is anterior and to the right of the LV.

Posterior

Right   Left

Right ventricle

Cross section of heart at fourth intercostal space level.

8. If conduction down the right bundle is blocked, what is the expected direction of the terminal forces, taking into consideration that the RV is anterior and to the right?

    ANS.: Anterior and to the right.

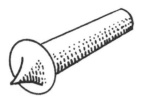

9. If the vector forces of the terminal part of the QRS in RBBB are pointing rightward, in which frontal plane semicircle must this terminal vector lie?
ANS.: The semicircle on the right, i.e., beyond ± 90°.

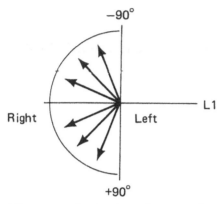

All vectors going 'to the right' are in this semicircle.

10. If the terminal vector of the QRS is pointing to the right in RBBB, which limb lead is the only one in which terminal negativity or an S wave must always be present? Proof?
ANS.: Lead 1 is the only lead where terminal negativity always means that the terminal vector is to the right of ± 90°.

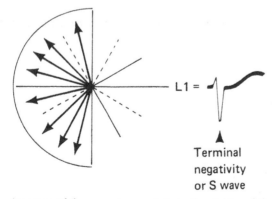

Any one of these vectors points to the right and therefore may be a terminal vector for RBBB.

Proof (a): If the terminal vector points to the right and *downward*, lead 2 does not have a terminal S, but lead 1 does.

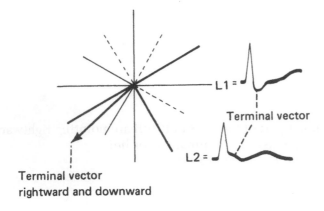

Terminal vector
rightward and downward

Proof (*b*): If the terminal vector points to the right and *upward*, aVL does not have a terminal S, but lead 1 does.

Terminal vector
rightward and upward

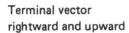
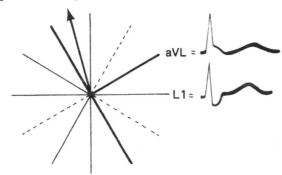

RULE 2 for RBBB. *Typical RBBB always produces an S or s in lead 1; i.e., terminal negativity need be present only in lead 1.*

11. If the terminal part of the QRS in RBBB points to the right and *anteriorly*, which chest leads have terminal positivity?
    ANS.: Right chest leads.

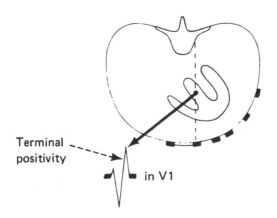

Terminal positivity

in V1

12. If the terminal vector of the QRS in RBBB points to the right and anteriorly, which routine chest lead has terminal negativity?
    ANS.: V6.

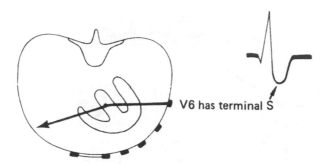

V6 has terminal S

13. If there is already a small septal r in V1, what is the terminal positivity called?
    ANS.: R prime (R').

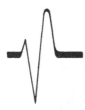

14. If there is no septal r in V1, what is a terminal positivity called?
    ANS.: A terminal R or, simply, terminal positivity.

    RULE 3 for RBBB. *Typical RBBB always has a terminal R or R' in V1.*

Terminal Slowing in RBBB

1. If the right bundle is blocked, does the RV depolarize through the normal conduction system?
   ANS.: It is assumed that the RV is depolarized through a combination of muscle and Purkinje fibers; i.e., conduction through the RV is abnormal.
2. What is the proof of abnormal conduction through the RV in RBBB?
   ANS.: The terminal vector is not only rightward and anterior, it also is prolonged, as if conduction through the RV were slowed. Conduction through ventricular muscle is one-tenth as fast as through the Purkinje system.
   Note: Another theory to explain terminal slowing in RBBB is that there is an unbalancing of forces. This concept implies that there is always slow velocity through the right ventricular conduction system but that it is not manifested on a normal ECG because there is fusion of simultaneous forces, canceling out the slowing effect.
3. How does slowing show on an ECG?
   ANS.: By widening or increased duration of the wave as well as by thickening of the line if recorded by a hot stylus on heat-sensitive paper.

Note: a. A heated stylus melts a wider pathway through waxed ECG paper if the stylus moves slowly
b. Thickening is referred to as 'slurring' by many cardiologists.

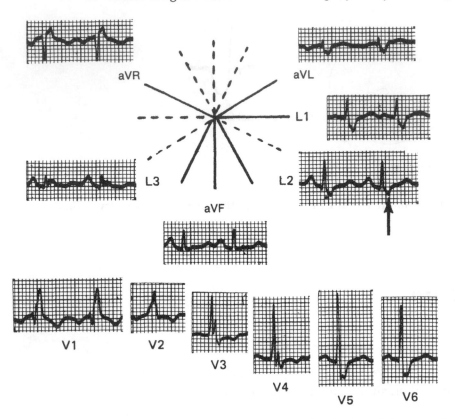

ECG 9. RBBB in a 69-year-old man with urinary retention due to prostatic hypertrophy. He sustained a myocardial infarction 6 years previously but was asymptomatic thereafter. The thickened end of the QRS in the leads that show a wide, large area terminal force represents slow conduction through the RV (see arrow).

RULE 4 FOR RBBB. *RBBB always has a wide S in lead 1 as well a wide R′ or terminal positivity in V1.*

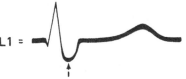

Wide terminal negativity or S wave

The new ink writers or writers that do not use heated wax paper do not show thickening when the writing mechanism moves more slowly.

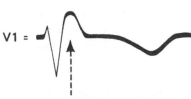

Wide terminal positivity or R′

Note: To simplify the diagnosis of typical RBBB, you need only look at leads 1 and V1. Simply look for the wide S in lead 1 and the wide terminal positivity in V1.

Complete and Incomplete RBBB

1. What is the usual width of a QRS?
    ANS.: It is usually 80 msec (0.08 sec) but is occasionally as long as 90 msec (0.09 sec) and, especially in young people, as short as 50 msec (0.05 sec).
2. What are the causes of a QRS wider than 90 msec?
    ANS.: A wide QRS implies a conduction defect that has caused slowed or delayed conduction. The slowed conduction may be in the initial, middle, or terminal third of the QRS. The commonest conduction defect is a bundle branch block. The next most common is a divisional block (discussed in Chap. 19). Initial slowing can similarly widen a QRS (discussed under preexcitation, in Chap. 18, p. 187). Uniform slowing of all three thirds is caused by hyperkalemia and by excessive doses of drugs such as quinidine or tricyclic antidepressants [36].
3. In which leads must one look for the widest QRS?
    ANS.: In any lead. Most textbooks state that only the limb leads should be used to measure the QRS width. This statement must be based more on tradition than on logic. If the QRS is thought of as a series of vectors, a piece of the beginning or end of the QRS may easily be perpendicular to the frontal or the horizontal plane and so make the QRS appear narrower in either the limb or the chest leads.

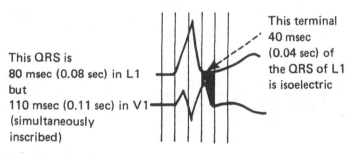

This QRS is 80 msec (0.08 sec) in L1 but 110 msec (0.11 sec) in V1 (simultaneously inscribed)

This terminal 40 msec (0.04 sec) of the QRS of L1 is isoelectric

Only V1 in the above example shows the true width of the QRS.

4. What is meant by 'complete' RBBB?
    ANS.: It is called complete if the QRS is widened to at least 120 msec (0.12 sec), or three small divisions.
    Note: Because RBBB in the QRS can be as wide as 160 msec (0.16 sec), 120 msec cannot be considered *really* complete. By convention, however, we use the term *complete* for a 120-msec RBBB.
5. What is meant by 'incomplete RBBB'?
    ANS.: It is called incomplete if the QRS is prolonged, but to less than 120 msec (0.12 sec).

6. What is the value of distinguishing between complete and incomplete RBBB?

ANS.: a. Incomplete RBBB is more likely to be a normal variation than is complete RBBB.

b. When it does reflect an abnormality, incomplete RBBB is more likely to be due to right ventricular hypertrophy (RVH) than is complete RBBB.

*7. How can you bring out normal conduction when an RBBB or LBBB appears to be fixed? Why does it work?

ANS.: By slowing the rate with vagal stimulation by means of carotid sinus massage. This measure allows time for recovery of conduction by the right or left bundle. It is known as rate-dependent bundle branch block (see p. 573). *Note:* Bradycardia-dependent RBBB has been reported but is rare [21].

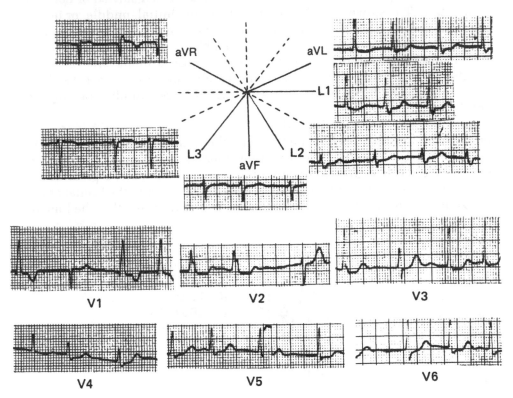

ECG 10. *An 80-year-old asymptomatic woman with an idiopathic cardiomyopathy has an irregular rhythm due to atrial fibrillation. It has produced short and long R-R intervals. After most long intervals the QRS is narrow; after short intervals the terminal changes of RBBB are evident. This abnormality is known as rate-dependent bundle branch block. Note that both the initial forces and the left axis deviation do not change when RBBB develops. Because the QRS widens only to 0.10 sec (100 msec), it is an incomplete RBBB.*

Summary of Rules for Recognizing RBBB

1. The initial vector is not affected.
2. There must be a wide S in L1.
3. There must be a wide terminal positivity in V1 (terminal R or R').

RBBB Pattern

1. What is meant by an 'RBBB pattern'?

   ANS.: The same terminal vectors as in RBBB (S in L1 with terminal R in V1) but without recognizable terminal widening, so that the QRS width is not beyond the upper limits of normal. In other words, any ECG with an S in L1 and an R′ in V1 without prolongation of the QRS has a RBBB pattern (see ECG 11).

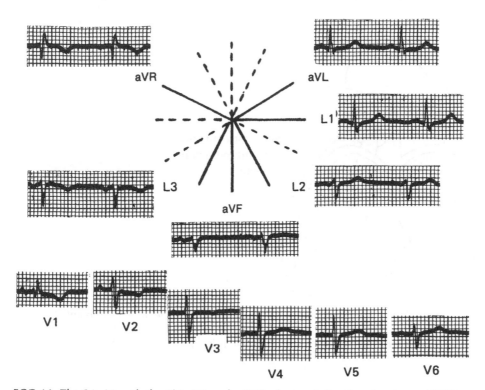

ECG 11. The S in L1 with the R′ in V1 and a QRS of normal duration denotes an RBBB pattern. This ECG is from a healthy 67-year-old woman with a normal heart and lungs. Note that the terminal forces (e.g., S waves in L1, L2, and L3) are not wide or slurred.

Note: Varying degrees of pressure by a catheter on the outflow tract of the RV (where the right bundle branch is superficial and subendocardial) can produce varying degrees of RBBB, so that a control QRS of 60 msec can become an incomplete RBBB with a QRS of only 80 msec. The latter would not be recognized as abnormally wide for that subject without a control tracing [28].

2. What is the value of recognizing an RBBB pattern?

   ANS.: a. Almost all patients with atrial septal defects (ASDs) have either an RBBB or an RBBB pattern. Without either one or the other appearing on an ECG, an ASD is unlikely. The reason for this pattern is presumably the RV volume overload, which may cause stretching of the right bundle.

   b. An RBBB or an RBBB pattern may be the only sign of acute dilatation of the RV, as in pulmonary embolism.

   c. A RBBB pattern may be the only sign of RVH, even though most patients with this pattern have normal ventricles.

d. An RBBB pattern is also a normal pattern and, even with a marked left axis deviation, may still be a normal variant (see ECGs 43A and 43B on pp. 213 and 214).

3. Where is the terminal conduction pathway in normal subjects with the RBBB pattern?

ANS.: Up the outflow tract, or infundibulum, of the RV [3].

Note: All newborns have RVH, and terminal forces may be controlled by a part of the RV for several decades and sometimes permanently.

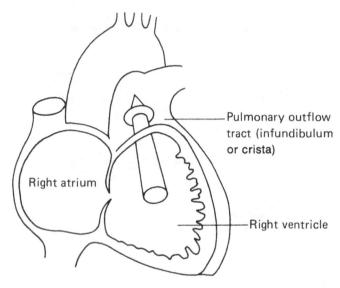

When the terminal force is up the outflow tract of the right ventricle, it tends to point in the direction of the infundibulum, which is usually slightly posterior and to the right. This situation tends to produce either a small terminal positivity or a shallow S in V1.

4. If the terminal conduction is up the right ventricular outflow tract, the terminal vector may not be anterior and to the right but slightly posterior and to the right. What does this do to the terminal portion of V1?

ANS.: Instead of a terminal R or R′ there is only a shallow S. This pattern may be called an atypical RBBB or, if the QRS is not wide, an atypical RBBB pattern (see ECG 3, p. 51, and ECG 12).

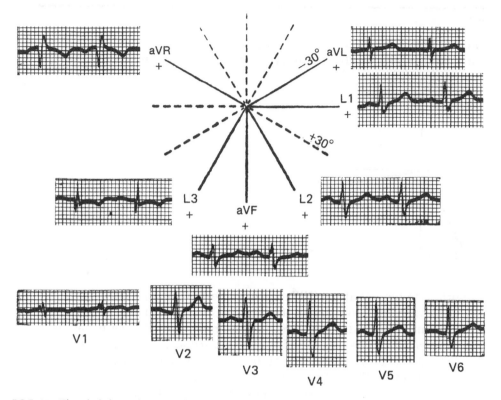

ECG 12. The slightly wide QRS of 100 msec (0.10 sec) with an S in L1 and a shallow S in V1 represents an atypical incomplete RBBB. If it were typical, there would be a terminal positivity in V1. An incomplete RBBB such as this is either a normal variant or a sign of right ventricular hypertrophy. This ECG is from a normal 48-year-old man. Note the slightly slurred (thick) S in L1, denoting slow conduction through the RV.

5. Why is the RBBB pattern with its terminal conduction up the outflow tract of the RV occasionally called the 'cristal pattern'?

ANS.: The outflow tract of the RV has a muscular ridge called the crista supraventricularis.

6. What percentage of normal subjects have RBBB, atypical or typical?

ANS.: About 95 percent of normal subjects under age 20 have at least an atypical RBBB pattern [3]. A typical RBBB pattern (R′ in V1) is found in about 5 percent of normal subjects under age 40 [34].

Note: A rare way of describing the various degrees of RBBB, e.g., RBBB pattern, incomplete RBBB, and complete RBBB, is by 'first-degree,' 'second-degree,' and 'third-degree' RBBB.

7. What problematic QRS axis may be produced if the initial forces arise from the LV and the terminal forces go up the outflow tract of the RV?

ANS.: This situation may produce an indeterminate axis; i.e., at least two limb leads may be equiphasic so that it is impossible to derive a frontal plane axis (see ECG 12). These terminal forces are superior, to the right, and usually slightly posterior so that there is an S1, S2, S3 pattern and V1 has a shallow S rather than a terminal positivity [11].

Axis in RBBB

1. What is a normal QRS frontal plane axis in RBBB?
    ANS.: From + 10° to about + 120°. (Without RBBB the normal range is 0° to 90°.)

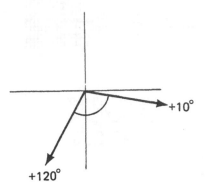

2. Why is it important to figure out the QRS axis in subjects with an RBBB?
    ANS.: Because marked left axis deviation with RBBB helps in the diagnosis of some congenital heart diseases; and in acquired heart disease it has been found empirically to be associated with myocardial infarction or scarring (see ECG 10, p. 114). (This subject is discussed under hemiblocks, or divisional blocks, in Chap. 19.)

3. What is the significance of an RBBB *pattern* with left axis deviation?
    ANS.: Some normal subjects have marked left axis deviation with only the RBBB pattern. In such patients, terminal conduction is up the infundibulum, which can shift the axis superiorly. With actual RBBB with terminal slowing, however, the terminal conduction is presumably into the body of the RV and should not shift the axis superiorly without an additional conduction defect such as anterior divisional block (see p. 204).

    Note: A left axis deviation with RBBB may signify the presence of an ASD of the endocardial cushion type. If a patient with an ASD has a left axis deviation (i.e., the QRS axis is 0° or more), the patient usually has a very low septal defect of the primum type. It is due to maldevelopment of the endocardial cushion and is often associated with a cleft mitral or tricuspid valve or with a ventricular septal defect. The more common secundum ASD, the mid-septal defect, does not usually show a left axis deviation.

    Although a primum ASD should be strongly suspected when there is a left axis deviation, it is never 100 percent certain on the basis of axis alone [17]. In several series the incidence of left axis deviation with either secundum or sinus venosus (high) defects was about 4 percent [4].

    Note: In one study of adults with a primum defect about 60% did not have a leftward axis [12A].

LEFT BUNDLE BRANCH BLOCK

Initial Vector in LBBB

1. If the left bundle is blocked and the forces propagated by the right bundle branch are unopposed, what part of the heart is depolarized first?
   ANS.: The right side, i.e., the RV and right side of the septum.
2. Do early right ventricular forces actually show themselves when LBBB leaves the right bundle branch unopposed?
   ANS.: Yes. The anterior part of the RV is depolarized first, and the initial vectors must include those due to RV depolarization.
3. If the RV and right side of the septum are depolarized first in LBBB, in what direction must the initial vector travel?
   ANS.: From right to left.

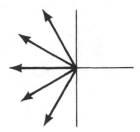

Possible normal initial
vectors

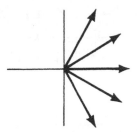

Possible initial vectors
in LBBB

4. If the septal vector is from right to left in LBBB, which leads ought always to have initial positivity?
   ANS.: L1 and V6 (see ECG 13).

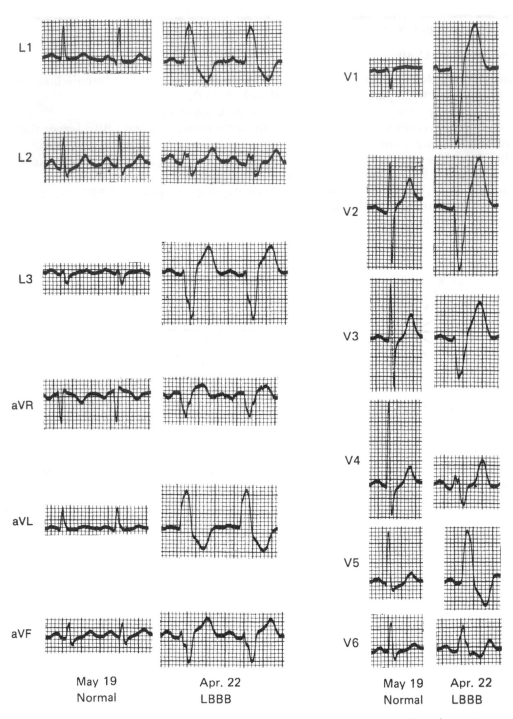

May 19	Apr. 22	May 19	Apr. 22
Normal	LBBB	Normal	LBBB

ECG 13. Serial ECGs from a 66-year-old normal man treated only with tranquilizers for anxiety. He had an intermittent LBBB. Note that the septal q in L1, as well as in V5 and V6, disappears when LBBB develops. Note also the negative S-T, T that developed in leads with wide QRS complexes (L1, aVL, and V5).

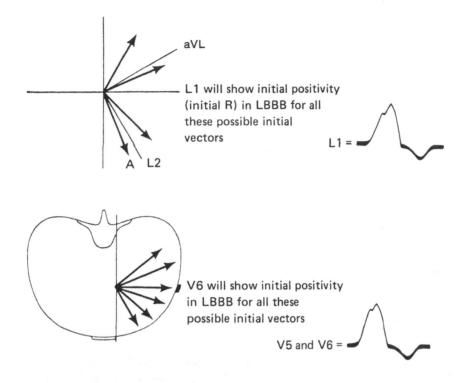

5. Can there be a q in aVL in LBBB?

   ANS.: Yes, the most inferior vectors in the frontal plane of the preceding figure (vector A) are going from right to left but are more than 90° to the lead line of aVL, resulting in initial negativity in that lead.

   Note: A q in aVF in the presence of LBBB suggests infarction because the initial forces of uncomplicated LBBB usually point at least slightly inferiorly.

   RULE 1 FOR LBBB. *In LBBB there should be no q wave or initial negativity in lead 1 or V6.*

*6. Why may LBBB allow a small septal R in V1 and V2 (i.e., a small left-to-right force shown only in the right chest leads) but no septal q in lead 1 or V6?

ANS.:

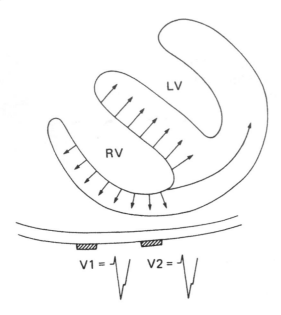

V1 and V2 are situated so close to the RV that they can pick up the small initial left-to-right forces in the wall of the RV. These forces are so small in the thin RV that they are not picked up by remote positive electrodes as in L1 and V6.

7. Is the height of the r in the right precordial leads in LBBB high or low?

ANS.: Low. They may even be absent. The initial anterior and left-to-right forces of the RV are small and may be picked up weakly or not at all in V1 and V2 if the chest wall is thickened or the anteroposterior diameter of the chest is increased. The first forces recorded may even be the initial septal right-to-left forces, which may result in absent R waves in V1 or V2.

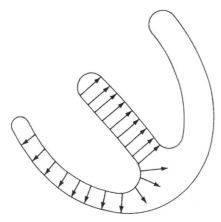

The thin RV has small left-to-right and anterior forces that produce a small r in V1 and V2 that may disappear with a thick chest or a chest with a large posteroanterior diameter.

*8. How is the duration of septal activation affected by loss of left-to-right forces?
   ANS.: Septal forces are prolonged because, instead of being simultaneously depolarized by the left and right bundle branches from both sides, the septum
   must depend entirely on right-to-left depolarization from the right bundle.
   Note: Septal activation proceeds at normal speed, but it lasts longer and
   contributes to much more of the QRS in LBBB than in normal conduction.
   Right ventricular activation and septal activation occur for about the first
   half of the QRS in LBBB.

Mid-QRS Forces in LBBB

1. How does the right-to-left wave front spread from the septum to the entire
   subendocardium and epicardium in LBBB?
   ANS.: It moves across the septum and free wall of the LV in a broad front from right
   to left [42].

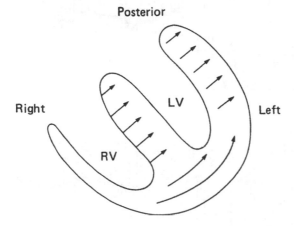

*2. What happens to the area of wave front as the broad septal front moves toward the
   free wall of the LV?
   ANS.: The area decreases [42].

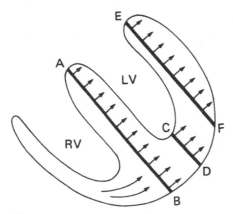

*The wave front CD is smaller than the fronts AB or EF, thereby causing a decreased
electromotive force in the middle of the QRS.*

3. What happens to the QRS when the wave front suddenly decreases in area?
   ANS.: A notch or slur occurs [42] (see ECG 14).
   > *Note:* Vector loops show marked slowing of the depolarization wave in the middle of the QRS loop in patients with LBBB.

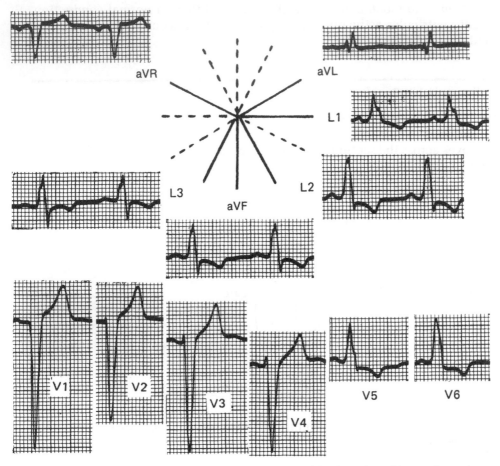

ECG 14. LBBB in a 41-year-old man in the hospital for a mild subarachnoid hemorrhage due to a congenital arteriovenous malformation. Fifteen years earlier an automobile dropped onto his chest without fracturing ribs. No ECG had ever been taken until this present one. He has no cardiac symptoms. Note the mid-QRS notch in L1 and the equivalent deep mid-QRS dip (s wave) in aVL.

Terminal QRS Forces and Intrinsicoid Deflections in LBBB

1. What happens to the QRS when the wave front suddenly increases as it continues laterally through the free wall of the LV (E-F in the wave front diagram on p. 123)?
   ANS.: Another peak is produced.

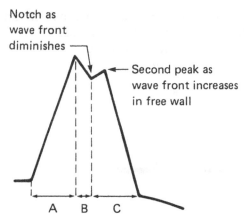

A = right ventricular and septal activation. B = notch during crossover into the free wall of the LV. C = depolarization of the free wall of the LV.

RULE 2 FOR LBBB. *In LBBB there is a change in vector magnitude in the first half of the QRS, usually shown by a mid-QRS notch or slur.*

2. What is meant by an exploring electrode?
   ANS.: It is a positive electrode of a lead whose other end either is at zero potential or is so far away from the positive end that it has been called an 'indifferent' electrode. When this positive electrode is placed on the heart or chest, it is an exploring electrode.
3. What kind of deflection does an exploring electrode on the LV produce as the usual endocardial-to-epicardial activation approaches the electrode?
   ANS.: It produces increasing positivity.

4. What happens to the increasing positivity when depolarization finishes at the epicardium directly under the electrode?
   ANS.: The ECG stylus returns to the baseline.

5. What is the final downstroke produced by this epicardial electrode called?
   ANS.: The intrinsic deflection.
6. If the exploring electrode is not placed directly on the heart but is placed on the chest wall, as in actual practice, what is the final downward deflection called?
   ANS.: The intrinsicoid deflection (-*oid* is Greek for 'similar to').

7. What is the time taken for the electrical activation of the septum plus activation from endocardium to epicardium under the exploring electrode called?

ANS.: Ventricular activation time. The QRS configuration up to the final downstroke is called the preintrinsicoid deflection.

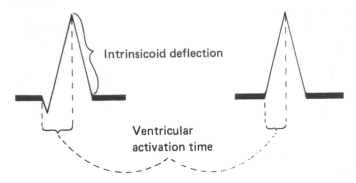

8. If an exploring electrode is placed directly over an exposed normal LV, what QRS complex is produced? Why?

ANS.: A qR or qRs. It is because the septal vector from left to right produces the q wave (initial negativity), followed by ventricular activation toward the electrode (depolarization of the LV from endocardium to epicardium), making an R wave upstroke. As the depolarization wave moves away from the epicardial electrode, the downstroke of the R wave is produced. In most adults a tiny s wave is produced by final depolarization of the high posterior part of the LV.

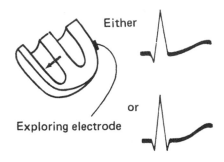

9. What is a QRS complex that is produced by an exploring electrode directly on a normal LV called? Which leads usually show this kind of complex?

ANS.: A left ventricular complex, usually seen in aVL and left precordial leads.

10. If ⋀ is a left ventricular complex, what is a right ventricular complex? Why?

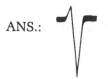

ANS.: is a right ventricular complex. If an exploring electrode is placed directly on an exposed normal RV, a complex with an r and a deep S is seen, usually in the right precordium and in aVR. The r is the septal vector, and the S is due to depolarization of the LV.

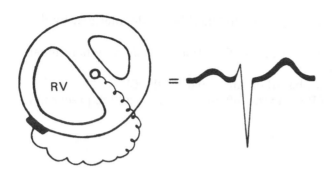

11. What is the maximum normal ventricular activation time or preintrinsicoid deflection in aVL or left precordial leads when they have left ventricular complexes?
     ANS.: Not more than 50 msec (0.05 sec).

12. What happens to the ventricular activation time in LBBB; i.e., how long is the preintrinsicoid deflection if prolonged conduction through the ventricle is produced by LBBB?
     ANS.: It depends on how marked the block or slowing of conduction is. It is prolonged to at least 70 msec (0.07 sec) in complete LBBB.

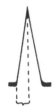

50 msec (0.05 sec)

The upper normal ventricular activation time is 50 msec (0.05 sec).

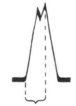

70 msec (0.07 sec)

The usual minimum ventricular activation time (preintrinsicoid deflection) in complete LBBB is 70 msec (0.07 sec).

13. What is usually meant by *complete* LBBB?
     ANS.: Enough slowing to produce a QRS of at least 120 msec (0.12 sec), or three small divisions, in duration.

*14. If there are several notches in the widened QRS of a patient with complete LBBB, which downstroke is the intrinsicoid deflection?
     ANS.: The final downstroke is considered to be the intrinsicoid deflection.

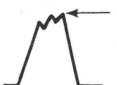

This is the final downstroke and therefore the intrinsicoid deflection

RULE 3 for LBBB. *In complete LBBB the ventricular activation time is 70 msec (0.07 sec) or more.*

15. If the left bundle branch is blocked, is terminal depolarization ever up the outflow tract of the RV?

ANS.: No. Every part of the RV has long since finished being depolarized by the time the LV's free walls are traversed.

16. If the terminal part of the QRS is not via the outflow tract of the RV, where must terminal depolarization occur in LBBB?
ANS.: In the high posterior (superior basal) or lateral part of the LV.
17. If the terminal part of the QRS in LBBB is to the left and posterior, which precordial leads never have terminal positivity or an R'?
ANS.: The right precordial leads, i.e., V1 and V2.

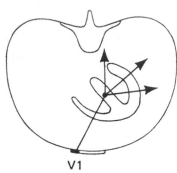

All these terminal vectors are possible with LBBB. Note that they are all more than 90° from V1. Therefore V1 never has terminal positivity in LBBB.

RULE 4 FOR LBBB. *In LBBB the right precordial leads do not have terminal positivity.*

Complete and Incomplete LBBB

1. What is the trouble with the term *complete* LBBB?
ANS.: As in RBBB, LBBB that is really complete can produce a QRS much longer than 120 msec; it may be as long as 200 msec (0.20 sec). Most lesions that produce bundle branch block are incomplete lesions. Therefore the ECG term *complete* does not imply a histological completeness. The term *marked* or *severe* LBBB might be more fitting.
2. What is meant by incomplete LBBB?
ANS.: LBBB is incomplete if the QRS is widened, but to *less than 120 msec* (0.12 sec), with *initial right-to-left conduction*, i.e., no Q or q in left ventricular leads such as L1, V5, and V6. In left ventricular leads R wave often has a hump, or shoulder, on the upstroke (see ECG 15).

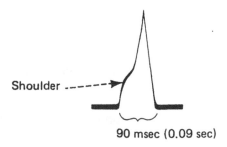

Shoulder ·------▶

90 msec (0.09 sec)

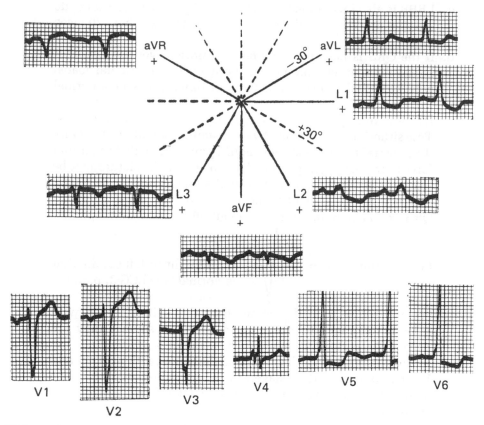

ECG 15. *This ECG is from a 68-year-old hypertensive man with severe coronary disease and an enlarged heart. Note the hump on the upstroke of V5 and V6, as in typical incomplete LBBB. The QRS is widened to 100 msec (0.01 sec). Incomplete LBBB is a common secondary sign of left ventricular hypertrophy. The patient died of an acute right coronary occlusion 2 weeks after this ECG.*

Note: a. An incomplete LBBB may be only 80 msec in duration if the preblock ECG showed that the normal width for that subject was 70 msec. This picture could be called 'incomplete LBBB pattern.'

b. Various degrees of LBBB can occur with changes of cycle length; i.e., with increasingly faster rates, the degree of slowing along the left bundle branches may increase from left bundle branch pattern to incomplete LBBB to complete LBBB. This condition is known as rate-dependent bundle branch block (see ECG 15A and p. 573).

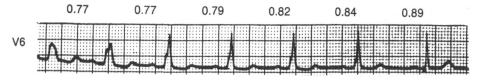

ECG 15A. *This ECG is from a 40-year-old woman with occasional paroxysmal tachycardias of short duration and a normal heart on physical examination and x-ray. The cycle length of 0.77 second produces complete or incomplete LBBB. A cycle length of 0.84 second produces an incomplete LBBB pattern, and at 0.89 second the Q wave of left-to-right conduction returns.*

c. LBBB is also incomplete if the QRS is 120 msec (0.12 sec) wide but the intrinsicoid deflection occurs at less than 70 msec (0.07).

d. If the QRS is *not prolonged* beyond normal yet has apparent initial right-to-left conduction (no q in left ventricular leads) with a normal ventricular activation time, it may be a normal variant. The initial forces may seem to be going from right to left but are actually going straight up or down and anteriorly. This situation is confirmed by a substantial septal r in V1. Only if the septal r in V1 is absent should you assume that the initial forces are really going from right to left. This picture can be found in about 5 percent of normal subjects under age 40 [8]. Very slight initial right-to-left conduction is expected if the QRS axis is more inferior than about 60°.

For example, if L1 = ⌄ initial right-to-left conduction is normal (see ECG 3, p. 51).

(Vector loops generally show that the initial forces with inferior axes are straight up and anterior, so that they are perpendicular to L1 rather than right to left.)

*e. In the presence of marked left axis deviation, although V5 and V6 may not show the delayed intrinsicoid deflection because of the deep S waves there, the high lateral position of aVL shows it well.

3. Why is it important to recognize a minor degree of incomplete LBBB?

ANS.: The loss of the normal septal vector may indicate three important conditions.

a. It may indicate septal fibrosis [2], which probably means that the septal fascicle of the left bundle has been damaged, so that it either slowed in its conduction or is completely blocked.

b. It may be the only secondary sign of left ventricular hypertrophy (LVH) that can be used in conjunction with voltage criteria.

c. It may mean that the Q waves in the right precordium do not indicate an infarct.

*4. What pathological condition has been found when an incomplete LBBB is seen?

ANS.: Incomplete fibrosis of the left bundle and of the summit and even the apex of the ventricular septum [2, 40]. Occlusive disease of one or both coronary arteries has been found to be the cause in some patients [40].

Note: a. Most of the blood supply to the main left bundle trunk is from the right coronary artery, with some help from the anterior descending coronary artery.

b. Any kind or degree of bundle branch block can result from a focal lesion or area of refractoriness within the bundle of His. It is probably due to longitudinal dissociation of parallel fibers in the His bundle with relatively few cross connections [23].

Summary of Criteria for LBBB

1. The initial vector must be from right to left (L1 and V6 have initial positivity).
2. The terminal vector points posteriorly and to the left. (The right precordial leads have terminal negativity.)
3. A notch or slur is seen in the first third or the middle of the QRS.
4. The intrinsicoid deflection is delayed in onset because the ventricular activation time is prolonged. In complete LBBB it is delayed to at least 70 msec.

SECONDARY S-T, T CHANGES

1. If a QRS is widened, are the S-T and T vectors affected; i.e., is repolarization affected?
   ANS.: Yes.
2. What does a large area enclosed by the QRS do to the S-T and T vectors?
   ANS.: The S-T and T vectors move in a direction opposite to the large-area QRS. They also increase in magnitude.

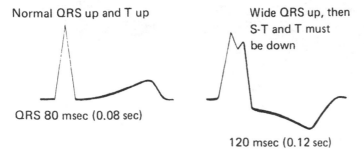

Normal QRS up and T up

QRS 80 msec (0.08 sec)

Wide QRS up, then S-T and T must be down

120 msec (0.12 sec)

3. Are the S-T, T changes seen in conjunction with large QRS areas to be considered normal or abnormal?
   ANS.: Normal.
4. What is the normal S-T, T change found with a large QRS called?
   ANS.: A secondary S-T, T change (see ECG 13, p. 120).
       Note: The normal secondary S-T, T changes seen in a left ventricular lead in LBBB have a characteristic configuration, as follows: a depressed J point; a slightly upward convex, down-sloping proximal limb to a negative T wave; and a shorter, up-sloping terminal limb. This pattern is similar to the one described later for the LVH strain pattern, which in LBBB does not signify left ventricular hypertrophy.
5. Can a T wave be negative in 'critical leads' (L1, L2, and aVF) with a wide QRS and still be normal?
   ANS.: Yes, it is what is meant by a *secondary* T change.
6. What is an *abnormal* S-T or T called in the presence of a wide QRS to identify those that would have been abnormal even before the wide QRS developed?
   ANS.: A primary S-T or T change; e.g., an upright T with a wide upright QRS is a primary T abnormality (see ECG 16).

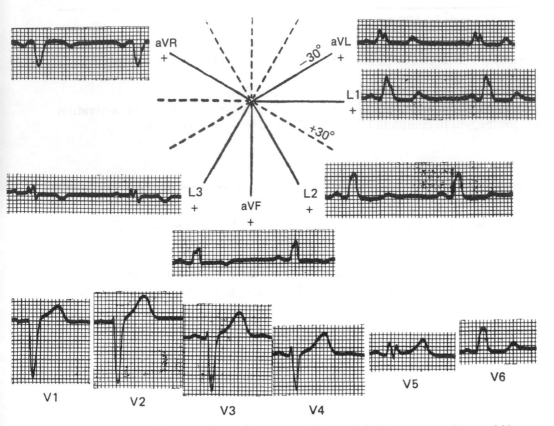

ECG 16. LBBB in a 67-year-old man with an infarct 5 years before. If the T were normal, it would be negative in L1, aVL, and V6 because the QRS in those leads is wide and positive. Therefore the positive T in those leads denotes a primary T abnormality.

7. If lead 1 looks like this [image: QRS and T complex] , is the T probably normal (second-
    arily changed) or abnormal primarily changed)?
    ANS.: Abnormal. It is probably a primary T abnormality because, despite a wide
    QRS, the T is going in the same direction as the QRS.
    Note: a. If a prebundle branch block T negativity is present only in the left
    precordial leads, when bundle branch block develops it does not
    show a primary T abnormality; i.e., the T does not become upright.
    The prebundle branch block T negativity must be in the right
    or mid-precordium (posteriorly turned) to show as a primary T
    abnormality when LBBB develops [19].
    b. In the presence of intermittent LBBB, the T may be abnormal (con-
    cordant with the QRS) simply owing to the intermittency. When
    the LBBB disappears, the T waves may be found to be temporarily
    abnormal, usually deeply negative in the right precordium and
    mid-precordium [32]. The cause of this T negativity is unknown. It
    may last only a few days, because it is not due to coronary or

myocardial disease; a permanent LBBB with concordant T waves is probably more indicative of myocardial disease.

8. What direction does the T take in the secondary change due to RBBB?

ANS.: It goes in a direction opposite to the terminal wide part of the QRS and not opposite to the early normal part of the QRS [28] (see ECG 9, p. 112).

9. Which bundle branch block has a secondary J point shift that is

a. Small?

b. Large?

ANS.: a. RBBB usually has a small shift.

b. LBBB usually has a large shift.

10. Can a wide QRS hide an abnormal S-T or T that was present in the preblock ECG?

ANS.: Yes, especially if the abnormal S-T or T was only in the left ventricular leads, V5 and V6.

SIGNIFICANCE OF RIGHT AND LEFT BUNDLE BRANCH BLOCK

1. When is RBBB suggestive of myocardial damage or a serious infarct?

ANS.: a. When there is marked left axis deviation, especially with a long P-R interval (see trifascicular blocks in Chap. 19, p. 230).

b. When it suddenly develops in the course of acute anterior infarction. It is then considered an indication for an immediate demand pacemaker, because complete atrioventricular (AV) block usually ensues. The risk is similar with or without accompanying first degree AV block [15].

c. If it develops suddenly, together with severe dyspnea. It then suggests a pulmonary embolus.

*d. Complete or incomplete RBBB was found in about 14 percent of 93 young patients (mean age 33) proved to be susceptible to malignant hyperthermia by caffeine contracture and ATP depletion studies on skeletal muscle biopsies. They had never had a known hyperthermic reaction and were selected because of family history. Abnormal ECGs were found in about 25 percent of such subjects including necrosis vectors, LVH voltage with secondary S-T, T changes, and anterior divisional blocks [24].

2. When is RBBB not indicative of myocardial damage when it develops during adulthood?

ANS.: When it is associated with a clinically normal heart [20].

Note: Incomplete RBBB is often a benign congenital variant, unassociated with signs or symptoms of heart disease throughout a long life. It has been shown that slight congenital hypertrophy of the right side of the septum and pulmonary outflow tract can produce an incomplete RBBB [22].

*3. What is the prognostic significance of LBBB during infarction?

ANS.: When LBBB is present during acute infarction, the prognosis is worse than with no bundle branch block [26]. However, there is no difference in infarction mortality whether LBBB develops during infarction or was established long before infarction occurred [9, 12, 25].

It is surprising that RBBB carries a worse prognosis than LBBB in acute infarction in view of the dual blood supply to both bundle branches. The proximal part of the right bundle is supplied by a branch of the left anterior descending artery as well as by the right coronary artery; the left bundle is supplied by septal branches of both right and left coronary arteries [26].

*4. What is the significance of chronic LBBB with a normal axis in the diagnosis and prognosis of coronary disease or myocardial damage?

ANS.: Follow-up data on asymptomatic patients with accidentally discovered LBBB have shown no cardiac abnormalities and no difference in morbidity or mortality over 10 years. The axes in this benign form of LBBB (i.e., with no other clinical disease) are almost always normal in any series in which coronary angiography has shown no coronary disease. A normal axis, however, does not exclude coronary disease or cardiomyopathy [13, 16, 18].

The prognosis of chronic bundle branch block (left or right) with or without a normal axis is determined mainly by the degree of associated cardiovascular disease [33]. In one study of patients with LBBB who had left main or three-vessel coronary disease or coronary disease with poor ventricular contraction, the mortality over 2 years was 55 percent. In patients with normal coronary arteries, there were no deaths over a 2-year follow-up period [29]. In one study asymptomatic men who developed LBBB at about age 50 had a 10 times greater 5-year incidence of sudden death as the first manifestation of heart disease than did asymptomatic men without LBBB [31].

Note: The cause of LBBB of a benign type in some patients has been thought to be an unusually short (less than 6 mm) main left coronary artery [16, 18].

5. What is the significance of *marked* left axis deviation in a patient with chronic LBBB?

ANS.: In patients with LBBB and with a left axis deviation of − 30° or more, the incidence of myocardial dysfunction and cardiovascular mortality is greater than in those with a normal axis [1, 5].

Note: a. In aortic stenosis, a combination of LBBB with marked pre-operative left axis deviation significantly increased the incidence of late postoperative left ventricular failure and death after valve replacement. Because there is no increased incidence of coronary disease in such patients, the combination of LBBB with marked left axis deviation probably reflects diffuse myocardial damage [39].

b. LBBB with right axis deviation is a marker for severe myocardial disease with a probable dilated cardiomyopathy [15].

*6. What is the danger of cardiac catheterization in a patient with LBBB?

ANS.: Pressure of the catheter against the right side of the septum can produce an RBBB, thus possibly producing complete atrioventricular block. Probably, it is likely only if the right bundle is already partly blocked, as shown by the presence of a long P-R [37].

7. Why would you expect RBBB to occur with less provocation or damage than LBBB?

ANS.: Because the right bundle branch has a long, narrow, vulnerable tract before it divides. The left bundle branch is broader and divides higher, making it less vulnerable to a local area of damage. Therefore more widespread damage is necessary to cause LBBB. Proof of vulnerability of the right bundle branch is seen when a cardiac catheter is pressed against the outflow tract of the RV and various degrees of RBBB are produced [28]. Damage to the left bundle can be produced experimentally only if there is severe damage to the bundle high in the septum.

8. What other than an infarct can cause the sudden occurrence of RBBB?

ANS.: a. A sudden pressure load on the RV, as in acute pulmonary embolism, can cause all degrees of RBBB. This subject is discussed in detail in Chap. 25.

b. A right ventriculotomy, as in operations for a ventricular septal defect or tetralogy of Fallot [8, 34, 35]. It may also be caused by direct damage to the main right bundle, as in operations for a membranous ventricular septal defect when the approach is through the atrium and tricuspid valve [27].

*Note: The most likely cause of postoperative RBBB in tetralogy of Fallot operations is disruption of the distal branches of the right bundle by a right vertical ventriculotomy. The block occurs at the time of the right ventricular incision [10].

c. Nonpenetrating chest trauma [16].

d. Tricyclic antidepressants in large doses can produce not only RBBB but also atrioventricular or divisional block.

Note: The duration of the QRS complex may be the most reliable sign of tricyclic antidepressant overdosage [36]. Doxepin, however, causes very little conduction delay.

*9. Do the various degrees of RBBB disappear after closure of an ASD and the resulting decrease in the size of the RV?

ANS.: The various degrees of RBBB regress and often disappear completely [28].

Note: The causes of bundle branch blocks are discussed further under bifascicular and trifascicular blocks (Chap. 19).

10. What is the significance of rate-dependent LBBB during an exercise test?

ANS.: The onset of LBBB at a heart rate of 125 or higher is highly correlated with the presence of normal coronary arteries despite the presence of chest pain during the exercise [41].

The left bundle branch block rarely becomes permanent and the prognosis is excellent [13A].

REFERENCES

1. Beach, T. B. et al. Benign left bundle branch block. *Ann. Intern. Med.* 70:269, 1969.
2. Burch, G. E. An electrocardiographic syndrome characterized by absence of Q in leads 1, V5 and V6. *Am. Heart J.* 51:487, 1956.
3. Camerini, F., and Davies, L. G. Secondary R-waves in right chest leads. *Br. Heart J.* 17:28, 1955.
4. Davia, J. E., Cheitlin, M. D., and Bedynek, J. L. Sinus venosus atrial septal defect: Analysis of fifty cases. *Am. Heart J.* 85:177, 1973.
5. Dhingra, R. C., et al. Significance of left axis deviation in patients with chronic left bundle branch block. *Am. J. Cardiol.* 42:551, 1978.
6. Dhingra, R. C., et al. The clinical significance of left axis deviation in patients with left bundle branch block. *Clin. Res.* 25:217A, 1977.
7. Egenberg, K. E. The electrocardiogram and the frontal vectorcardiogram in ostium secundum defect and endocardial cushion defect. *Acta Med. Scand.* 175:239, 1964.
8. Fisher, J. M., et al. Electrocardiographic sequelae of right ventriculotomy in patients with ventricular septal defects. *Circulation* 22:280, 1960.

9. Gann, D., et al. Prognostic significance of chronic vs acute bundle branch block in acute myocardial infarction. *Chest* 67:298, 1975.

10. Gelband, H., et al. Etiology of right bundle branch block in patients undergoing total correction of tetralogy of Fallot. *Circulation* 44:1022, 1971.

11. Goldberger, A .L. The genesis of indeterminate axis. *J. Electrocardiol.* 15:221, 1982.

12. Gould, L., Ramana, C. V., and Gomprecht, R. F. Left bundle-branch block prognosis in acute myocardial infarction. *J.A.M.A.* 225:625, 1973.

12A. Greenstein, R., Noaz, G., and Armstrong, W. F. Usefulness of electrocardiographic abnormalities for the detection of atrial septal defect in adults. *Am. J. Cardiol.* 88:1054–1056, 2001.

13. Haft, J. E., Herman, M. F., and Gorlin, R. Left bundle branch with block. *Circulation* 43:279, 1971.

13A. Heinsimer, J. A., et al. Underlying coronary disease in exercise-induced left bundle branch block. *Am. Coll. Cardiol.* 60:1065, 1987.

14. Herbert, W. Left bundle branch block and coronary disease. *J. Electrocardiol.* 8:317, 1975.

15. Hindman, M. D., et al. The clinical significance of bundle branch block in acute infarction. *Circulation* 58:689, 1978.

16. Kumpris, A. G., et al. Right bundle branch block: Occurrence following nonpenetrating chest trauma without evidence of cardiac contusion. *J.A.M.A.* 242:172, 1979.

17. Lee, Y.-C., and Scherlis, L. Atrial septal defect electrocardiographic, vectorcardiographic, and catheterization data. *Circulation* 25:1024, 1962.

18. Lewis, M. C., et al. Coronary arteriographic appearance in patients with left bundle branch block. *Circulation* 41:299, 1970.

19. Luy, G., Bahl, O. P., and Massie, E. Intermittent left bundle branch block. *Am. Heart J.* 85:332, 1973.

20. Massing, G. K., and Lancaster, M. C. Clinical significance of acquired right bundle branch block in 59 patients. *Aerospace Med.* 40:967, 1969.

21. Massumi, R. A. Bradycardia-dependent bundle branch block. *Circulation* 38:1066, 1968.

22. Moore, E. N., et al. Incomplete right bundle branch block: An electrocardiographic enigma and possible misnomer. *Circulation* 4:678, 1971.

23. Narula, O. S. Longitudinal dissociation in the His bundle. *Circulation* 56:996–1006, 1977.

24. Nikolic, G., and Marriott, H. J. L. ECG abnormalities associated with malignant hyperthermia susceptibility. *J. Electrocardiol.* 15:137, 1982.

25. Nimetz, A. A., et al. The significance of bundle branch block during acute myocardial infarction. *Am. Heart J.* 90:439, 1975.

26. Norris, R. M., and Croxson, M. D. Bundle branch block in acute myocardial infarction. *Am. Heart J.* 79:728, 1970.

27. Okoroma, E. P., et al. Etiology of right bundle branch block pattern after surgical closure of ventricular-septal defect. *Am. Heart J.* 90:14, 1975.

28. Penaloza, D., Gamboa, R., and Sime, F. Experimental right bundle branch block in the normal human heart. *Am. J. Cardiol.* 8:767, 1961.

29. Peter, R. H., Dixon, J., and Conley, J. J. The prognostic implication of left bundle branch block in patients with proven coronary artery disease. *Am. J. Cardiol.* 41:399, 1978.

30. Pryor, R., Woodward, G. M., and Blount, S. C. Electrocardiographic changes in atrial septal defects. *Am. Heart J.* 58:689, 1959.

31. Rabkin, S. W., Mathewson, F. A. L., and Tate, R. B. Natural history of left bundle branch block. *Br. Heart J.* 43:164, 1980.

32. Rosen, K., et al. A characteristic repolarization abnormality in intermittent left bundle branch block. *Circulation* 55, 56 (Suppl.3):244, 1977.

33. Rotman, M., and Triebwasser, J. H. A clinical and follow-up study of right and left bundle branch block. *Circulation* 51:477, 1975.

34. Said, S. I., and Bryant, J. M. Right and left bundle branch block in young healthy subjects. *Circulation* 14:993, 1956.

35. Scherlis, L., and Lee, Y.-C. Right bundle branch following open heart surgery. *Am. J. Cardiol.* 8:780, 1961.

36. Spiker, D. G., et al. Tricyclic antidepressant overdose: Clinical presentation and plasma levels. *Clin. Pharmacol. Ther.* 18:539, 1975.

37. Spurrell, R. A. J., Krikler, D. M., and Sowton, E. Apparently benign left bundle branch block. *Proc. R. Soc. Med.* 65:24, 1972.

38. Sung, R. J., et al. Analysis of surgically-induced right bundle branch block pattern using intracardiac recording techniques. *Circulation* 54:442, 1976.

39. Thompson, R., et al. Conduction defects in aortic valve disease. *Am. Heart J.* 98:3, 1979.

40. Unger, P. N., Greenblatt, M., and Lev, M. The anatomic basis of the electrocardiogram abnormality in incomplete left bundle branch block. *Am. Heart J.* 76:486, 1968.

41. Vasey, C., et al. Exercise-induced left bundle branch block. *Am. J. Cardiol.* 56:892, 1985.

42. Walston, A., II, et al. Relationship between ventricular depolarization and QRS in right and left bundle branch block. *J. Electrocardiol.* 1:155, 1968.

43. Zinsser, H. F., and Gurdarshan, S. T. Right bundle branch block after nonpenetrating injury to the chest wall. *J.A.M.A.* 207:1913, 1969.

17. Myocardial Infarction

GENERAL VECTOR RULES

1. If a dog's anterior descending coronary artery is clamped, what is the first change in its ECG lead 2?
   ANS.: The T inverts, reaching maximum inversion in about half a minute [7,8].

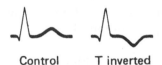

Control   T inverted

2. If the clamp on the coronary artery is immediately removed, what happens to the T?
   ANS.: It returns to normal; i.e., the T negativity is reversible [8].
3. What is this reversible T change called?
   ANS.: It is the state of ischemia, and the T is an ischemic T wave.
4. If the anterior coronary clamp is left on a minute longer, what is the next change that occurs in lead 2? Is it reversible?
   ANS.: The S-T segment rises. If the clamp is removed in less than 5 minutes, the S-T returns to the baseline [8].

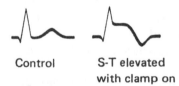

Control   S-T elevated
with clamp on

5. What is the preceding S-T change called?
   ANS.: A change due to *injury*. A 'current of injury' is said to have occurred (why it is called current of injury is explained on p. 245).
6. If the coronary clamp is left on still longer, what change occurs? Is it reversible?
   ANS.: If the clamp is left on for about 45 minutes, a deeper and wider q or Q wave develops at the expense of the R wave. It may be permanent.

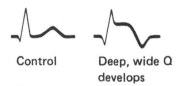

Control   Deep, wide Q
develops

   Note: In monkeys with anterior descending occlusion 3 cm beyond the circumflex, the immediate changes are S-T elevations [45].
7. What is the initial QRS change called? Why?

ANS.: The necrosis change. The vector is the necrosis, or dead zone, vector. This stage is the only one at which the usual histological studies reveal any abnormality. Necrotic muscle is seen at this stage.

Note: It actually requires at least 20 minutes of occlusion — and usually 45 minutes — before microscopic muscle necrosis can be shown at necropsy [11, 45, 76].

8. How do the changes described in animal studies compare with changes in human infarction?

ANS.: In human subjects as in monkeys
   a. The first change is often the injury current [54].
   b. The terminal part of the QRS also often changes direction.

Note: a. Even in dogs, an injury current can occur first if a branch of the anterior descending coronary artery, rather than the proximal anterior descending coronary artery, itself is occluded.
   b. When Q waves of infarction develop, they begin to show during about the second hour after the onset of pain and are fully developed by 12 hours [68].

9. Which of the QRS and T vectors may be affected by myocardial infarction?

ANS.: a. Initial part of the QRS.
   b. Terminal part of the QRS.
   c. S-T segment.
   d. T wave.

Note: Although the middle part of the QRS may also be affected and cause abnormal notchings, it is too difficult to analyze to be of much value unless high-frequency recordings or vector loops are used.

10. Which of these four vector changes may not be seen on the ECGs of patients with acute infarction?

ANS.: No abnormalities may be seen, or any permutation and combination of the four vector changes may be absent. ECG abnormalities may be absent because changes were so transient that the ECG had returned to normal by the time of the first recording or because the infarct was small and in an area that does not show on the ECG.

Note: As many as 25 percent of patients admitted to a coronary care unit with a confirmed first infarct have no ECG evidence of infarction [58].

11. How do each of the four vectors affected by transmural myocardial infarction (if they are affected at all) relate to the site of the infarction?

ANS.: a. The initial QRS vectors tend to point away from the area of infarction.
   b. The terminal QRS vectors tend to point toward the infarction.
   c. The S-T vector tends to point toward the infarction.
   d. The T vector tends to point away from the infarction, usually after a few minutes or hours.

Note: a. A subendocardial infarct (relatively rare) has opposite rules for the S-T and T vectors.
   b. The foregoing direction rules must be memorized, especially as only the initial and terminal vector changes have an easily understood explanation. Remember *A T T A* for initial, terminal, S-T, and T.
   c. If the S-T shows additional elevation with a positive T wave within the first hour of thrombolysis, this may be a sign of successful reperfusion.

* Material marked with an asterisk is included for reference and for advanced students in cardiology.

d. With successful spontaneous reperfusion the S-T returns to baseline with the T negative by the second day.

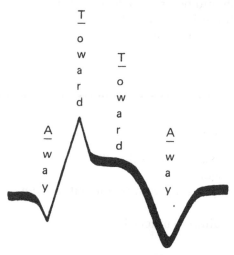

You may find it easier to memorize this QRST picture of an acute infarct with every
vector abnormality present, as seen by a positive electrode over a transmural infarct,
than to memorize A T T A.

12. Which of the above vector changes in addition to the necrosis vector are most often
permanent?
ANS.: Some T abnormality also commonly remains.
   Note: Barring any recurrence after a first infarction, about 10 percent of
   ECGs return to normal in 1 year, and about 20 percent in 4 years [17]. If the
   infarct developed q waves, only about 5 percent return to normal compared
   to about 50 percent of those with non-Q wave infarctions, i.e., with only S-T,
   T changes [24]. The long-term prognosis is not improved by the return of the
   ECG to normal [52].

*13. What do electrocardiographers mean by 'transmural' infarction?
ANS.: The term is often used:
   a. As a synonym for 'subepicardial plus subendocardial,' as distinct from
      subendocardial alone.
   b. To mean an infarct that produces a necrosis vector on an ECG.
   c. To mean an infarct that produces necrosis vectors plus S-T, T changes
      [52]. *Transmural* is used in this book to mean a through-and-through
      infarction involving subepicardium as well as subendocardium.
   Note: a. The term *nontransmural infarction* has been used to indicate that
               only S-T or T wave changes have occurred. However, it causes
               confusion because some call this 'subendocardial infarction.' (See
               p. 269 for a more likely ECG picture of subendocardial infarction.)
           b. Because subendocardial infarction can also produce necrosis
               vectors, the term *transmural* is misleading if used as a synonym
               for infarcts with Q waves of necrosis on the ECG [61]. When read-
               ing the literature other than this book you should interpret the
               word *transmural* strictly as an ECG description denoting the pres-
               ence of abnormal Q waves. Only in this book should you imbue
               the term with any pathological correlation. Clinically, however,

the absence of Q waves appears to confer a different immediate and late clinical course from those patients with Q waves [48]. The terms 'Q wave infarct' should be used instead of 'transmural,' and 'non-Q wave infarct' should be used instead of 'subendocardial,' 'non-transmural,' or 'S-T, T' infarction.

INITIAL QRS VECTOR CHANGES

Direction of Initial Forces in Myocardial Infarction

1. How much of the initial QRS is usually affected by an infarct?
   ANS.: The first 10 to 40 msec (0.01–0.04 sec).
2. In which direction is the left ventricle depolarized, from inside out or from outside in?
   ANS.: From inside out, i.e., from endocardium to epicardium.

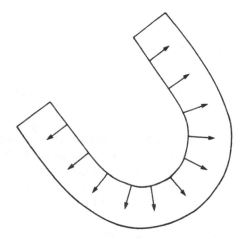

3. What is the usual resultant direction of the initial 30-msec vector through the entire subendocardium of the left ventricle (LV), which is depolarized nearly simultaneously?

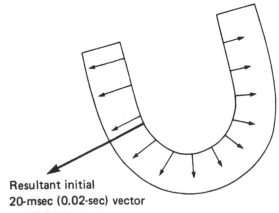

Resultant initial
20-msec (0.02-sec) vector

It is a resultant vector, i.e., the average of myriad directions of electrical activity during this period of time.

ANS.: From left to right; i.e., the septal forces dominate even though the impulse is spreading radially in all directions at about the same time.

4. If a portion of septum is infarcted, which initial forces then dominate?
   ANS.: Those of the apex and free wall of the LV.

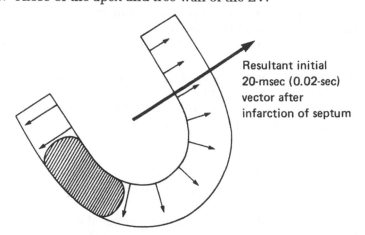

Resultant initial
20-msec (0.02-sec)
vector after
infarction of septum

5. If a portion of the free lateral wall is infarcted, which initial forces dominate?
   ANS.: The septal and apical forces.

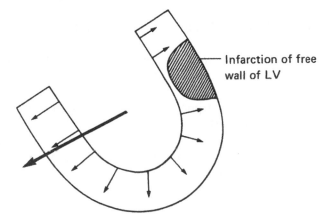

Infarction of free
wall of LV

Note: It is apparent from the above diagrams that the initial necrosis forces tend to point *away* from the site of the infarction.

6. How does the initial force produced by necrosis relate to the site of the infarct?
   ANS.: It is apparent from the above diagrams that the initial necrosis forces tend to point away from the site of the infarction.

7. What proof is there that the initial forces are produced not only by septal but also by lateral free-wall activation?
   ANS.: When the lateral free wall is infarcted, the initial 10-, 20-, and even 30-msec vectors may be affected.

Pathogenesis and Recognition of Necrosis Vectors

1. How severe must destruction of tissue be before an initial QRS vector change shows itself?

ANS.: There must be at least enough destruction to render the tissue unable to conduct normally. Tissue that cannot conduct electricity is not necessarily dead or necrotic. It may be only nonfunctional, as proved by the return of the initial vector to normal in about 30 percent of patients. Such regression or disappearance of the necrosis vector often occurs within about 1.5 years, so that eventually the diagnosis cannot be made by an ECG [52].

Note: It is not surprising that prognosis is not influenced by the disappearance of necrosis vectors in view of the reappearance of the abnormal necrosis vectors with acute ischemic episodes such as angina and shock. Nor is it surprising that after coronary bypass surgery preoperative anterior necrosis forces have returned to normal [77]. The three possible causes for such a return to normal are listed in the answer to the next question.

2. For how long does an initial vector abnormality remain? Why?

ANS.: Permanently, unless

    a. It was originally produced by only functionally dead tissue, and the development of collateral circulation of recanalization produces a return of function.

    b. An infarct of the opposite wall causes oppositely directed initial vectors. This situation may abolish the initial vector changes of the first infarct.

    *c. Left bundle branch block (LBBB), divisional block, or preexcitation bypass of an atrioventricular (AV) node changes the pathway of initial depolarization.

3. For how long must a coronary artery be occluded to cause irreversible initial QRS changes?

ANS.: In dogs it takes about 45 minutes. In humans the development of initial QRS changes begins within 6 hours after the onset of pain and is complete by 24 hours [68].

4. If the initial 40-msec vectors turn away from a positive electrode, what does the initial 40 msec of the QRS look like in that lead?

ANS.: It is negative and so produces a wide Q wave, lasting at least 40 msec (0.04 sec), or one small division on ECG paper. The normal septal q is not more than 30 msec (0.03 sec) in duration.

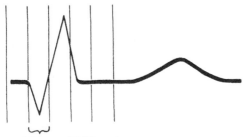

40 msec (0.04 sec)

*5. What part of the LV was once considered by some electrophysiologists to have no effect on the normal ECG? Why?

ANS.: The endocardial one-half or three-fourths (in dogs) [64, 70]. There is a possibility that in these layers depolarization occurs in such a way that all vectors cancel each other out.

Note: Despite these dog experiments, an infarct of the subendocardium can produce an abnormal initial QRS vector as well as abnormal S-T and T vectors [44, 75]. One possible explanation is that vectors from this area may be *balanced*, and an infarct may 'unbalance' them and produce resultant vectors that were not visible before. There is evidence that the subendocardial area is electrically active [16].

6. When does a necrosis vector occur in the absence of myocardial infarction?
   ANS.: a. When there is an area of confluent fibrosis, as in patients with idiopathic cardiomyopathies [67].
   b. When infiltrates replace the myocardium, as in metastatic carcinoma.
   Note: Long-standing constrictive pericarditis can infiltrate the epicardium enough to produce a necrosis vector [55].

Recognition of a Necrosis Vector in the Frontal Plane

1. Which limb leads may normally have a Q wave?
   ANS.: Any of the limb leads.

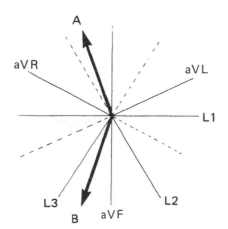

Vectors A and B could be normal septal vectors because they go from left to right. Vector A is beyond the perpendicular to L1, L2, aVF, and L3, thus producing normal Q waves in those leads. Vector B is beyond the perpendicular to aVL and aVR and produces normal Q waves in those leads.

2. If any limb lead can have a Q wave normally, how can you tell when a limb lead Q wave is abnormal?
   ANS.: If it is absolutely too wide or relatively too deep.
3. What is the range of duration of the usual normal septal vector?
   ANS.: 10 to 30 msec (0.01–0.03 sec).
4. When is a frontal plane Q wave diagnostic of a necrosis vector?
   ANS.: a. If it is at least 40 msec (0.04 sec) in duration and the abnormal duration is not due to the causes listed in question 5.
   b. If it is relatively deep, i.e., with respect to the R that follows it.

Note: In the horizontal plane a q wave may be abnormal if in addition to the above it is seen in the wrong places.

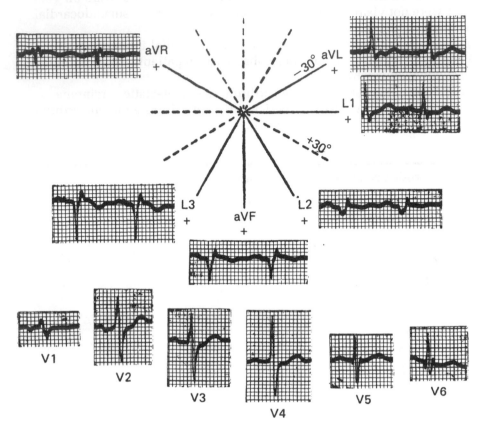

ECG 17. The wide Q in L2, L3, and aVF (60 msec [0.06 sec]) is diagnostic of a necrosis vector. It is too wide to be caused by left ventricular hypertrophy (LVH) alone. The ECG is from a 67-year-old man with a history of two infarctions. A radiograph showed a slightly enlarged heart and a bronchial carcinoma. (The deep q in L3 is not due to infarction but to LVH.)

5. Because the widest normal septal Q is 30 msec (0.03 sec), are all initial Q waves that last 40 msec caused by infarction, fibrosis, or infiltrates?
   ANS.: No. The wide Q may instead be caused by:
   a. An exceptionally thick septum, as in marked LVH [60].
   *b. An AV nodal bypass preexcitation problem, as in Wolff-Parkinson-White conduction (see p. 188).
   c. An initial vector pointing away from the AV valve area of the LV, i.e., away from aVR's positive electrode and toward the apex of the heart.
6. What is meant by a relatively deep Q wave?
   ANS.: One that is at least 30 percent of the R in whites and 25 percent of the R in blacks.

Note: If the R is followed by an S, the relative depth of the Q cannot be judged, as some of the terminal R force has been canceled out by the S wave; i.e., if the S wave were not present, the R wave might have been quite high.

7. In which limb leads is a relatively deep Q of no diagnostic help?

ANS.: In L3 or aVR.

> *Note:* a. The relative or absolute depth of the Q in L3 has no relation to infarction. It usually reflects the presence of LVH; i.e., a deep Q in L3 suggests LVH rather than infarction. The Q in L3 must be wide, i.e., at least 0.4 second (40 msec), before it can be considered due to infarction.
>
> b. The q in aVL should probably be at least 50 percent of the R wave before you can with confidence attribute it to infarction. It is in aVF (the Y axis of the ECG) in which the relatively deep Q is most sensitive and specific.

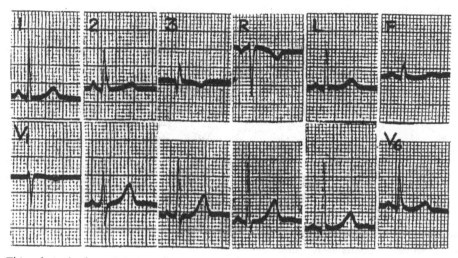

This relatively deep Q in L3 (about 75% of the R) in the absence of LVH voltage is a normal finding. This is from a normal 18-year-old girl.

Recognizing Sites of Infarction by Frontal Plane Necrosis Changes

1. How can you diagram a heart on the hexaxial system?

> *Note:* a. The electrical center is about one-third to one-half the way down from the base (where the septal activation begins).
>
> b. The apex points inferiorly and to the left.

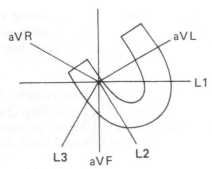

Only the LV need be shown because the right ventricle (RV) contributes little to the ECG in the absence of right ventricular hypertrophy (RVH) or right bundle branch block (RBBB).

2. If an infarct is on the diaphragmatic or inferior surface of the LV, in which direction does the initial QRS 'dead zone' vector point?
   ANS.: Superiorly and leftward.

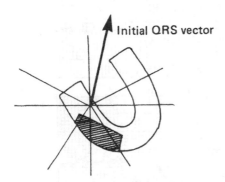

Dead zone inferior; therefore, the initial QRS vector points away from this area

Note: Always draw vectors as if they are originating from the center of the hexaxial system.

3. If an infarct is on the inferior surface of the LV, which limb leads have an initial Q wave?
   ANS.: Lead 3, aVF, and usually lead 2 as well (see ECGs 17 and 18). These leads are known as the 'inferior leads' because their positive electrodes are inferior in relation to the heart and to the center of the hexaxial system.
4. What determines whether lead 2 shows the infarction changes of an inferior infarct, i.e., similar to the changes in lead 3 and aVF?
   ANS.: If the right coronary is dominant but gives only small *branches beyond the inferior intraventricular groove*, the changes will be confined to L3 and aVF. If large inferior surface branches are given off from the right coronary instead of the circumflex, then L2 changes will be as marked as those in lead 3 and aVF [62].

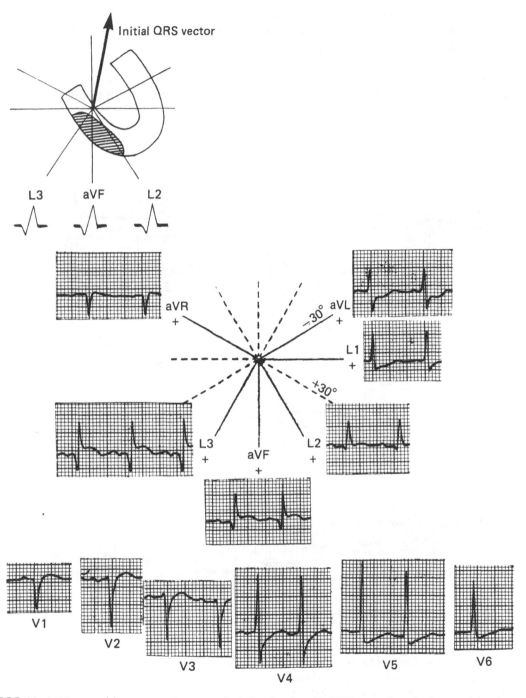

ECG 18. A 76-year-old normotensive man died shortly after this ECG was taken. It shows wide, deep Q waves in L2, L3, and aVF that reflect the old and new inferior infarction found at autopsy. If the Q waves in even one lead are due to necrosis, the initial forces in every lead are due to infarction; i.e., the R in aVL is also a necrosis vector.

5. Why may *diaphragmatic* be a poor word for an inferior infarct?
   ANS.: a. Seeing this word, surgeons have asked if we meant that the patient had an infarct in the diaphragm.
   b. It is longer and more difficult to spell than *inferior.*
   c. It has no vector direction connotation, as does the word *inferior.*
6. In an apical infarct, in which direction does the initial vector of the QRS point?
   ANS.: Toward the right shoulder, i.e., rightward and superiorly. It produces abnormal q waves in L1, L2, and aVF (see ECG 19).

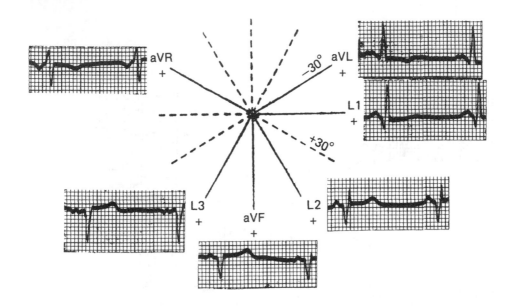

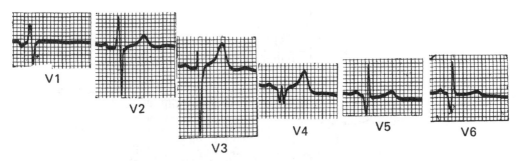

ECG 19. Old apical infarction in a 40-year-old man with partial occlusion of the left circumflex and anterior descending arteries plus complete occlusion of the right coronary artery. The initial negativity (Q waves) from aVL down to aVF denotes an apical site for the necrosis. (The Q in V4 to V6 is also due to apical necrosis and should not be read as 'lateral' infarction; see p. 167 for explanation.)

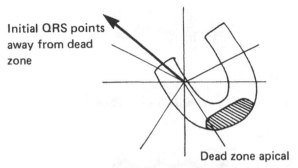

Initial QRS points away from dead zone

Dead zone apical

An apical infarction differs from an inferior infarct in that the latter has q waves in L2, L3, and aVF, whereas an apical infarct has Q waves not only in L2, L3, and aVF but also in L1; i.e., the necrosis vector not only points superiorly but also from left to right. Thus there must be a Q in L1 to differentiate an apical from an inferior infarction.

7. What word is more commonly used for an infarction on the upper surface of the left ventricle, superior or lateral?

   ANS.: *Lateral.* It is unfortunate because *superior* is a more specific frontal plane term; i.e., *lateral* can also refer to the horizontal plane.

8. If an infarct is on the high lateral surface of the left ventricle, in what direction does the initial QRS necrosis vector point?

   ANS.: Inferiorly and to the right.

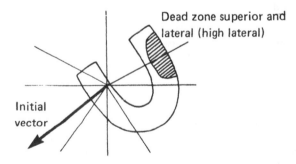

Dead zone superior and lateral (high lateral)

Initial vector

9. If an infarct is on the high lateral surface of the left ventricle, which limb leads have an initial negativity; i.e., which leads have a Q wave?

   ANS.: aVL and lead 1 (see ECGs 20 and 21).

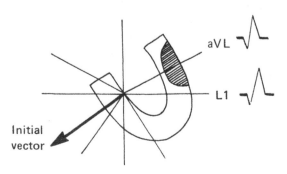

aVL

L1

Initial vector

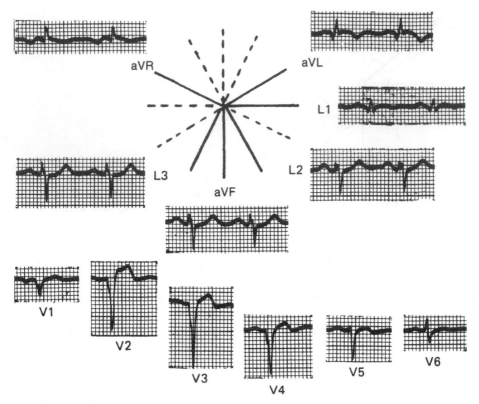

ECG 20. The slightly widened Q in aVL, which is also relatively deep (almost 50% of the R amplitude), is highly suggestive of a high lateral infarct. The q in L1 is usually also present with high lateral infarction. This ECG is from a 57-year-old man who had had a documented infarction 15 years before.

10. How is an anterior or posterior infarct seen in the limb leads?

   ANS.: A strictly anterior or posterior myocardial infarction is not seen in the limb leads. Remember that limb leads represent vectors only in the frontal plane. *Anterior* and *posterior* are horizontal plane terms.

   Note: Before the days of the vector approach to ECGs, all inferior infarcts were called 'posterior.' This terminology was based on empirical observation. Fortunately for the early ECG readers, who did not think in terms of vectors, most inferior infarcts are also found to be posterior at autopsy. The reason is that the right coronary artery usually supplies both posterior and inferior aspects of the LV. Pathologists often fail to distinguish between 'inferior' and 'strictly posterior,' which contributes to the confusion.

   There is documentation of deep, wide Q waves in L2 and L3 with definite infarction that was not at all posterior at autopsy [56].

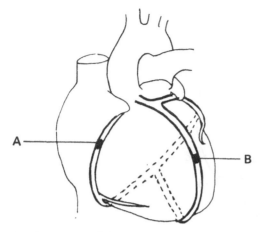

An obstruction of the right coronary artery at A can produce both posterior and inferior infarction. Before the vector approach, this abnormality was seen only as a posterior infarction. An obstruction at B can produce both anterior and inferior infarction in some subjects because the anterior descending coronary artery curves around the apex and around up the posterior intraventricular sulcus for a distance of 1 to 5 cm [50]. Before the vector approach, it was read as anterior and posterior infarction.
Note: An obstruction to the left circumflex artery can produce ECG changes indistinguishable from right coronary obstruction [37].

11. What has been found at autopsy when an anteroinferior infarct is diagnosed on ECG criteria?
    ANS.: a. Either extensive infarction of the septum, extending from anterior to posteroinferior aspects [3], or
    b. Apical infarction, extending into the anterior and posterior aspects of the ventricle [65].
    Note: a. It is not surprising that the initial necrosis vector may be a poor indicator of the exact site of an infarct in view of the findings in one study of more than one healed infarct in 90 percent of patients with a necrosis vector [72].
    b. Infarct changes in L1 and aVL are frequently caused by isolated first diagonal branch occlusion [49A].

Horizontal Plane Necrosis Changes

Anterior Infarction
1. How can a heart be diagramed on a horizontal plane six-lead system?

ANS.:

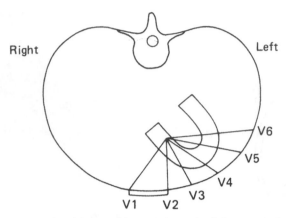

V6 may be drawn either straight to the left at 0° or slightly posteriorly.

2. If the infarct is anterior, in what direction do the initial QRS vectors point?
   ANS.: Posteriorly.

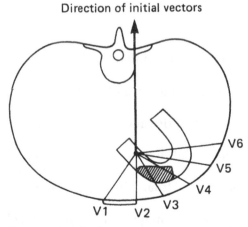

The cross-hatched area represents an anterior infarct.

    Note: All vectors are drawn as if radiating from the electrical center of the heart, i.e., from the site of the beginning of the bundle branches.

3. Where is an infarct Q wave (initial negativity) expected in the horizontal plane in a patient with an anterior infarct?
   ANS.: A Q wave can be expected anywhere in the precordial leads because a Q wave means initial negativity, and initial negativity means that the vector is pointing away from the site of the positive electrode placement on the chest wall (see ECG 21). A vector pointing away from an anterior electrode is also pointing away from the anterior surface of the left ventricle. To put it another way, an initial vector that has turned away from the anterior wall may mean an anterior infarct.

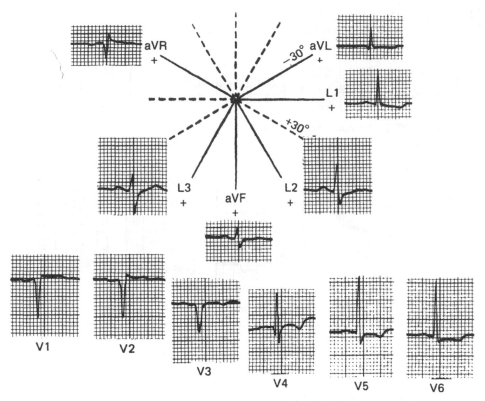

ECG 21. Anteroseptal and high lateral infarction. The Q in V1 to V4 is due to an anterior infarction because it means that the initial vector is going posteriorly, i.e., away from the anterior surface of the heart. (The q in aVL means that the infarct is also high on the anteroseptal surface. Plotting a spatial vector for the initial forces will prove this to you.)

4. When does a Q in V2 to V6 mean an infarction, and when may it be normal?
   ANS.: A V2 to V6 Q wave is probably due to an anterior necrosis vector if V2 is not a transitional lead (see ECG 22).

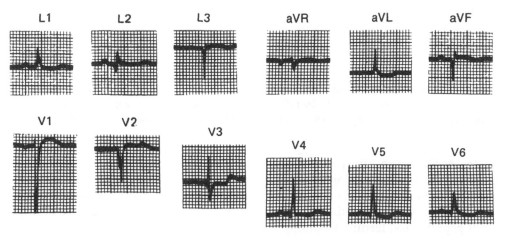

ECG 22. This patient had an anteroinferior infarction. Initial negativity from V2 to V6 suggests an anterior necrosis vector if V2 is not a transitional lead or if V2 is to the right (patient's right) of the transitional lead. Here the transitional lead is at V3; i.e., V2 is to the right of the transitional lead.

If V2 is at or nearly at the QRS transition area (i.e., nearly equiphasic), the Q in V2 to V6 is probably a normal septal vector (see ECG 23).

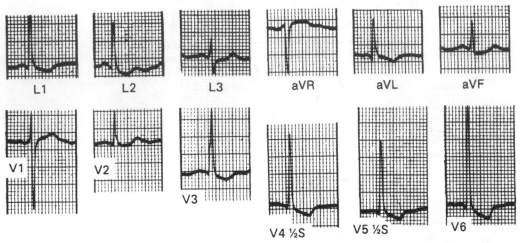

ECG 23. This patient had severe LVH due to rheumatic aortic regurgitation. (A prosthetic mitral valve was also present.) The Q in V2 to V6 is not due to infarction because the transition zone is to the right of V2, i.e., between V1 and V2. Therefore the Q in V2 is the normal septal Q. The S-T, T configuration is due to the LVH plus digitalis. Note that V4 and V5 are taken at half-standard.

5. Why is it usually abnormal to have a Q wave in V2 to V6?
   ANS.: Because it represents a posterior and rightward initial vector, which is almost always due to infarction unless the QRS is very anterior.

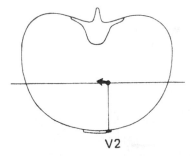

This rightward and posterior initial QRS vector might be a rare variation of a normal septal vector if there is a very anterior QRS, i.e., if the transition zone for the QRS was between V1 and V2. Usually, however, a q from V2 to V6 implies a necrosis vector.

Note: A Q in the mid-precordium with an R in both V1 and the left precordium should be diagnosed as an anterior area of necrosis. *The only known exceptions to this are in hypertrophic subaortic stenosis and in a child with tricuspid atresia. In the latter it is thought due to an absence of a right septal mass, leading to unopposed initial posterior forces [38].

6. How can an ECG in a patient with an anterior infarction show loss of anterior forces other than producing Q waves?

ANS.: By showing a lack of R/S progression across the precordium.

Note: a. This lack of R/S progression can also occur in early RVH, anterior divisional block, and severe LVH [78].

b. When poor R/S progression is the only QRS sign of infarction, the infarct is usually small [27] and contraction abnormalities on angiography are mild [78].

*7. When should you suspect that poor R/S progression means infarction?

ANS.: If the R in V3 is 1.5 mm or less, or the R in L1 is 4 mm or less. This reasoning is valid only if

a. The entire ECG does not show low voltage (every lead less than 10 mm).

b. The S in L1 is not more than 1 mm (seen in RVH patients) [78] (see ECG 24).

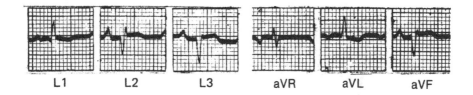

| L1 | L2 | L3 | aVR | aVL | aVF |

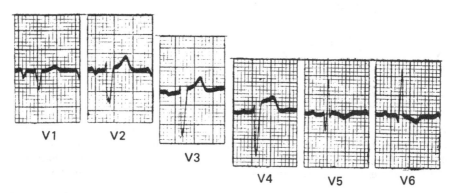

| V1 | V2 | V3 | V4 | V5 | V6 |

ECG 24. This 63-year-old man had a blood pressure of 240/120 mm Hg and a pulmonary infarction. Autopsy 7 days later showed marked LV enlargement and old infarctions in the mid-septum and lateral and posterior LV. A recent infarction involved the RV only, and a new thrombus was attached to its wall. The poor R/S progression from V2 to V3 represents loss of anterior forces, possibly due to the old septal infarct. There is a tiny r in L2, L3, and aVF. It may hide an inferior infarct because a wide Q resulting from functional loss of conduction during acute infarction may disappear in a few weeks owing to the return of a tiny r in these leads. A vectorcardiogram may uncover such an infarct.

Note: The literature does not use the concept of poor R/S progression but, instead, uses poor R wave progression. The latter concept is not as logical as that of poor R/S progression, for the following reasons:

a. The absolute height of the R waves in each chest lead depends on the proximity of the positive electrode to the heart (see ECG 5 on p. 75).

b. Definitions of poor R-wave progression and estimates of its ability to identify loss of anterior forces due to necrosis vary widely [79].

8. How can you tell the size of an infarct by the number of chest leads with abnormal Q waves?

ANS.: It seems that a small anterior infarct could produce a widespread Q from V1 to V6. In fact, only a large infarct has enough influence to change the intial forces to such a degree that it turns them 180° away from the site of infarction. Because the initial forces are a resultant of all the septal, apical, and free wall initial forces, it is not surprising that the degree to which an infarct can turn the initial forces away from itself depends on the infarction size.

*9. Does a purely subendocardial anterior infarct (up to one-half the inner myocardial thickness) cause an abnormal necrosis vector?

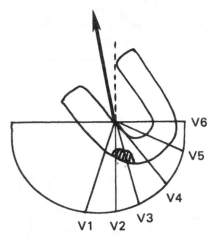

An infarct in this area turns the initial forces 180° from itself only if it is large enough to nullify all anterior forces completely. The small infarct in this illustration is not likely to be able to do this. It may simply reduce the size of the precordial r waves and produce a poor R/S progression or it may produce a small localized Q wave in the mid-precordial leads.

ANS.: Generally it only lowers the height of the R waves in the right and mid-precordium [23]. It can, however, cause pathological Q waves or necrosis vectors [75].

Note: A subendocardial infarction with papillary muscle necrosis in infants with severe aortic stenosis shows diminishing right precordial R wave amplitude in serial tracings as well as a qR in V3R.

10. What is always implied when the diagnosis of an infarct is made on the basis of only a necrosis vector without a history of infarction or angina?

    ANS.: In the absence of a history of infarction or angina, the diagnosis of a chronic infarct area always implies that only an imitation of an infarct may be present; i.e., the area may be either infiltrated or replaced by nonconducting material such as amyloid, tumor, or fibrous tissue, all of which can produce the identical necrosis vector. The cause of the necrosis vectors in idiopathic cardiomyopathies with marked LVH is probably at least partly due to focal fibrosis [3, 67].

    Note: a. Fibrosis is probably the cause of the infarction necrosis vectors in about one-third of patients with myotonia atrophica [34].

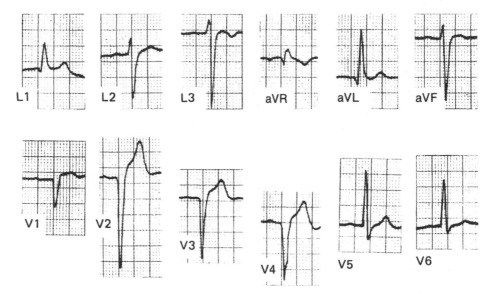

ECG 25. *This 23-year-old black man had a muscular dystrophy (myotonia atrophica) and 'blackouts.' The Q in V1 to V4 and the slightly wide Q in aVL is characteristic of anteroseptal and lateral infarction. The wide QRS with the marked left axis deviation suggests periinfarction block (see p. 226 for explanation).*

    *b. It is surprising that in one study none of the patients with dilated types of idiopathic cardiomyopathies had pathologically wide Q waves [13]. Other studies have not confirmed this finding [67].

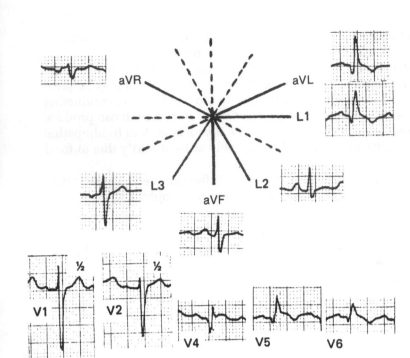

ECG 26. This 15-year-old boy had a chronic viral myocarditis. Despite the wide Q in L1 and aVL, autopsy 2 weeks later showed only diffuse fibrosis, which was especially marked laterally. The P-R segment elevation in aVR and the S-T elevation in L1 without reciprocal depression in L3 suggests that pericarditis may have been present at the time of this ECG.

11. Which congenital heart diseases are associated with a necrosis vector?
    ANS.: Foremost is an anomalous left coronary artery arising from the pulmonary artery. Next is endocardial fibroelastosis in those infants with the worst prognosis [25].

Posterior Infarction
1. What are the synonyms for a high posterior infarct?
    ANS.: a. Posterior.
           b. True posterior.
           c. Dorsal.
           d. Posterobasal.
2. If an infarct is on the posterior surface of the LV, how do the initial QRS vectors change?
    ANS.: Initial vectors are not usually affected by a high posterior infarct because the posterior parts of the ventricle are activated late, i.e., after about 30 msec [1A, 30, 31].

3. How may the loss of posterior QRS forces due to a posterior infarct affect the direction of the mean QRS vector?
   ANS.: The loss of posterior forces may cause a gain in anterior forces shown by an anterior shift of the QRS.
4. How can you recognize an anterior shift of the QRS due to a posterior infarct?
   ANS.: The transition zone shifts to the right.

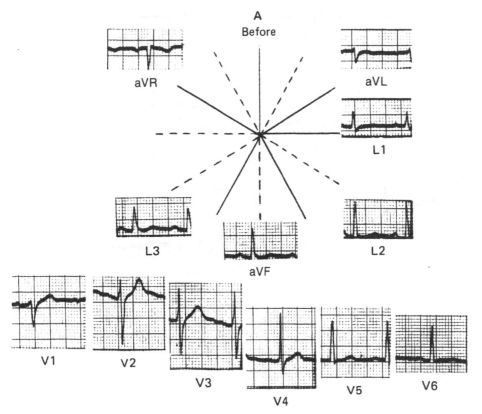

ECG 27A. *This 45-year-old man during the past 3 months had two episodes of brief resting chest pains with right arm paresthesias. The T in V6 is abnormally low (less than 10% of the R).*

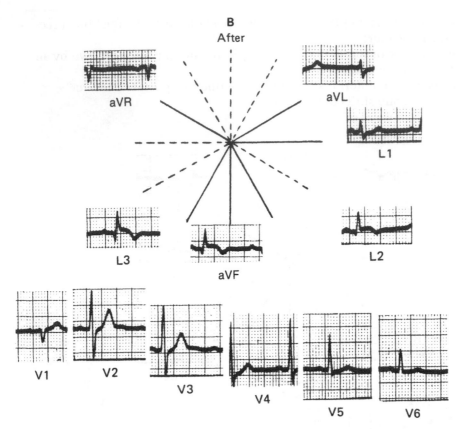

ECG 27B. This ECG was taken 3 days after ECG 27A, when chest pain recurred. The pain lasted for 2 days after this second ECG was taken. Not only are there new Q waves in L2, L3, and aVF(inferior necrosis), but there is also a shift in the transition zone from V3 to V2 due to loss of posterior forces. Therefore it is an acute posteroinferior infarction. Note that the T waves are upright in the right and mid-precordium. See p. 305 for a description of T waves in posterior infarction.

5. How do the delayed QRS changes of a posterior infarct usually show on the R wave of the right precordial leads?

    ANS.: Because the posterior LV is depolarized late, the initial QRS vectors should be normal. Then, owing to loss of mid and late posterior forces, the septal r in the right chest leads V1 to V3 may continue to rise to form a taller, wider R of 40 msec or more in duration. There is often a slur or notch high on the descending limb of the R [63]. A low notch may be a normal variant.

    Note: a. Most posterior infarcts are posteroinferior or posterolateral, so that additional initial and middle vector changes of inferior or lateral infarction are common.

    b. A posterior or posteroinferior infarct as shown by a wide, tall R in both V1 and V2 is highly predictive of both right and circumflex coronary obstruction [14].

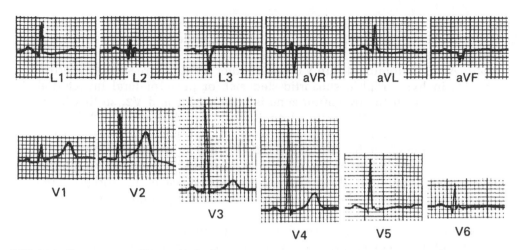

ECG 28A. This 48-year-old man had a history of acute posteroapical infarction 1 year before. The QRS is markedly anterior (dominant R waves across the precordium) owing to loss of posterior forces. The Q in L1, L2, and L3 means that the apex is also involved.

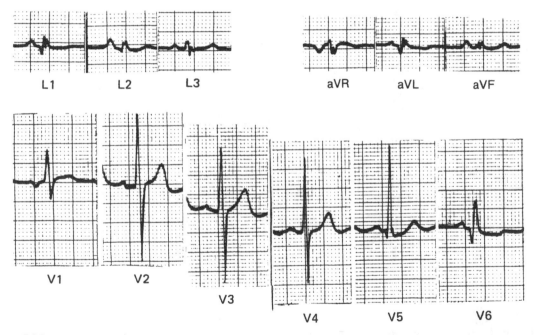

ECG 28B. An ECG from a 60-year-old man shows a wide R in V1 due to a posterolateral infarct. Note also the relatively deep Q in L1, aVL, and V6, which reflects the lateral location of the infarct.

*6. How may a small posterior infarct manifest if it is not large enough to increase late anterior forces?

    ANS.: It may show as a notching in the right precordial leads. New notching in V1 or V2 is just as suggestive of posterior infarction as is an increase of R height in those leads.

7. How may a posterolateral myocardial infarction manifest in chest leads?

   ANS.: A posterolateral infarction may show as a tall, wide R in V1, usually with upright T waves (see ECG 28B and 29B).

   Note: A tall or dominant R in V1 means either RVH, severe septal hypertrophy (as in hypertrophic subaortic stenosis), or posterolateral myocardial infarction [14]. If the transition zone is between V1 and V2, so that V2 is already a predominantly positive lead, it means that the QRS is slightly anterior, which commonly is a normal variation. If the transition zone is at V1, it is anterior enough so that the QRS should be read as an anterior QRS, and a posterior myocardial infarction should be ruled out. If, however, an inferior infarction is apparent in the frontal plane and the T waves are upright in the right precordial leads, the ECG is read as a definite posteroinferior infarction.

   Note: An anterior QRS has been shown in one study to occur also with only anterior LV wall damage [46]. It may be due to slowed conduction along a set of fibers that have been described as directed anteriorly and supplying the anterior wall of the LV [26].

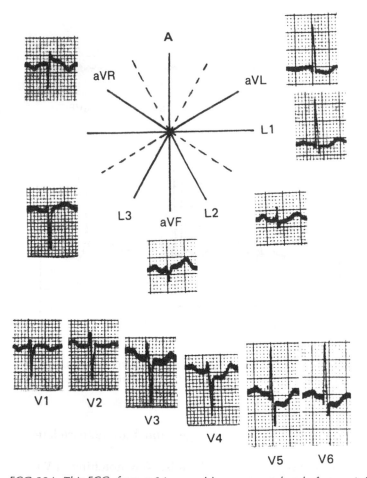

ECG 29A. This ECG, from a 64-year-old man, was taken before an infarction. The sagging S-T segments in V3 to V6 are due to digitalis. Both the initial and terminal QRS forces changed (see ECG 29B) after his infarction.

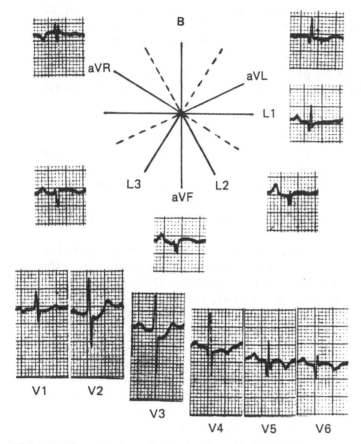

ECG 29B. The wide, large R that developed in V1 and V2 represents a loss of posterolateral forces. The enlarged Q in aVL and leads 1 and 2 also tells us that there is a lateral infarction. The Q waves in V4 to V6 represent the apical necrosis vectors. At autopsy there was a posterolateral and apical infarction.

Note: *If it had been a purely posterior myocardial infarction, the initial forces would not have changed.*

Normal Septal Versus Infarct Vectors in the Horizontal Plane

1. Where are there normally initial R waves in the precordium?

    ANS.: In the right precordial leads. The normal septal vectors points to the right and anteriorly.

2. What is this initial normal r in the right precordium called? Why?

    ANS.: The 'septal r' because it is dominated by the activation of the septum, i.e., by left-to-right forces.

    Note: Actually, the septal vectors in V1 and V2 are a resultant not only of septal activation but also of the subendocardial surface of at least the inner half of the LV free wall plus even some weak depolarization vectors of the anterior wall of the RV. (The V1 and V2 electrodes are so close to the right ventricular wall that they are probably the only routine leads that can pick up some right ventricular early vectors.)

3. How can a septal r be modified by the presence of a necrosis vector?

ANS.: a. The septal r may diminish in amplitude or may disappear and leave a QS or qR.

b. A tiny q may precede the septal r (see V2 in ECG 47, p. 228).

4. Where does the normal 'septal q' usually appear in the precordial leads?

ANS.: In the left chest leads, i.e., V4 to V6. It usually begins in the first or second lead with a predominantly positive QRS, i.e., usually at either V4 or V5. (Occasionally it appears normally in the transitional leads; i.e., it may appear in V2 or V3 if they are the first equiphasic leads.)

Note: a. A 'septal q' beginning at V2 is usually due to infarction unless it is a transitional lead.

b. If a terminal conduction defect is present, a q may be normal in V2 even if it is not a transitional lead. The reason is that if the terminal conduction defect were absent, the Q in V2 might have been a septal vector in an anteriorly turned QRS. The terminal conduction change masks the site of the normal transition zone.

5. When do Q waves in the right precordium imply an anterior infarct?

ANS.: A Q in V1 may be due to an anteroseptal infarction or to the right-to-left conduction of an incomplete LBBB pattern. A Q in V1 and V2 means the same two possibilities as above. A Q in V1, V2, and V3 means the same two possibilities as above. A Q in V1 to V4, however, nearly always implies an anteroseptal infarction. The occasional times that it does not mean infarction are when the Q is due to an inferior initial force that can be identified by seeing an r in aVF [73] or in the presence of complete LBBB.

Note: a. A purely septal infarction will show a disappearance of septal q waves in lateral leads, S-T depression in inferior leads, and loss of initial R waves in the medial precordial leads [73A].

b. RBBB can unmask a q wave in V1 of anterior or septal infarction. This is because surprisingly the initial left-to-right septal depolarization (initial r in V1) has a contribution from the right bundle; therefore blocking the right bundle will eliminate its contribution and unmask a necrosis Q wave [34A].

6. When does a Q in the left pericordium almost always mean an infarct rather than the normal septal vector?

ANS.: a. When there is an LBBB.

b. When it is 40 msec wide.

c. When it is relatively deep, i.e., at least 25 percent of the R wave height.

Note: a. Both b and c above can be present without myocardial infarction if there is LVH due to a hypertrophic cardiomyopathy, as in hypertrophic subaortic stenosis [3]. It is thought due to the long distance necessary to travel through the thickest part of the hypertrophied septum. In patients with hypertrophy, pathological Q waves are usually confined to those whose hypertrophy is localized to the

mid-septum [41]. A reciprocal tall R may be present in V1 and
V3R. That it is not due to RVH in these patients is shown by its
disappearance after the thickest part of the septum is surgically
excised [15].

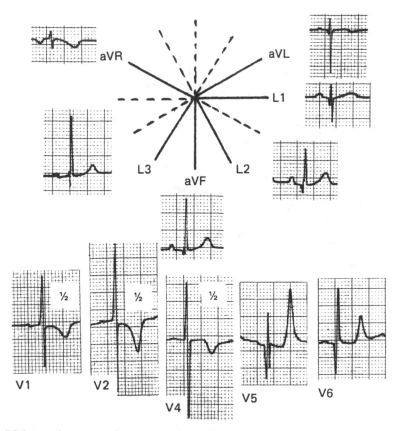

*ECG 30. This ECG is from an 8-year-old boy with hypertrophic subaortic stenosis. The right axis
deviation and T negativity in V1 to V4 are probably due to the RVH found at autopsy after his
sudden death a few months later. The deep Q in V5 and V6, which is suggestive of infarction,
is probably due to the septal hypertrophy, which is also reflected in the tall R in V1.*

    *b. A QR in V3R in an infant or child is abnormal and signifies either
marked RVH, myocardial infarction, or ventricular inversion
(corrected transposition [51]).

7. Does an abnormal Q in the left precordium mean that there is a lateral infarct?
ANS.: Not necessarily. Inferior infarcts also produce a Q wave in the left precordial
leads V4, V5, and V6. If the left precordial leads are at or above the electrical
center, however, they may show what is in L1 and aVL and therefore show a
lateral infarct. If, instead, the left precordial leads are below the electrical
center, they may represent what is in L2, L3, and aVF. In the latter situation,
the left precordial leads may be thought of as inferolateral leads. They
become 'infero' because of the eccentric manner in which their electrodes
are placed by convention (see ECG 30A).

Even if the lateral leads aVL and L1 have infarction vectors, if the V5 and 6 also have those changes, V5 and 6 may be below the electrical center enough to represent an apical infarct. See illustration below [74A].

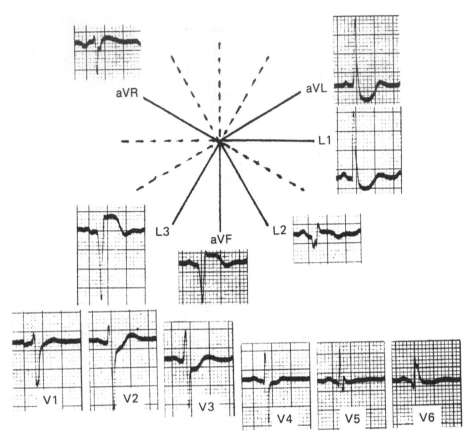

ECG 30A. This ECG is from a 68-year-old hypertensive woman with angina who died in shock shortly after an attack of severe pain. In addition to concentric hypertrophy, she had a large recent posteroinferior infarction that included about one-third of the right ventricle. A ventricular septal rupture near the apex was also present. There was no lateral or apical infarction. The q wave in V5 and V6 reflects the q waves in leads 2, 3, and aVF; i.e., the superior initial forces pointing away from the inferior infarct are seen in V5 and V6.

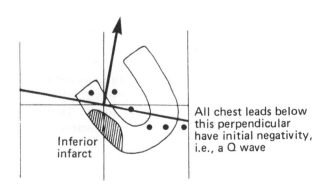

*8. Does exploring the chest for a Q wave of 40 msec (0.04 sec) help to diagnose an infarct if the wide Q is not found in the usual precordial leads? Defend your answer.

ANS.: No, because there is normally a large area of the chest wall in which a Q of 40 msec can be found. It is called the normal Q area. The following illustration shows the normal Q area, which is in the right anterior chest, occasionally as close to the midline as the V1 electrode and as close to the left posteriorly as the left scapula.

Note: It means that a Q can occasionally normally appear in V1. Also, if the Q area extends to the left scapula, it produces a wide septal R of 40 msec in V1, as is indeed observed in some young people.

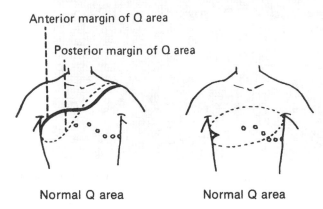

Anterior margin of Q area

Posterior margin of Q area

Normal Q area   Normal Q area

*9. What condition can *transiently* cause all the ECG changes of acute infarction, including a necrosis vector, in the presence of normal coronary arteries? Why?

ANS.: Acute pancreatitis [22]. One theory to account for it is that some enzymes released by the inflamed pancreas might produce sublethal damage to myocardial cells. A local potassium leak might then change depolarization and repolarization in enough cells to cause necrosis, injury, or an ischemic vector [22, 39, 71].

Note: a. A syndrome characterized by chest pain with transient loss of initial anterior forces within 2 to 6 days and normal isoenzymes has been thought due to a transient conduction block of the septal fascicle of the left bundle [43].

b. A wide Q in V9 (left paraspinal area) has the best predictive accuracy for diagnosing old posterior infarction, and if used together with a T in V1 higher than the T in V6 by as little as 0.5 mm, the specificity is 98 percent [64A].

c. An S-T elevation of even slight degree in a posterior chest lead can detect acute circumflex occlusion [6A].

Uncovering Hidden Necrosis Vectors

1. What can bring out a necrosis vector that may not show in the normal complexes?

ANS.: a. An ectopic ventricular beat or ventricular tachycardia [10, 66]. Either can also bring out the S-T, T changes of acute infarction that may be absent in the sinus beats [20, 21].

b. Intermittent LBBB.

c. Coronary insufficiency and myocardial ischemia due to shock, anemia, exercise, or angina [6, 58A].

Note: a. Temporary myocardial ischemia can bring out a necrosis vector, presumably because the area of true necrosis was too small to manifest until an area of surrounding 'functional necrosis' made the total area large enough for the initial vector abnormality to become apparent [40].

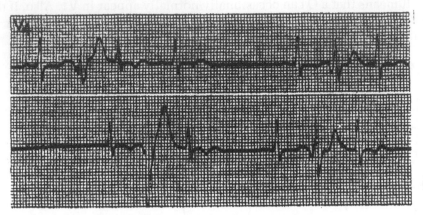

This is from a 52-year-old man who has had an anterior infarction two years previously. Note that only the PVCs show the wide necrosis Q waves.

*b. There is a possibility that hyperkalemia, by slowing conduction, can either unmask an infarct or cause a normal Q to widen and so mimic a necrosis vector [2].

2. What configuration of a QRS in a ventricular ectopic or pacemaker-induced ventricular beat is suggestive of a myocardial infarct?

ANS.: A qR or Qr in any lead except aVR [10] (see ECG 31). The infarct usually involves the lower septum [18, 36, 69].

3. Where on the precordium has the qR or Qr been seen if an ectopic premature ventricular contraction (PVC) is from the

a. Right ventricle?
b. Left ventricle?

ANS.: a. When the PVC is from the RV (i.e., when it looks like LBBB), the qR or Qr is seen in the left precordial leads.

b. When the PVC is from the LV (i.e., when it looks like RBBB), the qR or Qr is seen in the right precordial leads [18].

4. What are the indications for taking precordial leads one interspace higher to pick up q waves of infarction that are not present at the normal precordial sites?

ANS.: When a high lateral infarct is suspected from an aVL that shows a negative T and a questionable q [35].

Note: In the presence of anterior divisional block, anterior chest Q waves have been said not to mean infarction. This statement may be true for a Q in V1 to V3, but if the Q is from V1 to V4 this author has seen no necropsy proof that it does not denote infarction. Because an anterolateral infarct can produce an anterior divisional block, it is unlikely that a Q in V1 to V4 does not mean an infarct simply because a divisional block is present.

*5. What are the indications for taking V3R and V4R in acute myocardial infarction?

    ANS.: If a posteroinferior infarction is suspected, a QS in V3R or V4R and/or an S-T elevation of even 1 mm not only suggests the presence of right ventricular infarction as well as involvement of the septum but also indicates with high probability that AV block of varying degrees will develop [5].

       Note: a. In normal subjects an rS pattern is always present in V3R and frequently (91%) in V4R. A QS or QR in both V4R and V3R is 100% specific for right ventricular necrosis [59A].

          b. The S-T elevation in V4R may be absent with RV infarction if the right coronary artery is obstructed proximal to the first RV branch causing concomitant posterior as well as inferior LV infarction [53A]. Only if the S-T elevations in V4R are greater than those in V1, V2, and V3 is it reliable for RV infarction [56B].

          c. Another sign of RV infarction is finding the S-T elevation in L_3 greater than that in L2 in the presence of acute inferior infarction [1A]. When combined with S-T elevation in V1 it strongly predicts occlusion of the proximal or mid portion of the right coronary artery [79A].

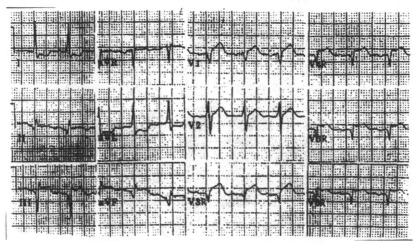

If in the presence of an inferior infarction the S-T elevation in L3 is greater than the S-T elevation in L2 and/or there is an S-T elevation in V3R or V4R (as in the ECG below), there is a right ventricular infarction.

Infarction in the Presence of LBBB

1. If the left bundle branch is blocked, which part of the ventricle is depolarized for the first half of the QRS?

    ANS.: Because the right bundle branch then controls early depolarization, approximately the first half of the QRS in LBBB is dominated by depolarization of the RV and septum. Thus the RV manifests its forces early in LBBB and late in RBBB.

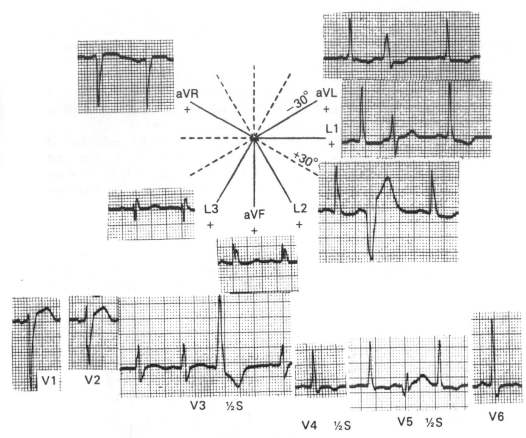

ECG 31. *This subject had had documented old inferior infarction many years before, shown here only by the Qrs in the PVC in V5, and the qR in the PVC in V3. (The infarct usually involves the septum if it is seen in a PVC's initial vector.)*

2. If, in LBBB, initial left ventricular depolarization is controlled almost entirely by the activation of a thin RV and a thick septum, where should the infarct be if the initial vector in LBBB is abnormal?

    ANS.: In the septum. However, the infarct can be found anywhere in the ventricle except in the high anterior and high mid-septum [48].

        Note: If a septal infarct is present with LBBB, the 'septal' R waves in the right precordium may become larger than normal because early right ventricular forces are unopposed. It may even cause a regression of the R/S ratio of V1 to the transition zone [19] (see ECG 32). Remember that normally the R/S ratio increases from V1 to the transition zone (see ECG 32).

3. What is meant by an abnormal initial vector in LBBB?

    ANS.: The initial vector is abnormal if

        a. It points superiorly to make a qR or QR in aVF [48].

        b. The R in V1 is tall.

        c. It goes from left to right (←) instead of from right to left (→).

        Note: In the presence of LBBB, infarction may not show a q in leads 1 and V6 unless the inferior surface of the heart is pulled downward and perhaps rotated by a deep inspiration.

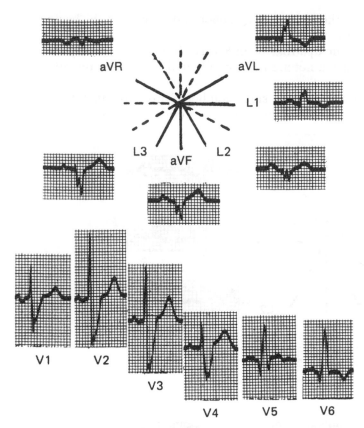

ECG 32. LBBB with wide notched R in L1 and aVL with a q in L1 (i.e., initial left-to-right conduction due to diffuse myocardial fibrosis) in a 36-year-old man. (The tall R in V1 is very unusual in the presence of LBBB. Because it is due to initial depolarization of the right ventricle, it is tall either from RVH or from unopposed forces due to loss of septal vectors by fibrosis or infarction.)

*4. Where is the infarct site if, with a LBBB, the q, instead of being lateral (i.e., in L1), is inferior, producing some variation of a qR in aVF?

ANS.: The infarct is almost always either apical, inferior, or posterolateral. When the infarct is in the septum, the posteroinferior lower two-thirds is often involved [48]. The reason is that although the Q in leads 2, 3, and aVF of an inferior infarction with normal conduction is usually obliterated by the development of LBBB, it is not invariably so [9, 57].

Note: a. If a qR is seen in aVF with LBBB, an infarct is present more often than when a lateral q with LBBB is seen [47, 48].

b. If an LBBB is produced by a pacemaker in the apex of the RV, an inferior infarct may show as a QR in inferior leads [4].

*5. How can an extensive anterolateral and apical infarction with aneurysm change an LBBB QRS other than by producing abnormal initial vectors?

ANS.: a. It can produce an rsR' or a deeply notched R in left ventricular leads (lead 1, aVL, or V6) [19] (see ECG 33). This pattern is even more likely due to infarction if the LBBB is incomplete or if there is no block at all [33].

b. It can produce a deep notch of the S in the precordial lead just to the right of the transition zone. This lead is of low amplitude, and the notch is usually on the downstroke of the S or QS, about 30 msec from the beginning of the complex [19].

Note: A notch low on the upstroke of an R wave in LBBB is usually due to infarction. The expected notch in uncomplicated LBBB is in the middle of the QRS [19].

Note: The specificity of Cabrera's sign (notched S upstroke in V3, V4, V5) as a sign of myocardial infarction (usually anterior) in the presence of left bundle branch block is about 90 percent [52A].

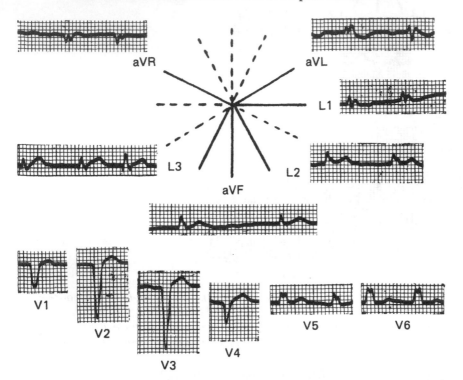

ECG 33. *LBBB in a 62-year-old woman with a history of infarction and with marked cardiomegaly on x-ray. The deep notch in L1 and aVL suggests a large area of infarction. The upright T waves in L2, V5, and V6 are abnormal and suggest that without a bundle branch block the waves would be inverted in the right precordium or mid-precordium.*

*6. What are the major differential diagnoses of LBBB with a septal infarct?

ANS.: It may not be a LBBB at all but a lateral infarct with the anterior divisional block variant known as periinfarction block. (This phenomenon is explained in Chap. 19.)

Note: When a chronic LBBB masks the ECG signs of acute infarction, a PVC may bring out all the vectors of infarction (including S-T and T vectors) [27].

LBBB Initial Vectors Versus Infarct Vectors

1. What abnormality can cause a Q from V1 to V3 without an infarct?

ANS.: An incomplete or complete LBBB or an LBBB pattern; i.e., if the initial forces are from right to left due to block or delay along the septal fascicle or left bundle branches, an infarct cannot be diagnosed merely from Q waves in V1 to V3 (see ECG 34).

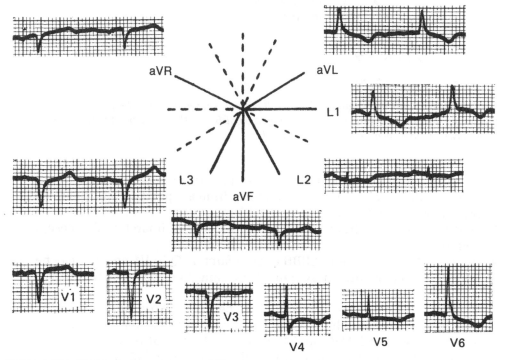

ECG 34. This ECG is from an 80-year-old hypertensive woman, with cardiomegaly on chest x-ray, in the hospital for chronic syncopal attacks. There is no history of infarction or angina. The QS in aVF and L3 does not necessarily mean that infarction is present because the width of the Q is really unknown. The absence of a septal q in L1 and V6 makes the Q in V1 to V3 a possible right-to-left septal vector of incomplete LBBB. Therefore a definite infarction should not be read here. A QS should be thought of as containing a Q of unknown width and depth. (Note that the QRS voltage in V6 is larger than that in V5, which is a sign of cardiac dilatation [see p. 384].)

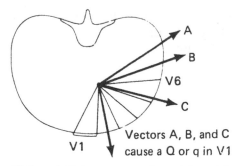

All these initial vectors are from right to left and are therefore possible initial vectors in LBBB, complete or incomplete.

2. How can you tell anteroseptal infarct Q waves in the right precordium from those due to complete LBBB, incomplete LBBB, or merely the LBBB pattern?

   ANS.: LBBB or an LBBB pattern initial vectors are rarely as posterior as septal infarct vectors can be. The most posterior LBBB initial vector is about − 45°, i.e., about perpendicular to V4.

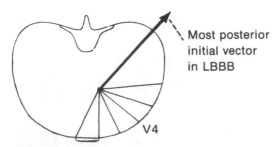

The initial vector in incomplete LBBB or LBBB pattern is rarely beyond the perpendicular to V4; i.e., V4 should not have a Q in incomplete LBBB or LBBB patterns. It may, however, have a Q in patients with complete LBBB.

3. On the basis of the facts about LBBB initial vectors just stated, what pattern rule can help you recognize that Q waves in the right precordium are posterior enough to be due to an infarct and not to LBBB?

   ANS.: Only if the Q extends from V1 to at least V4 may an infarct be diagnosed. Therefore

   a. A Q in V1 may be due to LBBB or an infarct. A Q in V1 and V2 may be due to LBBB or an infarct. A Q in V1, V2, and V3 may be due to LBBB or an infarct, but

   b. A Q in V1, V2, V3, and V4 *is likely to be due only to infarction.* If the LBBB is incomplete, the Q V1 to V4 almost certainly means infarction (see ECGs 44A and 44B, pp. 216 and 217). If the LBBB is complete, an occasional V1 to V4 Q can be seen without infarction [48, 57].

   Note: For some inexplicable reason, the site of the infarct in complete LBBB with Q V1 to V4 is often the high posterolateral area [47].

4. If the initial vector in LBBB moves from right to left, what happens to the height of the 'septal' R waves in the right precordium?

   ANS.: They become lower in amplitude.

   Note: A subendocardial myocardial infarction can also lower the R waves in the right precordium.

*5. What is implied about the site of infarction if a bundle branch block develops during an acute infarction, and which artery is likely to be involved?

   ANS.: The septum is most probably involved [56]. Because the anterior descending artery supplies at least two-thirds of the septum (in some patients 90–100%), a septal infarction is usually caused by occlusion of the anterior descending coronary artery [50].

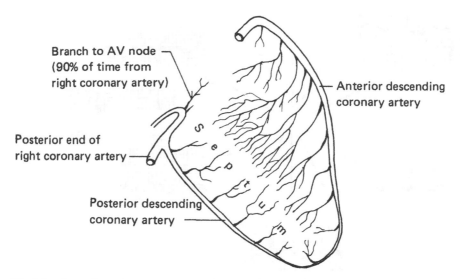

The blood supply to the septum is predominantly supplied by the anterior descending artery. Note also the U turn of the right coronary artery, at whose apex the artery to the AV node is given off.

Right Ventricular Overload Initial Vectors Mimicking Necrosis

1. How can a pulmonary embolus cause an initial frontal plane vector abnormality?
   ANS.: Sudden dilatation and an increase in pressure in the RV can cause both an initial and a terminal vector change. When the initial vector is changed, it often goes more superiorly, producing a Q in lead 3 and, less often, in aVF.
   Note: a. An S in a lead 1 or aVL, as well as Q in lead 3, is considered a classic pulmonary embolus change, but these changes are usually seen only in massive embolism. They resemble somewhat the changes seen in posterior divisional block, which is discussed in detail in Chap. 19 (see ECGs 35A–C.)
   b. If before the embolism lead 3 looked like this

   after the embolism the initial small r may disappear, and it therefore looks like this

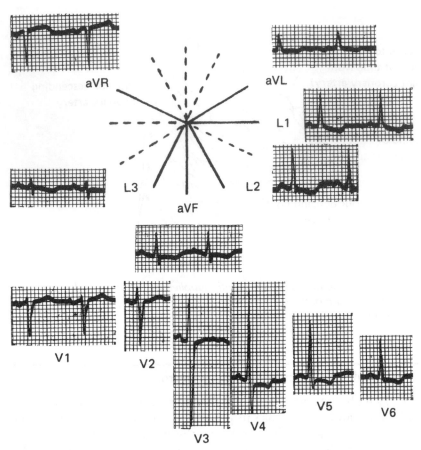

ECG 35A. Preoperative ECG of a moderately hypertensive 60-year-old woman admitted for a hysterectomy for endometrial cancer. The lack of a Q wave in L1 and V6 represents loss of the normal left-to-right septal forces. This LBBB pattern is commonly seen as a secondary sign of LVH.

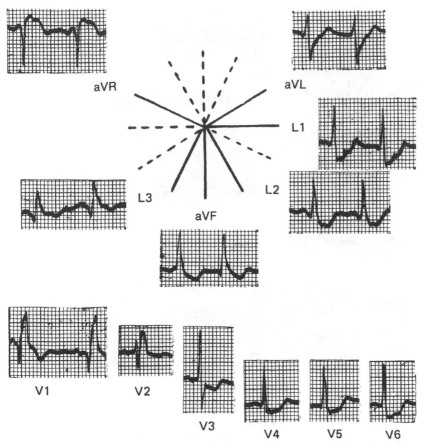

ECG 35B. Twenty days postoperatively the same patient as in ECG 35A had this ECG, showing a RBBB on the same day an acute pulmonary embolism was diagnosed. (A q has developed in L3 and an S in L1, which can be explained by a posterior divisional block, discussed in Chap. 19.)

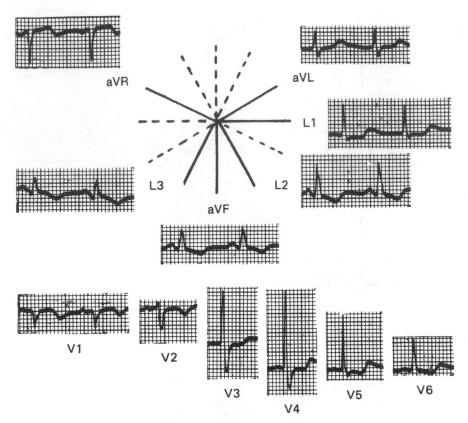

ECG 35C. The patient of ECGs 35A and 35B showed a terminal inferior vector (S in L1 and aVL) and a superior initial vector (q in aVF and L3) even when the RBBB disappeared a day later. (Note the negative T waves in V1 and V2. Their presence is often a sign of right ventricular overload [see p. 418].)

*2. How can a pulmonary embolism produce Q waves in the right precordium and so imitate an anteroseptal myocardial infarction?
    ANS.: There are two possible explanations:
        a. If the patient already has RVH and an initial right-to-left vector, an embolus can shift the electrical center to the left by expanding the right atrium and RV. This situation produces negativity farther to the left.
        b. If a posterior divisional block is actually produced, it can produce initial negativity in the right precordial leads. (For an explanation, see the section on posterior divisional blocks in Chap. 19.)

*3. How can a Q in lead 3 due to an embolus be distinguished from an inferior infarction Q if there are no other abnormal ECG findings except in the initial QRS vector?
    ANS.: a. If there is no Q in lead 2 or aVF, an infarct is unlikely.
        b. The q resulting from embolism is more likely to be transient than is the Q of an inferior infarction.

*4. How can a myocardial infarct be imitated by emphysema?

ANS.: In some emphysema patients there is a QS from V1 to the mid-precordium without any anteroseptal infarct [49]. One possible explanation is that the initial vector does not point posteriorly but straight down, away from the right precordial electrodes. This inferior orientation in emphysema may be due to

a. Downward displacement of the electrical center, so that electrodes are placed relatively high on the chest.

b. Posterior or backward rotation of the apex of the heart.

Note: If the R in V3 one interspace lower is less than 2 mm, compared with the conventional electrode placement, there is probably an associated anterior infarction. If the R one interspace lower is more than 3 mm high, an anterior infarction in addition to chronic obstructive pulmonary disease (COPD) is unlikely [42].

Normal Q Wave in Lead 3 Versus Inferior Infarction

1. Is there normally a Q in lead 3?

ANS.: Normally, there may be a Q in any limb lead because the septal vector can travel either superiorly or inferiorly (as well as from left to right) (see p. 145).

2. What can produce a slightly wide Q in lead 3 without infarction?

ANS.: LVH; i.e., the 'septal vector' may be prolonged if the septum is hypertrophied.

3. What is more significant for a necrosis Q wave in lead 3, its width or its depth?

ANS.: Its width. In the absence of marked LVH, a Q of 40 msec in lead 3 is highly likely to be due to necrosis. However, even moderate LVH can produce a deep Q in lead 3.

Note: If the Q in L3 is questionable in width or even absent, an inferior infarction is likely if there is regression of initial inferior forces from L3 to L2. This pattern means

(1) A deeper Q in L2 than L3, or

(2) A Q in L2 and no Q in L3, or

(3) An initial R in L3 and a simultaneous isoelectric segment in L2, or

(4) A taller initial R in L3 than a simultaneously recorded R in L2.

All the above assumes no counterclockwise QRS rotation in the frontal plane; i.e., the maximum deflection of the QRS in L3 must not precede the maximum QRS deflection in L2 [74].

4. When a deep or wide Q is seen in lead 3 or aVF, what else would you look for to help you decide whether an old infarct is present?

ANS.: Look for

a. Signs of LVH. A wide Q is more likely to be due to infarction if there is no LVH [63].

b. A Q in lead 2. If no Q is present in lead 2, an infarct is less likely. The deeper and wider the Q is in lead 2, the more likely it is that Q waves in leads 3 and aVF are due to infarction (see ECG 19, p. 150).

c. A notched or splintered Q in leads 3 and aVF [32]. (Running the paper at double speed when in doubt often brings out Q wave notchings.)

  d. A negative T in leads 3 and aVF. (The T vector points away from transmural infarcts.)

  e. An abnormal Q in the chest leads. Remember that, if the initial vector in the horizontal plane is recognizably due to infarction, so is every initial vector in the frontal plane.

  f. A relatively deep Q in aVF, i.e., more than 25 percent of the R wave (see ECG 36).

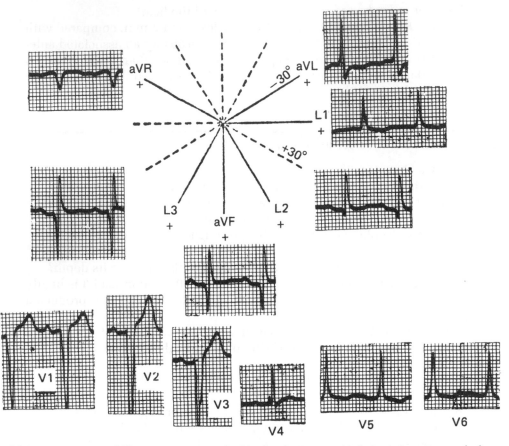

ECG 36. A 68-year-old hypertensive man had had a documented inferior infarct 7 years before this ECG was taken. The absolute depth of the Q waves in L3 and aVF is due to LVH. The width and relative depth of the Q in aVF are virtually diagnostic of inferior infarction.

  Note: a. A common beginner's error is to call a QS in lead 3 and aVF a wide necrosis Q, when in fact you cannot tell where the Q ends and the S begins (see ECG 34, p. 175).

    b. It used to be thought that only a normal Q wave in L3 could be decreased in depth or duration by inspiration. This idea is not true. Inspiration can also decrease the amplitude and duration of a pathological Q wave in L3 [12, 59].

    c. In treadmill testing it is common to place arm electrodes in the infraclavicular fossae and the foot electrode in the anterior axillary line just above the left iliac crest. This measure not only shifts a QRS axis so that it may be as much as 60° downward, but it may eliminate the deep, wide Q of an inferior infarct and also may exaggerate the Q in aVL enough to mimic a lateral infarct [53].

REFERENCES

1. Andersen, H. R., Nielsen, D., and Falk, E. Right ventricular infarction: diagnostic value of ST elevation in lead 3 exceeding that of lead 2 during inferior/posterior infarction and comparison with right-chest leads V3R to V7R. *Am. Heart J.* 117:82–86, 1989.
1A. Abildskov, J. A., and Boyle, R. S. Further studies of the electrocardiographic effects of experimental myocardial lesions. *Am. Heart J.* 69:49, 1965.
2. Arensdorf, M. F. Electrocardiogram in hyperkalemia. *Arch. Intern. Med.* 136:1161, 1976.
3. Banta, H. D., and Estes, E. H., Jr. Electrocardiographic findings in patients with idiopathic myocardial hypertrophy. *Am. J. Cardiol.* 14:218, 1964.
4. Barillon, M., et al. Premonitory sign of heart block in acute posterior myocardial infarction. *Br. Heart J.* 37:2, 1975.
5. Barold, S. S., Ong, L. S., and Banner, R. L. Diagnosis of interior wall myocardial infarction during right ventricular apical pacing. *Chest* 69:232, 1978.
6. Bateman, T., Gray, R., and Berman, D. Transient Q waves during exercise ECG. *Am. Heart J.* 104:182, 1982.
6A. Battle, R., Capeless, M., Langburd, A., Ditchey, R., et al. Posterior leads detect myocardial injury during circumflex coronary artery occlusion. *J.A.C.C.* 17:311A, 1991.
7. Bayley, R. H., and LaDue, J. S. Electrocardiographic changes of impending infarction and the ischemic-injury pattern produced in the dog. *Am. Heart J.* 28:54, 1944.
8. Bayley, R. H., LaDue, J. S., and York, D. S. Electrocardiographic changes (local ventricular ischemia and injury) produced in the dog by temporary occlusion of a coronary artery, showing a new stage of the evolution of myocardial infarction. *Am. Heart J.* 27:164, 1944.
9. Befeler, B., et al. Changes in the pattern of old inferior wall myocardial infarction produced by acute left bundle branch block and hemiblock. *Chest* 63:18, 1973.
10. Bisteni, A., Medrano, G. A., and Sodi-Pallares, D. Ventricular premature beats in the diagnosis of myocardial infarction. *Br. Heart J.* 23:521, 1961.
11. Blumgart, H. L., Gilligan, D. R., and Schlesinger, M. J. Experimental studies on the effect of temporary occlusion of coronary arteries. *Am. Heart J.* 22:374, 1941.
12. Bodenheimer, M. M., Banka, V. S., and Helfant, R. H. Determination of lead III Q waves significance: utility of deep inspiration. *Arch. Intern. Med.* 137:437, 1977.
13. Bodenheimer, M. M., Banka, V. S., and Helfant, R. H. Q waves and ventricular asynergy: Predictive value and hemodynamic significance of anatomic localization. *Am. J. Cardiol.* 35:615, 1975.
14. Bough, E. W., and Koor, K. S. Prevalence and severity of circumflex coronary artery disease in posterior infarction. *J. Am. Coll. Cardiol.* 7:990, 1986.
15. Braudo, M., Wigle, E. D., and Keith, J. D. Distinctive electrocardiogram in muscular subaortic stenosis due to ventricular septal hypertrophy. *Am. J. Cardiol.* 14:599, 1964.
16. Brusca, A., et al. Process of activation of the ventricular wall in experimentally induced chronic cardiac infarction. *Mal. Cardiovasc.* 7:23, 1966.
17. Burns, C. J. Return to normal of the ECG after myocardial infarction. *Lancet* 1:1194, 1967.
18. Castellanos, A., Jr., et al. ST-qR pacing. *Br. Heart J.* 35:1161, 1973.
19. Chapman, M. G., and Pearce, M. L. Electrocardiographic diagnosis of myocardial infarction in the presence of left bundle branch block. *Circulation* 16:558, 1957.
20. Chiche, P., and Haiat, R. Transient Q waves: An anamnestic response of an old myocardial infarction. *Am. J. Cardiol.* 38:544, 1976.

21. Cohen, J. Acute myocardial infarction early and objectively diagnosed through ventricular extrasystoles. *Am. J. Cardiol.* 7:882, 1961.

22. Cohen, M. H., et al. Electrocardiographic changes in acute pancreatitis resembling acute myocardial infarction. *Am. Heart J.* 82:672, 1971.

23. Cook, R. W., Edwards, J., and Pruitt, R. D. Electrocardiographic changes in acute subendocardial infarction. *Circulation* 18:603, 1958.

24. Cox, C. J. Return to normal of the electrocardiogram after infarction. *Lancet* 1:1194, 1967.

25. Danilowicz, D. A. Prognostic value of the electrocardiogram in endocardial fibroelastosis. *Br. Heart J.* 38:516, 1976.

26. Demoulen, J. C., and Kulbertus, H. E. Histopathological examination of conception of left hemiblock. *Br. Heart J.* 34:807, 1972.

27. DePace, N. L., et al. Poor R wave progression in the precordial leads *J. Am. Coll. Cardiol.* 2:1073, 1983.

28. Dressler, W. A case of myocardial infarction marked by bundle branch block but revealed by PVCs. *Am. J. Med. Sci.* 206:361, 1943.

29. Dunn, W. J., Edwards, J. E., and Pruitt, R. D. The electrocardiogram in infection of the lateral wall of the left ventricle. *Circulation* 14:540, 1956.

30. Durrer, D. Electrical aspects of human cardiac activity. *Cardiovasc. Res.* 2:1, 1968.

31. Durrer, D., et al. Total excitation of isolated human heart. *Circulation* 41:899, 1970.

32. Dwyer, E. M., et al. Inferior myocardial infarction and right coronary artery occlusive disease: A correlative study. *Br. Heart J.* 37:464, 1975.

33. El-Sherif, N. The rR' pattern in left surface leads in ventricular aneurysm. *Br. Heart J.* 32:440, 1970.

34. Fearrington, E. L. Gibson, T. C., and Churchill, R. E. Vectorcardiographic and electrocardiographic findings in myotonia atrophica: A study employing the Frank lead system. *Am. Heart J.* 67:599, 1964.

34A. Fisch, C. Septal myocardial infarction: Q waves unmasked by right bundle branch block. *Am. Coll. Cardiol.* Current Journal Review 1998; 68–69.

35. Fletcher, E., et al. Indications for high chest leads in ischaemic heart disease. *Br. Heart J.* 31:623, 1969.

36. Freundlich, J., and Kavanagh-Gray, D. The significance of ventricular premature beats in the diagnosis of septal infarction. *Can. Med. Assoc. J.* 91:1145, 1964.

37. Fuchs, R. M., et al. ECG localization of coronary artery narrowings. *Circulation* 66:1168, 1982.

38. Gamboa, R., Gersony, W. M., and Nadas, A. S. The electrocardiogram in tricuspid atresia and pulmonary atresia with intact ventricular septum. *Circulation* 34:24, 1966.

39. Gottesman, J., Casten, D., and Beller, A. J. Changes in the electrocardiogram induced by acute pancreatitis. *J.A.M.A.* 120:892, 1943.

40. Haiat, R., and Chiche, P. Transient abnormal Q waves in ischemic heart disease. *Chest* 65:140, 1974.

41. Harmjanz, D., Bottcher, D., and Schertlein, G. Correlations of electrocardiogram pattern in obstructive cardiomyopathy. *Br. Heart J.* 33:928, 1971.

42. Hart, G. J., Barrett, P. A., and Burke, J. J. Diagnosis of old anterior infarction in emphysema. *Br. Heart J.* 45:522, 1981.

43. Hassett, M. A., Williams, R. R., and Wagner, G. S. Transient QRS changes simulating acute infarction. *Circulation* 62:975, 1980.

44. Hellerstein, H. K., and Katz, L. N. The electrical effects of injury at various myocardial locations. *Am. Heart J.* 36:184, 1948.

45. Hill, J. D., et al. Experimental myocardial infarction in unanesthetized monkeys. *Am. Heart J.* 84:82, 1972.

46. Hoffman, I., et al. Anterior conduction delay: A possible cause for prominent anterior QRS forces. *J. Electrocardiol.* 9:15, 1976.

47. Horan, L. G., Flowers, N. C., and Johnson, J. C. Significance of diagnostic Q waves of myocardial infarction. *Circulation* 43:428, 1971.

48. Horan, L. G., et al. The significance of diagnostic Q waves in the presence of bundle branch block. *Chest* 58:214, 1970.

49. Ishikawa, K., Eddleman, E. E., Jr., and Pipberger, H. V. Electrocardiograms in pulmonary emphysema mimicking myocardial infarction. *Med. Ann. D.C.* 39:20, 1970.

49A. Iwasaki, K., Kusachi S., Kita T., Taniguchi, G. Prediction of isolated first diagonal branch occlusion by 12-lead electrocardiography: ST segment shift in leads 1 and aVL. *J. Am. Coll. Cardiol.* 23:1157–1561, 1994.

50. James, T. N., and Burch, G. E. Blood supply of the human interventricular septum. *Circulation* 17:391, 1958.

51. Kangos, J. J., et al. Electrocardiographic changes associated with papillary muscle infarction in congenital heart disease. *Am. J. Cardiol.* 23:801, 1969.

52. Kaplan, B. M., and Berkson, D. M. Serial electrocardiograms after myocardial infarction. *Ann. Intern. Med.* 60:430, 1964.

52A. Kindwall, K. E., et al. Predictive accuracy of criteria for chronic myocardial infarction in left bundle branch block. *Am. J. Cardiol.* 57:1255, 1986.

53. Kleiner, J. P., Nelson, W. P., and Boland, M. J. The 12-lead electrocardiogram in exercise testing: A misleading baseline? *Arch. Intern. Med.* 138:1572, 1978.

53A. Kosuge, M., Kimura, K., Ishkawa, Hongo, Y., et al. Implications of the absence of ST-segment elevation in Lead V_{4R} in patients who have inferior wall acute myocardial infarction with right ventricular involvement. *Clin. Cardiol.* 24:225–230, 2001.

54. Lamb, L. E. Electrocardiographic changes noted at the onset of coronary occlusion and myocardial infarction. *Am. J. Cardiol.*

55. Levine, H. D. Myocardial fibrosis in constrictive pericarditis: Electrocardiographic and pathologic observations. *Circulation* 48:1268, 1973.

56. Levine, H. D., and Phillips, E. An appraisal of the newer electrocardiography: Correlations in one hundred and fifty consecutive autopsied cases. *N. Engl. J. Med.* 245:833, 1951.

56A. Lopez-Sendon, J., Coma-Canella, I., Alcasena, S., Seoane. J., Gamallo, C. Electrocardiographic findings in acute right ventricular infarction: Sensitivity and specificity of electrocardiographic alterations of right precordial leads V_{4R}, V_{3R}, V_1, V_2, and V_3. *J. Am. Coll. Cardiol.* 6:1273–1279, 1985.

57. Luy, G., Bahl, O. P., and Massie, E. Intermittent left bundle branch block: A study of the effects of left bundle branch block on the electrocardiographic patterns of myocardial infarction and ischemia. *Am. Heart J.* 85:332, 1973.

58. McGuiness, J. B. First electrocardiogram in recent myocardial infarction. *Br. Med. J.* 2:449, 1976.

58A. Meller, J., Conde, C. A., Donoso, E., Dack, S. Transient Q waves in Prinzmetal's angina. *Am. J. Cardiol.* 35:691–695, 1975.

59. Mimbs, J. W., deMello, F., and Roberts, R. The effect of respiration on Q waves. *Am. Heart J.* 94:579, 1977.

59A. Morgera, T., Alberti, E., Silvestri, F., Pandullo, Mea, M. T. D., Camerini, F. Right precordial ST and QRS changes in the diagnosis of right ventricular infarction. *Am. Heart J.* 108:13–18, 1984.

60. Myers, G. B. QRS-T patterns in multiple precordial leads that may be mistaken for myocardial infarction. *Circulation* 1:844, 1950.

61. Myers, G. B. The electrocardiogram in subendocardial infarction with pathological correlations. *Am. J. Med. Sci.* 222:417, 1951.

62. Nemate, M., et al. The influence of constitutional variables on orthogonal electrocardiograms of normal women. *Circulation* 56:989, 1977.

62A. Papouchado, M., et al. Simple basis for surface ECG changes during angiography. *E. Heart J.* 8:254, 1987.

63. Perloff, J. K. The recognition of strictly posterior myocardial infarctions by conventional scalar electrocardiography. *Circulation* 30:706, 1964.

64. Prinzmetal, M., et al. Intramural depolarization potentials in myocardial infarction. *Circulation* 7:1, 1953.

64A. Rich, M. W., Imburgia, M., King, T.R., et al. Electrocardiographic diagnosis of remote posterior wall myocardial infarction using unipolar posterior lead V_9*. *Chest* 96:489–493, 1986.

65. Roesler, H., and Dressler, W. An electrocardiographic pattern of infarction of the interventricular septum. *Am. Heart J.* 38:817, 1947.

66. Rubin, I. L., Gross, H., and Arbeit, S. R. Transitory abnormal Q waves during bouts of tachycardia. *Am. J. Cardiol.* 11:659, 1963.

67. Rubler, S., et al. Cardiomyopathy simulating myocardial infarction. *N.Y. State J. Med.* 73:1111, 1973.

68. Selwyn, A. P., et al. Loss of electrically active myocardium during inferior infarction in man. *Br. Heart J.* 40:1019, 1978.

68A. Shalev, Y., Fogelman, R., Oettinger, M., Caspi, A. Does the electrocardiographic pattern of 'anteroseptal' myocardial infarction correlate with the anatomic location of myocardial injury? *Am. J. Cardiol.* 1995: 75:763–766.

69. Silverman, J. J., and Salomon, S. Myocardial infarction pattern disclosed by ventricular extrasystoles. *Am. J. Cardiol.* 4:695, 1959.

70. Sodi-Pallares, D., et al. Unipolar QS morphology and Purkinje potential of the free left ventricular wall. *Circulation* 23:836, 1961.

71. Spritzer, H. W. Electrocardiographic abnormalities in acute pancreatitis and coronary angiography. *Milit. Med.* 134:687, 1969.

72. Sullivan, W., et al. Correlation of ECG and pathologic findings. *Am. J. Cardiol.* 42:724, 1978.

73. Surawicz, B., et al. QS and QR patterns in leads V3 and V4 in absence of infarction. *Circulation* 12:391, 1955.

73A. Tamura, A., Kataoka, H., Mikuriya, Y. Electrocardiographic findings in patients with pure septal infarction. *Br. Heart J.* 65:166–167, 1991.

74. Warner, R., et al. Improved electrocardiographic criteria for the diagnosis of inferior myocardial infarction. *Circulation* 66:422, 1982.

74A. Warner, R. A., Hill, N. E., Mookherjee, S., Smulyan, H. Diagnostic significance for coronary artery disease of abnormal Q waves in the 'lateral' electrocardiographic leads. *Am. J. Cardiol.* 58:431–435, 1986.

75. Wilkinson, R. S., Jr., Schaefer, A. J., and Abildskov, J. A. Electrocardiographic and pathologic features of myocardial infarction in man: A correlative study. *Am. J. Cardiol.* 11:24, 1963.

76. Yabuki, S., et al. Time studies of acute, reversible, coronary occlusions in dogs. *J. Thorac. Cardiovasc. Surg.* 38:1, 1959.

77. Zeft, H. J., et al. Reappearance of anterior QRS forces after coronary bypass surgery. An electro-vectorcardiographic study. *Am. J. Cardiol.* 36:163, 1975.

78. Zema, M. J., and Klingfield, P. ECG poor R wave progression. *J. Electrocardiol.* 12:11, 1979.

79. Zema, M. J., and Klingfield, P. ECG poor R wave progression. *Arch. Intern. Med.* 142:1145, 1982.

79A. Zimetbaum, P. J., Krishnan, S., Gold, A., Carrozzall, J. P., et al. Usefulness of ST-segment elevation in lead III exceeding that of lead II for identifying the location of the totally occluded coronary artery in inferior wall myocardial infarction. *Excerpta Med.* 918–919, 1998.

18. Initial Vector Abnormalities in Preexcitation Syndromes

CLASSIC WOLFF-PARKINSON-WHITE SYNDROME

1. What produces the P-R interval?

    ANS.: The P-R interval consists of three parts:
    a. The depolarization of the atrium, which inscribes the P wave.
    b. The time spent traveling through the atrioventricular (AV) node, which inscribes part of the isoelectric line known as the P-R segment.
    c. Time spent traveling through the bundle of His and bundle branches, which inscribes the last part of the P-R segment.

    Note: The time through the AV node, the bundle of His, and bundle branches is mostly indicated by an isoelectric segment between the P and the QRS. This interval is the P-R segment. More than one-half of the P-R segment, however, consists of conduction through the AV node.

2. Where on an ECG does a P-R interval begin and end?

    ANS.: It is measured from the beginning of the P wave to the beginning of the QRS, even if the QRS begins with a q wave.

3. What is meant by the Wolff-Parkinson-White (WPW) syndrome?

    ANS.: It generally refers to conduction from atrium to ventricles via accessory bundles that bypass both the AV node and bundle of His, resulting in a short P-R, a wide QRS, and a tendency to paroxysmal tachycardias [41]. These anomalous pathways have in the past been called the bundles of Kent. Paroxysmal supraventricular tachycardias (atrial flutter, fibrillation, or tachycardia) occur in about 10 percent of adults with WPW conduction followed for an average of 20 years [2]. When paroxysmal tachycardias occur in patients with such accessory bundles, the term *WPW syndrome* is appropriate. When there are no tachycardias the ECG should be described as showing AV preexcitation. (See p. 556 for discussion of atrial tachycardias in the WPW syndrome.)

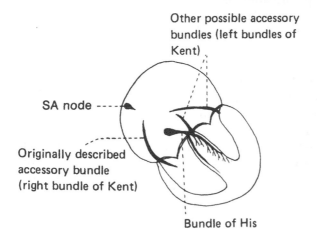

Other possible accessory bundles (left bundles of Kent)

SA node

Originally described accessory bundle (right bundle of Kent)

Bundle of His

Note: It has been suggested by a working party of the European Society of Cardiology that the bundles of Kent be called accessory AV bundles [1].

4. What happens to the P-R interval if the AV node is bypassed?

   ANS.: It is shortened, because the AV node has one-fifth the conduction velocity of atrial conduction (200 versus 1000 mm/second); i.e., conduction is slowed considerably at the AV node. This slowing produces most of the pause between the P wave and the QRS known as the P-R segment.

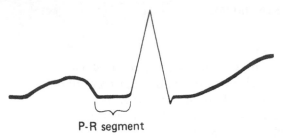

P-R segment

The P-R segment is the isoelectric interval caused mainly by slow conduction through the AV node.

5. What part of the P-R interval is encroached on if the AV node is bypassed?

   ANS.: The P-R segment. It is shortened when there is AV preexcitation.

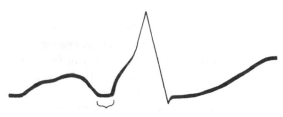

Short P-R segment

6. What tells us that the bypass fibers in AV preexcitation do not link up the atrium directly with the ventricular conduction system?

   ANS.: The initial ventricular depolarization is always slow for a short period before it begins to travel at its normal speed through the ventricular conducting tissue. Therefore it must be initially traveling through muscle.

7. If bypass fibers go through ventricular muscle first, what does it do to the initial part of the QRS?

   ANS.: It produces a wide initial vector. Conduction through ventricular muscle is 10 times slower than through the conduction system (400 versus 4000 mm/second). Because of slow conduction, the initial vector is darker or thicker than the rest of the QRS unless the ECG machine uses an ink writer.

   Note: That conduction down the accessory AV bundle does not contribute to the initial slowing in AV preexcitation is also suggested by the fact that the bypass pathway has the histologic appearance of specialized atrial conduction tissue.

* Material marked with an asterisk is included for reference and for advanced students in cardiology.

8. What is the initial slow conduction in the QRS with AV preexcitation called?
   ANS.: A delta wave, because when it is positive in a left ventricular lead it reminds
   you somewhat of the Greek letter delta.

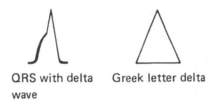

QRS with delta   Greek letter delta
wave

9. Because the delta wave is slowly inscribed, how is the duration of the QRS affected?
   ANS.: It is prolonged (see ECG 37).
10. What, then, is the entire ECG picture of AV preexcitation?
    ANS.: a. Shorter-than-normal (less than 120 msec) P-R interval owing to a short
    P-R segment.
    b. Delta wave.
    c. Prolonged QRS.
    Note: A right-sided accessory pathway has a short distance to go between
    the SA node and ventricle. Therefore it easily beats the AV node to the ven-
    tricle and produces a wide delta wave. A left-sided accessory pathway, on
    the other hand, has a relatively small delta wave.
*11. Is an accessory AV bundle ever acquired?
    ANS.: An accessory AV bundle has been seen to occur for the first time in adults
    after the development of an infarct, hypertrophic subaortic stenosis, idio-
    pathic cardiomyopathies, or thyrotoxicosis [27]. Because these conditions
    may merely have suppressed normal AV conduction or favored bypass
    conduction, and the bypass fibers may have been present at birth, the use of
    the term *acquired* is debatable.
    Note: a. Reports of the syndrome in members of the same family indicate
    that a bundle of Kent conduction can be familial [8, 35].
    b. About 0.3 percent of U.S. Air Force applicants between ages 18
    and 24 have a delta wave [37].
    c. The mortality in adults with the WPW syndrome is about three
    times that of normal subjects without WPW syndrome [20A]. This
    high mortality rate is probably due to the development of atrial
    fibrillation followed by ventricular fibrillation because the bundle
    of Kent cannot block the rapid impulses to the ventricles [14].
    Ventricular fibrillation has been documented in the WPW syn-
    drome [17].
    d. Ebstein's anomaly of the tricuspid valve is frequently associated
    with AV preexcitation.
*12. Are T waves ever normally negative in V5 and V6 with the wide QRS of accessory
    AV bundle preexcitation?
    ANS.: No. The maximum normal secondary T change is an isoelectric T in V5 or
    V6. However, a negative T has been found when left ventricular overloading
    was also present [39] (see ECG 37).

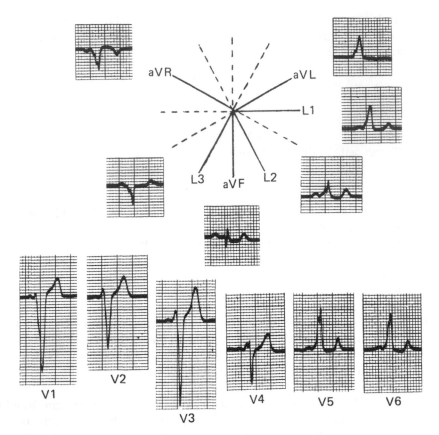

ECG 37. Type B AV preexcitation in a 36-year-old asymptomatic man. A right-sided accessory bundle has produced a delta wave that is anterior enough to produce an initial r in V1. However, the QRS is posterior as seen by the deep S in V1.

*13. When is the P-J interval after bundle of Kent preexcitation the same as before the preexcitation?

ANS.: When the terminal part of the QRS is produced by depolarization via the AV nodal pathway. (P-J = from P to J point).

Note: If the depolarization is entirely by the accessory pathway, the P-J interval is prolonged.

CLASSIFYING WPW TYPES

1. What did Kent originally describe; i.e., what was the original 'bundle of Kent'?

ANS.: Kent, in his first article on the subject, described a muscular connection between the lateral right atrium and right ventricle across the AV sulcus. He called it 'the right lateral AV node' [22]. We, however, use the term *bundle of Kent* in its more general meaning, i.e., any nodal bypass pathways between atrial and ventricular muscle. (In his later writings Kent described AV connections in many sites around the AV sulcus.)

2. If both the delta wave and the QRS point anteriorly (positive in V1), what type of preexciation has it been called? Where is the accessory AV bundle (bundle of Kent) in this type?

ANS.: Type A [33]. It has usually been associated with a left-sided accessory AV bundle.

Note: a. That type A is due to a left-sided AV accessory bundle has been shown in many ways. By electrically stimulating the left and right atrium at equal rates in type A, the greatest amount of pre-excitation is seen after left atrial stimulation. Also, when there is a tachycardia with anterograde AV node conduction, left atrial excitation precedes right atrial activation by a considerable time.

V1 =

b. If a patient has a left-sided accessory AV bundle and a right bundle branch block (RBBB) is present, the terminal changes of RBBB are seen. If, however, the patient has a right-sided AV bundle, no terminal changes occur [19, 34]. This difference has been used to confirm that in type A the left ventricle (LV) is depolarized first, and in type B the right ventricle (RV) is depolarized first [3].

3. If the delta wave is anterior but the QRS is posterior so that V1 has an rS configuration, what is this type called, and where is the accessory bundle?

ANS.: Type B. The accessory pathway is in the free wall of the RV (see ECG 37).

Note: a. If V1 shows a QS or QR and the QRS is posterior, it has been called type C, and the accessory pathway is thought to be in the posterior septum (see ECG 38) [40]. However, in the classic terminology of Rosenbaum et al., even the posterior QRS with a QS in V1 is called type B [33]. This distinction is easy to remember because if the QRS is anterior it is called type A (A for anterior) and if posterior it is type B (B for backward).

Type C has also been described as one with a positive delta wave in V1–V4 and rS or QS in V5 and V6, and is thought to begin in the posterolateral wall of the left ventricle [42].

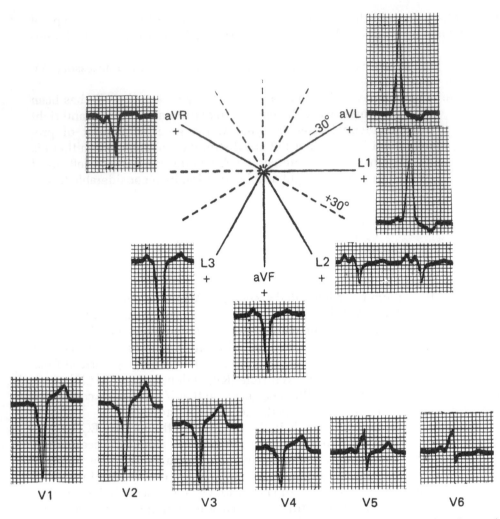

ECG 38. WPW type B or C. The delta wave causing a QS in L3, aVF, and V1 to V4 may be read as an anteroinferior infarct by the unwary. The absence of a q in L2 should make an inferior infarct unlikely.

b. A right-sided accessory AV bundle has never been known to produce an anterior QRS, i.e., a classic type A.

c. One group found that if a delta wave is anterior but the QRS is posterior, five of six such patients had a left ventricular overload [39].

d. The vector of the delta wave corresponds well with the initial direction of depolarization of the ventricle into which the bundle of Kent enters; i.e., it tells you roughly where the bundle of Kent is. For example, if the 20-msec QRS vector goes to the right and anteriorly and inferiorly, the accessory bundle was always in the LV. If it goes to the left and inferiorly, it was in either the RV or the pulmonary outflow tract. A superior initial force strongly suggests a septal accessory bundle [38].

*4. What suggests that at least some subjects have accessory AV nodal bypass fibers that travel close to the bundle of His?

ANS.: His bundle recordings have occasionally shown a spike from the bypass pathway in subjects with bundle of Kent types of ECG; i.e., there are both septal and parietal accessory AV bundles.

Note: Some subjects have bilateral anomalous pathway, with one conducting anterogradely and the other able to conduct only retrogradely, which permits the production of reentry arrhythmias [12].

*5. What is the value of knowing that a right-sided or left-sided bundle of Kent type of pathway is producing the preexcitation?

ANS.: a. Intractable paroxysmal tachycardia may require an operation to cut the accessory bundle [36]. However, even when electrical mapping of surgically exposed hearts has shown where initial ventricular activation begins, surgical transection of this area has not always abolished the delta wave [10].

b. A permanent pacemaker in the right atrium to pace it intermittently in order to interrupt a supraventricular tachycardia can be expected to work only with a right-sided bundle of Kent-like pathway. (The implanted power can be activated at will by placing a magnet over it [31].)

c. Prolapsed valve syndromes are usually associated with Type A [17]. Ebstein's anomaly is usually associated with type B and left axis deviation [23].

d. Atrial flutter, atrial fibrillation, and ventricular fibrillation tend to occur mostly with left-sided AV bundles.

Note: Atrial fibrillation tends to result in ventricular fibrillation if the patient is on digitalis because digitalis may shorten the conduction time through the accessory pathway [9, 13].

e. A cyanotic child with a type B bundle of Kent and a left axis deviation very likely has Ebstein's anomaly, tricuspid atresia, or tetralogy of Fallot. With a normal axis, consider a complete transposition as most likely.

*6. How can you recognize a posteroseptal accessory pathway by ECG?

ANS.: The delta wave is superiorly directed (negative in aVF) [32A].

ELICITING THE ACCESSORY AV BUNDLE TYPE OF PREEXCITATION

1. What brings out the accessory pathway mode of conduction in a subject with intermittent preexcitation?

ANS.: a. Vagal stimulation.
b. Atrial pacing at rapid rates [7].
c. Isoproterenol [32].

2. Why do vagal stimulation, atrial pacing, and isoproterenol tend to bring out a nodal bypass pathway?

ANS.: Conduction is divided between the normal AV node-bundle of His pathway and the bundle of Kent. Vagal stimulation or atrial pacing depresses the normal AV nodal conduction pathway and so allows the bypass pathway to take over. Isoproterenol shortens the refractory period of the accessory pathway more than that of the AV node.

Note: A *very* early premature beat can block the accessory pathway more than it blocks the AV node. If the focus for the premature beat were much closer to the AV node than to the accessory pathway, it could also produce normal conduction [28]. A long diastole can also normalize a preexcitation QRS because it can result in faster AV nodal conduction than accessory bundle conduction.

3. What is meant by saying that the accessory AV bundle type of conduction produces a fusion beat?

ANS.: Although the initial ventricular activation is through the anomalous pathway, conduction through the AV node proceeds as usual and may help to depolarize part of the LV through normal conduction pathways [11].

Note: The proof that most WPW QRS complexes are fusion beats that combine the depolarization effects of the bypass pathways with the depolarization of the AV node–His pathway consists of the following:

a. If the AV node–His conduction time is prolonged by atrial pacing at increasingly faster rates, the QRS becomes longer and longer, until conduction is entirely by the bypass pathway.

b. Bundle of His recordings can show the His deflection after the QRS has begun [7].

4. Why is it helpful to think of the QRS with the accessory AV bundle type of conduction as a fusion beat?

ANS.: It explains the hour-to-hour or day-to-day variation in the configuration of the QRS. Because the two pathways are always changing their relative ability to conduct, they may be always showing variable degrees of fusion due to variable conduction rates.

DELTA WAVE MASKING AND MIMICKING EFFECTS

1. The usual range of directions in the frontal plane for a delta wave is about − 30° to + 100°.

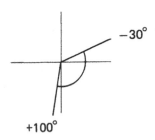

Which of the frontal delta waves in the figure imitates the necrosis vector of
a. An inferior infarct?
b. A lateral infarct?

ANS.: a. The one that goes superiorly imitates an inferior infarct (see ECG 38).
  b. The one that goes inferiorly can imitate a lateral infarct.

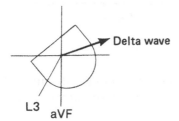

L3 aVF

Like an inferior infarct

The above superior delta wave produces a wide Q in L3 and aVF.

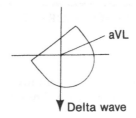

Like a lateral infarct

The above inferior delta wave produces a wide Q in aVL.

2. The usual range of directions of the delta wave in the horizontal plane is about the same as in the frontal plane, i.e., from about $-30°$ to $+100°$. Which chest lead almost always has a positive (upright) delta wave if the above ranges are considered? Why is this fact important?
    ANS.: V6. It means that AV preexcitation with a Q in V6 is uncommon.

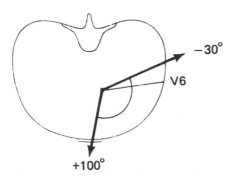

Most delta waves in this range produce a positive initial QRS vector in V6.

3. How can a delta wave be a serious obstruction to the interpretation of an ECG other than imitating an old infarction with wide initial negativity?
    ANS.: a. It can eliminate the initial necrosis vector of the infarct.
          b. It can imitate incomplete or complete left bundle branch block (LBBB).
          c. It can mask RBBB if the accessory pathway enters the RV directly, as in type B, thus depolarizing it early and nullifying the delaying effect of a proximal RBBB.
          d. It can produce false-positive exercise S-T changes suggesting ischemia [18].
4. If the delta wave masks the initial necrosis vector of an infarct, how can one unmask it; i.e., what can eliminate preexcitation, at least temporarily?
    ANS.: a. Sympathetic stimulation, e.g., by exercise or inhalation of amyl nitrite.
          b. Sympathetic release, e.g., by atropine.
          c. Depressing the bypass fibers, e.g., by quinidine, procainamide, or lidocaine.
         Note: Propranolol has no effect on an accessory AV bundle.

NONATRIOVENTRICULAR ACCESSORY BUNDLE PREEXCITATION

Mahaim Fibers

1. What are Mahaim fibers?

    ANS.: There are two main types—nodoventricular and fasciculoventricular [1]. Nodoventricular fibers arise from the AV node and fasciculoventricular arise from the bundle of His and/or upper bundle branches.

    Note: The P-R may be short or normal depending on the level of takeoff. The QRS will be wide with a delta wave. They may insert into the septum in such a way as to produce a LBBB pattern.

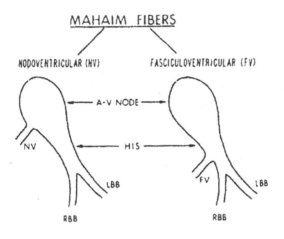

SITE OF ORIGIN :	A·V NODE	HIS BUNDLE ~ BUNDLE BRANCHES
P-R :	SHORT OR NORMAL	NORMAL (ISOLATED FV)
QRS :	ANOMALOUS ~ FUSION	ANOMALOUS

James Fibers and Short P-R, Normal QRS Preexcitation

1. What happens to the QRS width if the AV nodal bypass fibers go to the bundle of His? What have these bypass fibers been called?

    ANS.: Nothing happens to the QRS. These accessory pathway fibers are sometimes called 'James fibers' [21]. They are part of the posterior internodal tract (first described by Thorel in 1909), one of the three connections between the sinoatrial (SA) node and AV node [29].

    Note: a. There are three specialized conduction tracts between the SA and AV nodes (see p. 475 for details).

      *b. Because electrical stimulation near the SA node can reproduce the ECG picture of a short P-R and normal QRS, the presence of specialized conduction pathways to the His bundle is strongly suggested. (James described these bypass fibers in hearts that had normal ECGs. Therefore the use of these fibers may be intermittent.) These accessory pathways usually bypass only the upper part of the AV node. Only occasionally has a complete bypass been proved by atrial pacing and His bundle techniques [5]. Internodal fibers that completely bypass the AV node have not been seen on histologic examination [1]. Atrio–His accessory fibers bypassing the AV node have sometimes been found to be unrelated to any internodal tract [4].

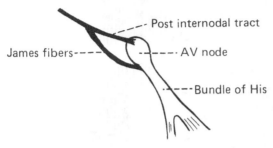

James fibers pass from right atrium to the lower AV node or bundle of His.

2. What happens to the P-R interval if the nodal bypass fibers go to the bundle of His?
   ANS.: It shortens.
3. What, then, is the total P, QRS picture if an atrio–His nodal bypass occurs?
   ANS.: A short P-R with a normal QRS.
       Note: a. If the atrio–His preexcitation is intermittent, the P wave vector is often up to 30° different in direction when the preexcitation is present from when it is not present. This finding suggests that the pacemaker is not usually in the SA node when James fibers are used.
       b. Another possible cause for a short P-R and a normal QRS would be specialized AV node conduction pathways that have the property of accelerated conduction.
4. Which terms have commonly been used to refer to the ECG resulting from nodal bypass fibers to the bundle of His?
   ANS.: a. Short P-R, normal QRS preexcitation.
       b. Coronary nodal rhythm [15].
       c. Atypical WPW syndrome.
       d. Lown-Ganong-Levine (LGL) syndrome [24].
       e. Atrio–His preexcitation.
       Note: The following questions are an attempt to defend 'atrio–His pre-excitation' as the description of choice.
*5. Why is *coronary nodal rhythm* a poor term?
   ANS.: It implies the presence of a 'coronary node,' which has never been described. It actually refers to the upper AV node near the coronary sinus.
6. What single term can encompass all the syndromes that bypass the AV node?
   ANS.: Preexcitation.
7. What do all the preexcitation syndromes have in common in addition to either a short P-R interval or a delta wave?
   ANS.: They all have a tendency to have paroxysms of supraventricular tachycardia.
8. When does atrio–His preexcitation become the LGL syndrome?
   ANS.: Only when the atrio–His preexcitation is associated with episodes of tachycardia is it the LGL syndrome (see ECG 39).
       In only about 10 percent of patients with atrio–His preexcitation is the bypass pathway used to produce a reentry type of tachycardia [5, 30].

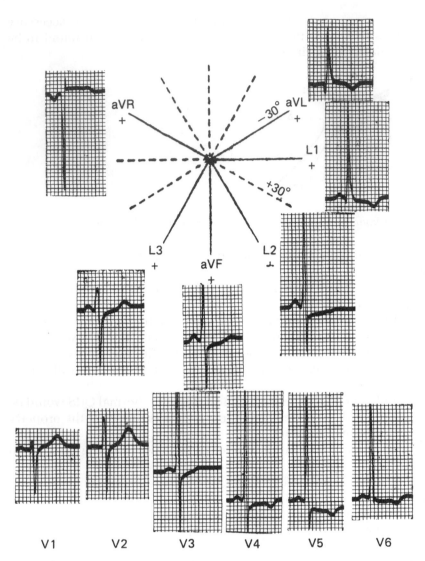

ECG 39. This ECG should be read as 'atrio–His preexcitation.' The P-R interval is 100 msec
(0.10 sec). Even without measuring the P-R interval you can guess that it is short by noting the
absence of a P-R segment. The AV node appears to be bypassed, presumably by James fibers
passing to the bundle of His. This ECG is from a 60-year-old hypertensive patient who has no
history of palpitations. Therefore the patient does not have the LGL syndrome.

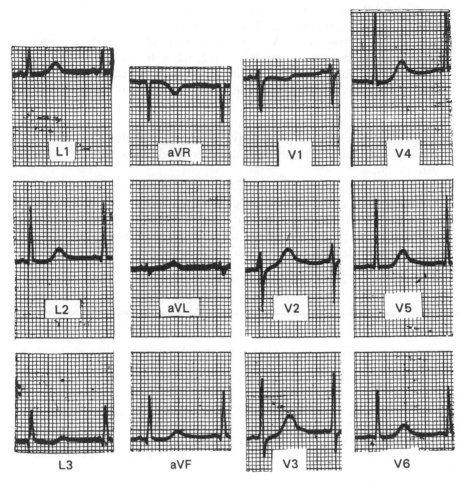

ECG 40. This ECG is from a 26-year-old woman with a normal heart except for the short P-R interval of about 100 msec (0.10 sec) and absent P-R segment compatible with atrio–His preexcitation. Because she also had episodes of rapid heart palpitations, she probably has the LGL syndrome.

9. What can exactly imitate a bundle of Kent type of preexcitation, i.e., with no accessory AV pathways actually being present?

   ANS.: a. A combination of atrio–His fibers (to bypass the AV node and produce the short P-R interval) and Mahaim or His-ventricular fibers (to bypass the proximal conduction system [16]).

   b. A nodo-ventricular accessory conduction from the middle of the AV node. This situation would produce a short P-R (because only a short piece of compact node is traversed) and then a delta wave as the conduction passes directly into ventricular septal muscle [1].

   Note: a. Atrial pacing can differentiate bundles of Kent, Mahaim, and James preexcitation. Atrial pacing at progressively faster rates causes more and more AV nodal delay, i.e., AV block. Therefore progressively faster atrial pacing, by prolonging AV nodal conduction, would cause more and more initial conduction through the bundle of Kent, making the QRS progressively wider and earlier, with the P-R interval remaining about the same. Because Mahaim fibers (His–ventricular bundles) cannot be activated until after conduction through the AV node, increasing rates of atrial pacing produce longer and longer P-R intervals without affecting the QRS. James fiber conduction often shows no effect from atrial pacing at relatively fast rates because the AV node may not be used at all [6].

b. Some patients with atrio–His preexcitation respond normally to atrial pacing, i.e., with progressively longer P-R intervals. Others have prolonged P-R intervals only after a critically rapid pacing rate [5, 26].

c. An imitation of a slight degree of AV preexcitation is seen in some patients with hypertrophic subaortic stenosis. It is not known whether the slow initial conduction in some of these patients is due to a bypass pathway or to conduction through the thick septum with its fiber disarray [20].

REFERENCES

1. Anderson, R. H., et al. Ventricular preexcitation: A proposed nomenclature for its substrates. *Eur. J. Cardiol.* 3/1:27, 1975.
2. Berkman, N. L., and Lamb, L. E. The Wolff-Parkinson-White electrocardiogram. *N. Engl. J. Med.* 278:492, 1968.
3. Boineau, J. P., and Moore, E. N. Evidence for propagation of activation across an accessory atrioventricular connection in types A and B pre-excitation. *Circulation* 41:375, 1970.
4. Brechenmacher, C. Atrio-His bundle tracts. *Br. Heart J.* 37:853, 1975.
5. Caracta, A. R., et al. Electrophysiologic studies in the syndrome of short P-R interval, normal QRS complex. *Am. J. Cardiol.* 31:245, 1973.
6. Castellanos, A., Jr., et al. His bundle electrocardiograms in patients with short P-R intervals, narrow QRS complexes, and paroxysmal tachycardia. *Circulation* 43:667, 1971.
7. Castellanos, A., Jr., et al. His bundle electrocardiograms in two cases of Wolff-Parkinson-White syndrome (pre-excitation). *Circulation* 41:399, 1970.
8. Chia, B. L., et al. Familial Wolff-Parkinson-White syndrome. *J. Electrocardiol.* 15:195, 1982.
9. Chung, K.-Y., Walsh, T. J., and Massie, E. Wolff-Parkinson-White syndrome. *Am. Heart J.* 60:116, 1965.
10. Cobb, R. F., et al. Successful surgical interruption of the bundle of Kent in a patient with Wolff-Parkinson-White syndrome. *Circulation* 38:1018, 1968.
11. Cole, J. S., et al. The Wolff-Parkinson-White syndrome. *Circulation* 42:111, 1970.
12. Denes, P., et al. Electrophysiologic demonstration of bilateral anomalous pathways in patients with Wolff-Parkinson-White syndrome (type B preexcitation). *Am. J. Cardiol.* 37:93, 1976.
13. Dreifus, L. S., et al. Ventricular fibrillation: A possible mechanism of sudden death in patients with Wolff-Parkinson-White syndrome. *Circulation* 43:520, 1971.
14. Durrer, D., Schuilenburg, R. M., and Wellens, H. J. J. Pre-excitation revisited. *Am. J. Cardiol.* 26:690, 1970.
15. Eyring, E. J., and Spodick, F. H. Coronary nodal rhythm. *Am. J. Cardiol.* 5:781, 1960.
16. Ferrer, M. I. New concepts relating to the pre-excitation syndrome. *J.A.M.A.* 201:162, 1967.
17. Gallagher, J. J., et al. Wolff-Parkinson-White syndrome: The problem, evaluation, and surgical correction. *Circulation* 51:767, 1975.
18. Gazes, P. C. False-positive exercise test in the Wolff-Parkinson-White syndrome. *Am. Heart J.* 78:13, 1969.

19. Gersony, W. M., and Ekery, D. D. Concealed right-bundle branch block in the presence of type B ventricular pre-excitation. *Am. Heart J.* 77:668, 1969.
20. Harmjanz, D., Bottcher, D., and Schertlein, G. Correlations of electrocardiographic pattern, shape of ventricular septum, and isovolumetric relaxation time in irregular hypertrophic cardiomyopathy (obstructive cardiomyopathy). *Br. Heart J.* 33:928, 1971.
20A. Hecht, H., et al. Anomalous AV excitation. *Ann. N.Y. Acad. Sci.* 65:826, 1956.
21. James, T. N. Morphology of the human atrioventricular node, with remarks pertinent to its electrophysiology. *Am. Heart J.* 62:756, 1961.
22. Kent, A. F. S. Illustrations of the right lateral auriculo-ventricular junction in the heart. *J. Physiol. (Lond.)* 48:63, 1914.
23. Lev, M., et al. Mahaim and James fibers as a basis for a unique variety of ventricular preexcitation. *Am. J. Cardiol.* 38:880, 1975.
24. Lown, B., Ganong, W. F., and Levine, S. A. The syndrome of short P-R interval, normal QRS complex and paroxysmal rapid heart action. *Circulation* 5:693, 1952.
25. Mahaim, I. Kent's fibers and the A-V paraspecific conduction through the upper connections of the bundle of His-Tawara. *Am. Heart J.* 33:651, 1947.
26. Mandel, W. J., Danzig, R., and Hayakawa, H. Lown-Ganong-Levine syndrome: A study using His bundle electrograms. *Circulation* 44:696, 1971.
27. Massumi, R. A. Familial Wolff-Parkinson-White syndrome with cardiomyopathy. *Am. J. Med.* 43:951, 1967.
28. Massumi, R. A., and Vera, Z. Patterns and mechanisms of QRS normalization in patients with Wolff-Parkinson-White syndrome. *Am. J. Cardiol.* 28:541, 1971.
29. Merideth, J., and Titus, J. L. The anatomic atrial connections between sinus and A-V node. *Circulation* 37:566, 1968.
30. Monahan, J. P., Denes, P., and Rosen, K. M. Portable electrocardiographic monitoring: Performance in patients with short P-R intervals without delta waves. *Arch. Intern. Med.* 135:1188, 1975.
31. Preston, T. A., and Kirsh, M. D. Permanent pacing of the left atrium for treatment of Wolff-Parkinson-White tachycardia. *Circulation* 42:1073, 1970.
32. Przybylski, J., et al. Unmasking of ventricular preexcitation by vagal stimulation of isoproterenol administration. *Circulation* 61:1030, 1980.
32A Rodriguez, L. M., et al. *J. Am. Coll. Cardiol.* 19:311A. (Abstract), 1992.
33. Rosenbaum, F. F., et al. Potential variations of the thorax and the esophagus in anomalous A-V excitation. *Am. Heart J.* 29:281, 1945.
34. Schamroth, L., and Krickler, D. M. Location of pre-excitation areas in Wolff-Parkinson-White syndrome. *Am. J. Cardiol.* 19:889, 1967.
35. Schneider, R. G. Familial occurrence of Wolff-Parkinson-White syndrome. *Am. Heart J.* 78:34, 1969.
36. Sealy, W. C., et al. Surgical treatment of Wolff-Parkinson-White syndrome. *Ann. Thorac. Surg.* 8:1, 1969.
37. Sears, G. A., and Manning, G. W. The Wolff-Parkinson-White pattern in routine electrocardiography. *Can. Med. Assoc. J.* 87:1213, 1962.
38. Tonkin, A. M., et al. Initial forces of ventricular depolarization in the Wolff-Parkinson-White syndrome. *Circulation* 52:1030, 1975.
39. Tranchesi, J., et al. Vectorial interpretation of the ventricular complex in Wolff-Parkinson-White syndrome. *Am. J. Cardiol.* 4:334, 1959.
40. Ueda, H. Electrocardiography of the Wolff-Parkinson-White syndrome. *Jpn. Heart J.* 23:7, 1982.
41. Wolff, L., Parkinson, J., and White, P. D. Bundle branch block with short P-R interval in healthy young people prone to paroxysmal tachycardia. *Am. Heart J.* 5:685, 1930.
42. Zipes, D. P. and McIntosh, H. D. In: Conn, H., Horwitz, O., eds. *Cardiac and Vascular Diseases*. Philadelphia: Lea and Febuger, 1971.

19. Terminal QRS Changes in Myocardial Infarction

HEMIBLOCKS OR DIVISIONAL BLOCKS

1. Into how many major branches does the bundle of His divide, and what are the branches called?

   ANS.: There are two major branches, the right and left bundle branches. The left bundle branch divides into two major divisions, the anterior-superior and the posterior-inferior. Thus, finally, there are three large divisions.

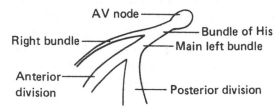

Conduction system viewed from the left side of the septum.

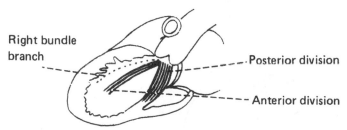

Anterior and posterior divisions of the left bundle, viewed through the left ventricle. The right bundle branch (dotted line) cannot be seen from the left side.

2. What recognizable ECG patterns are produced by a block in
   a. The right bundle?
   b. The main left bundle?
   c. The anterior division of the left bundle?
   d. The posterior division of the left bundle?

   ANS.: a. Right bundle branch block (RBBB).
   b. Left bundle branch block (LBBB).
   c. Anterior hemiblock (or divisional block).
   d. Posterior hemiblock (or divisional block).

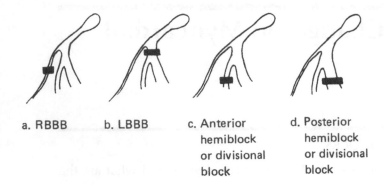

a. RBBB   b. LBBB   c. Anterior hemiblock or divisional block   d. Posterior hemiblock or divisional block

3. Why does a block or delay in one of the divisions of the left bundle rotate the QRS axis?

   ANS.: The anterior division travels superiorly over the septum and free wall of the left ventricle (LV) to supply the superior and anterolateral parts of the LV. If this division is interrupted, the area it supplies is reached last via the posterior division. Therefore the last area to be depolarized is the anterolateral, lateral, and superior parts of the LV. With the terminal forces pointing superiorly and laterally, the mean QRS is shifted upward to produce various degrees of left axis deviation. If the posterior division is blocked, by the same reasoning the terminal forces must be inferior and to the right, producing inferior or right axis deviations.

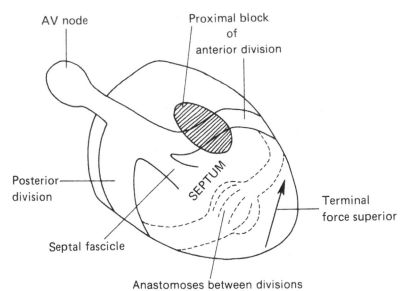

Left bundle and its divisions viewed from the right side with the right ventricle (RV) removed. The right bundle branch is also not depicted, although it runs down the right side of the septum. Note that a proximal block of the anterior division caused the initial forces to have a compulsory pathway downward mostly along the posterior division. This situation makes a septal r in inferior leads.

4. What is the classic pattern of
   a. Anterior hemiblock or divisional block?
   b. Posterior hemiblock or divisional block?

ANS.: a. Some degree of leftward axis deviation with an initial inferior and right-ward septal vector. Therefore there is a qR in aVL and an rS in L3 and aVF (see serial ECGs 41A and 41B).

   b. Some degree of rightward axis or right axis deviation with an initial superior and leftward septal vector.

5. Why is it important to remember that the anterior division of the left bundle con-ducts current mainly superiorly (from mid-septum to the high anterior and lateral aspect of the LV) and that the posterior division conducts current mainly inferiorly down the posterior wall?

ANS.: Because the vector changes seen in divisional blocks are apparent almost entirely in the frontal plane; i.e., the superior and inferior aspects are the only important ones. The only reasons for using the terms *anterior* and *posterior* divisional block are

   a. In deference to the common usage initiated by Rosenbaum et al. [53], the originators of the concept, who used the expression *anterior* and *posterior* hemiblock.

   b. To conform to the usual diagrams of the divisions. In these diagrams the superior division is actually shown as anterior (and slightly inferior) because its distal pathway along the ventricular wall is not shown.

   Note: a. The terms anterosuperior or posteroinferior divisional block are too cumbersome for routine use.

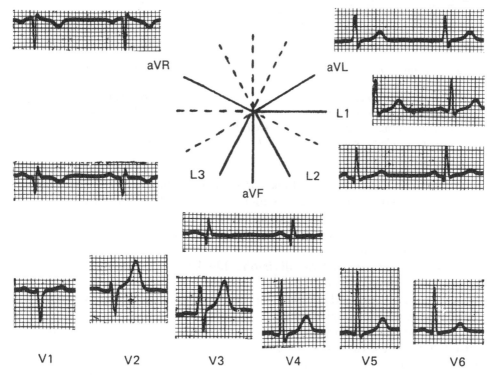

ECG 41A. The first of two tracings on a 38-year-old man with severe angina and cardiomegaly due to atherosclerotic obstruction of both right and anterior descending coronary arteries. The Q in L2 and L3 is due to old inferior infarction, which is strongly indicated by the relatively deep Q in aVF (about 50% of the R wave's height).

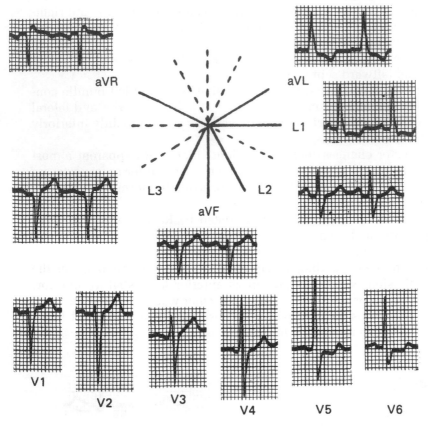

ECG 41B. The same patient as in ECG 41A, made after the patient had a double coronary bypass graft. There is now a marked left axis deviation (deep S in L2) because of the development of a terminal superior vector due to an anterior divisional block. Note that the Q in the inferior leads has disappeared owing to the change in initial vector; i.e., it has turned inferiorly. (The slurred R in aVR and S in L1 suggest a slight degree of RBBB as well. The lack of a slurred R' in V1, however, makes you suspect another possible cause of the terminal slowing. [See periinfarction blocks, p. 235.])

     b. The anterior hemiblocks or divisional blocks were formerly called 'anterolateral or superior parietal blocks' and the posterior blocks 'inferior parietal blocks.' They were both also sometimes called 'arborization blocks' or simply 'intraventricular conduction defects.'

6. Why are the terms *anterior* and *posterior* divisional blocks adequate to describe left anterior and left posterior hemiblocks?

    ANS.: a. The word left is redundant, because there are no clinically known right hemiblocks or divisional blocks.

         b. If the abbreviation LAH is used for left anterior hemiblock, it can be confused with left atrial hypertrophy. The abbreviation ADB for anterior divisional block is not confused with known abbreviations.

         c. A 'division' is more understandable anatomically than a 'hemi.'

         d. Because the anterior division is usually much smaller than the posterior division, a block of one division is not really a block of one-half of the main left bundle. 'Hemi' implies a block of one-half.

e. Because a septal fascicle has been shown to be another significant division of the left bundle branch, a block of one of three divisions cannot be said to be a block of half the left bundle.

7. What is usually seen histologically when an anterior or posterior divisional block is present in an ECG?

ANS.: Usually there is infarction or fibrosis in the anterior or posterior division of the left bundle.

Note: Some pathologists have been unable to find discrete anterior and posterior divisions [46A].

*8. What happens to the duration of the QRS when a divisional block develops?

ANS.: It is prolonged by an insignificant 10 msec or to as long as 120 msec. A very wide QRS may be due to terminal slowing, as in the classic periinfarction block. (See p. 236 for an explanation of the relation between divisional blocks and periinfarction blocks.)

Note: The wide QRS with a divisional block is presumably due to the slowing that occurs where the unblocked terminal fibers anastomose with the terminal fibers of the blocked opposite division. Anastomoses between the anterior and posterior divisions are probably between the anterior and posterior papillary muscles, where the divisions end. The interpapillary conduction time is about 10 to 20 msec (0.01–0.02 sec). Therefore it is not surprising that divisional blocks have been shown to prolong the QRS by at least 10 to 20 msec [11].

If the anastomotic area is damaged by fibrosis or infarction, the QRS is markedly prolonged. Consistent with this theory is the fact that when a divisional block disappears the wide QRS may narrow. (See the section on periinfarction blocks, p. 235, for another explanation for a wide QRS with a divisional block.)

Anterior Divisional Blocks

Definitions of Left Axis Deviation

1. What was originally meant by left axis deviation? How does it differ from a leftward axis?

ANS.: The original meaning of left axis deviation was an axis that would produce predominant negativity in lead 3 and predominant positivity in lead 1. This terminology was formulated in the days before there were unipolar leads and the only limb leads available were leads 1, 2, and 3. Today, with the hexaxial system, we know that negativity in lead 3 may mean an axis of about + 20° or more leftward. Unless a QRS axis is superior to 0°, we do not consider it abnormal. Therefore it is more appropriate to describe the axes from + 30° to 0° by the benign term *leftward axis.*

Note: Although a leftward axis is usually normal, in a long-chested or very young person such an axis may represent left ventricular hypertrophy (LVH) or a very minor degree of terminal conduction defect.

---

* Material marked with an asterisk is included for reference and for advanced students in cardiology.

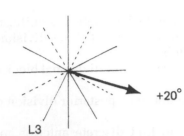

L3

This pattern was called left axis deviation when only the triaxial system was available. A + 20° vector should be called a 'leftward axis.'

2. What is meant by a marked left axis deviation?
   ANS.: More than – 30° superiorly and to the left.

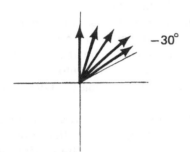

All these vectors are more than – 30° superior and therefore have a marked left axis deviation. Beyond – 90° is 'no-man's land,' i.e., between marked left and marked right axis deviation.

3. What terminology can distinguish an axis of merely less than 30° from either an abnormal left axis of between 0° and – 30° or a marked left axis of more than – 30°?
   ANS.: We should call an axis between 0° and – 30° a left axis deviation and an axis more leftward than – 30° a *marked left axis deviation*.
   Note: There are many cardiologists who consider up to – 30° as normal. We have been unable to confirm this idea in the absence of an RBBB pattern. (See p. 210 for further explanation.)

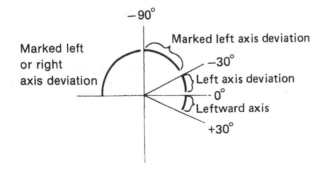

Significance of Left Axis Deviation

1. Why is it useful to distinguish between a marked left axis deviation and a mere leftward axis or left axis deviation?

    ANS.: A marked left axis deviation is almost always due to a terminal conduction defect caused by divisional block or delay. A leftward axis or left axis up to − 30°, on the other hand, may be the result of a mid-QRS conduction change as in some patients with LVH, although even here it is often also caused by a minor degree of divisional block or delay. (The evidence that the left axis deviation in some patients with LVH is not due to a divisional block is presented on p. 217.)

    Note: a. Acute and chronic anterior divisional block (ADB) has been shown by epicardial mapping (during coronary artery surgery) to cause delayed activation of the basal portion of the anterolateral left ventricle [43].

    b. About one-third of asymptomatic subjects with marked left axis deviation of unknown etiology have ischemic S-T changes on exercise testing. It is not surprising, as the most frequent cause of an ADB is atherosclerotic heart disease. However, one-third of subjects with marked left axis deviation probably have primary degeneration of the conduction system [28].

    c. Although in subjects with ADB diffuse fibrosis is found in all three divisions of the left bundle, there is usually a greater degree of fibrosis in the anterior than in the posterior division [13]. Often it is difficult to tell that there is more damage to the anterior than to the posterior division [55].

2. What is the usual direction of the *terminal* force of an ADB?

    ANS.: Usually, between − 60° and − 90°.

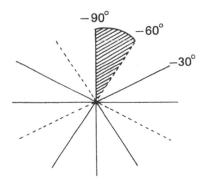

    Note: a. If it goes rightward enough to be beyond − 90°, it is not necessarily depolarizing the LV; i.e., it may be going up the infundibulum or outflow tract of the RV and so may not be an ADB (see illustration on p. 116).

    *b. In the presence of RBBB with marked terminal *slowing*, the terminal force may then go beyond − 90° with an ADB. The reason probably is that with complete RBBB the terminal force is depolarizing the *body* of the RV and not the outflow tract, so that the terminal force is the resultant of a markedly rightward as well as a superior and leftward force.

3. If the terminal force of an ADB is from − 60° to − 90°, what should always be expected in aVR?

ANS.: Terminal positivity.

> *Note:* Lack of terminal positivity in aVR may occur in ADB, although this pattern cannot be read as an ADB with any degree of certainty. However, with simultaneous leads, using a three-channel ECG machine, it is often seen that the terminal forces are isoelectric in aVR. This finding implies a − 60° terminal vector, and an ADB can be identified.

4. How can you tell if a terminal force is going up the outflow tract of the RV and therefore cannot be read as an ADB?

ANS.: There is an S in lead 1. Remember that the perpendicular to lead 1 separates 'rightness' from 'leftness' of a vector on the hexaxial system. Therefore an S in lead 1 means that the terminal force is not only superior (if there is also an S in lead 2) but it is also going from left to right.

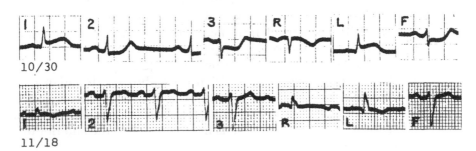

These limb leads show the frontal plane ECG of a 60-year-old man who had an acute anterolateral infarction on October 30. On November 18 an ADB with an axis of about − 70° developed. Note the absent S in L1 and the terminal positivity in aVR when the block developed.

*5. What is the maximum left axis deviation that can be caused by an ADB alone?

ANS.: About − 85°; i.e., lead 1 is always predominantly positive.

6. Why may an RBBB pattern or slight degree of RBBB produce a marked left axis deviation with an R' in aVR?

ANS.: The RBBB pattern or slight degree of RBBB implies that terminal conduction is up the outflow tract or infundibulum of the RV, which is a superior and rightward structure.

7. How can you tell that a marked left axis deviation with terminal positivity in aVR is not due to an ADB but, instead, to an RBBB pattern or to a minor degree of RBBB?

ANS.: If the left axis deviation is due to an RBBB pattern, there is an S in lead 1 and a terminal positivity or shallow S in V1. The significance of a marked left axis deviation with an RBBB pattern or minor degree of RBBB (i.e., no, or only slight, widening of the QRS) is unknown and should be considered a variation of normal.

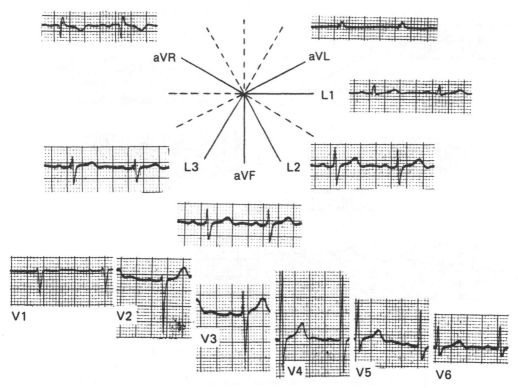

ECG 42A. This ECG is from a 17-year-old boy with a normal heart. The QRS in lead 3 is 95 msec (0.095 sec). The small S in lead 1, terminal positivity in aVR, and shallow S in V1 suggest that this picture is an atypical RBBB of a very minor degree. Therefore the left axis deviation may be a variation of normal and not an ADB; i.e., the terminal forces are superior and to the right, pointing up the outflow tract of the RV. See ECG 42B for proof that the terminal forces are due to superior and rightward forces despite the absent R' in V1; i.e., the terminal forces were not anterior enough or the V1 electrode was not placed high enough to produce positivity in V1, and this pattern is therefore not a typical incomplete RBBB. Note that the S in lead 2 is deeper than the S in lead 3.

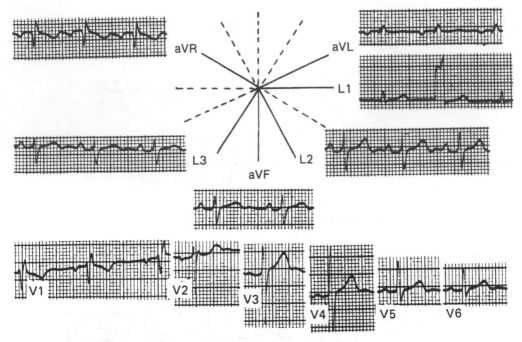

ECG 42B. This ECG is from the same boy as in the preceding tracing, taken a day later by a differ- ent technician, who had not been taught properly how to find the fourth right interspace. Instead of counting from below the sternal angle, she counted from below the clavicle. Therefore the V1 electrode was placed too high, i.e., in the third right interspace. It picked up terminal positivity in V1, giving the typical picture of an incomplete RBBB. Note the + 90° P wave on this tracing due to an ectopic pacemaker that shifted from a normal site the day before. (There is a misplaced standardization in lead 1. It should have been done before the ECG was switched to a lead.)

Note: a. A terminal force superior and to the right of necessity makes a deeper S in lead 2 than in lead 3. This point has been suggested as a means of recognizing that a left axis deviation is not due to a divisional block. However, the presence of an S in lead 1 is a faster way of recognizing an RBBB pattern or a minor degree of RBBB.

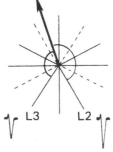

Because a terminal force that is superior and rightward is more parallel to lead 2 than to lead 3, the S is of greater amplitude in lead 2 than in lead 3.

b. Although an RBBB *pattern* with a *narrow* or only slightly widened QRS and a marked left axis deviation should not be read as an ADB, an actual complete RBBB with left axis deviation should be interpreted as an RBBB plus an ADB. The reason is that if there is an actual block in the right bundle the terminal forces are presumably due to depolarization of some part of the body of the RV and should not produce a superiorly directed force unless there is another conduction defect as well.

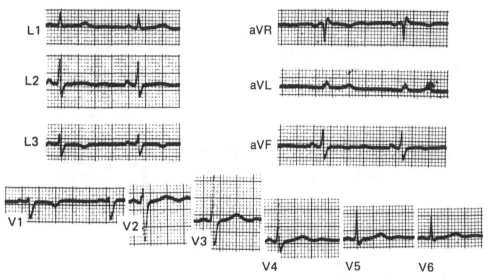

ECG 43A. Pseudo-ADB in a tall 24-year-old woman with a normal heart. The marked left axis deviation without an S in L1 suggests an ADB. However, an atypical RBBB pattern should be suspected because of the narrow QRS in L1 and the shallow notched S in V1. The terminal QRS forces are isoelectric in L1; i.e., they are pointing straight up. (On a Burger triangle they are pointing to the right, i.e., up the outflow tract of the right ventricle. See pp. 214 and 215 for an explanation of the Burger triangle.)

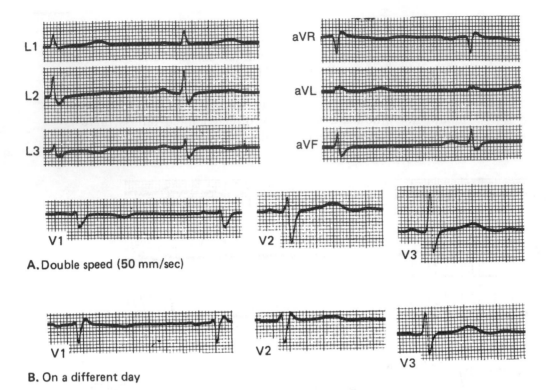

A. Double speed (50 mm/sec)

B. On a different day

ECG 43B. This ECG is from the same subject as in 43A, but the ECG was taken at double speed. Leads 1, 2, and 3 are simultaneous leads to demonstrate that the terminal forces of the QRS in L1 are isoelectric. B. Further proof that this patient has a type of RBBB pattern is seen here, where, a day later, a terminal positivity of a classic RBBB pattern is seen in V1 although her limb leads were identical to those in A. The terminal vectors were simply shifted about 5° more anteriorly for unknown reasons, or the electrical center shifted down one interspace, and superior forces became manifest in the right precordium. A frontal plane vectorcardiogram displayed a QRS loop with the major portion showing a mean axis of + 60° and a terminal small superior and rightward force.

    c. A terminal QRS force may be at exactly – 90° and still be going up the outflow tract of the RV because – 90° on the Einthoven triangle is actually more than – 90° on the true triangle (Burger triangle) made by limb leads. On this triangle the perpendicular to lead 1 really points slightly to the right because the true direction of lead 1 slopes upward toward the left shoulder.

    The true relative magnitudes and directions of leads 1, 2, and 3 have been determined by filling a model of the human torso with conducting solution and placing a simple electrical generator (dipole) in the region of the model where the heart would lie [10]. This triangle of true directions and magnitudes is called the Burger triangle.

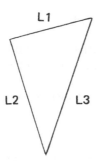

In the Burger triangle, lead 3 has greater magnitude than the other axes. Also, lead 1 is at − 10° and has the least magnitude.

8. What proof is there that there are degrees of ADB?
    ANS.: a. Various degrees of aberrant conduction in premature atrial beats have shown various degrees of ADB from a control direction of, say, + 60° to various leftward, left axis, and marked left axis deviations up to − 60° [11, 26].
    b. Occasionally, an ADB varies in degree from moment to moment in response to minor muscular movements such as a change in posture or even protrusion of the tongue [11].
    Note: If you think of a normal QRS as a fusion beat resulting from anterior and posterior divisional conduction, it helps to explain how various degrees of delay in conduction along one division could produce various degrees of anterior or posterior divisional block patterns.
9. When should you suspect that a leftward axis of, say, + 5° is a minor degree of ADB?
    ANS.: If there is an R′ or terminal positivity in aVR. It means that the leftward axis results from a marked superior and leftward turning of the terminal part of the QRS and is probably due to an 'incomplete' ADB. (An RBBB pattern must be ruled out by making sure there is no S in lead 1.)
    Note: Although the above explanation is contrary to Rosenbaum's classic teaching, he has shown all degrees of divisional block with axes from + 30° to − 90° in the same patient with different degrees of aberrant conduction [11, 26; 54].

Anterior Divisional Blocks and Left Precordial S Waves
1. Why does a left axis deviation often produce S waves in the left precordium?
    ANS.: In most patients the left precordial leads are below the electrical center of the heart; i.e., they are like modified inferior leads 2, 3, and aVF. If leads 2, 3, and aVF have deep S waves, as in left axis deviation, so do the left precordial leads V4, V5, and V6 (see ECGs 41B, 42A, and 42B).

2. What disease of the chest can cause S waves in the left precordium without a divisional block?

   ANS.: Emphysema, or chronic obstructive pulmonary disease (COPD). The S waves then are due to late rightward forces secondary to right ventricular hypertrophy (RVH).

   Note: S waves in V4, V5, and V6 may also represent either the rightward forces of an RBBB or the superior forces of an ADB.

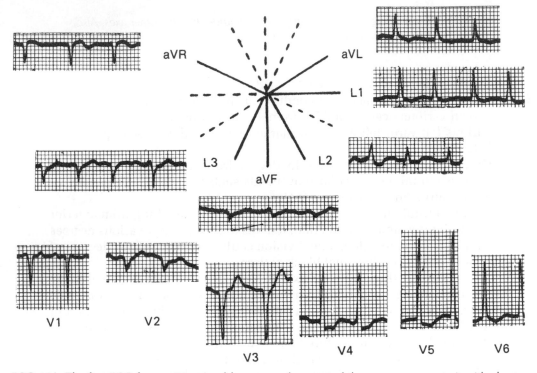

ECG 44A. *The first ECG from a 67-year-old woman who entered the coronary care unit with chest pain. There is an axis of about 0°, probably due to LVH. The sagging S-T segments and the low amplitude of the T waves in the left ventricular leads (L1, L2, V4, V5, and V6) are due to digitalis. The Q in V1 to V4 represents a recent necrosis vector. The tiny q in V4 is seen only in the first complex. The rhythm is irregular owing to atrial fibrillation.*

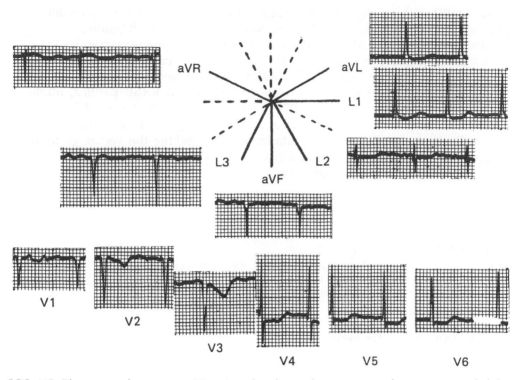

ECG 44B. The same subject as in ECG 44A, 2 days later. The axis is now about − 35° (L2 slightly predominantly negative) due to an ADB. Note the new r' in aVR due to the terminal conduction's being so superior. Note also the new S in V5 and V6 because these leads reflect events in inferior leads. Also see ECG 21 (p. 155) for an ADB associated with the initial forces of infarction and a mean QRS axis of only 5°.

*3. If an ADB and COPD can each produce deep S waves in the left precordium, what do the left precordial leads look like when both COPD and an ADB coexist? Why?

ANS.: The S waves tend to disappear. It is because in ADB the terminal superior forces tend to go slightly from right to left, producing terminal positivity in high left chest leads. Because the electrical center tends to shift lower than normal in COPD patients, V5 and V6 tend to be relatively high and to resemble leads 1 and aVL; i.e., they are at the level of the electrical center.

Left Axis Deviation with No Divisional Blocks

1. What other than a divisional block can cause a marked left axis deviation (more than − 30°)?

ANS.: a. A rightward superior force, as in some RBBB patterns in normal subjects.

b. COPD. Even in this condition it may often be an ADB that causes the marked left axis deviation.

*2. How could you account for severe hyperkalemia's causing a marked left or right axis deviation?

ANS.: Excess potassium may depress conduction along one or several divisions and produce a divisional block or a bundle branch block [3, 4, 19, 22, 53]. However, in patients on dialysis there may be normal conduction during hyperkalemia and ADB with normal potassium levels [12].

3. How may COPD with emphysema cause marked left axis deviation without actual interference with conduction along the anterior division of the left bundle?

ANS.: Because of poor electrical conduction through the emphysematous lung, all X-axis vectors tend to be minimized, and vertical vectors (i.e., Y-axis vectors) tend to be exaggerated. Therefore a minor degree of leftward turning of the axis, e.g., to about – 10° due to LVH or an RBBB pattern, might be exaggerated into – 50° or – 60° by 'verticalizing' the terminal leftward vector. Here 'verticalizing' does not imply going downward but merely implies the opposite of 'horizontalizing,' i.e., making the vector go more along the Y axis than along the X axis.

If before emphysema the vector looks like

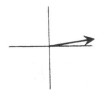

after emphysema the vector looks like

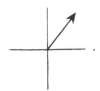

Therefore a terminal vector can be raised so superiorly that there is a marked left axis deviation without intracardiac conduction abnormalities. Similarly it can be made so inferior that there is a marked inferior axis without an intracardiac conduction abnormality.

LVH and Anterior Divisional Blocks

*1. How can a dilated LV cause an ADB?

ANS.: The anterior division may be stretched enough to cause a relative delay in comparison with the posterior division. By elongating the anterior division more than the posterior division, various degrees of ADB may be produced. About 30 percent of patients with severe aortic regurgitation have an ADB. It can also occur with severe mitral regurgitation [27].

2. Why should LVH be expected to cause an ADB?

ANS.: The LVH in patients with hypertension is often associated with fibrosis of the upper part of the septum. This fact may explain why the incidence of hypertension is five times higher in patients with marked left axis deviation than in matched controls with normal axes [18]. Endocardial thickening over the conduction system has been seen in LVH in which there were conduction problems.

Note: About 10 percent of patients with the LVH of hypertrophic subaortic stenosis have marked left axis deviation, possibly due to some effect of the abnormal septal hypertrophy on the anterior division [28].

3. How can you tell the difference between the leftward axis of a divisional block and the leftward axis of LVH without a divisional block?

ANS.: It is often impossible. However, in LVH without divisional block there is often only a 'middle-of-the-QRS' conduction defect, as shown by the absence of terminal positivity in aVR. That is, there is not a marked enough superior turning of the *terminal* vector to produce terminal positivity in aVR.

Congenital Heart Disease with Possible ADBs

*1. List the congenital cardiac abnormalities that are often associated with some degree of left axis deviation.

ANS.: a. Endocardial cushion defects, e.g.,
   (1) Ostium primum atrial septal defects (ASDs) (see ECG 45).
   (2) Ventricular septal defects (VSDs) in the endocardial cushion location [44], or when multiple [23].
   b. Corrected transposition [48].
   c. Persistent ductus arteriosus with the rubella syndrome, often with peripheral pulmonary artery stenosis [29].
   d. Anomalous origin of the left coronary artery from the pulmonary artery.
   e. Single ventricle with the infundibular chamber on the right.
   f. Tricuspid atresia, except with transposition of the great vessels.

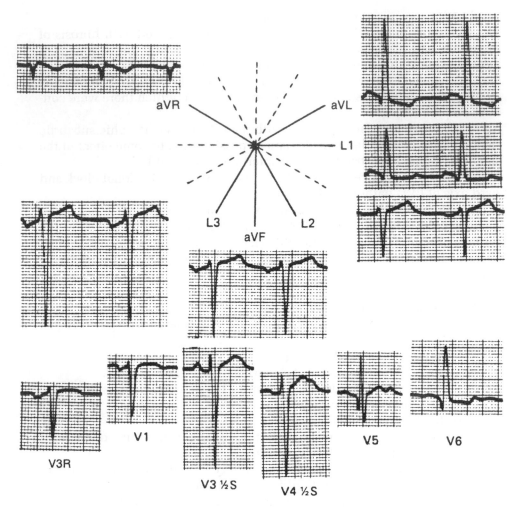

Tricuspid atresia in a 2.5-year-old cyanotic boy with a large left ventricle, a small ventricular septal defect, and a hypoplastic right ventricle. There was also infundibular and valvular pulmonary stenosis. The ECG was taken at double speed (50 mm/second). Note the marked left axis deviation due to ADB. The P waves are low atrial or junctional (negative in aVF).

Note: a. Pulmonary atresia also requires that the LV do all the work of both ventricles, yet there is no left axis deviation in pulmonary atresia. It may be because there is usually a significant right ventricular muscle mass to counteract any left ventricular forces [25].

b. A short posterior division has been found in a dog with a congenital ostium primum defect. There was no delay along the anterior division of the left bundle. Therefore the left axis deviation may not be due to an ADB but to earlier completion of conduction along a short posterior division [7].

c. The presence of RVH does not make less left axis deviation with an ostium primum defect but may even make the axis more superior, as shown by the less superior axis that results when the preoperative RVH is relieved by surgery [8].

d. Because about 5 percent of patients with ordinary secundum ASDs have left axis deviation, and the occasional patient with a primum defect has a normal axis, it is useful to strengthen the diagnosis of a primum defect by looking for the combination of a Q in V6 and a long P-R interval [9].

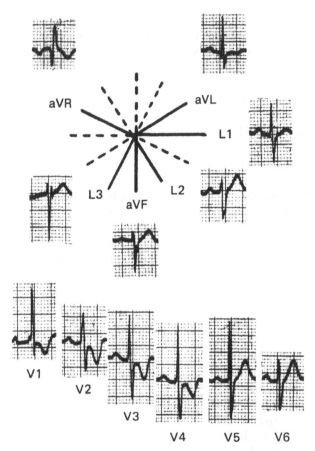

ECG 45. A 6-year-old boy had an ASD due to an ostium primum type of endocardial cushion defect. There was a 2.5:1.0 pulmonary-to-systemic flow ratio and moderate mitral regurgitation. The right ventricular pressure was 40 mm Hg (normal is 25 mm Hg). Note the marked left axis deviation (deep S in L2 and L3) and the atypical RBBB pattern (S in L1 and shallow S in V1). The P-R of 0.2 sec (200 msec) is slightly prolonged for a 6-year-old child.

*2. What suggests that the left axis deviation of tricuspid atresia is not due to the left ventricular overload predominating over the hypoplastic RV?

ANS.: In pulmonary atresia with a similarly hypoplastic RV there is not necessarily a left axis deviation.

Posterior Divisional Blocks

1. Why does a block or slowed conduction along the posterior branch of the left bundle produce a right axis deviation?

   ANS.: For the same reason that interference with conduction along the anterior branch of the left bundle produces a left axis deviation (see p. 204).

   *Note: In contrast to pathologic findings in ADB, the fibrosis underlying posterior divisional blocks (PDBs) is often less disseminated and more often limited to the posterior radiation [13]. However, in a patient with known coronary disease the presence of a PDB is usually associated with extensive coronary obstructions [47].

2. What is the chief imitator of a PDB?

   ANS.: RVH, because it also turns the mean QRS rightward by way of the terminal vector.

3. For what kind of patient is an inferior axis abnormal and should therefore be suggestive of a minor degree of PDB?

   ANS.: a. A squat, stocky, or obese patient [30].

   b. A patient 45 years of age or more.

   *Note: a. Do not diagnose PDB when you see an inferior axis in the absence of some other evidence of left ventricular disease [30, 54].

   b. Although PDBs are usually not diagnosed by most cardiologists unless a right axis deviation of at least + 120° is present, in fact a PDB axis can be anywhere from + 70° to 120° [54, 63]. If the axis is less than 120° we may call it a minor degree of PDB.

4. What axes suggest a PDB?

   ANS.: Any axis that is more inferior than expected for the patient's age and body build may represent a minor degree of PDB. This definition, of course, refers to patients without RVH [30] and with a terminal rightward force.

   Note: In one series of patients with acute infarction and PDB by vector-cardiographic criteria, almost one-third had no right axis deviation [49].

5. Which is commoner, anterior or posterior divisional block? Why?

   ANS.: Anterior. The reason is that the posterior division of the left bundle is less vulnerable to damage than the anterior division, not only because it is broader but also because it is fed by both the anterior descending and right coronary artery septal branches (though mostly by the latter). The anterior division, on the other hand, has only a single blood supply, the anterior descending coronary artery.

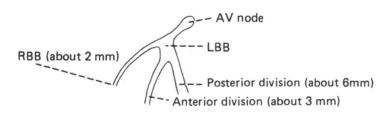

*6. When can notching of the QRS suggest a divisional block?

ANS.: Although it is normal to have a notch low on the downstroke of a left ventricular lead's R wave or high on the upstroke of a right ventricular lead's S wave, a notch nearly halfway up the R upstroke or halfway down the S downslope strongly suggests a divisional block if the axis is abnormally inferior or superior. If the axis is normal, it suggests some focal fibrosis or posterolateral myocardial infarction. It is described as an intraventricular conduction defect.

Note: a. Complete PDB is more serious than complete ADB. The reason is that the former implies occlusion of arteries to both anterior and posterior parts of the septum. Minor degrees of PDB, however, may occur with only a right coronary occlusion.

b. In the setting of acute infarction, a PDB carried a mortality of 86 percent in one study, and most of the septum was involved at necropsy [51].

*7. How often will acute inferior infarction manifest a minor degree of posterior divisional block?

ANS.: In one series all of 10 consecutive patients developed an increase in the R in lead 3 and aVF, as well as an S in aVL [3A].

---

*Initial Vector in Divisional Blocks

*1. If a proximal ADB is present, which fascicles must carry the initial depolarization forces of the septum and LV?

ANS.: They must travel initially down the posterior division of the left bundle as well as the septal fascicle. Remember that the posterior division is also an inferior division. See illustration for question 3, page 224.

2. What must the initial vector direction be if the initial forces travel down the posteroinferior division of the left bundle as well as the septal fascicle?

ANS.: The direction is inferior and from left to right. It produces initial positivity in inferior leads and tends to produce a Q or q in the lateral leads aVL and lead 1 (see ECGs 44A and 44B, pp. 216 and 217).

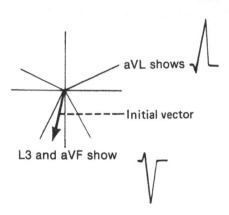

3. When is the initial vector of a divisional block not always dominated by a compulsory pathway along the opposite division?

ANS.: When the block is in a distal portion of the division.

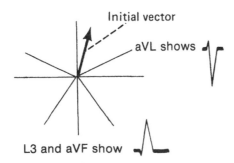

AV node   Anterior division

2.

1.   3.

SEPTUM

Posterior division   Terminal force superior

Septal fascicle   Anastomoses between divisions

Note that when the block is in the distal portion of the anterior division, the initial 'septal' forces are due to a resultant of three pathways (1, 2, and 3), so that there is no compulsory pathway only along the opposite division.

Note: a. Divisional blocks produced by selective coronary arteriography show almost no change in initial forces, suggesting that the block is in the periphery of the division [21]. Therefore a divisional block should be diagnosed by terminal vector changes alone [32].

    *b. Only in about 30 percent of elderly hospitalized patients with a normal axis is there a q wave in lead 1, aVL, or both. This exceptionally high incidence (70%) of right-to-left conduction with normal axes suggests slow conduction along a fibrosed septal fascicle in an older population. If a left axis deviation is present, however, about 60 percent have a q in lead 1, aVL, or both. This finding suggests that with a delay along the anterior division the compulsory pathway along the posterior division is not only inferior but also often from left to right as well, probably because part of the compulsory initial pathway also involves the septal fascicle [45].

4. What should the initial vector direction be if a proximal PDB is present? Why?

  ANS.: Superior (and usually to the left) [6, 65]. Remember that the anterior division runs superiorly shortly after it leaves the septum.

Initial vector

aVL shows

L3 and aVF show

Note: ADBs are not diagnosed from chest leads because the anterior division produces almost no anterior forces. It produces mostly superior ones.

5. Why is it important to know that the initial vector may have a compulsory pathway in some divisional blocks?

ANS.: a. The necrosis vector of a myocardial infarct can be masked by the initial vector of a divisional block; e.g., a Q in L3 and aVF due to inferior infarction can disappear in the presence of the initial inferior forces of an ADB.

  b. An ADB can also eliminate the Q waves of an anteroseptal infarct if the chest leads are slightly below the electrical center of the heart.

  c. An ADB has been said to be able to produce q waves in the right and mid-precordium and imitate an infarct [20]. The reason is that if the chest electrodes are high (i.e., above the electrical center) the initial inferiorly pointing forces point away from the electrodes and thus produce Q waves. This concept can be proved by placing the electrodes one interspace lower and noting the disappearance of Q waves.

  Note: a. It has yet to be established that an ADB alone can produce Q waves from V1 to V4 in the absence of infarction. In some case reports in which transient ADB brought out q waves in the right precordium, the patients had had known infarction [24], whereas in other reports where no history of infarction was recorded there was no angiographic or necropsy proof of the presence or absence of infarction [41]. Therefore an ADB may bring out infarction rather than produce a false picture (see p. 217). If an ADB is seen in patients under age 20 with no cardiomyopathy or is produced experimentally in a normal heart, no q waves are produced in leads V1 to V4. These findings suggest that patients with ADB associated with small, narrow q waves in the right or mid-precordial leads have unmasked infarction or fibrosis rather than falsely produced abnormal necrosis vectors.

  *b. A PDB may have its right axis deviation attenuated by the initial superior necrosis forces of inferior infarction. If the initial superior and leftward forces (Q in lead 3 and R in aVL) of the necrosis vector are large, they enlarge the R wave in lead 1 and thus turn the axis more leftward [65].

  *c. On the other hand, a relatively deep Q in aVF of an inferior myocardial infarction can be masked by the tall R wave in that lead produced by a PDB. The initial forces remain the same, but the middle and terminal forces that produce the R increase, so that one of the signs of inferior infarction may be missing (a relatively deep Q in aVF) [5]. It is as if the tall R waves in leads 2, 3, and aVF are pulling the QRS upward at the expense of the Q wave amplitude.

  *d. In PDB there should be initial superior forces (Q waves in leads 2, 3, and aVF). If these forces are absent, suspect high lateral infarction [54].

*6. How can you diagnose an inferior infarct initial vector abnormality in a subject with a left axis deviation due to an ADB?

ANS.: The peak of the R in aVL must occur before the peak of the terminal positivity in aVR (simultaneous leads are assumed); then look for

  a. Any Q in L2 [66]. (In uncomplicated ADB, L2 has an initial r and L1 has a Q.)

  b. A notched R in L2.

  c. The initial r in L2 is smaller than the r in L3 and aVF.

  d. The initial r in L3 and aVF is less than 3 mm high.

  Note: The presence of ADB in a patient with an inferior infarct suggests obstruction of both the right and anterior descending coronary arteries [42].

*7. What abnormal ECG changes can anterior divisional block obscure besides the Q waves of inferior myocardial infarctions?

  ANS.: a. The right axis deviation of RVH will disappear.

   b. The T negativity in inferior leads may become upright.

   c. The LVH strain pattern may be diminished or obliterated in the chest leads.

*8. How can a large posterior pericardial effusion affect the initial and terminal vectors of the QRS?

  ANS.: It can rotate the heart in such a way that all QRS forces tend to point posteroinferiorly [56]. This situation can cause initial negativity that can

   a. Uncover an old anterolateral infarction, or

   b. Mimic old anterolateral infarction. The terminal inferior force can mimic RVH or PDB.

*9. Does the initial vector of ostium primum defects with left axis deviations act like the usual ADB initial vector?

  ANS.: Yes. It is usually inferior and slightly rightward (see ECG 45, p. 221). When epicardial excitation was studied in patients with endocardial cushion defects, it was found that the posterior and inferior surface of the LV was excited earliest [17].

*10. How can we account for an anterior or posterior divisional block sometimes producing prominent initial anterior R precordial initial forces?

  ANS.: Histopathological studies of patients with marked left axis deviation have often shown a block in the septal fascicle [31A, 31B, 43A]. This could unbalance the initial forces. If some subjects have the septal forces directed mostly posteriorly and the posterior fascicle is small, then if the septal fascicle were blocked, the *anterior division* would dominate the initial forces and produce a prominent initial anterior vector.

*11. What is the significance of an axis shift (divisional block) produced by an exercise test in patients with and without coronary disease?

  ANS.: a. It has not been seen in heart with normal coronary arteries.

   b. A left axis shift predicts anterior descending disease, and a right axis shift predicts right coronary or circumflex disease [45A].

Bifascicular and Trifascicular Blocks

Bifascicular Blocks

1. What is meant by a fascicle?

  ANS.: The literal meaning of *fascicle* is 'small bundle.' In electrocardiography a fascicle is one of the four divisions coming off the bundle of His; i.e., the right bundle, anterior and posterior divisions of the left bundle, and septal branches are all fascicles.

2. What should a block in two fascicles be called?

  ANS.: A bifascicular block.

Note: When the right bundle branch is also involved, it has been called bilateral bundle branch block. This term is poor because it literally means complete AV block.

3. What should result from a simultaneous block in both the right bundle and the anterior branch of the left bundle, i.e., the right fascicle and the anterior fascicle?
   ANS.: An RBBB with left axis deviation (see ECG 47).

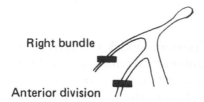

Right bundle

Anterior division

4. What should result from a simultaneous block in the right bundle and the posterior branch of the left bundle?
   ANS.: An RBBB with right axis deviation, i.e., more than + 90°.

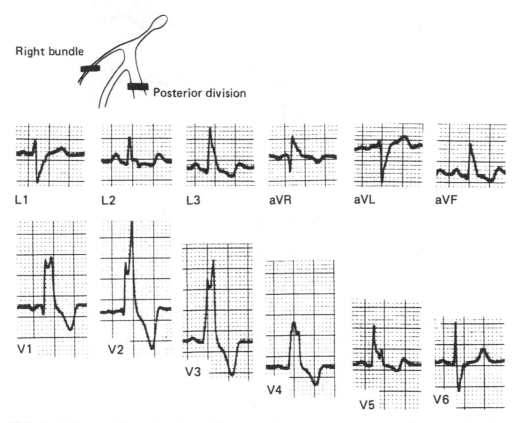

Right bundle

Posterior division

L1   L2   L3   aVR   aVL   aVF

V1   V2   V3   V4   V5   V6

ECG 46. A 55-year-old man had heart failure secondary to coronary disease. The terminal wide S in lead 1 and wide positivity in V1 make this RBBB. The marked right axis deviation of about 125° tells you that this patient has either right ventricular overload or a PDB. It is often impossible to say which of the two possibilities is the true one without much more pertinent clinical or laboratory data.

*5. What happens to the mean QRS axis when RBBB develops?

ANS.: a. In the frontal plane it depends on the preblock axis. A preblock leftward or superior axis is made more leftward or superior, but not superior and rightward unless there is an ADB. The intermediate or inferior axis is shifted more rightward, to as much as + 120°. A preblock extreme right axis deviation is not affected.

   b. In the horizontal plane in some patients with ADB and RBBB, the axis may turn so anteriorly (due to the loss of an S wave in V1) as to suggest loss of posterior forces wrongly; i.e., it may suggest posterior myocardial infarction [35].

Note: Because an RBBB alone with no divisional block can turn the mean axis far to the left or right, a posterior or anterior divisional block should be diagnosed in the presence of RBBB not by using the mean QRS but by using only the axis of the first one-third or one-half of the QRS, which is not as much affected by the RBBB. It is much more easily done with vector loops.

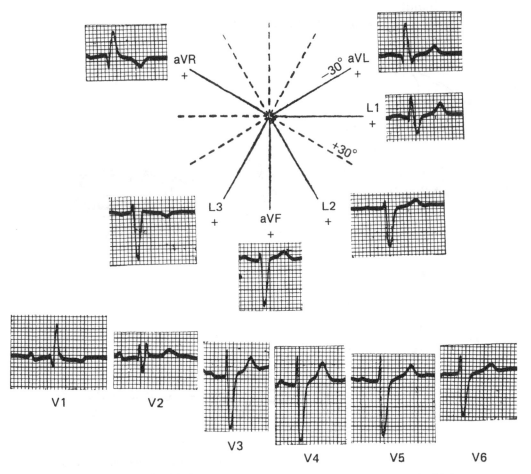

ECG 47. This ECG is from a 71-year-old man after a second infarction. The marked left axis deviation (mean axis of about − 100°) and RBBB signify a bifascicular block. If the P-R of 210 msec (0.21 sec) in V1 represents first-degree AV block, the impulse may be traveling with difficulty down the remaining fascicle (the posterior division of the left bundle). It, then, might be a partial trifascicular block. However, if the AV block is due to slow conduction through the AV node, it is only a bifascicular block.

*Masquerading Bundle Branch Block

*1. When does the combination of RBBB and ADB cause the S wave to disappear in lead 1?

ANS.: When the ADB is extreme. When there is a *marked* delay in depolarization of the anterior division, there is then probably simultaneously delayed depolarization of both the LV and RV. The terminal forces are not dominated by the usual rightward vectors of the RBBB but by the delayed superior (and anterior) vectors of the anterolateral portion of the LV.

*2. Why does the ECG look confusing if there is no terminal S in lead 1 in the presence of an RBBB in the chest leads?

ANS.: It looks like RBBB in the chest leads and LBBB in the limb leads. This picture has been called 'LBBB masquerading as RBBB' and 'RBBB masquerading as LBBB,' or simply 'masquerading bundle branch block.'

Note: These patients often have severe but noncoronary cardiomyopathy with arteriolar narrowing [64].

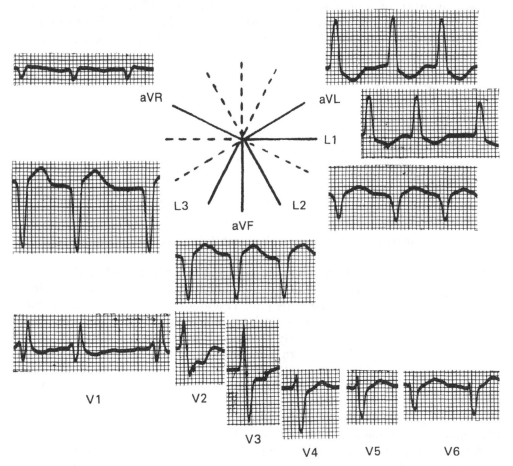

ECG 48. Masquerading bundle branch block. This ECG is from a 70-year-old diabetic woman in intractable failure but with no history of angina or infarction. There is an apparent LBBB in the limb leads (wide QRS with no S in L1) and an RBBB in the precordium. Note the marked left axis deviation (L2 negative) due to an ADB. The Q in L2, L3, and aVF probably represents inferior infarction. (It is so unusual to have a QS in L2 that one should assume the presence of infarction.)

*3. How can an RBBB horizontal plane QRS be modified by an ADB?
   ANS.: In two opposite ways:
      a. It may exaggerate the terminal positivity in the right precordium [64]. A similar RBBB anterior QRS can be produced by electrical stimulation of the low posterior division [37]. This situation suggests that in some patients with ADB and RBBB the lower posterior division is reached early.
      b. It may eliminate the terminal positivity in the right precordium, probably due to powerful left ventricular posterior forces caused by LVH. If a QRS is more than 20 msec wider than normal with an ADB, suspect RBBB and place the precordial electrodes one interspace higher as well as in the V3R position to try to pick up the terminal forces of RBBB [54].

Postdivisional LBBB and QRS Axis
1. How could you explain an LBBB with left axis deviation by fascicular block theory?
   ANS.: If conduction along the posterior branch of the left bundle is delayed an arbitrary quantity of, say, 2 +, but the anterior branch of the left bundle is blocked 4 +, the LBBB may have a left axis deviation; i.e., a form of postdivisional block and not a block of the *main* left bundle is suggested [48].

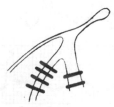

Anterior
division with 4+ block

This diagram illustrates an arbitrary grading of 1 to 4 degrees (shown as black bars) of conduction delay or block.

2. By how much can an axis turn leftward with a postdivisional type of LBBB? What is its significance?
   ANS.: Up to − 60°. In one retrospective study of patients with LBBB and marked left axis deviation, an earlier ECG without LBBB showed a left axis deviation in only about one-fifth of patients [40]. Therefore a marked left axis deviation (more than − 30°) in a patient with LBBB does not mean that the marked left axis deviation was necessarily present in the preblock tracing.
   Note: Because the axis may turn inferiorly as far as + 70° with a postdivisional LBBB, an inferior axis with LBBB does not imply a PDB prior to the development of LBBB. However, it often does imply the possibility of RVH.

Trifascicular and Quadrifascicular Blocks or Delays
1. What is a block in all three major fascicles usually called?
   ANS.: A trifascicular block. If complete, it implies complete AV block. If partial or incomplete, the term *partial* or *incomplete trifascicular block* may be used.
      Note: a. The term *bilateral bundle branch block* is often used to mean partial trifascicular block, but because a bifascicular block and a complete AV block may also be a bilateral bundle branch block, the term should be avoided.

b. The term *quadrifascicular block* is more accurate than trifascicular block. Some pathologists are unable to find two distinct fascicles or divisions of the left bundle in human subjects. Indeed, the fibers fan out not only posteriorly and anteriorly, but also into the septum. However, others have clearly demonstrated (by Lugol's staining within 1.5 hours after death) the anterior and posterior divisions as distinct bundles. Also, the septal fascicle has been clearly delineated and the refractory period of its fibers and its action potential duration have even been shown to be shorter after a premature impulse than the refractory period and action potential duration of the posterior division [55]. Considering the septal branches of the left bundle as a fourth functional fascicle provides another explanation of incomplete LBBB patterns; i.e., damage to the septal fascicles may obliterate or slow left-to-right septal activation.

c. Further proof of a trifascicular left bundle is the finding that in human hearts the initial electrical activity occurs simultaneously at three points in the left ventricular myocardium: the central left side of the ventricular septum; the posterior LV near the septum between the apex and base; and anteriorly, just below the mitral valve [16]. This does not refer to the initial breakthrough into the epicardium, which is almost always over the anterior RV [68].

2. What conduction problems occur if all fascicles but one are completely blocked and the remaining fascicle has a partial block or delay; i.e., if an incomplete trifascicular or quadrifascicular block is present?

ANS.: There is a first-degree AV block due to the incompletely blocked fascicle, as well as the conduction defect produced by the complete block of the other fascicles.

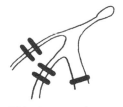

This diagram shows a 2 + block in the right bundle (RBBB) and anterior division of the left bundle (left axis deviation). The 1 + block in the remaining fascicle results in a first-degree AV block.

3. What is the clinical significance of a first-degree AV block with an RBBB and an anterior or posterior divisional block?

ANS.: It may mean that

a. All four fascicles are involved, with three markedly involved and one only moderately so; i.e., it may be due to an incomplete quadrifascicular block.

b. The first-degree A-V block may be at the AV node and not in an incompletely blocked fascicle.

Note: a. A long P-R interval occurs with chronic ADB in less than 5 percent of patients, and with ADB plus RBBB in about 10 percent. However, a long P-R interval occurs with chronic PDB plus RBBB in about 90 percent of patients. This finding suggests that PDB with

RBBB is usually part of an incomplete trifascicular or quadri-fascicular block and therefore signifies more serious disease and a greater chance of developing complete AV block than does ADB.
  b. If during acute infarction a partial trifascicular block is seen (first-degree AV block plus bifascicular block) the risk of developing syncope or sudden death during the first year of follow-up is about 50 percent when no permanent pacemaker is inserted [67].

Diagnosis of Divisional Blocks
1. Anterior divisional block
   a. A leftward QRS axis or left axis deviation due to a terminal superior force.
   b. Terminal positivity in aVR (or if not, simultaneous leads show that the terminal force is exactly at − 60°).
   c. No S in L1 (unless the S is wide because of an RBBB).
2. Posterior divisional block
   a. An inferior axis or right axis deviation due to a terminal rightward force not due to RVH, a young age, or a long chest.

Etiologies and Prognoses of Bifascicular and Trifascicular Blocks
*1. What is more common, an RBBB with anterior or with posterior divisional block? Why?
   ANS.: An RBBB with ADB is much more common, which is expected because the right bundle and anterior branch of the left bundle are fed by the same arteries and are anatomically closer together; they are in close proximity near their origin from the bundle of His. A small, high lesion can therefore cause both RBBB and an ADB [1].

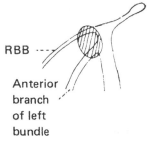

RBB

Anterior branch of left bundle

Note: a. The His bundle is partitioned longitudinally by fine collagen septa [23, 33], which suggests that the fascicles of the conduction system are already separated within the bundle of His. Therefore divisional or bifascicular blocks may occur when there is damage only to the bundle of His.
   b. In one study the development of a bifascicular block involving the right bundle and either anterior or posterior divisions of the left bundle during acute infarction was invariably associated with an anterior myocardial infarction. The death rate was 10 times higher in those in whom this type of bifascicular block developed. This type of bifascicular block occurs in about 5 percent of patients with acute infarction [62].
   c. On rare occasions, a right coronary occlusion can also produce an RBBB with ADB. The reason is that the right coronary artery in

some subjects may feed the proximal part of the right bundle just as it bifurcates from the bundle of His, where the right bundle is still in close proximity to the anterior division of the left bundle. (See the illustration for question 6.)

*2. How many fascicles are likely to be damaged by occlusion of
   a. An anterior descending coronary artery?
   b. A posterior descending coronary artery?
   c. The circumflex artery?

   ANS.: a. Because most of the right bundle and the anterior division of the left bundle are supplied by the anterior descending artery, we would expect these two fascicles to be affected primarily. However, a massive anterior infarct could produce at least a partial PDB as well.

   b. Because the posterior descending artery supplies most of the posterior division of the left bundle and often the initial segment of the right bundle, a PDB together with RBBB may occur [24]. Because the anterior descending artery also feeds the posterior division, however, only a moderate degree of PDB should result from a posterior descending artery occlusion alone.

   Note: An RBBB plus PDB is much rarer and means much more severe disease than RBBB together with ADB. The reason is that the right bundle branch is mostly supplied by the anterior descending artery and the posterior division is supplied primarily by the right coronary or circumflex artery, so that at least two-vessel disease is likely.

   c. Injection of the left circumflex artery during coronary angiography routinely produces an ADB.

*3. Which coronary artery occlusion is most likely to produce a first-degree AV block due to

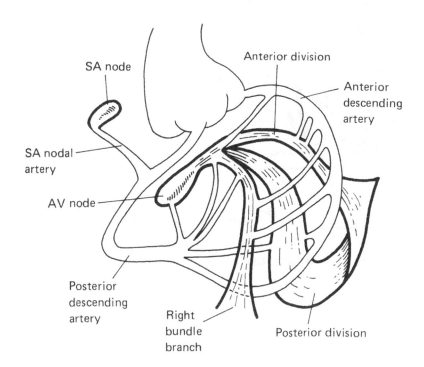

a. AV node damage?

b. Incomplete quadrifascicular block?

ANS.: a. A right coronary occlusion is most likely to damage the AV node because this artery supplies the AV node in 90 percent of subjects.

   b. An anterior descending occlusion is most likely to cause quadrifascicular damage because it supplies all four fascicles, at least to some extent.

   Note: Partial bifascicular, trifascicular, and quadrifascicular blocks are often transient and intermittent. On one day, there may be an RBBB with left axis deviation, and the next day there may be an LBBB with first-degree AV block or any permutation and combinations of blocks in the three fascicles.

4. What are the chances that a complete AV block will develop if the diagnosis of RBBB with bifascicular block is made?

ANS.: Outside the context of acute infarction, complete AV block develops in only about 10 to 15 percent of patients with an RBBB and either a posterior or anterior divisional block [14]. Even if the patient is under anesthesia, a pacemaker need not be inserted for a chronic bifascicular block [38]. However, if a partial trifascicular block is present, succinylcholine may prolong conduction along the incompletely blocked fascicle and produce complete AV block [57].

   If seen during an acute infarct, however, complete AV block develops in about 30 to 60 percent of patients, irrespective of whether the RBBB is associated with anterior or posterior divisional block [52, 58].

   Note: Mortality in patients with RBBB and bifascicular block with acute infarction depends more on the heart failure classification than on the presence of the block [50].

   *Note: The aortic and tricuspid valves are close to the beginning of the right bundle where it touches the anterior division of the left bundle.

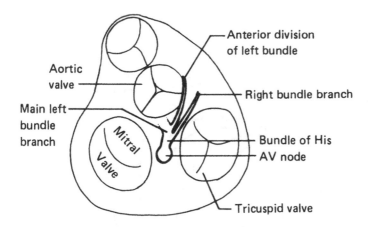

From the diagram it can be seen that calcification of the aortic valve or replacement of the tricuspid valve by a prosthetic valve could cause an RBBB, an ADB, or even complete AV block [2].

*5. What should you think of as a cause of RBBB with left axis deviation in a subject under age 20?

ANS.: a. A congenital heart problem, especially a low ASD, as part of the abnormality known as endocardial cushion defect. In this defect the AV node and bundle of His are displaced posteriorly [36]. Occasionally, the cause is a familial conduction abnormality, and no ASD is present.

b. Muscular dystrophy [5].

6. What may account for a divisional or bundle branch block without coronary or myocardial disease?

ANS.: Mitral annular calcification near the bundle of His and left bundle. Conduction disturbances are more prevalent in such patients than in matched controls [63A].

Lev's Disease and Lenegre's Disease

1. What processes are thought to be more common than coronary disease as the cause of damage to the proximal part of the bundle branches?

ANS.: Two processes are postulated:

a. Degenerative processes of the upper part of the ventricular septum, resulting in sclerosis of the left side of the cardiac skeleton. Lev [39] included in this process the central fibrous body, the summit of the ventricular septum, the mitral annulus, and the aortic valve, the latter two only when infiltrated with calcium. This sclerosis has been called Lev's disease.

b. Idiopathic sclerosis, specifically of the bundle of His, its divisions, or both. This combination has been called Lenegre's disease. (A neurotropic virus has been postulated as the cause.)

2. What suggests that Lenegre's disease is not due to an aging process?

ANS.: RBBB, LBBB, and divisional blocks have been seen to develop in the age group 21 to 45, with no apparent disease and with normal coronary angiograms [15, 61].

3. About what proportion of patients coming to autopsy who had chronic complete AV block showed either Lev's or Lenegre's disease as a cause for the block? What is its significance in the etiology of complete AV block?

ANS.: About one-half. Because many of the remainder had myocardial or valve calcification problems, coronary disease causes only a few of the cases of chronic complete AV block.

PERIINFARCTION BLOCKS

1. What is meant by periinfarction block?

ANS.: It is the ECG picture of a wide QRS with an initial necrosis vector followed by a wide, terminal force that travels in the opposite direction.

Note: The terminal slowing is much better seen on a vector loop than on an ECG.

2. What has been postulated to cause a terminal QRS vector to point toward an infarct without a divisional block?

ANS.: One theory is that some of the fibers in or around the necrosed muscle conduct current more slowly than do the normal fibers. Therefore depolarization of this area is delayed, resulting in a slow vector at the end of the QRS. That is, the normal ventricle is depolarized first and the area in or around the infarct last. Those who believe that the slowing is *inside* the infarcted area would like to call it intrainfarction block. Those who believe the slowing is around the infarct call it periinfarction block [22].

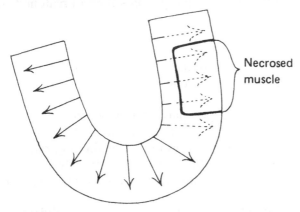

The broken arrows are slowed terminal vectors either <u>in</u> or <u>around</u> the necrosis area. Conduction through normal tissue finishes first.

*3. How can a divisional block be brought into a theory to explain periinfarction block?

ANS.: Let us assume that the infarct is transmural and therefore involves the subendocardium. Because depolarization is from endocardium to epicardium, if endocardial conduction is blocked, conduction to the overlying subepicardium must be by way of the alternative pathways, i.e., the division opposite to the one that would normally supply that subepicardium. The result, then, is a divisional block type of terminal conduction. Then, if slow activation of the subepicardium occurs because of a damaged division, the ECG picture of periinfarction block results.

Note: a. Terminal slowing is seen with some divisional blocks in both humans and, when the posterior division is cut, dogs [68]. The terminal slowing in healthy dogs is, however, at the most, extremely slight [46].

b. The terminal vectors of periinfarction blocks generally show well only in the frontal plane just as in divisional blocks (see ECG 49).

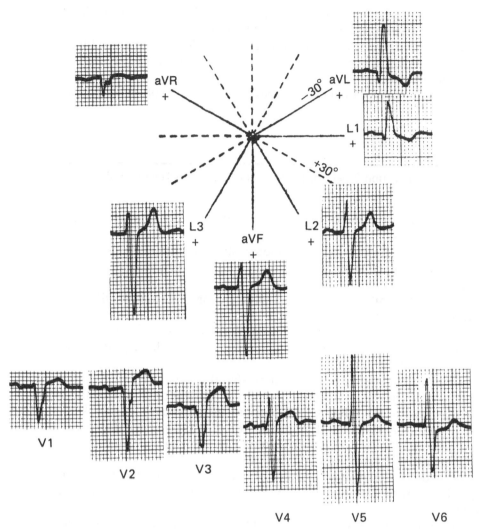

ECG 49. The wide QRS of 130 msec (0.13 sec) with the Q in aVL, L1, and V2 to V5 is due to either LBBB with infarction or an anterolateral infarct with periinfarction block (ADB with terminal slowing). The Q in V2 to V5 represents the anterior necrosis vector. The periinfarction block (initial and terminal vectors in opposite directions) shows only in the frontal plane. (A vector loop can help rule out LBBB by showing absence of mid-slowing.)

Periinfarction blocks may really represent divisional blocks with terminal slowing, and the only major difference from a divisional block is the marked widening of the QRS plus a necrosis vector. Also, as in divisional block, the usual direction of the terminal vector in a classic anterolateral periinfarction block is superior and to the left (and slightly anterior), as in ADB. The usual direction of the terminal vector in a classic inferior periinfarction block is inferior and slightly posterior, i.e., as in a PDB.

c. The necrosis vector of the classic periinfarction block has been seen to disappear when the divisional block type of terminal conduction defect disappears, again telling us that a classic periinfarction block is a type of divisional block.

4. What, then, is the most widely accepted total picture of classic periinfarction block?
   ANS.: a. A necrosis vector is present; i.e., there is a wide initial vector pointing away from the site of the infarct.
   b. The terminal vectors widen the QRS beyond 80 msec (0.08 sec) and point toward the infarct—and therefore in a direction opposite to the necrosis vector.

Imitators of Classic Periinfarction Block, or Divisional Blocks with Terminal Slowing plus a Necrosis Vector

*1. Does the classic ECG picture of periinfarction block always correlate with a myocardial infarction at autopsy?
   ANS.: No. Diffuse fibrosis of both the conduction system and the myocardium has been found on more than one occasion with the classic ECG pattern of periinfarction block.

2. When can LVH imitate the initial and terminal wide vector angle abnormality seen in classic periinfarction block?
   ANS.: LVH may cause a slightly widened Q. Therefore any divisional block with LVH looks like a classic periinfarction block, as the wide 'septal Q' may resemble a necrosis Q.

*3. What drug can cause an imitation of a classic periinfarction block? How?
   ANS.: Quinidine. Toxic doses can slow ventricular conduction and diffusely widen every part of the QRS, so that normal initial vectors can look like necrosis vectors, and the normal terminal vectors may look like the slowed, oppositely directed vectors of a periinfarction block. The maximum widening with therapeutic doses is by 20 msec [31].

*4. When does LBBB become the greatest imitator of classic periinfarction block; i.e., when does it produce a wide necrosis vector with initial and terminal vectors going in opposite directions?
   ANS.: When LBBB is associated with an infarct. It can produce Q waves of 40 msec (0.04 sec) or more in aVL and even in leads 1, V5, and V6. It looks exactly like a lateral infarct with classic periinfarction block (see ECG 49, p. 237). The difference is often apparent if one sees terminal positivity in the right precordium because LBBB never produces terminal positivity in the right precordium, whereas commonly the terminal vectors of a classic periinfarction block point anteriorly.

*5. How can periinfarction block imitate RBBB?
   ANS.: When an ADB occurs, the terminal forces are not only superior but may also be slightly anterior or slightly posterior, or have no tilt at all. If terminal slowing occurs, anterior forces can give the appearance of RBBB. If the terminal forces are slightly posterior or not tilted at all, the usual V1 shows no terminal positivity. If, however, the V1 electrode is placed one or two interspaces higher than usual, the terminal wide positivity may become apparent and look like a RBBB. This pattern has been described as an actual RBBB obscured by the ADB [59].

REFERENCES

1. Alboni, P., et al. Right precordial q waves due to anterior fascicular block. *J. Electrocardiol.* 12:41, 1979.
2. Aravindakshan, V., Elizari, M. D., and Rosenbaum, M. B. Right bundle branch block and left anterior fascicular block following tricuspid valve replacement. *Circulation* 42:895, 1970.
2A. Aron, L., et al. Prolonged P-R interval associated with an abnormal frontal QRS axis. *Int. J. Cardiol.* 19:327, 1988.
3. Bahl, O. P., Walsh, T. J., and Massie, E. Left axis deviation. *Br. Heart J.* 31:451, 1969.
3A. Barnhill, J. E., et al. Localization of ischemia by analysis of terminal QRS changes. *Circulation* 72:111–162, 1985.
4. Bashour T., et al. Atrioventricular and intraventricular conduction in hyperkalemia. *Am. J. Cardiol.* 35:199, 1975.
5. Befeler, B., et al. Changes in the pattern of old inferior wall myocardial infarction produced by acute left bundle branch block and hemiblock. *Chest* 63:18, 1973.
6. Bobba, P., Salerno, J. A., and Casari, A. Transient left posterior hemiblock: Report of four cases induced by exercise test. *Circulation* 46:931, 1972.
7. Boineau, J. P., Moore, E. N., and Patterson, D. F. Relationship between the ECG, ventricular activation, and the ventricular conduction system in ostium primum ASD. *Circulation* 48:556, 1973.
8. Borkon, A. M., et al. The superior QRS axis in ostium primum ASD: A proposed mechanism. *Am. Heart J.* 90:215, 1975.
9. Burchell, H. B., DuShane, J. W., and Brandenburg, R. O. The electrocardiogram of patients with atrioventricular cushion defects (defects of the atrioventricular canal). *Am. J. Cardiol.* 6:575, 1960.
10. Burger, H. C., and VanMilaan, J. B. Heart-vector and leads, part II. *Br. Heart J.* 9:154, 1947.
11. Das, G. Left axis deviation: A spectrum of intraventricular conduction block. *Circulation* 53:917, 1976.
12. Deliyannis, A. A., and Symvoulidis, A. D. ECG QRS axis shift with left anterior hemiblock. *J.A.M.A.* 217:341, 1971.
13. Demoulin, J.-C., and Kulbertus, H. E. Histopathologic correlates of left posterior fascicular block. *Am. J. Cardiol.* 44:1083, 1979.
14. Dhingra, R. C., et al. Chronic right bundle branch block and posterior hemiblock. *Am. J. Cardiol.* 36:867, 1975.
15. Dianzumba, S. B., Singer, D. H., and Smith, J. M. Lenegre's disease in youth. *Am. Heart J.* 94:479, 1977.
16. Durrer, D., Roos, J. P., and VanDam, R. T. The genesis of the electrocardiogram of patients with ostium primum defect. *Am. Heart J.* 71:642, 1966.
17. Durrer, D., VanDam, R. T., and Freud, G. E. Total excitation of the isolated human heart. *Circulation* 41:899, 1970.
18. Eliot, R. S., Millhon, W. A., and Millhon, J. The clinical significance of uncomplicated marked left axis deviation in men without known disease. *Am. J. Cardiol.* 12:767, 1963.
19. Ewy, G. A., Karliner, J., and Bedynek, J., Jr. Electrocardiographic QRS axis shift as a manifestation of hyperkalemia. *J.A.M.A.* 215:429, 1971.
20. Farnham, D. J., and Shah, P. M. Left anterior hemiblock simulating anteroseptal myocardial infarction. *Am. Heart J.* 92:363, 1976.
21. Fernandez, F., Scebat, L., and Lenegre, J. ECG study of hemiblock in man during arteriography. *Am. J. Cardiol.* 26:1, 1970.
22. First, S. R., Bayley, R. H., and Bedford, D. R. Peri-infarction block; electrocardiographic abnormality occasionally resembling bundle branch block and local ventricular block of other types. *Circulation* 2:31, 1950.
23. Fox, K. M., et al. Multiple and single ventricular septal defect. *Br. Heart J.* 40:141, 1978.
24. Gambetta, M., and Childers, R. W. Rate-dependent right precordial Q waves: 'Septal focal block.' *Am. J. Cardiol.* 32:196, 1973.
25. Gamboa, R., Gersony, W. M., and Nadas, A. S. The electrocardiogram in tricuspid atresia and pulmonary atresia with intact ventricular septum. *Circulation* 34:24, 1966.

26. Gooch, A. S., and Crow, R. S. Labile variations of intraventricular conduction unrelated to rate changes. *Circulation* 38:480, 1968.

27. Grant, R. P. Architectonics of the heart. *Am. Heart J.* 46:405, 1953.

28. Grayzel, J., and Neyshaboori, M. Left-axis deviation: Etiologic factors in one-hundred patients. *Am. Heart J.* 89:419, 1975.

29. Halloran, K. H., Sanyal, S. D., and Gardner, T. H. Superiorly oriented electrocardiographic axis in infants with the rubella syndrome. *Am. Heart J.* 72:600, 1966.

30. Halpern, M. S., et al. Intermittent left posterior hemiblock. *Chest* 60:499, 1971.

31. Heissenbuttel, R. H., and Bigger, J. T., Jr. The effect of oral quinidine on intraventricular conduction in man: Correlation of plasma quinidine with changes in QRS duration. *Am. Heart J.* 80:453, 1970.

31A. Heraga, T., et al. Histopathological study of marked left axis deviation. *Jpn. Heart J.* 23:181, 1982

31B. Hoffman, I., et al. Anterior conduction delay: A possible cause for prominent anterior QRS forces. *J. Electrocardiol.* 9:15, 1976.

32. Jacobson, L. B., LaFollette, L., and Cohn, K. An appraisal of initial QRS forces in left anterior fascicular block. *Am. Heart J.* 94:407, 1977.

33. James, T. N., and Sherf, L. Fine structure of the His bundle. *Circulation* 44:9, 1971.

34. Kossmann, C. E., et al. The electrocardiogram in ventricular hypertrophy and bundle-branch block. *Circulation* 26:1337, 1962.

35. Kulbertus, H. E., Collignon, P., and Humblet, L. Vectorcardiographic study of QRS loop in patients with left superior axis deviation and right bundle-branch block. *Br. Heart J.* 32:386, 1970.

36. Kulbertus, H. E., Coyne, J. J., and Hallidie-Smith, K. A. Electrocardiographic correlation of anatomical and haemodynamic data in ostium primum atrial septal defects. *Br. Heart J.* 30:464, 1968.

37. Kulbertus, H. E., deLeval-Rutten, F., and Casters, P. Vectorcardiographic study of aberrant conduction: anterior displacement of QRS: Another form of intraventricular block. *Br. Heart J.* 38:549, 1976.

38. Kunstadt, D., et al. Bifascicular block: A clinical and electrophysiologic study. *Am. Heart J.* 86:173, 1973.

39. Lev, M. Anatomic basis for atrioventricular block. *Am. J. Med.* 37:742, 1964.

40. Lichstein, E., et al. Significance of complete left bundle branch block with left axis deviation. *Am. J. Cardiol.* 44:239, 1979.

40A. Massing, G. K., and James, T. N. Anatomical configuration of the His bundle and proximal bundle branches in the human heart. *Circulation* (Suppl) XLIII & XLIV:218, 1971.

41. McHenry, P. L., et al. Right precordial qrS pattern due to left anterior hemiblock. *Am. Heart J.* 81:498, 1971.

42. McKeever, L., et al. The meaning of VCG left anterior hemiblock and inferior myocardial infarction. *Circulation* 55/56:181, 1977 (Abstract).

43. Meeran, M., et al. Comparison of epicardial activation in patients with normal conduction and left anterior fascicular block. *Circulation* 55/56:111, 1977 (Abstract).

43A. Nakaya, Y., et al. Prominent anterior QRS force in left septal vascicular block. *J. Electrocardiol.* 11:39, 1978.

44. Neufeld, H. N., et al. Isolated ventricular septal defect of the persistent common atrioventricular canal type. *Circulation* 23:685, 1951.

45. Nevins, M. A., Das, D., and Saranathan, K. Normal initial vectors on the ECG. *Am. Heart J.* 97:130, 1970.

45A. Ogino, K., et al. The usefulness of exercise-induced QRS axis shifts. *Clin. Cardiol.* 11:101, 1988.

46. Okuma, K. ECG and VCG changes in experimental hemiblock and bifascicular block. *Am. Heart J.* 92:473, 1976.

47. Papa, L. A., et al. Coronary angiographic assessment of left posterior hemiblock. *J. Electrocardiol.* 16:297, 1983.

48. Pryor, R., and Blount, G. S. The clinical significance of true left axis deviation. *Am. Heart J.* 72:391, 1966.

49. Ribeiro, C., Bordalo, A., and Longo, A. Left-posterior 'hemiblock' associated with acute myocardial infarction: Incidence and clinical significance. Abstracts, VIII World Congress of Cardiology, 1978, p. 146.

50. Riley, C. P., et al. Partial bilateral bundle branch block in acute myocardial infarction. *Chest* 63:342, 1973.
51. Rizzon, P. Left posterior hemiblock in acute myocardial infarction. *Br. Heart J.* 37:711, 1975.
52. Roos, J. C., and Dunning, A. J. Right bundle-branch block and left axis deviation in acute myocardial infarction. *Br. Heart J.* 32:847, 1970.
53. Rosenbaum, M. B., Elizari, M. W., and Lazzari, J. O. *The Hemiblocks.* Oldsmar, Fla: Tampa Tracings, 1970.
54. Rosenbaum, M. B., et al. Left anterior hemiblock obscuring the diagnosis of right bundle branch block. *Circulation* 48:298, 1973.
55. Rossi, L. Histopathology of conducting system in left anterior hemiblock. *Br. Heart J.* 38: 1304.
56. Salem, B. E., et al. Electrocardiographic pseudo-infarction pattern: appearance with a large posterior pericardial effusion after cardiac surgery. *Am. J. Cardiol.* 42:681, 1978.
57. Santini, M., et al. Effects of anaesthetic agents in patients with A-V conduction disturbances. Abstracts, IX World Congress of Cardiology, 1982, p. 447.
58. Scanlon, P. J., Pryor, R., and Blount, S. G., Jr. Right bundle branch block associated with left superior or inferior intraventricular block. *Circulation* 42:1135, 1970.
59. Sclarovsky, S., et al. Left anterior hemiblock obscuring the diagnosis of right bundle branch block in acute myocardial infarction. *Circulation* 60:26, 1979.
60. Shadaksharappa, K. S., et al. Recognition and significance of intraventricular block due to myocardial infarction (peri-infarction block). *Circulation* 37:20, 1968.
61. Smith, R. F., et al. Acquired bundle branch block in a healthy population. *Am. Heart J.* 80:746, 1970.
62. Stephens, M. R., et al. The clinical features and significance of bifascicular block complicating acute myocardial infarction. *Eur. J. Cardiol.* 3/4:289, 1975.
63. Strickland, A. W., Horan, L. G., and Flowers, N. C. Gross anatomy associated with patterns called left posterior hemiblock. *Circulation* 46:276, 1972.
63A. Takamoto, T., and Popp, R. L. *Am. J. Cardiol.* 51:1664, 1983.
64. Unger, P. N., et al. The concept of 'masquerading' bundle-branch block. An electrocardiographic-pathologic correlation. *Circulation* 17:307, 1958.
65. Varriale, P., and Kennedy, R. J. Right bundle branch block and left posterior fascicular block. Vectorcardiographic and clinical features. *Am. J. Cardiol.* 29:459, 1972.
66. Warner, R., et al. ECG criteria for the diagnosis of inferior infarction and left anterior hemiblock. *Am. J. Cardiol.* 51:718, 1983.
67. Waugh, R. A., Wagner, G. S., and Morris, J. J., Jr. Immediate and remote prognostic significance of fascicular block during acute myocardial infarction. *Circulation* 47:765, 1973.
68. Wyndham, C. R., et al. Epicardial activation of the intact human heart. *Circulation* 59:161, 1979.

20. S-T Vector of Myocardial Infarction and Injury

NORMAL REPOLARIZATION PROCESS

1. What is the S-T segment? That is, where does it begin and end?

   ANS.: It begins at the end of the QRS and ends at the beginning of any change of slope of the T wave.

   Note: If there is no definite change of slope, as in perfectly normal ECGs, there is really no S-T segment. It merely becomes equivalent to the 'first part' of the T wave.

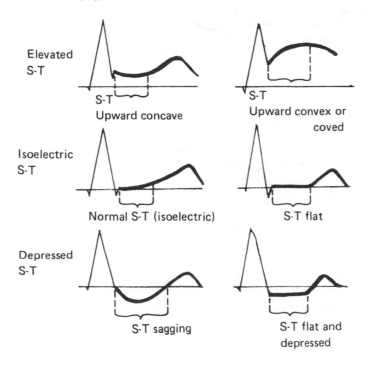

Elevated S-T — Upward concave — Upward convex or coved

Isoelectric S-T — Normal S-T (isoelectric) — S-T flat

Depressed S-T — S-T sagging — S-T flat and depressed

2. What is the end of the QRS called at the point where it joins the S-T segment?

   ANS.: The J point.

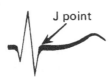

J point

   Note: It is often called the J junction, but because *J* stands for 'junction,' a J junction equals a 'junction junction.'

3. What did those who originally tried to standardize ECG nomenclature call the S-T segment?

ANS.: The RS-T segment (because the end of the QRS may be either an R or an S).

> *Note:* We do not find it necessary to call the P-R interval the P-QR interval simply because the QRS may start with either a Q or an R. Therefore it is inconsistent to call the S-T segment the RS-T segment.

4. To what do we usually refer to determine whether an S-T is elevated or depressed; i.e., where is the baseline?

ANS.: To the T-P segment, which, when isoelectric, is the baseline portion of the ECG; e.g., an S-T below the level of the T-P segment is depressed. When tachycardia or U waves eliminate the T-P segment, the P-R segment becomes the reference or assumed baseline.

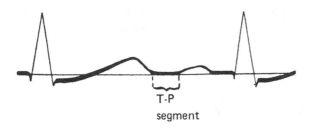

T-P
segment

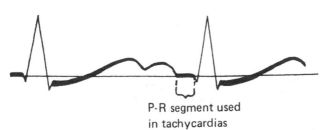

P-R segment used
in tachycardias

In the presence of a tachycardia, the T-P segment may be absent. The P-R segment then must be used as the baseline.

5. What part of the repolarization process does the S-T segment represent?

ANS.: It represents the middle part of the repolarization process of the ventricle; it does not represent the beginning, which is inside the QRS.

GENESIS AND DIRECTION OF THE INJURY CURRENT

*1. What is meant by the 'dielectric property' of a membrane?

ANS.: The ability of the membrane to keep ions or electrons more on one side of the membrane than on the other.

> *Note:* Injuries such as those caused by ischemia can destroy the dielectric properties of a cell membrane, so that potassium may flow out during both depolarization and repolarization. Sodium may continue to flow in during repolarization. (The preceding ionic flow abnormalities are only unproved possibilities.)

* Material marked with an asterisk is included for reference and for advanced students in cardiology.

2. If the dielectric property of a cell is destroyed, how may ionic flow be changed so that it can affect the baseline of the ECG?

   ANS.: Because it is ionic flow that produces the electrical phenomena that make an ECG, an abnormal movement of ions produces an electrical current. This current depresses the baseline of the lead with its positive electrode over the injured muscle and is known as the 'injury current.'

   Note: During the earliest phase of repolarization, when there is no important movement of ions, the loss of dielectric properties should not produce much effect on ionic flow. Because this early phase represents the S-T segment, it is not much affected by an injury current. If an injury current is suddenly produced experimentally, the baseline suddenly drops in any lead with its positive electrode on the epicardium. Only the S-T segment appears to remain at a level of the original baseline. In addition to a baseline shift, there is experimental evidence for a true S-T segment shift [83].

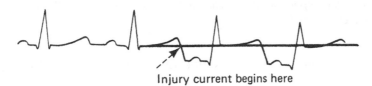

Injury current begins here

Note that the R wave also becomes taller in leads that show an epicardial injury current.

3. If a transmural infarction occurs, where is the injured area in relation to the necrotic area?

   ANS.: Around the necrotic area.

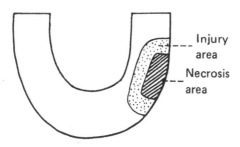

Injury
area

Necrosis
area

4. If the S-T is the only part of the entire ECG that is not affected by an injury current, how does the S-T segment appear?

   ANS.: It appears to be either depressed if the rest of the baseline is elevated or elevated if the rest of the baseline is depressed; i.e., the S-T is always opposite in direction to the baseline shift. The illusion is that the S-T has become elevated or depressed.

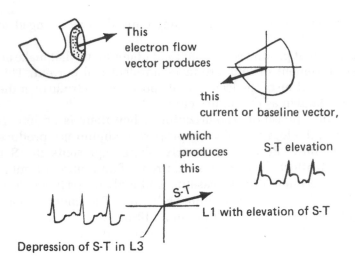

This electron flow vector produces

this current or baseline vector,

which produces this

S-T elevation

L1 with elevation of S-T

Depression of S-T in L3

In order to understand the upper part of the diagram, you must remember that current flow is opposite in direction to electron flow.

5. What are some of the adjectives used to describe the characteristic S-T injury contours or morphology?

ANS.: Convex, concave, arched, bowed, or cove plane; i.e., the elevated S-Ts are convex upward and the depressed S-Ts are concave upward. This elevated S-T, when associated with an inverted T, has also been called a 'Pardee wave.'

*6. What physiologic state complicating infarction can exaggerate an injury current?

ANS.: Hypotension [26], presumably due to decreased coronary perfusion during diastole.

HOW THE INJURY VECTOR LOCATES INFARCTS

Frontal Plane Sites of Infarction

1. How does the S-T injury vector relate to the site of the injury?

ANS.: *It tends to point toward* the site of transmural injury. (The reason is that the baseline vector points away from the site of transmural injury.)

2. If a transmural infarct produces an injury current from the *lateral* area of the left ventricle (LV), which leads have elevated S-Ts and which have depressed S-Ts?

ANS.: Leads with positive electrodes facing the lateral surface of the LV have elevated S-Ts, i.e., aVL and lead 1; aVF and lead 3, in contrast, have depressed S-Ts (see ECG 63A, p. 301).

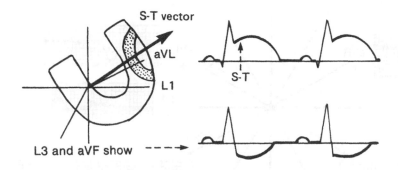

3. If a transmural infarct is on the *inferior* area of the LV, which leads have an elevated S-T and which a depressed S-T?

   ANS.: Lead 3 and aVF have elevated S-Ts and lead 1 and aVL have depressed S-Ts (see ECG 50).

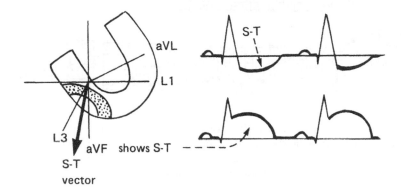

4. Of the three frontal plane sites of an infarct (i.e., lateral, apical, and inferior), where are the vast majority of transmural infarcts found?

   ANS.: They are either lateral or inferior.

   Note: Because most infarctions are either inferior or high lateral, the S-T tends to point inferiorly or superiorly; i.e., pure apical injury currents are rare.

5. Because most infarctions are either lateral or inferior, and S-Ts are elevated or depressed in leads on opposite sides of the heart and of the hexaxial system, what has this opposite S-T effect been called?

   ANS.: 'Reciprocal changes'; i.e., if the S-T is elevated in the superior leads (leads 1 and aVL), they are depressed in the inferior leads (aVF and lead 3), or vice versa (see ECG 50; see also ECG 63A, p. 301).

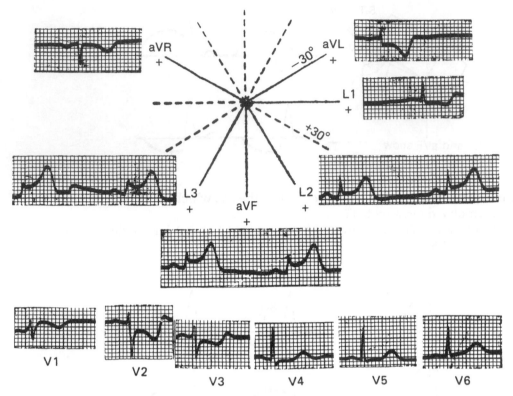

ECG 50. Acute posteroinferior infarction. The S-T elevation in L2, L3, and aVF tells us that there is an acute inferior injury current. Note the reciprocal S-T depressions in the high lateral leads aVL and L1. The S-T depressions in V2 to V4 show that the S-T vector points away from those positive electrodes; i.e., it points posteriorly. Therefore a posteroinferior injury current is present.

> *Note:* An apical infarct would have its injury current pointing toward the apex of the heart; i.e., it would point equally toward leads 1 and aVF, so that there would be no reciprocal changes. Almost all infarcts that show an injury current in the frontal plane, however, manifest reciprocal changes, which implies that either
> a. Apical infarcts are rare, or
> b. Apical infarcts have an eccentric injury vector that points either laterally or inferiorly. Because apical infarcts are common, b is the more likely explanation.

*6. Is the S-T in lead 2 elevated or depressed in the presence of a lateral myocardial infarction?

> ANS.: With low lateral infarction, the S-T in lead 2 may be elevated. This direction of injury is very uncommon.
> *Note:* Lead 2 tends to show inferior rather than lateral vectors and reflects whatever is seen in L3 and aVF rather than in L1 and aVL.

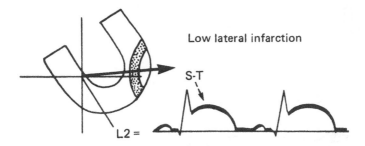

Low lateral infarction

If the infarction is high lateral, the S-T in lead 2 is depressed, as are the S-Ts in leads 3 and aVF. A high lateral infarction site is more common than a low lateral infarction site, so that with most infarctions lead 2 tends to look like the inferior leads 3 and aVF.

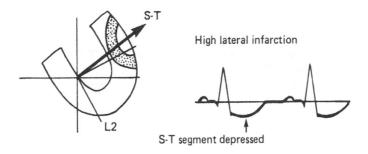

High lateral infarction

7. Is the S-T in lead 2 elevated or depressed with inferior myocardial infarction?
   ANS.: It is usually elevated; i.e., the S-T vector points toward lead 2 because lead 2 is situated slightly inferiorly. It is at + 60° and tends to follow the configuration of leads 3 and aVF.

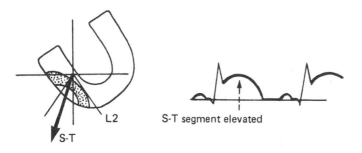

Horizontal Plane Sites

1. In which leads does an anterior myocardial infarction show an injury current?
   ANS.: In any or all precordial leads. All precordial leads except V6 are anterior to the electrical center of the heart.

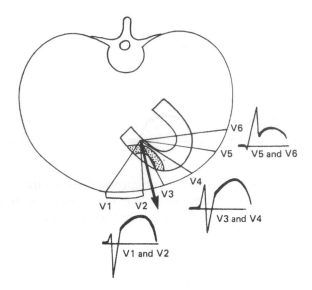

2. In which leads does a posterior myocardial infarction show an injury current? How do these leads show this S-T abnormality?

ANS.: In the right and mid-precordial leads, shown by the S-Ts being depressed.

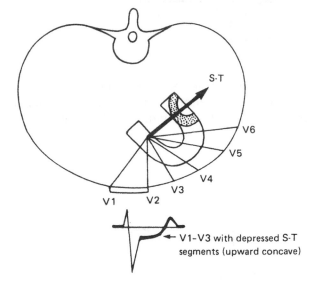

Note: a. S-T depressions of at least 1 mm in the precordial leads in a patient with an inferior infarction implies a larger infarct and severe left ventricular dysfunction and more likely postinfarction angina [66]. It does not usually represent anterior subendocardial ischemia [20] but is usually associated with a posterolateral infarction [38].

b. Occasional posterior injury currents as well as wide Q waves may be seen only in extra leads taken in the posterior axillary line V7, mid-scapular line V8, or between the mid-scapular line and the spine V9 [60].

*3. When can an S-T vector suggest a right ventricular infarction?

ANS.: When a patient with an acute inferior infarction has an elevated S-T segment in V4R, probably more than 25 percent of the right ventricle (RV) is damaged. There is a high likelihood of hypotension, atrioventricular (AV) block, and heart failure, and the prognosis for short-term survival is poor [29].

Note: Because in right bundle branch block (RBBB) the terminal forces are due to right ventricular depolarization, infarction of the RV should decrease the wide S in lead 1 and the terminal wide positivity in V1. (This hypothesis has yet to be confirmed.)

Note: If, with symptoms of acute infarct, the S-T segment elevation in aVR is equal to or greater than the elevation in V1, it is 80% specific for left main obstruction [97A].

4. Can the S-T vector of infarction overcome the S-T changes secondary to RBBB?

ANS.: Yes. The S-T secondary to RBBB goes in a direction opposite to the terminal wide force of the QRS. The S-T injury current could either summate with this secondary S-T change or nullify it (see ECG 51).

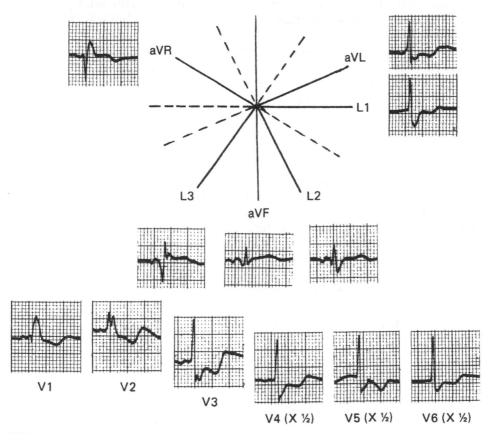

ECG 51. An 86-year-old man had an acute inferior infarction. (The negative P waves in leads 2 and 3 imply either a low atrial or a junctional pacemaker.) The wide S in L1 and large-area terminal positivity in V1 are diagnostic of RBBB. The S-T secondary to the RBBB should be elevated in L1, aVL, and V3 to V6. Instead, the S-T is depressed in these leads. The S-T shows the usual reciprocal S-T changes of an acute inferior infarct (S-T elevated in aVF and depressed in aVL). It also shows in the precordium the S-T depressions of a posterior infarction. Therefore this ECG shows an acute posteroinferior infarction in the presence of RBBB. The wide Q in leads 3 and aVF represents the inferior necrosis vector.

Significance of the Injury Current

*1. What S-T changes suggest that the septum has ruptured?

ANS.: A further rise in S-T elevation, together with an increase in P wave size suggesting right atrial overload (due to a right-sided overload) [47].

    Note: a. In one study an S-T elevation that continued to rise in subsequent ECGs (with the T still upright as in the hyperacute stage) was highly predictive of ventricular rupture, especially with protracted pain and elevated blood pressure as well as AV block [62].

    b. During the course of infarction, an increase in S-T elevation (or depression) with the T in the opposite direction may be due to pericarditis, angina without reinfarction, the sequelae of a tachyarrhythmia, or an infarct extension.

*2. What is the significance of a marked S-T elevation in acute myocardial infarction?

ANS.: The more marked the S-T elevation, the more frequent is ventricular tachycardia, cardiac arrest, and cardiogenic shock, especially with anterior infarction and with the first infarction. However, patients with multiple infarctions can have serious arrhythmias, cardiac arrest, or shock with a minor S-T elevation [67].

    Note: If the J point of the S-T segment was elevated to more than 50% of the R wave, the prognosis for hospital mortality was almost double that for those with J points lower than that [5A]. If the J point was as high or higher than the R wave it was called 'tombstoning', and was associated with obstruction in the left anterior descending together with circumflex or right coronary artery or both [43A].

3. When is an injury current permanent?

ANS.: Only if a very large scar (akinetic area) or aneurysm (dyskinetic area) develops. The reason is unknown.

    Note: The word *aneurysm* once meant only a dyskinetic area, i.e., an area that bulged outward while the rest of the ventricle was contracting. Today the word is used to include a large akinetic area; i.e., a persistent injury type of S-T vector can be produced at the edge of a very large infarct. Akinetic areas may be even more likely to have S-T elevation than are those with paradoxical outward movement.

4. What kind of S-T vector shape and direction is seen in the presence of a ventricular aneurysm?

ANS.: The same as in acute myocardial infarction (see ECG 52).

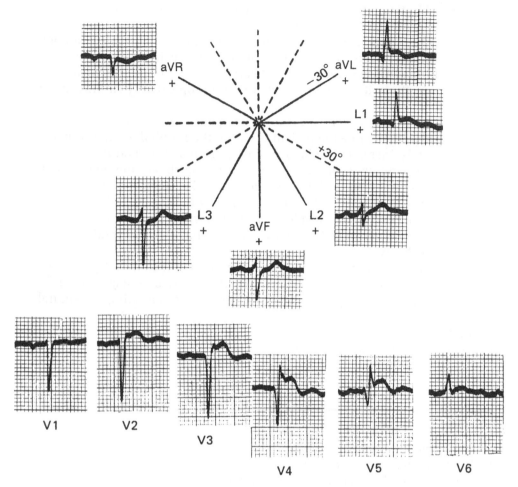

ECG 52. A ventricular aneurysm was observed by fluoroscopy in this 67-year-old man who had had a myocardial infarction 1.5 years before. The slightly wide Q in L1 and aVL together with the Q in V3 and V4 tells us that the necrosis is anterolateral. The upward convex S-T elevation in L1 and aVL and from V2 to V6 is a persistent injury current that tells us that the patient has an anterolateral aneurysm. A Q wave seen only in mid-precordial leads cannot be a septal Q (a septal Q is seen only in left precordial leads) or an incomplete LBBB Q (seen only in right precordial leads). Therefore these Q waves must be due to infarction.

5. In the absence of a clinical history, how can you tell if an S-T vector is due to an aneurysm or to an acute myocardial infarction?

   ANS.: It is impossible to tell except by serial ECGs. If the S-T abnormality remains for a longer time than expected, an aneurysm is probable.

   *Note: Two cases have been reported where an injury current had persisted for 3 weeks before death but neither showed an aneurysm at autopsy. In both cases the infarcts were due to occlusion of a dominant right coronary artery [49].

6. What is the maximum time the S-Ts of an acute infarct are expected to remain elevated before returning to baseline or to control levels?

   ANS.: If they remain elevated for more than a week, an aneurysm is probably present, and the S-T will probably never return to the baseline [61].

Note: a. About two-thirds of patients with ventricular aneurysms have persistent S-T elevation [61].

    *b. After aneurysmectomy or encircling endocardial ventriculotomy [28] S-T segments tend to remain elevated in all patients, with little relation to reduction in heart size or clinical improvement. In one study it was less elevated than preoperatively in only about one-fourth of postaneurysmectomy patients [39].

    *c. If a transient S-T *elevation* accompanies angina occurring after infarction while the patient is still in the hospital, there is a statistically increased incidence of early reinfarction and death when compared with the incidence in early postinfarction angina with either transient S-T *depression* or no S-T change at all (88).

    *d. The commonest QRS change seen with the chronic S-T vectors of aneurysms is a marked left axis deviation of the anterior divisional block or periinfarction block type, so that aVR has good terminal positivity.

    *e. An rsR′ or rSr′ with a normal or prolonged QRS in left precordial leads L1 or aVL is also suggestive of a ventricular aneurysm [27].

7. What noncardiac conditions may produce an injury current imitating transmural infarction?

ANS.: a. Acute pancreatitis.

    b. Subarachnoid hemorrhage [41].

THE BRUGADA SYNDROME

1. What is meant by the Brugada syndrome?

ANS.: RBBB of any degree with S-T elevation in V1 to V3 associated with sudden death despite no demonstrable structural heart disease.

    Note: a. Amiodarone and/or beta blockers are not protective. Only an implantable pacemaker can help [7A].

    b. Only the 'pattern' of RBBB need be present, i.e., S L1 and R′ or shallow S V1 need be present.

    c. The S-T segment may be either coved (upward convex) or saddlebacked, and is elevated 0.1 mv or more [2A].

    d. It is familial. The Brugada-type ECG is much more prevalent than the manifest syndrome [90A].

2. For what cardiac abnormalities is the Brugada syndrome most likely mistaken? Why?

ANS.: Arrhythmogenic right ventricular cardiomyopathy or dysplasia. They both have the RBBB-S-T elevation pattern and propensity to sudden death [90A].

    Note: a. The syndrome is also mimicked by Chagas disease, mediastinal tumor, and RV infarction.

    b. Procainamide can reproduce the abnormal ECG if it is transiently normalized as well as in family members with normal ECGs [2A].

    c. Beta blockade and alpha stimulation can normalize the abnormal ECG [60A].

d. The S-T segment elevation can change from a coved-type into a saddleback shape. When both shapes were combined in a study, the incidence was about 0.7%.

PERICARDITIS VERSUS INFARCTION

1. Why does pericarditis affect the S-T vector at all?
   ANS.: Probably because myocardium underneath the pericardium is injured in some way.
*2. How can you distinguish localized pericarditis with some subepicarditis beneath it from a transmural infarction S-T vector?
   ANS.: You cannot tell the difference. Fortunately, it is a rare occurrence because most pericarditis patients have generalized pericarditis.
   Note: Localized inferior pericarditis is occasionally seen with pancreatitis (see p. 169, question 9). Therefore on the ECG it may imitate an inferior myocardial infarction.
3. If, as in most cases, the pericarditis is generalized, what S-T vector direction can be expected?
   ANS.: If all the pericardium is affected, all the subepicardium is affected. This situation produces an injury current from all of the subepicardium. The sum of all the injury current vectors is merely one that points toward the main muscle mass, i.e., in the same direction as the mean QRS (in the absence of a conduction defect).

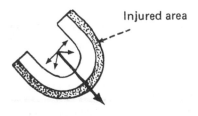
Injured area

   Note: Because the S-T points toward the mean mass of the LV in generalized pericarditis, the S-T vector tends to point toward the mean QRS vector, so that the mean S-T is almost the same as the mean QRS vector; i.e., it is parallel to the mean QRS vector. Therefore for a normal QRS axis the S-T tends to be elevated in all limb leads except aVR, and there are usually no reciprocal changes as with acute infarction. If, however, the QRS has a left axis deviation and lead 3 is predominantly negative, there may be S-T depression in lead 3 and elevation in aVL; i.e., there may be reciprocal types of change [42].
4. How does the S-T, T of pericarditis differ from that of an infarct? How can the Q-T interval help differentiate the two?
   ANS.: a. Early in the course of the evolution of pericarditis, the S-T is upward concave, despite being elevated. In infarction it is usually upward convex when elevated.
   b. The T often does not become inverted in pericarditis until the S-T has returned to the baseline. With infarction the T usually becomes inverted while the S-T is still elevated.

c. The Q-T (beginning of Q to end of T) is normal or even short in pericarditis [92]. In infarction it is prolonged (see serial ECGs 53A and 53B).

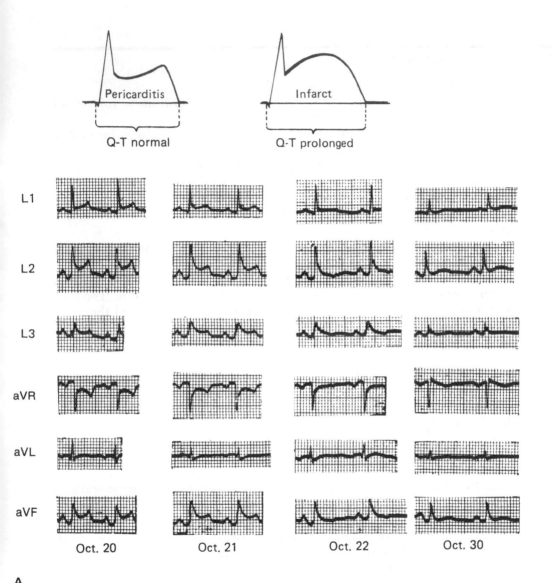

A

ECG 53. Limb (A) and chest (B) leads of a patient with evolving viral pericarditis. The S-T elevations of the first day are similar to those of the normal variant known as early repolarization except that they are too high. (Early repolarization rarely causes a 3-mm S-T elevation in V4 to V6.) The beginning of T negativity as the S-Ts become lower tells you that early repolarization is not the cause of the S-T elevation. Note that the S-Ts point in the same direction as the QRS; i.e., they are elevated in L1, L2, and L3 and in the mid-precordium and left precordium. A notched T commonly occurs in the late evolution, as seen on October 30 (the tenth day) in V4, V5, and V6. Note also that the P-R segment is depressed in L2, L3, and aVF and elevated in aVR. This picture is characteristic of pericarditis.

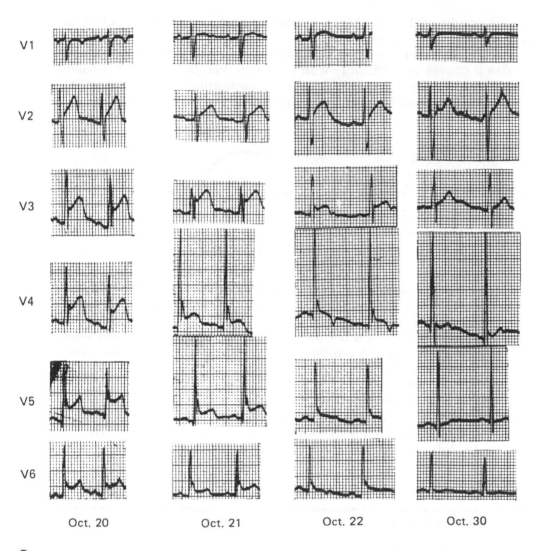

| V1 | V2 | V3 | V4 | V5 | V6 |

Oct. 20   Oct. 21   Oct. 22   Oct. 30

B

*5. Why is the pericarditis S-T more likely to be upward concave, and the infarct S-T is more likely to be upward convex?

ANS.: If the T tends to become inverted, it pulls down on the end of the S-T and makes it convex upward. Only with infarction does the T tend to become inverted while the S-T is still elevated. In pericarditis the T tends not to become inverted until the S-T has returned nearly to the baseline.

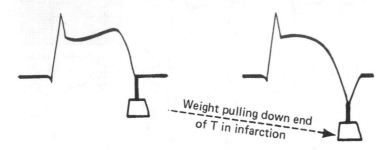

Note: a. There is often a stage in pericarditis at which the S-T has returned to the baseline and the T has not yet become inverted, resulting in a transiently normal S-T, T.

b. An injury current not due to infarction or pericarditis has been described in many patients with septic shock during dopamine infusion [93].

6. How does the P-R segment help to diagnose pericarditis?

ANS.: The P-R segment is elevated in aVR and is depressed in L2 and 3.

Note: The P-R shifts are probably due to subepicardial myocarditis, which may explain their absence in pure uremic pericarditis in which the pericardial inflammation does not penetrate the myocardium [87A].

EARLY REPOLARIZATION VERSUS PERICARDITIS

1. Is there a normal S-T vector?

ANS.: Yes.

2. In what direction is the normal S-T vector compared with the QRS?

ANS.: In nearly the same direction as the QRS but slightly more anterior in the horizontal plane, so that the lead with the transitional QRS may have an elevated S-T.

Note: The normal S-T also has the same direction as the normal T wave; i.e., wherever the T is upright, the S-T is elevated.

3. What is the magnitude of the normal S-T vector; i.e., is it large or small?

ANS.: It is usually small (1–2 mm), but it may be large. In V2 or V3, where the electrodes are closest to the heart, it may be as high as 5 mm, but it is rarely more than 3 mm [44].

4. What is meant by 'early repolarization'?

   ANS.: A normal S-T elevation due to an S-T vector that points toward the T. In pattern language it means that all leads with an upright T have elevated S-T segments, and all with negative Ts have depressed S-T segments. The S-T has an upward concavity and often begins with a notch. It is especially large in the mid-precordium (V2 to V5) and is commonly associated with a slightly anterior QRS (transition zone at V2 or V3) [44, 95] (see ECG 54).

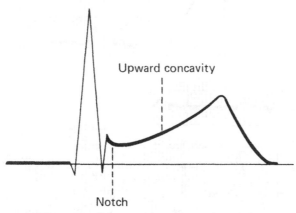

Upward concavity

Notch

A notch where the S-T joins the QRS is common with early repolarization but is rarely seen with the S-T segment elevation of pericarditis. The notch is not part of the QRS and should not be included in its width.

5. What age group and race tend to have early repolarization?

   ANS.: Although marked S-T elevations occur predominantly in the young black man, white subjects of all ages, even those over age 60, may show at least some early repolarization [44, 95].

   Note: a. Early repolarization may persist for decades [44].

   b. Although early repolarization is usually seen in healthy young hearts, it can also occur in subjects with significant coronary disease [2].

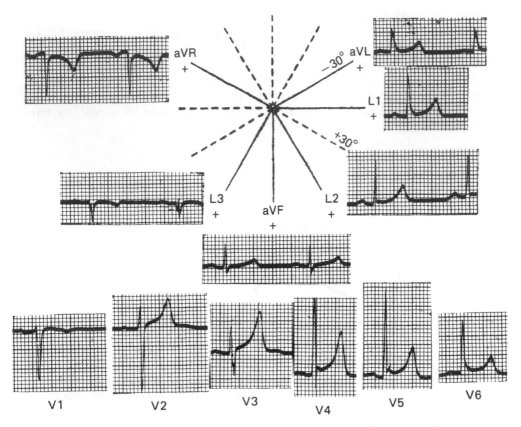

ECG 54. Early repolarization in a 52-year-old black man with a normal heart and blood pressure hospitalized for a leg injury. The S-T elevations in V2 to V6 with the tall T waves are a normal variation, usually seen in younger subjects. (There is no known upper normal value for the height of a T wave over mid-precordial leads.)

6. How does the early repolarization S-T elevation differ from that due to pericarditis?
   ANS.: a. In early repolarization the S-T is always associated with a tall T wave. In pericarditis the T becomes lower as the hours pass. Therefore only in the earliest hours of pericarditis, when the T has not yet been affected, may they look alike [95]. In early repolarization, however, the T is relatively tall in comparison with the S-T elevation. If the S-T elevation is more than 25 percent of the total T height (from baseline to peak), pericarditis is the more likely diagnosis [37].
   b. The S-T segments are almost always elevated in both limb and chest leads in early pericarditis. In early repolarization the S-T elevation may be seen in the chest leads alone [87]. (Early repolarization is rarely, if ever, seen in limb leads alone [44].)
   *c. The S-T in pericarditis tends to be slightly posterior, so that in V6 it is positive, and in V1 it is negative. In early repolarization the S-T is more likely to be to the right of both the QRS and T in the frontal plane. In the precordial leads, it is more anterior than in pericarditis; i.e., it may be positive in V1 and isoelectric in V6 [87].

d. The P-R segment shifts in both limb and chest leads with pericarditis. (With early repolarization, P-R segments shifts are rare, especially in the precordial leads [87].)

Note: About 80 percent of patients with acute pericarditis have a P-R segment shift of 180° away from the main P vector, probably due to subepicardial atrial injury. It is often best seen as an elevation in aVR [11, 87] (see ECG 26, p. 160).

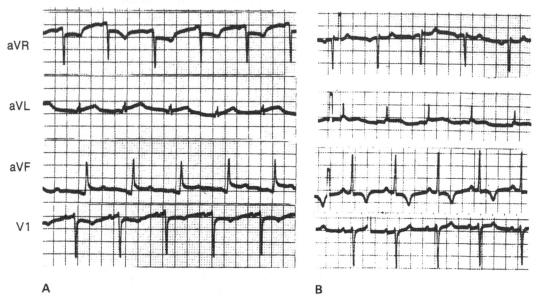

A   **B**

ECG 55A. This ECG is from a 35-year-old black man with pleuritic chest pain. A. Note the elevated S-T in aVL without reciprocal changes in aVF; i.e., the S-T is also elevated in aVF and so is not the S-T direction of infarction. The S-T is upward concave in aVF, also more a characteristic of pericarditis than of infarction. Note also the depressed P-R segment in aVF and the elevated P-R segment in aVR. (Also see ECG 53 for P-R segment changes in pericarditis.) B. ECG of the same patient taken 2 weeks later. Note that the T is now negative in aVF, but the S-T has not only returned to baseline but also is even slightly below it.

*7. How may exercise differentiate the early repolarization S-T from that due to pericarditis?

ANS.: Exercise often brings the early repolarization S-T back to the baseline, but it does not affect the S-T due to pericarditis. However, this test is unreliable because exercise can sometimes exaggerate rather than normalize early repolarization [95].

8. Why may the normal S-T elevation be greater in the right than in the left precordium? What is the maximum normal S-T elevation in the right precordium?

ANS.: Because the right precordial electrodes are closer to the heart (proximity effect). The maximum normal S-T elevation in V1 to V3 is about 3 mm.

*9. What can hyperventilation do to the S-T, T of early repolarization? What is the significance of this effect?

ANS.: The T often becomes inverted. Together with the S-T elevations, the negative T waves then look like those of an acute infarction [95]. Exercise may also invert the T in these subjects.

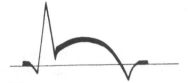

Note: Athletes, especially black athletes, are most likely to show the preceding combination of early repolarization and T negativity that mimics infarction. The T abnormalities seen in athletes are due to autonomic differences (decreased sympathetic tone) from the general population. Any autonomic imbalance can cause the same S-T, T changes as in athletes (see ECG 56).

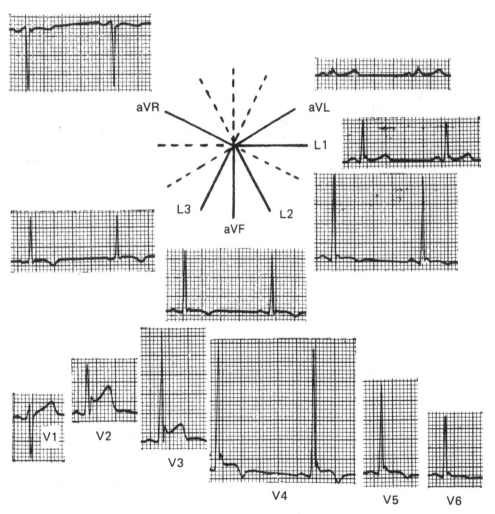

ECG 56. This asymptomatic 41-year-old black man had a blood pressure of 160/60 mm Hg with normal myocardial function and coronary arteries on angiography. The elevated S-T (early repolarization) and negative T waves in anterior and inferior leads are normal variations that together mimic acute infarction. The same ECG findings had been observed in this subject a year before. Note that the transition zone is between V1 and V2 (anterior QRS), a common finding when these S-T, T variants are seen together. (He was not an athlete.)

10. What conditions can cause S-T elevations that may mimic infarction, pancreatitis, pericarditis, or early repolarization?

ANS.: a. Cerebral hemorrhage has occasionally caused S-T elevations of a marked degree, suggestive of pericarditis, i.e., without reciprocal depressions [74]. However, reciprocal depressions may also occur and exactly imitate acute infarction [21]. However, the presence of a long Q-T interval caused by the cerebral abnormality makes the diagnosis of pericarditis unlikely [3].

      b. An S-T elevation also occurs in some severely hyperkalemic uremic patients on dialysis. This picture is unlike pericarditis and is more like an infarction injury current because there are reciprocal changes [10, 12].

      c. Carcinoma of the lung with neoplastic infiltration of the myocardium can produce an infarction-like injury current with characteristic reciprocal changes [45].

Note: Acute infarction with abnormal Q waves and injury vectors reverting completely to normal with no infarction at autopsy may occur in elderly women receiving blood transfusions for anemias secondary to gastrointestinal bleeding or cancer. Disseminated intravascular coagulation causing fibrin thrombi followed by lysis was assumed to be the cause in one report [48].

LEFT VENTRICULAR HYPERTROPHY STRAIN PATTERN VERSUS AN INJURY CURRENT

1. What is the general direction of a left ventricular hypertrophy (LVH) strain pattern S-T, T vector relative to the QRS direction?

ANS.: The LVH strain pattern S-T vector points away from the mean QRS. (For ease of remembering, it happens to be the converse of the direction of the early repolarization or the pericarditis S-T vector, which points *toward* the QRS. (See p. 374 for details of LVH strain pattern.)

*2. When may the reciprocal changes in LVH strain patterns mimic an injury current?

ANS.: When the QRS is very rightward or very leftward.

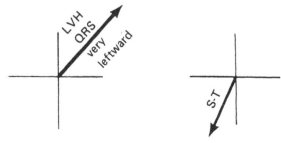

If there is a left axis deviation and the S-T due to LVH is about 180° away from a superiorly directed QRS, the 'inferior' leads 2, 3, and aVF show elevated S-T segments, and the 'superior' leads 1 and aVL show reciprocally depressed S-T segments.

Note: An infarct is more likely if the S-T is nearly perpendicular rather than 180° to the QRS.

DIGITALIS S-T VECTOR VERSUS THE LVH STRAIN PATTERN

1. What is the direction of the digitalis S-T vector?
   ANS.: Opposite to that of the QRS (as is the strain pattern S-T vector).
2. How can you tell a digitalis S-T vector from an LVH strain pattern S-T vector if they both go in the same direction?
   ANS.: a. The contour of the digitalis S-T vector shows *sagging* in the left ventricular leads. These S-T changes have also been called 'saucering,' 'scooping,' and 'cupping.' Put another way, the S-T of the LVH strain pattern is upward convex, whereas it is upward concave with the digitalis effect.
       b. Digitalis shortens the Q-T interval and lowers the amplitude of the T wave (see ECG 57).
           Note: a. That the T amplitude is made low by digitalis is shown by the fact that if you find an upright T wave in a lead with a large, predominantly positive QRS, you have practically excluded the possibility of a toxic digitalis level [43].
              b. About 15 percent of normal pregnant women show S-T segments that sag as much as 1 mm below the baseline, and, as with digitalis, the T amplitude is often low. The cause is unknown but is probably at least partly autonomic [69].
              c. Hypokalemia may modify the LVH strain pattern so that it looks like the digitalis effect. It does this by causing the upward convex S-T to sag slightly. Hypokalemia is not unusual in patients with LVH who are on diuretics for hypertension.
3. Why is it difficult to distinguish hypokalemia from digitalis effect on the S-T segment?
   ANS.: Both can produce sagging S-T segments, low T waves, and relatively high U waves.
           Note: a. A meal of 100 g of glucose can exaggerate the S-T sagging of digitalis after about 1 to 2 hours [71]. It may be due to the movement of potassium with the glucose into cells.
              b. A beta blocker can normalize the S-T, T changes of digitalis effect [31A].

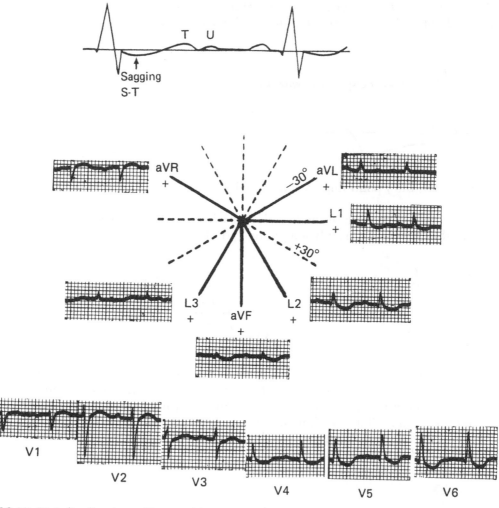

ECG 57. Digitalis effect in an 89-year-old woman with metastatic malignant melanoma, ascites, and questionable heart failure. The S-T segments sag in all left ventricular leads. The T is so small in amplitude that the S-T, T is one rounded segment in which the components cannot be separated from one another. It is therefore difficult to see that the T is actually negative in V4, V5, and V6. (The Q-T is probably short by inspection alone, as shown by the fact that the end of the T is less than halfway between R waves despite a tachycardia; see p. 320 for explanation.)

4. What happens to the J point with digitalis?

   ANS.: Ordinarily, it is unaffected by digitalis when conditions are fairly basal. However, digitalis can cause a J point depression in the presence of tachycardia, coronary insufficiency, or LVH.

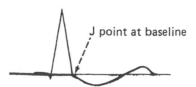

5. What happens to the J point with the LVH strain patterns?
   ANS.: It is displaced in the same direction as the S-T and T.

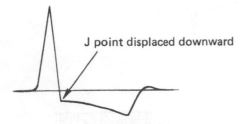

J point displaced downward

6. How can you tell the J point depression of digitalis from the J point depression of LVH?
   ANS.: Try to extend the line of the S-T slope backward. If it crosses the baseline near the QRS, it is probably a digitalis J point.

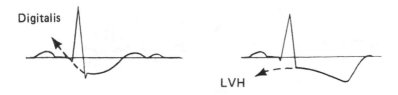

Digitalis

LVH

Note: The resistance to J point depression by digitalis causes the proximal end to be held up like one end of a hammock while the rest of the S-T becomes negative. It is as if a heavy ball had rolled down the R wave, landing on the S-T and making it sag. The S-T in the strain pattern has been said to look as though a heavy weight were hung by a rope from the T wave, pulling it downward.

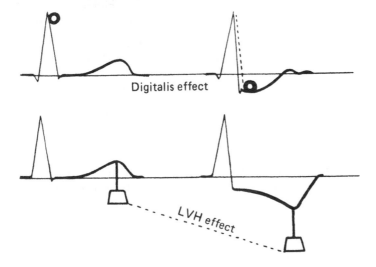

Digitalis effect

LVH effect

7. When does the digitalis effect mimic the injury current of a transmural infarct?
   ANS.: When it produces a marked elevation of the S-T in the right precordium [64]. The upward convexity on the right precordium is the reciprocal of the S-T

sagging in the left precordium. This exaggerated S-T elevation occurs in the presence of LVH because both digitalis and LVH produce S-T vectors that point away from the mean QRS. Because the right precordial leads show negativity of the QRS (often with great amplitude if LVH is present), the S-T is expected to be elevated [64]. This sequence follows the rule that a large-area QRS causes the S-T, T to go in the opposite direction.

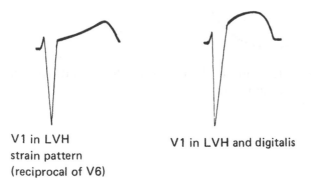

V1 in LVH
strain pattern
(reciprocal of V6)

V1 in LVH and digitalis

SUBENDOCARDIAL CURRENT OF INJURY

1. If the S-T of a transmural infarct points *toward* the site of an infarct, in what direction does the S-T of a subendocardial infarct point?

   ANS.: Away from the infarct, i.e., in the direction opposite to that of a transmural infarct [50, 99].

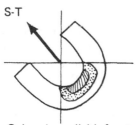

Subendocardial infarct

2. What are the commonest imitators of a subendocardial current of injury due to acute infarction?

   ANS.: a. Coronary insufficiency, as in a positive exercise ECG test.

   b. Subendocardial fibrosis.

3. Which layer of the heart is most affected by coronary insufficiency?

   ANS.: The subendocardial part, because during systole the pressure inside the ventricle is higher than outside, and thus the pressure on the subendocardial coronary vessels is greater than on the subepicardial vessels. Any decrease in blood supply to the coronary arteries therefore affects the subendocardial vessels more because there is greater resistance to flow through them due to pressure inside the ventricle.

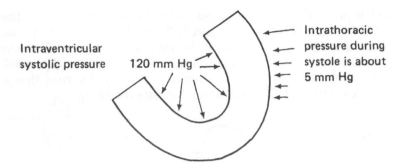

4. In which direction does the S-T vector point in the precordial leads in the presence of an anterior subendocardial current of injury?

   ANS.: The S-T points posteriorly [16].

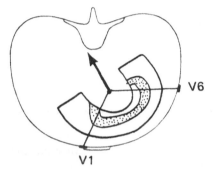

The S-T vector points away from all precordial leads from V1 to V6, thus producing S-T depression across the chest.

5. When is the subendocardium of the left ventricle affected enough to produce an injury current from all the subendocardial layers?

   ANS.: a. In severe coronary insufficiency, when all the subendocardial area of the LV tends to become deficient in blood supply. It occurs in such states as severe angina, severe hypotension, or severe anemia, and then all mid-precordial and left precordial leads show depressed S-Ts.

   b. In circumferential subendocardial infarction [76].

6. In what direction does the S-T vector point if an injury is produced from all the subendocardium, as in circumferential infarction or coronary insufficiency?

   ANS.: Posteriorly and to the right, toward the AV valve area, i.e., the mean of all the vectors pointing away from the subendocardial surface. It imitates the vector of a strictly anterior subendocardial as well as of a posterior transmural infarction [50, 51].

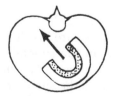
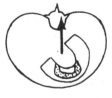
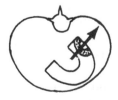

Total subendocardial injury current, as in angina   Anterior subendocardial infarct   Posterior transmural infarct

Note: You can distinguish the precordial S-T depression of an anterior or total subendocardial injury current from a posterior transmural infarct injury current only by the QRS and T changes that either one or the other produces.

7. When coronary insufficiency or an anterior subendocardial injury current is present, what do the precordial leads look like?

   ANS.: All the mid-precordial and left precordial leads have depressed S-Ts.

   Note: This ECG picture is especially likely with non-Q wave infarction as in the ECG 58 [68A].

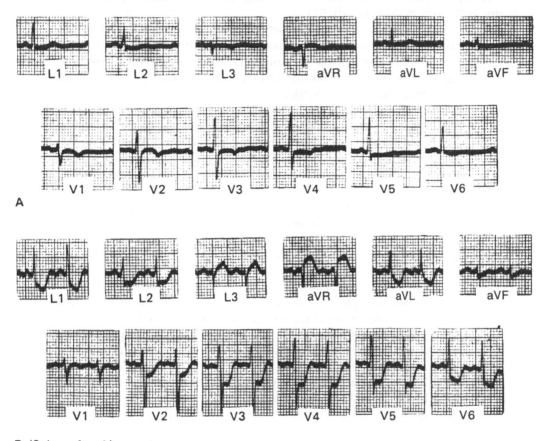

B (2 days after A)

ECG 58. A 64-year-old man had a 10-year history of angina and no heart failure or cardiomegaly. A. This ECG was taken 1 day before a transurethral prostatectomy and showed only a minor S-T, T abnormality. After spinal anesthesia the patient's blood pressure fell from a preoperative level of 150/95 to 80/60 mm Hg. For a few hours after surgery he had severe anginal attacks. B. The same patient as in A, 2 days later, showing marked S-T negativity across the mid-precordium and left precordium compatible with acute coronary insufficiency, subendocardial ischemia, or infarction. The patient died one-half hour after the tracing. No autopsy was done.
Note: *The absence of S-T elevation in aVF is evidence against the diagnosis of posteroinferior transmural infarction.*

*8. What does anterior subendocardial myocardial infarction do to the normally upright T wave in the precordium?

ANS.: Nothing, as a rule, although sometimes it makes the T taller [16, 50, 73]. It allows it to stay positive because the T points toward the area of subendocardial infarction. (This direction is opposite to that taken by the T vector of transmural infarction.) Therefore with anterior subendocardial infarction the ECG looks much like the ECG of coronary insufficiency as in a positive exercise test (see p. 277). In the limb leads the S-T tends to be depressed in all leads (except aVR) because subendocardial myocardial infarction tends to occur when there is an impairment of total coronary blood supply (often associated with cardiogenic shock) causing a pansubendocardial injury current [50, 51].

Note: a. The literature is full of references to precordial T inversions as a sign of anterior subendocardial infarction. This pattern can occur when the septum is involved [17]. Experimentally, however, anterior subendocardial infarctions do not invert the T in anterior precordial leads [65, 73, 99].

b. The term *nontransmural myocardial infarction* has been used to describe S-T depressions, T wave negativity, or both, associated with the clinical signs and symptoms of acute infarction if no initial vector abnormalities are present (see ECG 56). However, this term must be taken as a purely electrocardiographc description because

(1) Transient coronary ligation ischemia in animals has produced transient Q waves; i.e., no transmural infarct was produced despite Q wave production.

(2) Transmural infarction without abnormal Q waves can occur.

(3) S-T depressions thought to be due to pure subendocardial infarction, and T wave negativity thought due to nontransmural infarction have not always been found to be either purely subendocardial or nontransmural at autopsy. In fact, one study showed that both types of infarct pattern are associated with a high incidence of transmural infarctions at autopsy [1].

(4) The necrosis vector of a myocardial infarction can be masked by divisional blocks and old infarction of the opposite wall.

(5) Q waves present at the onset of infarction have disappeared within a few days.

From the preceding considerations, it is not surprising that the long-term prognosis in patients with only S-T or T wave changes (non-Q wave infarction) has been found to be the same as or even worse than that for patients with necrosis vector changes [8, 54, 85]. However, death due to cardiac rupture in one study occurred exclusively in those with a Q wave infarction [68]. Also pericarditis during acute infarction usually indicates a transmural lesion even without necrosis Q waves.

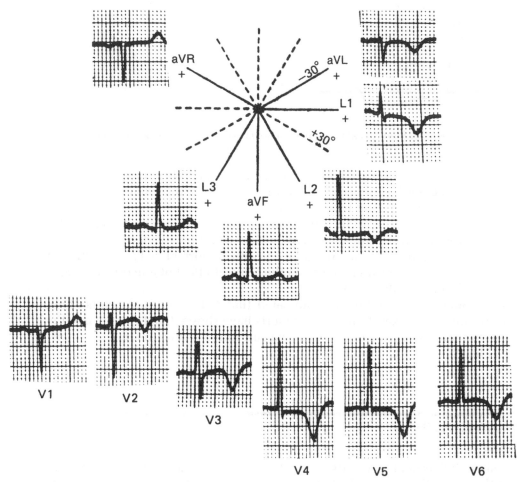

ECG 59. The T in V4 shows 7 mm of negativity. This deep T is expected only in acute ischemia due to infarction or in cerebrovascular accidents. The T in this case is due to acute infarction in which the necrosis vector is absent. When a necrosis Q wave is absent, the infarct has been called nontransmural by some and subendocardial by others; but there is no pathologic confirmation that such diagnoses are justified. Such T inversions have been known to persist for months after the acute episode.

9. What other than posterior transmural injury is the commonest imitator of the S-T depression of total subendocardial injury?

   ANS.: Subendocardial fibrosis, especially of the LV at the base of papillary muscles.

   Note: a. The S-T depression that is commonly associated with widespread subendocardial fibrosis is one with an upward convexity of an S-T segment downsloping to a negative T. It differs from the LVH strain pattern only in that it occurs in leads with a good S wave, i.e., not in the usual left ventricular leads but in those that are more toward the mid-precordium [72].

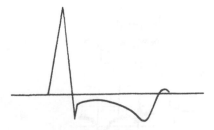

This S-T pattern, if chronic, is almost always associated with subendocardial fibrosis.

      b. Acute carbon monoxide poisoning may also depress the S-T segment in the mid-precordial and left precordial leads, as in subendocardial infarction [18].

10. What physiologic state can produce in a normal resting subject an abnormally depressed and flat S-T even with a negative T? How can it be avoided?

      ANS.: The digestion of glucose. An ECG with an abnormal S-T, T should be repeated a few hours after a meal, as the greatest effect of glucose can occur about 1 hour after its ingestion.

      Note: Some early studies had indicated that only abnormal hearts show postprandial changes. Subsequent reports have shown that this statement is not true, although a decrease in T wave amplitude is more marked in abnormal hearts after glucose ingestion [22].

*J WAVE AND HYPOTHERMIA

*1. What is a J wave?

      ANS.: A slow deflection that occurs during the terminal deflection of the QRS and in the same direction as the QRS, found during hypothermia of under 25°C [94]. It has also been called an 'injury potential.'

      Note: a. It has been recorded in cases of brain death as well but with temperatures between 26° and 34°C.

              b. A slight J wave type of deflection is occasionally seen in young patients with the S-T elevation of early repolarization [80] (see ECG 56, p. 262).

              c. It has been seen in patients with acute cardiac ischemia and is thought to be due to focal injury [97].

              d. Hypercalcemia has also caused a J wave [55].

              e. Subarachnoid hemorrhage has caused a J wave [22A].

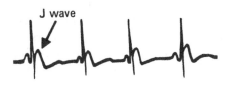

J wave

*2. Does the J wave have prognostic significance for ventricular fibrillation during hypothermia?

ANS.: Although a prolonged QRS is usually a more reliable sign of imminent ventricular fibrillation during hypothermia, when a J wave occurs during rapidly induced hypothermia or heart surgery, ventricular fibrillation develops in almost all patients [31].

Note: Ventricular fibrillation in hypothermia appears to depend primarily on the presence of acidosis [19].

*3. What is the probable mechanism of the 'injury potential'?

ANS.: In some hypothermic dogs a short period of greatly increased excitability (about 80-fold) occurs at the QRS–S-T junction [19].

THE EXERCISE ECG

1. How can an exercise ECG suggest the site of an old infarction?

   ANS.: If a patient has single vessel disease, S-T elevation and increased T amplitude in V1 with no or left axis shift indicates left anterior descending disease is likely. If the S-T is depressed in V1, it indicates circumflex disease and a rightward axis shift indicates right coronary or circumflex disease [40A].

2. What is the significance of exercise-induced S-T elevation in survivors of infarction under age 45?

   ANS.: It predicts an ejection fraction of about 50 percent and severe left ventricular wall motion abnormalities [29A].

3. What is the significance of exercise-induced transient Q waves?

   ANS.: In patients without coronary disease the mechanism is unknown. With coronary disease, they may or may not be due to ischemia.

   Note: Rate-dependent precordial Q waves occurring after anteroinferior infarction has been thought due to intermittent block of the septal fascicle of the left bundle [39A].

4. How can an exercise ECG help diagnose proximal stenosis of the right coronary artery?

   ANS.: The finding of any S-T elevation or depression in V3 to V6 [95A].

   Note: Prominent U waves in the precordial leads, especially after exercise, are a marker for significant narrowing of the circumflex or right coronary artery [12B].

TREADMILL TESTING AND THE MASTER TWO-STEP

Methods and Purposes

1. How can you very often produce the ECG changes of coronary insufficiency in a patient with a normal ECG but with poor coronary circulation?

   ANS.: By taking the ECG either during or after exercise.

2. What are the three major purposes of an exercise ECG?

   ANS.: a. To diagnose the presence and degree of coronary obstruction.

b. To predict the risk of future coronary events, e.g., angina, infarction, or sudden death.

c. To give an exercise prescription so that a patient with coronary disease can be told how much exercise he or she can do before symptoms or abnormal ECG findings such as S-T abnormalities or arrhythmias develop.
   Note: Testing to give an exercise prescription requires a monitored, progressive treadmill or bicycle test.

3. What is meant by a standard Master two-step test?

   ANS.: The patient walks up and over two 9-in. steps for either 1.5 minutes (single Master) or 3 minutes (double Master) for a number of trips according to weight, age, and sex tables. (A trip is once over the steps.) A postexercise ECG is then taken every 2 minutes for at least 6 minutes. Only some chest and limb leads are taken.

   Note: Master's tables allow fewer trips for heavier and older subjects. Master's assumption that a heavier subject does more work over a fixed distance than a subject of lighter weight disregards the increase in muscle mass and stroke volume that compensates for increased weight.

   When using Master's tables to determine the number of trips, the oxygen requirements per kilogram of body weight are much higher for lighter-weight subjects who do more trips (and approach their maximum oxygen uptake) than for heavier subjects, who may be as much as 50 percent from their maximal oxygen uptake [5, 82]. Also, there is no decreased mechanical efficiency with age in response to a fixed task, up to about age 70 [80]. You can overcome the faults of the Master tables if all subjects do 20 trips for a single and 40 trips for a double Master. It turns out to be the number of trips for a 150-pound, 50-year-old man, according to Master's tables. If this procedure is done, there is much less variation in oxygen consumption per kilogram than when a different number of trips is used for different ages and weights, as in Master's tables.

4. Is the double Master two-step test as specific as bicycle or treadmill tests in diagnosing the presence of coronary disease?

   ANS.: There is no difference in specificity between the usual double Master test and a progressive treadmill or bicycle test [14]. (Specificity tells you how often a group of patients without the disease have a negative test; i.e., it tells you how good the test is at avoiding false positives.)

5. Is a double Master two-step test as sensitive as a bicycle or treadmill test in diagnosing the presence of coronary disease?

   ANS.: Sensitivity tells you how often a test is positive in a group of patients with the disease; i.e., it tells you how well the test avoids false negatives. When one double Master study eliminated patients with postexercise rates of less than 110, it had a sensitivity of 84 percent, which was more sensitive than four of five bicycle tests and seven of ten treadmill studies [13, 14].

   Note: a. If multiple-vessel disease is present, a double Master test becomes even more sensitive if the postexercise rate is 110 or more, because then it has a sensitivity of 91 percent [14]. If there is a more than 2-mm S-T depression, there is a 95 percent chance of finding two-vessel or three-vessel disease [14]. This feature is important if you believe that if more than one vessel is involved bypass surgery is more likely to prolong life than medical management.

*b. Although myocardial oxygen consumption correlates better with S-T changes during exercise than during recovery from exercise [23], in one study of more than 5000 double Master and 200 submaximal treadmill or bicycle tests, only 3 percent of the patients had ischemic S-T changes only during exercise [14].

6. Is the double Master two-step test as sensitive and specific as a treadmill test in predicting future coronary events?

ANS.: The treadmill is almost twice as sensitive as the double Master in predicting future events in asymptomatic subjects, but it is not necessarily more specific; i.e., there are just as many or more false positives [14, 24, 25, 58]. In one study it was found that with maximum treadmill exercise, the degree of S-T depression did not correlate with either the severity of coronary disease or future events. However, with less strenuous exercise, the degree of S-T depression gave a fair correlation [14]. Therefore a test somewhere between the routine double Master and the maximum treadmill test might be a suitable compromise. An augmented double Master test may serve this role. Master himself went as far as an augmented double Master test (i.e., 15 percent more trips than his original protocol) because he found that there was no apparent increase in false positives with such tests.

Note: When the risk ratios of the double Master and progressive stress tests are compared, there is little difference between them [14]. (Risk ratio means the number of patients with a positive test in whom the disease develops compared with the number of patients with a negative test in whom it develops.)

7. How can you regulate the timing of the patient's pace in order to be sure that the required number of steps are done in 1.5 minutes for a single Master and in 3 minutes for a double?

ANS.: Set a metronome at a rate of 66, and the subject then achieves 20 trips in 1.5 minutes, or 40 trips in 3 minutes. If an augmented double Master test is desired, simply have the patient do 46 trips.

Note: If you wish the patient to achieve a low normal workload of at least 5 to 6 METS (a MET = metabolic equivalent and is the oxygen consumption per body surface area at rest), you must have the patient try to do 46 trips.

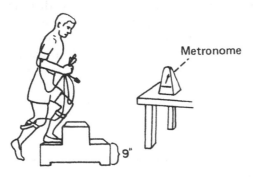

Metronome

9"

Safety Measures

1. What is the purpose of safety measures during an exercise test?

ANS.: They prevent acute infarction or ventricular fibrillation during the test.

2. What are Master's safety preparations for a Master two-step test?
   ANS.: The patient must
   a. Be fasting for at least 3 hours. For as long as 1 to 2 hours after a meal, the ECGs of even normal subjects can have slight false-positive S-T depressions and flattening [71].
   b. Not have had cigarettes or coffee for at least 3 hours before the test.
   c. Not have a history or an ECG suggestive of an infarction less than 2 months prior to testing.
   d. Not have an ischemic S-T depression on an ECG just before exercise.
   e. If the patient has known coronary disease, do a single-step test of 20 trips first. If it is negative, a double-step test may be done.
   f. Stop the test at the first sign of chest discomfort or dyspnea.
   Note: When the test was done with all these precautions, Master claimed that there was no untoward reaction in 20,000 consecutive tests [14].
3. When is it safe to do an augmented double Master immediately in order to save time?
   ANS.: When the patient's history suggests that the test is likely to be negative, i.e., if you can elicit a nonanginal symptom.
4. How can you prevent a patient from having vertigo and from having a tripping accident?
   ANS.: a. Have the patient turn toward you at the end of each descent. Thus the patient must turn in a different direction each time, so that dizziness is avoided.
   b. Always hold onto the patient's arms until you are sure that unsteadiness is not a problem.
5. What is the disadvantage of some of the strict safety factors prescribed by Master, e.g., fasting and no cigarettes or coffee?
   ANS.: Master did not use these precautions primarily for safety but in order to use the test as a measure of cardiac efficiency by using the ratio of the number of trips necessary to have the postexercise pulse and blood pressure return to within 10 points of the resting values by 2 minutes after exercise over the expected number of trips according to his tables [57].
   When the patient fasts before a test, the test tends to be negative. Because fasting also tends to make the test safe if coronary disease is strongly suspected from the history and physical findings, however, you should do a single Master (20 trips) first with the patient in the fasting state.
   Note: If done improperly, the Master two-step test can result in myocardial infarction, ventricular fibrillation, and even death because it is usually done without monitoring either blood pressure or ECG. Therefore only if the history suggests that angina is not present should you immediately do a 46-trip test.

Criteria for Positivity for an Ischemic S-T Response

1. What is usually meant by an ischemic S-T response to exercise?
   ANS.: A classic ischemic response is a flat or downsloping S-T depression.

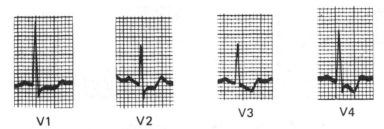

V1   V2   V3   V4

Examples of various types of ischemic S-T depressions seen in different patients or in subsequent tracings on the same patient. The S-T not only may be flat but, even worse, it may also be downward sloping. A negative T by itself is not a sign of a positive exercise test. In V3 and V4, the S-T cannot be separated from the T; i.e., it is an S-T, T.

2. What is the baseline from which you measure the S-T segment depression?

   ANS.: The baseline is the P-R segment, because with exercise the T-P segment, which is the baseline for slow rates, is obliterated by superimposition of the P on the T.

   Note: One study showed that with occlusion of a coronary artery in dogs potassium loss from the myocardium correlated best with the S-T changes [9].

3. How much S-T depression is considered to be significant for the diagnosis of coronary disease?

   ANS.: With a unipolar system, as with the Master two-step chest lead, a 0.5-mm flat or downsloping S-T depression is generally considered significant for an ischemic S-T depression. (Some treadmill and bicycle protocols also use a unipolar system for the chest leads.) For prognostic significance, any degree of flat S-T depression in a unipolar system is probably significant. With a bipolar system, as in many treadmill studies, a 1-mm S-T depression is usually considered necessary before significant ischemia of diagnostic or prognostic value is suggested.

   Note: One study suggested that if a premature ventricular contraction (PVC) induced by exercise has a superior axis, it is indicative of significant coronary disease even if there are no S-T changes [57]. S-T changes during chest pain suggestive of left main disease are S-T depressions in six or more leads with the maximal depression in V4 or 5 [5A].

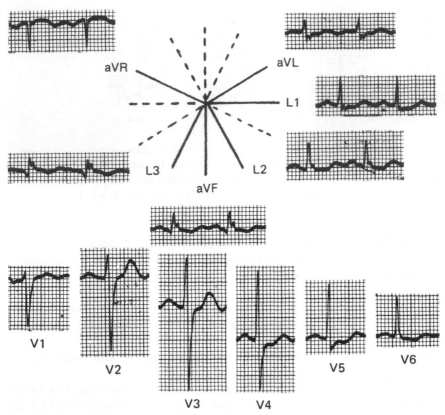

ECG 60A. Control tracing for a Master two-step test in an asymptomatic 58-year-old man with a history suggestive of infarction 2 months before. The wide Q in L3 is probably due to inferior necrosis. The slightly wide QRS is due to a periinfarction block type of divisional block type (confirmed by vectorcardiogram). A single Master two-step test was done, with the results seen in ECG 60B.

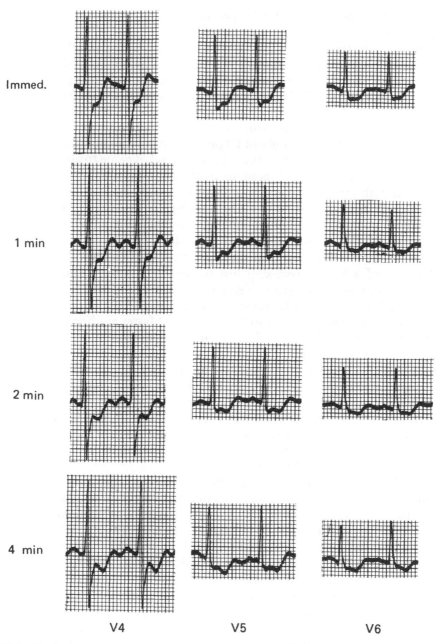

Immed.

1 min

2 min

4 min

V4   V5   V6

ECG 60B. A positive single Master's two-step test in the patient of ECG 60A. Note the following:
a. Although the immediate postexercise V4 shows only a slightly up-sloping S-T depression, subsequently the S-T not only flattens out in 1 minute but actually slopes downward by 2 minutes.
b. There is no effect on the T wave.
c. The most marked effect is seen in V4.
d. Exercise produced an adequate heart rate increase (125 beats/minute).
e. The extreme positivity of the single test despite the absence of pain during the test could have made a double Master two-step test dangerous.

4. What is the incidence of false-negative and false-positive exercise tests for the diagnosis of coronary disease?

ANS.: The ordinary double Master two-step had a false-negative incidence of 45 percent when five studies were averaged [14]. However, when tests that reached a postexercise rate of at least 110 were used, there was only a 15 percent false-negative incidence [13]. (No augmented double Master tests were done.) The average incidence of false negatives in 14 progressive stress tests was about 30 percent [14]. The incidence of false positives when seven double Master studies were averaged was about 20 percent. When the incidence of false positives in 12 progressive stress tests was averaged, it came to about 10 percent. Even with triple-vessel disease, as many as 25 percent of false negatives occurred with maximal exercise testing. Therefore the incidence of false positives and false negatives is significant enough with every kind of exercise test to make one question whether any exercise test should be used for diagnostic purposes. The preangiographic diagnosis of coronary disease should be based on the history, physical findings, resting ECG, and chest x-ray film. The use of a Master two-step test to predict future coronary events holds much more promise than its use for diagnostic purposes.

5. How can a Master two-step be used to predict future coronary events?

ANS.: Compare risk ratios. The average risk ratio for 11 double Master studies was 11:1. For coronary deaths, it was 40:1 [14]. (The average risk ratio for a progressive stress test was 12:1.)

Robb and co-worker, in a double Master study of 3300 men (one-half with atypical pain and one-fourth with no pain but an abnormal ECG), found that over an average of 9 years the risk ratio for an S-T depression from 0.1 to 0.9 mm was 2:1; for an S-T depression of 1.0 to 1.9 mm, it was 3:1; and for an S-T depression of 2.0 mm, it was 10:1. For coronary deaths alone the risk ratios were three to four times higher than for other coronary events for every category of S-T depression [14, 78].

6. How can a treadmill test be used for prognosis early after myocardial infarction?

ANS.: A flat or downsloping S-T of 1 mm or more within a few weeks after infarction predicts between 20 and 50 percent of coronary events over the next 2 years. If no S-T depressions are found, the incidence of coronary events (severe angina, infarction, or sudden death) over the next 2 years ranges from only 1 to 6 percent. If no S-T depression is combined with no frequent PVCs, the 2-year mortality is only 1 percent [15A].

7. How can a treadmill test be used for prognosis in patients with chronic angina?

ANS.: The incidence of future events, i.e., progression of angina, myocardial infarction, and death, over a period of 6 years, increases with the magnitude of S-T depression only when analyzed at low workload (about 4 METS). An S-T depression of 2 mm or more predicts a 60 to 80 percent probability of subsequent coronary events. Even a 4-mm S-T depression at high workload has only barely significant prognostic powers [15].

Note: a. S-T elevations with exercise usually denote the presence of an aneurysm or large akinetic area in patients with chronic angina. Early after infarction, however, S-T elevations usually indicate a low ejection fraction and a poor prognosis [89].

b. Deep T wave inversions (equal to or over 8 mm) during or after an exercise test with a modified Bruce protocol are almost 100 percent specific for three-vessel or left main trunk disease [12B].

How to Avoid False Positives

1. Which kind of control ECG makes it difficult to interpret a postexercise S-T depression as signifying ischemia?

    ANS.: An LVH strain pattern, either secondary to LVH or left bundle branch block (LBBB). (See p. 374 for a description of the LVH strain pattern.) Any wide QRS, as with Wolff-Parkinson-White preexcitation, can produce markedly depressed S-T segments with exercise [33].

    Note: If in the presence of LVH strain pattern or LBBB the S-T becomes depressed in leads with an equiphasic or negative QRS (usually in the mid-precordial leads), a true ischemic S-T depression is most likely. There are studies suggesting that in the presence of LBBB a further S-T depression of 1 mm means a true positive [17] but some require an S-T depression of 2 mm [30, 52]. It is difficult to confirm that even this is a true positive with all treadmill studies [70]. One study found that in RBBB and Wolff-Parkinson-White preexcitation a positive test is significant, although this judgment is controversial [33, 86]. In RBBB, if you avoid false positives by ignoring the S-T depressions in V1 to V3, you may achieve a sensitivity of about 60 percent and a specificity close to 100 percent [91].

2. How can a U wave help to confirm a true positive S-T depression?

    ANS.: A postexercise inverted U may be the only sign of ischemia, although it usually appears with significant S-T depression.

    Note: It usually indicates significant proximal anterior descending coronary obstruction [34].

3. When does a change in T waves signify coronary disease?

    ANS.: Negative T waves alone are not to be considered a sign of ischemia because autonomic effects can produce this change in normal subjects [7]. However, a markedly negative T that becomes upright should make you suspect an old infarction.

    Note: T wave abnormalities at rest not secondary to electrolyte abnormalities, drugs, or wide QRS conduction defects do not modify the interpretation of the exercise ECG, suggesting that T waves may often be generated by components different from those of S-T segments [4].

4. How does digitalis administration affect the interpretation of an S-T depression?

    ANS.: Although digitalis can cause up to 50 percent false positives and can make a slightly positive test more strongly positive, it is not so much a contraindication to doing the test as a warning not to interpret S-T depressions as being necessarily abnormal.

    Note: It takes about 2 weeks to rid the tissues of digoxin. However, usually there are no changes on exercise due to digitalis unless the resting ECG shows S-T depressions. Therefore, it is probably not always necessary to wait until all the digitalis is out of the body before an exercise test can be interpreted [41A].

5. Which electrolyte disorder can cause false positives?
   ANS.: Hypokalemia.
6. Which sex has the higher incidence of false positives?
   ANS.: The female sex. However, not all studies have confirmed that women have a greater incidence of false positives than do men.
7. What is the significance of postexercise premature ventricular or atrial contractions for the diagnosis of coronary disease?
   ANS.: None [7].
8. What other than coronary disease can give positive tests by limiting coronary flow?
   ANS.: Any valvular, myocardial, or pulmonary disease severe enough to limit cardiac output with exercise, e.g., mitral or aortic stenosis.
9. How can anxiety cause a false-positive test?
   ANS.: Hyperventilation not only can cause an ischemic S-T depression but also can prolong the corrected Q-T. Therefore with an anxious patient a resting ECG should be taken with forced hyperventilation to see if the changes are reproducible [59].

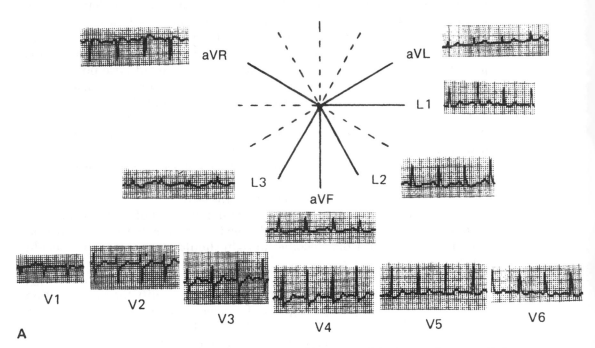

A

ECG A was taken on an anxious and depressed 49-year-old woman while she was hyperventilating enough to have carpopedal spasm. She was admitted to a coronary care unit because of chest heaviness and the 1-mm S-T depression in V4. ECG B was taken 2 hours later and is perfectly normal.

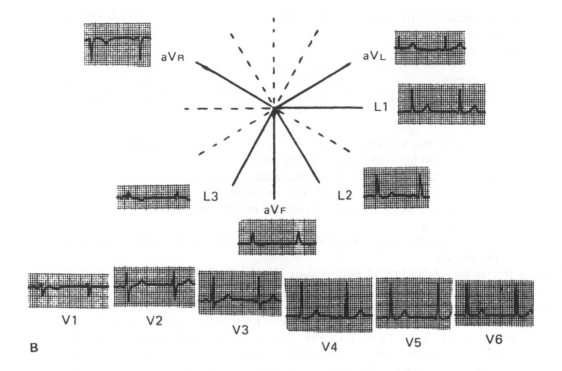

B

Note: In the patient who hyperventilates, the Q-T is less likely to be prolonged in the *immediate* postexercise tracing than in the patient with ischemic heart disease.

*10. In neurasthenic patients, what is the effect on the falsely positive S-T depressions of
   a. Standing?
   b. Postexercise heart rate changes?
   ANS.: a. Standing reproduces the S-T changes without chest pain [11].
        b. As the postexercise heart rate slows, the S-T changes may recur [32].

11. Does an ECG taken during chest discomfort always show an ischemic S-T depression?
   ANS.: Not always, although it is much more likely to do so than if there are no symptoms while the ECG is being recorded. If exercise is continued to the point of pain, the Master two-step test is positive in about 90 percent of subjects [96].

12. What is the significance of exercise-induced transient Q waves?
   ANS.: In patients without coronary disease the mechanism is unknown. With coronary disease, they may or may not be due to ischemia.
   Note: Rate-dependent precordial Q waves occurring after anteroinferior infarction has been thought due to intermittent block of the septal fascicle of the left bundle [32A, 39A].

How to Avoid False-Negative Tests for Ischemia

1. Which leads are most likely to show ischemic changes?
   ANS.: Chest leads V4, V5, and V6 and limb leads 2, 3, and aVF.

Note: Occasionally, among these leads, only one shows significant S-T depressions.

2. How soon must the postexercise ECG be done?

ANS.: As soon as possible because some patients' S-T depressions are limited to the first minute. If you are doing the test to determine prognosis, it is not necessary to obtain an immediate postexercise ECG because if the test is negative a minute or two after exercise the prognosis is probably good. Patients with a poor prognosis due to severe coronary obstructions usually have persistence of the S-T abnormalities for at least 1 to 2 minutes after exercise.

3. What drugs can lead to false-negative exercise tests?

ANS.: a. The antianginal drugs, e.g., nitrates and propranolol.

   Note: It takes at least 2 days to rid the tissue of propranolol.

   b. Diuretics can decrease preload (venous return) and thus decrease oxygen consumption.

   Note: Diuretics may also produce false-positive tests by decreasing body potassium.

4. What is meant by a false J point depression? How can a P wave be responsible for this finding?

ANS.: If the J point is depressed and the S-T has a rapid upslope, this kind of S-T depression can be at least partly caused by repolarization of the P wave, which is called the Ta or Tp wave. (See p. 443 for a description of the Ta wave.) The repolarization vector of the P wave is long enough to be superimposed on the end of the QRS and the beginning of the S-T segment. The taller the P wave, the deeper the Ta wave. During tachycardia the height of the P increases, and the Ta wave can then deepen enough to cause depression of the S-T segment. It is especially true when a bipolar lead system is used for the chest leads, as in many progressive exercise protocols. It is less likely with the unipolar system of a Master two-step test, where the P waves in the left precordial leads are rarely very large.

5. When can a slowly upsloping S-T be interpreted in such a way that it is as significant as a flat S-T?

ANS.: There are several methods of recognizing a significant upsloping S-T. The upsloping S-T is probably ischemic

   a. If the T wave begins below the baseline.

   b. If the S-T is still below the baseline at 80 msec (0.08 sec) after the J point.

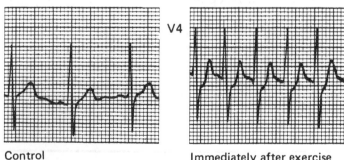

Control   Immediately after exercise

This 2-mm J point depression has a steep slope upward and represents a negative exercise test. The baseline is the P-R segment, where the QRS begins.

6. Where is the ischemic or infarcted area when the T waves become normal with exercise?

   ANS.: They point away from the site of myocardial ischemia or infarction.

VASOSPASTIC ANGINA PECTORIS S-T ABNORMALITIES

1. What is peculiar about the S-T vector in vasospastic angina (Prinzmetal's variant form of angina or angina inversa)? What is the prognosis in this form of angina?

   ANS.: Instead of diffuse ischemic S-T depression, the ECG during pain (which occurs at rest and often at about the same time each day or night) shows a localized elevation of the S-T segment with reciprocal changes, as in a transmural infarction. Occasionally, the pain and S-T elevation are precipitated by emotion [75].

   Note: a. Continuous monitoring has shown that unless the S-T changes reach a certain degree, they may occur without chest symptoms [40]. The S-T elevation may occur during sleep without relation to rapid eye movements and without awakening the patient [6].

   b. Arrhythmias occur in about 50 percent of subjects during the S-T changes [36, 39].

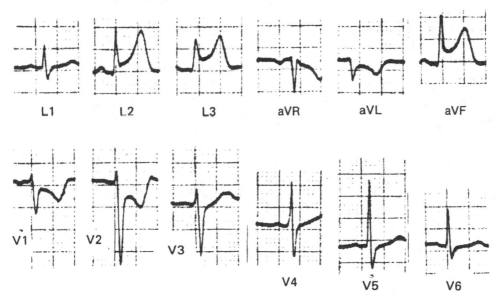

ECG 61. *Acute transient injury current during an episode of variant angina pectoris in a 51-year-old man with recurrent lower retrosternal pressure at rest, mostly nocturnal and awakening him from sleep. The posteroinferior injury vector was caused by spasm associated with a 90 percent obstruction of the circumflex artery, diffuse right coronary disease, and a dominant left coronary artery. He occasionally had short runs of ventricular tachycardia with the angina.*

   c. Myocardial infarction usually occurs subsequently at the site indicated by the ECG during the angina. Most often the angina disappears after the infarction, but it has worsened on occasion [40].

2. What other than elevation, rather than depression, is peculiar about the S-T vector in variant angina?

ANS.: The S-T elevation is often markedly exaggerated. There are usually reciprocal changes, as with acute infarction.

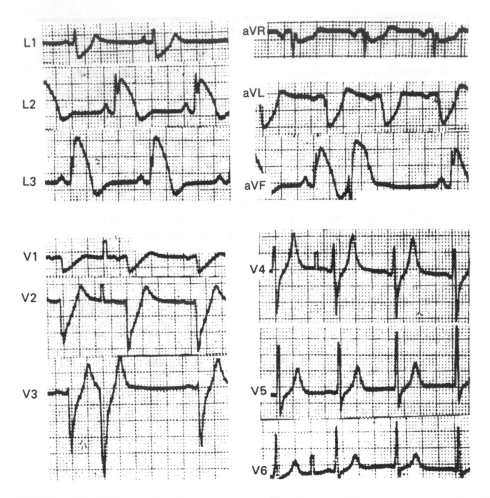

ECG 62A. This ECG was taken during chest pain in a 40-year-old black man who had had 6 years of nocturnal crushing retrosternal pain, increasing to as many as 10 attacks per night, as well as attacks at rest during the day, with faintness and diaphoresis. The chest leads are at half-standard. Note the marked S-T elevation in L3 and aVF that is even higher than the R wave, producing an almost monophasic contour.

> *Note:* a. Although the vasospastic type of S-T segment elevations usually occur at rest, they can occur even with exercise or pacing in some patients. One patient with obstruction plus spasm was reported to have had alternating S-T depressions and elevations with treadmill testing [46].

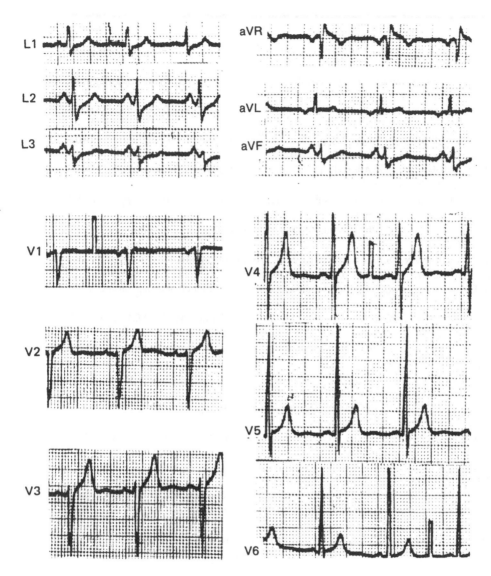

ECG 62B. This ECG is from the same patient as in ECG 62A, taken 10 minutes later. Angiograms showed no fixed obstructions. He had pain and diffuse spasm of the right coronary artery during contrast injections, rapidly relieved by nitroglycerin.

    b. On coronary angiography, patients with vasospastic angina pectoris may have normal coronary arteries, or single-, two-, or three-vessel coronary obstruction with spasm.

    c. The R wave often becomes taller during the S-T elevation. Whenever an S-T segment shows a marked injury vector, as during the first few hours of an infarction, R wave amplitude often increases [53]. This increase probably does not last for more than an hour, so that the R height is usually no longer increased by the time the patient reaches the hospital. (In dogs the relative increase in R height over control levels can predict the extent of necrosis [77].)

REFERENCES

1. Abbott, J. A., and Scheinman, M. M. Nondiagnostic electrocardiogram in patients with acute myocardial infarction. *Am. J. Med.* 55:608, 1973.
2. Alimurung, B. N., et al. The influence of early repolarization on the exercise electrocardiogram. *Am. Heart J.* 99:739, 1980.
2A. Alings, M., Wilde, A. Brugada syndrome. Clinical data and suggested pathophysiological mechanism. *Circulation* 99:666–673, 1999.
3. Anderson, G. J., Woodburn, R., and Fisch, C. Cerebrovascular accident with unusual electrocardiographic changes. *Am. Heart J.* 86:395, 1973.
4. Aravindakshan, V., Surawicz, B., and Allen, R. D. ECG exercise test in patients with abnormal T waves at rest. *Am. Heart J.* 93:706, 1977.
5. Astrand, P. O., et al. Cardiac output during submaximal and maximal work. *J. Appl. Physiol.* 19:268, 1964.
5A. Atie, J. ECG finding during an outside chest in patients with left main disease. *Circulation* 80:11–39, 1989 (Abstract).
5B. Birnbaum, Y., Herz, I., Sclarovsky, S., Zlotikamen, B., et al. Prognostic significance of the admission electrocardiogram in acute myocardial infarction. *J. Am. Coll. Cardiol.* 27:1128–1132, 1996.
6. Bodenheimer, M. D., et al. Prinzmetal's variant angina: A clinical and electrocardiographic study. *Am. Heart J.* 87:304, 1974.
7. Brody, A. J. Master two-step exercise test in clinically unselected patients. *J.A.M.A.* 171:1195, 1959.
7A. Brugada, J., Brugada, R., Brugada, P. Right bundle-branch block and ST-segment elevation in leads V1 through V3. *Circulation* 97:457–460, 1998.
8. Cannon, D., Levy, W., and Cohen, L. S. The short- and long-term prognosis of patients with transmural and nontransmural myocardial infarction. *Am. J. Med.* 61:452, 1976.
9. Case, R. B., Roselle, H. A., and Crampton, R. S. Relation of S-T depression to metabolic and hemodynamic events. *Cardiologia* 48:2, 1966.
10. Castleman, L. Selected electrocardiographic changes during hemodialysis. *Am. J. Cardiol.* 2:841, 1963.
11. Charles, M. A., Bensinger, T. A., and Glaser, S. P. Atrial injury current in pericarditis. *Arch. Intern. Med.* 141:657, 1973.
12. Chawla, K. K., et al. Electrocardiographic changes simulating acute myocardial infarction caused by hyperkalemia: Report of a patient with normal coronary arteriograms. *Am. Heart J.* 95:5, 1978.
12A. Chikamori, T., Doi, Y., Yonezawa, Y., Kuzume, O., Furuno, T., Ozawa, T., Hamashige, N. [Clinical significance of prominent negative T waves induced by exercise test]. *J Cardiol.* 19(3):741–8, 1989 (Japanese).
12B. Chikamori, T., Takata, J., Furuno, T., Toshikozu, Yobe, et al. Usefulness of U-wave analysis in detecting significant narrowing limited to a single coronary artery. *Am. J. Cardiol.* 75:508–511, 1995.
13. Cohen, P. F., et al. Diagnostic accuracy of two-step post-exercise electrocardiogram. *J.A.M.A.* 220:501, 1972.
14. Constant, J. Master two-step test: Present status. *N.Y. State J. Med.* 80:39, 1980.
15. Constant, J. Exercise testing in chronic angina: Its prognostic vs its diagnostic value. *Pract. Cardiol.* 10:53, 1984.
15A. Constant, J. Prognostic information from early post-infarction exercise testing. *Am. J. Med.* 81:655, 1986.
16. Cook, R. W., Edwards, J., and Pruitt, R. D. Electrocardiographic changes in acute subendocardial infarction. *Circulation* 18:603, 1958.
17. Cooksey, J. D., Parker, B. M., and Bahl, O. P. The diagnostic contribution to exercise testing in left bundle branch block. *Am. Heart J.* 88:482, 1974.
18. Cosby, R. S., and Bergeron, M. Electrocardiographic changes in carbon monoxide poisoning. *Am. J. Cardiol.* 11:93, 1963.

19. Covino, B. G., and Hegnauer, A. H. Ventricular excitability cycle: Its modification by pH and hypo-thermia. *Am. J. Physiol.* 181:553, 1955.
20. Croft, C. H., et al. Significance of 'reciprocal' anterior S-T segment depression in acute inferior infarction. *Circulation* 64:86, 1981 (Abstract).
21. Cropp, G. J., and Manning, G. W. Electrocardiographic changes simulating myocardial ischemia and infarction associated with spontaneous intracranial hemorrhage. *Circulation* 22:25, 1960.
22. Dear, D., Buncher, C. R., and Sawayama, T. Changes in electrocardiogram and serum K following glucose ingestion. *Arch. Intern. Med.* 124:25, 1969.
22A. de Sweit, J. Changes simulating hypothermia in the electrocardiogram in subarachnoid hemor-rhage. *J. Electrocardiol.* 5(2):193–195, 1972.
23. Detry, J.-M., Piette, F., and Brasseur, L. A. Hemodynamic determinants of exercise ST-segment depression in coronary patients. *Circulation* 42:593, 1970.
24. Diamond, G. E. The exercise test and prognosis of coronary heart disease. *Circulation* 24:736, 1961.
25. Doyle, J. T., and Kinch, S. H. The prognosis of an abnormal electrocardiographic stress test. *Circulation* 41:545, 1970.
26. Ekmerci, A., et al. Angina pectoris. *Am. J. Cardiol.* 7:412, 1961.
27. El-Sherif, N. The rsR' pattern in left surface leads in ventricular aneurysm. *Br. Heart J.* 32:440, 1970.
28. Engel, T. R., et al. ST segment elevation with ventricular aneurysm: Results of encircling ventriculotomy. *J. Electrocardiol.* 17:75, 1982.
29. Erhardt, L. R., Sjogren, A., and Wahlberg, I. Single right-sided precordial lead in the diagnosis of right ventricular involvement in inferior myocardial infarction. *Am. Heart J.* 91:571, 1976.
29A. Erikson, S. V., et al. Exercise-induced S-T elevation after infarction. *Circulation* 84:11–154, 1991 (Abstract).
30. Feil, H., and Brofman, B. L. The effect of exercise on the electrocardiogram of bundle branch block. *Am. Heart J.* 46:665, 1953.
31. Fleming, P. R., and Muir, F. H. Electrocardiographic changes in induced hypothermia in man. *Br. Heart. J.* 19:59, 1957.
31A. Frick, M. H., et al. Modification of digitalis changes. *Ann. Clin. Res.* 4:213, 1972.
32. Friesinger, G. C., et al. Vasoregulatory asthenia: A cause for false-positive exercise electrocardio-grams. *Circulation* 31–32 (Suppl.):90, 1965.
32A. Gambetta, M., et al. Rate-dependent right precordial Q waves. *Am. J. Cardiol.* 32: 1973.
33. Gazes, P. C. False-positive exercise test in the presence of the Wolff-Parkinson-White syndrome, *Am. Heart J.* 78:13, 1969.
34. Gerson, M. C., et al. Exercise-induced U wave inversion as a marker of stenosis of the left anterior descending coronary artery. *Am. J. Cardiol.* 43:353, 1979 (Abstract).
35. Gibson, R. S., et al. Precordial S-T depression in patients with acute inferior infarction. *Circulation* 64:IV-86, 1981 (Abstract).
36. Gillilan, R. E., Hawley, R. R., and Warbasse, J. R. Second degree heart block occurring in a patient with Prinzmetal's variant angina. *Am. Heart J.* 77:380, 1969.
37. Ginzton, L. E., and Laks, M. M. The differential diagnosis of acute pericarditis from the normal variant. *Circulation* 65:1004, 1982.
38. Goldberg, H. L., Borer, J. S., and Scheidt, S. S. Anterior segment depression in acute inferior infarction. *Am. J. Cardiol.* 48:1009, 1981.
39. Gooch, A. S., Patel, A. R., and Maranhao, V. Persistent ST segment elevation in left ventricular aneurysm before and after surgery. *Am. Heart J.* 98:11, 1979.
39A. Greenspan, M., et al. The significance of exercise-induced Q waves. *Am J Med* 67:454, 1979.
40. Guazzi, M., et al. Continuous electrocardiographic recording in Prinzmetal's variant angina. *Br. Heart J.* 32:611, 1970.
40A. Halon, D. A., Mevorach, D., Rodeanu, D., Robinson, M., Lewis, B. S. New insights into localization of coronary artery disease. *J.A.C.C. (Abstracts)* 17:192A, 1991.
41. Hammer, W. J., Luessenkop, A. J., and Weintraub, A. M. Observations on the ECG changes associated with subarachnoid hemorrhage. *Am. J. Med.* 59:427, 1975.
41A. Hirsch, E. Z. The effects of digoxin on the ECG after strenuous exercise. *Am. Heart J.* 70:196, 1965.

42. Hull, E. The electrocardiogram in pericarditis. *Am. J. Cardiol.* 7:21, 1961.
43. Joubert, P. H., et al. A correlative study of serum digoxin levels and electrocardiographic measurements. *S. Afr. Med. J.* 49:1177, 1975.
44. Kambara, H., and Phillips, J. Long-term evaluation of early repolarization syndrome (normal variant RS-T segment elevation). *Am. J. Cardiol.* 38:157, 1976.
45. Katz, L. N., et al. Symposium: Pitfalls in diagnosing coronary artery disease. *Circulation* 28:274, 1963.
46. Kemp, G. L. Value of treadmill stress testing in variant angina pectoris. *Am. J. Cardiol.* 30:781, 1972.
47. Kerr, F., and Haywood, L. J. Electrocardiographic changes produced by interventricular septal rupture. *Br. Heart J.* 38:1098, 1976.
48. Kuramoto, K., Matsushita, S., and Murakami, M. Acute reversible myocardial infarction after blood transfusion in the aged. *Jpn. Heart J.* 18:191, 1977.
49. Leon-Sotomayor, L., and Hampton, J. R. Ominous electrocardiographic signs in posterior myocardial infarction: A report on three cases. *South. Med. J.* 62:437, 1969.
50. Levine, H. D., and Ford, R. V. Subendocardial infarction: Report of six cases and critical survey of the literature. *Circulation* 1:246, 1950.
51. Levine, H. D., and Phillips, E. An appraisal of the newer electrocardiography: correlations in one hundred and fifty consecutive autopsied cases. *N. Engl. J. Med.* 245:833, 1951.
52. Lewis, C. M., et al. Coronary arteriographic appearance in patients with left bundle-branch block. *Circulation* 41:299, 1970.
53. Madias, J. E. The earliest electrocardiographic sign of acute transmural myocardial infarction. *J. Electrocardiol.* 10:193, 1977.
54. Madias, J. E., et al. A comparison of transmural and nontransmural acute myocardial infarction. *Circulation* 49:498, 1974.
55. Marandapalli, R., et al. Electrocardiographic J wave of hypercalcemia. *Am. J. Cardiol.* 54:672, 1984.
56. Mardelli, T. J. Superior QRS axis of VPCs in exercise testing. *Am. J. Cardiol.* 45:236, 1980.
56A. Marin, J. J. Significance of T wave normalization during exercise. *Am. Heart J.* 114: 1342, 1987.
57. Master, A. M., Friedman, R., and Dack, S. The electrocardiogram after standard exercise as a functional test of the heart. *Am. Heart J.* 24:777, 1942.
58. Mattingly, T. The postexercise electrocardiogram, its value in the diagnosis and prognosis of coronary arterial disease. *Am. J. Cardiol.* 9:395, 1962.
59. McHenry, P. L., et al. False positive electrocardiographic response to exercise secondary to hyperventilation: Cineangiographic correlation. *Am. Heart J.* 79:683, 1970.
60. Melendez, L. J. Usefulness of three additional ECG chest leads (V7, V8, and V9) in the diagnosis of acute infarction. *Can. Med. Assoc. J.* 119:745, 1978.
61. Mills, R. M., Jr., et al. Natural history of S-T segment elevation after acute myocardial infarction. *Am. J. Cardiol.* 35:609, 1975.
62. Mir, M. A. M-complex: The electrocardiographic sign of impending cardiac rupture following myocardial infarction. *Scott. Med. J.* 17:319, 1972.
63. Mirvis, D. M. The electrogenesis of terminal QRS notches in normal subjects. *J. Electrocardiol.* 16:113, 1983.
63A. Miyazaki T, Mitamura H, Miyoshi S, Soejima K, et al. Autonomic and antiarrhythmic drug modulation of ST segment elevation in patients with Brugada syndrome. *J. Am. Coll. Cardiol.* 27:1061–1070, 1996.
63B. Morphet, J. A. M. Cardiac markers for decision making 'Tombstoning.' *A.C.C. Curr. J. Rev.* 115, 2000.
64. Myers, G. B. QRS-T pattern in multiple precordial leads that may be mistaken for myocardial infarction. *Circulation* 1:844, 1950.
65. Myers, G. B., Sears, C. H., and Hiratzka, T. Correlation of electrocardiographic and pathologic findings in ring-like subendocardial infarction of the left ventricle. *Am. J. Med. Sci.* 222:417, 1951.
66. Nasmith, J., et al. Clinical outcomes after inferior infarction. *Ann. Intern. Med.* 96:22, 1982.

67. Nielsen, B. L. ST-segment elevation in acute myocardial infarction: prognostic importance. *Circulation* 48:338, 1973.
68. Ogawa, H., Hiramori, K., and Ikeda, M. Comparison of clinical features of non-Q wave and Q wave infarction. *Am. Heart J.* 111:513, 1986.
68A. Ogawa, H., Kiramori, K., Haze, K., Saito, M., Sumiyoshi, T., et al. Classification on non-Q-wave myocardial infarction according to electrocardiographic changes. *Br. Heart J.* 54:473–478, 1985.
69. Oram, S., and Hold, M. Innocent depression of the S-T segment and flattening of the T-wave during pregnancy. *J. Obstet. Gynecol.* 68:765, 1961.
70. Orzan, F., et al. Is the treadmill exercise test useful for evaluating coronary artery disease in patients with complete left bundle branch block. *Am. J. Cardiol.* 42:36, 1978.
71. Ostrander, L. D., Jr., and Weinstein, B. J. Electrocardiographic changes after glucose ingestion. *Circulation* 30:67, 1964.
72. Phillips, J. H., DePasquale, N. P., and Burch, G. E. The electrocardiogram in infarction of the anterolateral papillary muscle. *Am. Heart J.* 66:338, 1963.
73. Pinto, I. J., et al. Tall upright T waves in the precordial leads. *Circulation* 36:708, 1967.
74. Poliakoff, H. Basilar artery thrombosis: Electrocardiogram simulating acute infarction. *N.Y. State J. Med.* 72:2891, 1972.
75. Rakov, H. L. Exotic angina pectoris. *N.Y. State J. Med.* 68:567, 1968.
76. Raunio, H., et al. Changes in the QRS complex and ST segment in transmural and subendocardial myocardial infarctions: A clinicopathologic study. *Am. Heart J.* 98:176, 1979.
77. Ribeiro, L. G. T., et al. Early augmentation of R voltage after coronary occlusion. *J. Electrocardiol.* 12:89, 1979.
78. Robb, G. P., and Marks, H. H. Postexercise electrocardiogram in arteriosclerotic heart disease. *J.A.M.A.* 200:918, 1967.
79. Robinson, S. Experimental studies of physical fitness in relation to age. *Arbeitsphysiologie* 10:251, 1938.
80. Rothfield, E. L. Hypothermic hump. *J.A.M.A.* 213:626, 1970.
82. Rowell, L. B., et al. The physiologic fallacy of adjusting for body weight in performance of the Master two-step test. *Am. Heart J.* 70:461, 1965.
83. Samson, W. E., and Scher, A. M. The nature of acute ST changes in experimental coronary occlusion. *West. Soc. Clin. Res.* 7:97, 1959.
84. Sandler, G. Comparison of radiocardiography and conventional electrocardiography in the exercise tolerance test. *Br. Heart J.* 29:71, 1967.
85. Scheinman, M. M., and Abbott, J. A. Clinical significance of transmural vs nontransmural electrocardiographic changes in patients with acute myocardial infarction. *Am. J. Med.* 55:602, 1973.
86. Smith, J. E., Harper, C. R., and Kidera, G. J. Wolff-Parkinson-White syndrome simulating myocardial infarction. *Aerospace Med.* 41:328, 1970.
87. Spodick, D. H. Differential characteristics of the electrocardiogram in early repolarization and acute pericarditis. *N. Engl. J. Med.* 295:523, 1976.
87A. Spodick, D. H. Mechanisms of acute epicardial and myocardial injury in pericardial disease. *Chest* 113 (Number 4):855–856, 1998.
88. Stenson, R. E., et al. Transient ST-segment elevation with postmyocardial infarction angina: Prognostic significance. *Am. Heart J.* 89:449, 1975.
89. Sullivan, I. D., Davies, D. W., and Sowton, E. Submaximal exercise testing early after infarction. *Br. Heart J.* 52:147, 1984.
90. Surawicz, B., Lepeschkin, E., and Herrlich, H. C. Effect of magnesium on the electrocardiogram, action potential and contractility of the mammalian ventricle. *Circulation* 20:776, 1959.
90A. Surawicz B. Brugada syndrome: manifest, concealed, 'asymptomatic,' suspected and simulated. *J. Am. Coll. Cardiol.* 38:775–777, 2001.
91. Tanaka, T., et al. Diagnostic value of exercise-induced S-T segment depression in patients with right bundle branch block. *Am. J. Cardiol.* 41:670, 1978.
92. Taran, L. M., and Ordorico, D. Electrical systole (Q-T intervals) in acute rheumatic pericarditis in children. *Pediatrics* 5:947, 1950.

93. Terradellas, J. B., Bellot, J. F., and Garriga, J. R. Acute, transient S-T elevation during bacterial shock. *Chest* 81:444, 1982.

94. Trevino, A., Razi, B., and Bellet, B. M. The characteristic electrocardiogram of accidental hypo-thermia. *Arch. Intern. Med.* 127:470, 1971.

95. Wasserburger, R. H., and Alt, W .J. The normal RS-T elevation variant. *Am. J. Cardiol.* 8:184, 1961.

95A. Wellens, H. J. J. The value of the right precordial leads of the the electrocardiogram. *N. Engl. J. Med.* 340:381–383, 1999.

96. Wood, P., et al. The effort test in angina pectoris. *Br. Heart J.* 12:363, 1950.

97. Wynn, N. A., Fuller, J. A., and Szekely, P. Electrocardiographic changes in hypothermia. *Br. Heart J.* 22:642, 1961.

97A. Yamaji, H., Iwasaki, K., Kusachi, S., et al. Prediction of acute left main coronary artery obstruction by 12-lead electrocardiography. *J. Am. Coll. Cardiol.* 38:1348–1354, 2001.

98. Yeh, B. K., and Rogers, C. M., Jr. Prinzmetal angina. *Chest* 58:396, 1970.

99. Zakopoulos, K. S., Herrlich, H. C., and Lepeschkin, E. Effect of subendocardial injury on the elec-trocardiogram of intact dogs. *Am. J. Physiol.* 213:143, 1967.

21. T Wave of Myocardial Infarction and Ischemia

DIRECTION OF THE NORMAL T VECTOR

1. What does the T wave represent?
   ANS.: Repolarization of the ventricles.
2. The direction of ventricular depolarization is from endocardium to epicardium. In which direction is ventricular repolarization? Is it from endocardium to epicardium, or vice versa?
   ANS.: Epicardium to endocardium.
3. What would the T wave look like if depolarization proceeded from endocardium to epicardium and repolarization occurred in the same direction, i.e., from endocardium to epicardium?
   > ANS.: The T would be in a direction opposite to the QRS, because whatever the electrical charge of the excitation from that advanced from endocardium to epicardium to produce the QRS, an oppositely charged excitation front would now proceed in the same direction during repolarization.
   >
   > If ▭➡ represents depolarization from endocardium to epicardium with a positive front facing the positive electrode of a lead, the QRS would look like

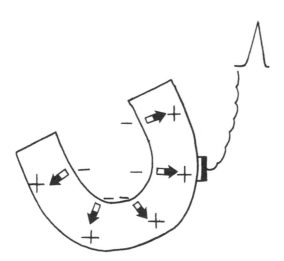

> and if ◼▷ represents repolarization also from endocardium to epicardium, with a negative charge the positive electrode of a lead, the T wave would look like

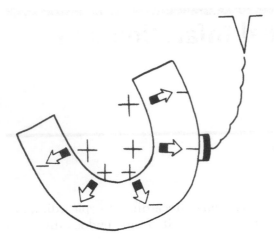

i.e., if depolarization looks like

repolarization should look like

i.e., exactly the opposite and equal.
4. What direction of repolarization must occur to produce an upright T wave in a lead with an upright QRS, i.e., the normal QRS-T relation?
   ANS.: Epicardium to endocardium, i.e., the opposite of the preceding diagram.
5. Why does repolarization occur from epicardium to endocardium and take about five times longer than depolarization?
   ANS.: Repolarization occurs during ventricular systole, surprising as it may seem.

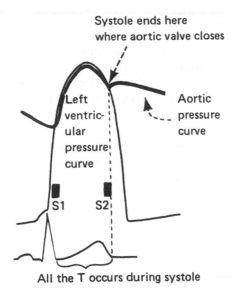

Systole ends here
where aortic valve closes

Left ventric-ular pressure curve

Aortic pressure curve

S1   S2

All the T occurs during systole

The ventricular pressure is highest during repolarization. Because the pressure is higher against the subendocardium than against the subepicardium, the subendocardial blood vessels are compressed, and the muscle there is relatively ischemic in comparison with that of the subepicardium. This situation results in a relatively delayed repolarization in the subendocardial region, and thus epicardial repolarization occurs first. The refractory periods of the ventricular muscle become longer as you measure them from epicardium to endocardium [1].

*6. What effect is produced on the T vector by the unexpected epicardium-to-endocardium repolarization?

ANS.: It turns the T in the same direction as the QRS; i.e., the T tends to be in the same direction as the QRS vector. (Opposite directions of repolarization and depolarization, plus opposite directions of advancing electrical fields, equal the same direction of electrical vector.)

Note: If repolarization *were* in the same direction as depolarization (as would happen in an isolated muscle strip), and each was considered a vector quantity, the sum of the vector quantity of the QRS and the T of an isolated muscle strip would be zero. If, however, some physiologic change should cause one portion of the isolated muscle strip to remain in the excited state of depolarization longer than another portion, the direction of the electrical field of repolarization could not be the same as that of depolarization. The sum of the two vectors of the QRS and the T would then add up to some sum that is not zero. *Ventricular gradient* is the term used for the sum of a QRS + T vector that reflects the degree to which the heart differs from an isolated muscle strip and repolarizes relatively slowly from epicardium to endocardium.

* Material marked with an asterisk is included for reference and for advanced students in cardiology.

SHAPE AND DURATION OF THE ISCHEMIC T

1. What is the abnormal T vector called in acute myocardial infarction?

    ANS.: An *ischemic T*. This term is derived from the experimental production of infarction in dogs. If a clamp is placed on a dog's anterior descending coronary artery, the first change that takes place in lead 1 of the ECG is sometimes a negative T wave, called the ischemic T. It is reversible if the clamp is removed in a few minutes [5].

    Note: In human subjects the first ECG changes of coronary occlusion appear to be S-T injury changes [19]. The reason for the difference between humans and the dog experiments is discussed on page 140.

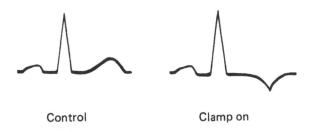

| Control | Clamp on |

2. How long does an ischemic T remain if the coronary artery remains occluded?

    ANS.: Many weeks, months, or years, but it becomes less deep as time goes on and may even become normal.

    Note: It may become transiently normal during an episode of angina, possibly due to the development of ischemia on the opposite of the heart, opposing the chronically abnormal T forces [13, 21]. In 50 percent of subjects with negative T waves following a first infarction, the T becomes upright during mild to moderate exercise [20].

3. What is the shape of an ischemic T?

    ANS.: a. It is usually symmetrical, with a sharp peak.

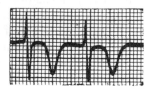

V4

It may be likened to a bird on the wing and has been called a 'seagull' T wave.

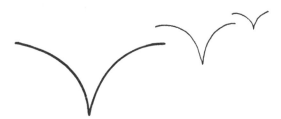

b. It may be only terminally inverted; i.e., it may be + −.

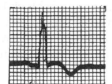 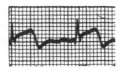

c. It tends to have a wide base.

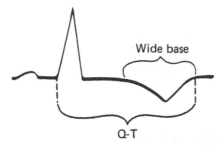

The Q-T prolongation makes a wide base for the T.

Note: The downslope of an ischemic T does not begin at the J point. There is invariably a short S-T segment at, above, or below the baseline.

4. What are the two commonest imitators of the ischemic T wave?

ANS.: a. The T inversion of myocardial infiltrates or fibrosis (cardiomyopathies). The ischemic T is especially common in fibrosis secondary to severe left ventricular hypertrophy or coronary disease.

b. The normal T inversion in the right precordium of some adults, known as the juvenile T pattern.

Note: About 20 percent of patients with either hypertension or a history of atherosclerotic heart disease have new ischemic changes following major surgery. (About two-thirds of the 20 percent have permanent changes, and about one-tenth have probable infarction [6].)

*5. List the rare imitators of ischemic T waves, excluding infiltrates or fibrosis.

ANS.: a. The T inversion seen in cerebrovascular accidents, e.g., subarachnoid hemorrhage or unilateral carotid occlusion [14].

b. The T negativity in the right precordium in severe right ventricular overloads.

c. The T inversion of schizophrenic and neurotic patients, the latter especially on standing or with hyperventilation.

d. The deep T negativity following Stokes-Adams attacks in complete atrioventricular (AV) block.

e. The deep T negativity following removal of an electronic pacemaker.

f. The giant T negativity seen in patients with the type of hypertrophic cardiomyopathy in which there is asymmetric apical (not septal) hypertrophy [28]. (This type of hypertrophic cardiomyopathy usually has absent septal Q waves in leads 1 and V1 owing to initial right-to-left

conduction. These T wave inversions (often as deep as 10 mm) can improve either with exercise or spontaneously [18, 27].

g. The giant T negativity seen in intermittent left bundle branch block [7].

h. The labile T negativity that occasionally occurs with early repolarization.

Note: The vagotonia in subjects with reflex bradycardia due to severe gall-bladder disease with stones can exaggerate the ischemic T wave due to coronary disease. These T waves can be improved by atropine [17].

6. How many millimeters of T negativity strongly suggest ischemia?

ANS.: If the T is 5 mm or more in depth, it is probably due to either a recent infarction or cerebral damage if the rarer causes of giant T negativity are excluded.

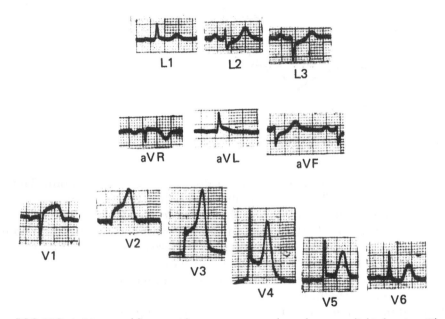

ECG 62C. A 64-year-old man with an acute anterolateral myocardial infarction. The gigantic T waves in V3 and V4 are associated with marked S-T elevations.

7. When may an ischemic T be tall and peaked in the precordium; i.e., when can the 'seagull' be upside down?

ANS.: a. In anterior infarction if the S-T is markedly elevated.

b. In posterior ischemia caused by a posterior infarct (explained in the next section).

T DIRECTION IN MYOCARDIAL INFARCTION

1. In what direction does the T vector point relative to the site of a transmural infarction?

   ANS.: The T tends to point away from the site of the transmural infarction.

   Note: The T direction is a resultant of the repolarization forces of the noninfarcted and infarcted myocardium. Therefore although the local reversal of repolarization due to ischemia tends to turn the T, the rest of the normal repolarization also controls the T wave and tends to turn it toward its normal direction; i.e., the T is the resultant of a patient's normal T and of the T turning away from the site of the infarct. Therefore you should not expect the T to point exactly away from the infarct.

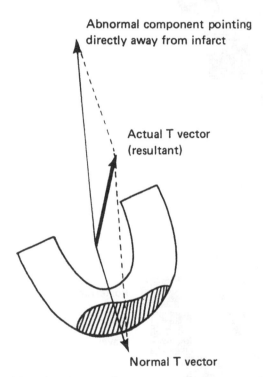

Abnormal component pointing
directly away from infarct

Actual T vector
(resultant)

Normal T vector

Note that the actual T vector resultant is somewhat eccentric in relation to the infarct; i.e., it does not point exactly 180° away from the infarct.

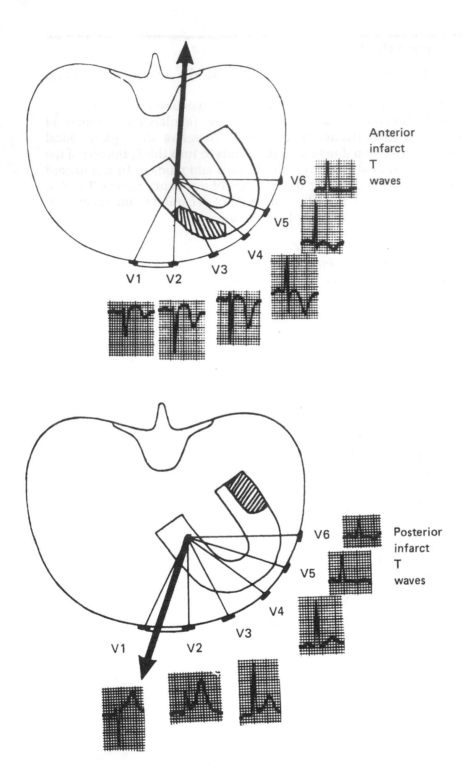

2. Can a resultant T ever point toward a transmural infarct?
ANS.: Yes, it usually does in the hyperacute stage (see serial ECGs 63A, B, C and 64).

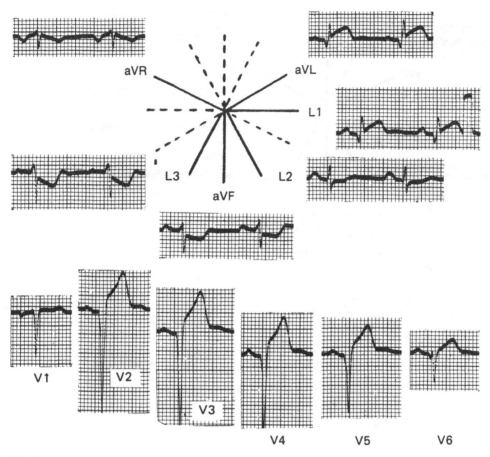

ECG 63A. Anterolateral myocardial infarction. Note that the T is still elevated in the anterolateral leads where the S-Ts are elevated. These T waves, still pointing toward the site of the infarct, signify the hyperacute stage.

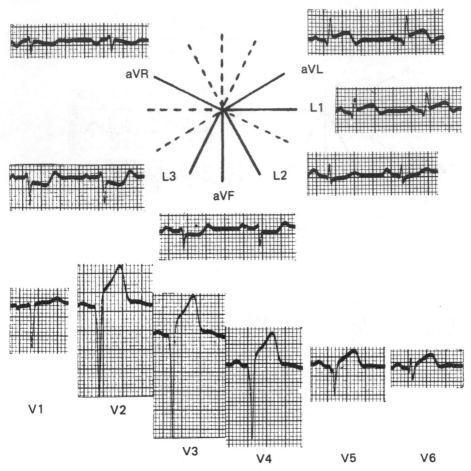

ECG 63B. Evolving infarction. It is the second day of the acute infarction. Now the T is terminally inverted in the limb leads but still in the hyperacute stage in the chest leads.

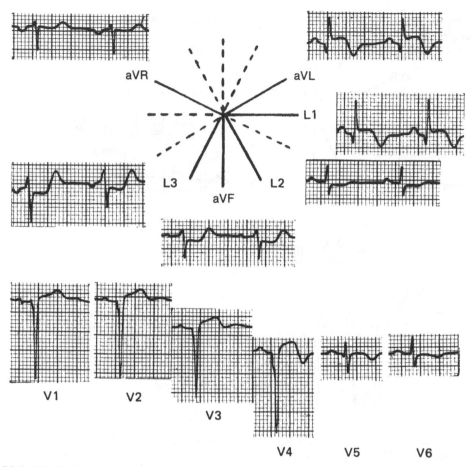

ECG 63C. *Evolving infarction a day later. The T is now more inverted, in both the lateral limb and left precordial leads. Note the reciprocal changes (mirror images) between the lateral leads 1 and aVL and the inferior leads 3 and aVF. Lead 2 tends to reflect inferior lead changes.*

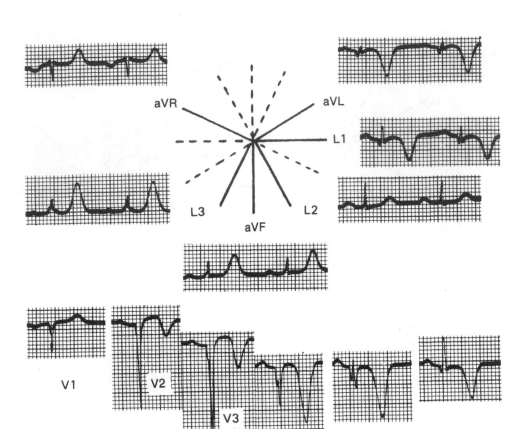

ECG 64. *Evolving anterolateral infarction. Two weeks later the T waves are deeply inverted in the anterior chest and high lateral limb leads. Such deeply negative T waves in the mid-precordium and left precordium are usually due to either a myocardial infarction or a cerebrovascular accident.*

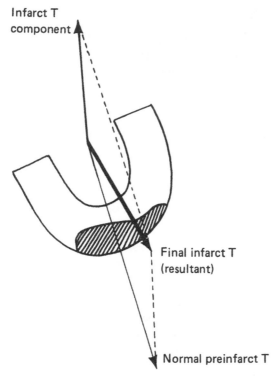

Infarct T
component

Final infarct T
(resultant)

Normal preinfarct T

Note that in this diagram the infarct T points toward the transmural infarct, which is what is seen in the hyperacute phase. It can be explained by the preinfarct T pointing toward the infarct and the infarct vector being small in magnitude. As the infarct T component increases, inspection of the diagram of question 1 shows that the final infarct T increasingly points away from the site of transmural infarction.

3. How can a T positivity in the right precordium predict the probability of a posterior infarction due to left circumflex occlusion?
   ANS.: A T in V2 that is 5 mm or more higher than the T in V6 is 90 percent specific for posterior infarction [8A].
4. How long does the hyperacute stage of infarction last?
   ANS.: A few hours to a few days.
5. What is the least accurate vector for determining the site of an acute infarct: initial QRS, terminal QRS, S-T, or T? Why?
   ANS.: The T is the least accurate. It is because the T may point away from an infarct in one plane, e.g., the frontal plane, and toward it in the horizontal plane, depending on the direction of the preinfarct T in each plane. Also, as the infarct evolves, the T often changes from upright to negative and back again every few days (the 'seesaw' T waves of myocardial infarction).
   Note: The T may change completely to normal for a day or two during the evolution of an acute infarction. This transiently normal T has been called by some the 'intermediate phase' of myocardial infarction [21]. The cause is unknown.

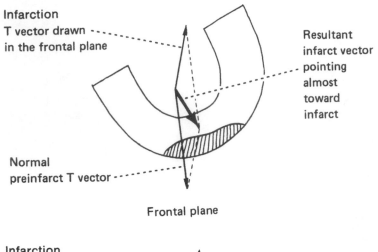

Infarction
T vector drawn
in the frontal plane

Resultant
infarct vector
pointing
almost
toward
infarct

Normal
preinfarct T vector

Frontal plane

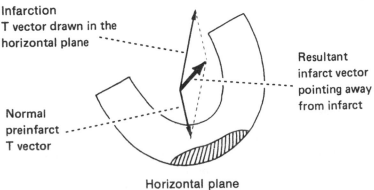

Infarction
T vector drawn in the
horizontal plane

Resultant
infarct vector
pointing away
from infarct

Normal
preinfarct
T vector

Horizontal plane

This horizontal plane infarct T vector points away from the site of the infarct despite the fact that it is the same vector as in the frontal plane of the preceding diagram.

6. What is the direction of the T in subendocardial myocardial infarction?

   ANS.:   It tends to point toward the infarct; i.e., the vector rules for *subendocardial* infarction are opposite to those for transmural infarction for both the S-T and T [31] (see ECG 58, p. 269).

7. Where would you expect T positivity in the precordium of a patient with a transmural infarction if the hyperacute stage has passed and the infarction is

   a. Anterior?

   b. Posterior?

   ANS.:   a.   T positivity is not expected in an anterior infarction because the T vector points away from the anterior chest.

   b.   Posterior infarct T waves are expected to be upright in the right and mid-precordium. A wide r at least 0.04 sec (40 msec) in duration with an upright T in V1 is highly correlated with posterior infarction, especially if the R/S ratio in V1 or V2 is 1 or more [2] (see ECGs 27B, 28A, 28B, and 65).

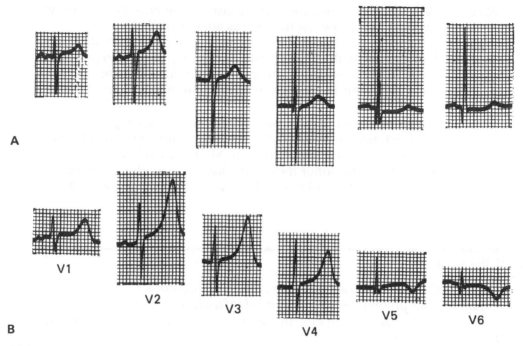

A

V1

V2

V3

V4

V5

V6

B

ECG 65. A. This ECG was taken 5 weeks before this 66-year-old man had an acute posteroinferior infarction. B. The ninth day of the infarct's evolution. Note the tall T waves with the wide base (long Q-T). The heart rate in A is 60 and the Q-T is 440 msec, or about 10 msec prolonged beyond normal. The heart rate in B is 50 and the Q-T is 520 msec, or about 60 msec prolonged. (The transition zone in A is at V4; in B it is at V2. This difference implies an anterior shift of the mean QRS due to loss of posterior forces.)

8. Does a deepening of the T wave during the first week of an acute infarction mean that more infarction is occurring?

   ANS.: No. Because the area of injury causing the S-T vectors can become smaller either by becoming a larger area of necrosis or a larger area of ischemia, a deepening T may mean that a larger area of ischemia has developed. Because it is preferable to enlargement of the necrosis area, you might say that a deeper T means that the more favorable of the two alternatives is occurring. Thus we merely report the deeper T as '*evolving* myocardial infarction,' giving no hint as to whether things are getting better or worse.

9. What is the earliest sign on an ECG that a precordial upright T is abnormally anterior, i.e., may be due to ischemia?

   ANS.: The T in V1 may become taller than the T in V6 [30]. This relation is found in only a small percentage of normal subjects. A clue that it is abnormal is the finding of

   a. Low T voltage in the limb leads, because the ischemic T often tends to turn away from the frontal plane into the horizontal plane [12].

   b. A negative T in aVL.

   c. The presence of a transition QRS complex shifted to V4 or V5; i.e., the QRS is slightly posterior [16]. This finding really implies that the QRS-T angle is abnormally wide.

Note: a. When coronary disease is the cause of the anterior T, men are twice as likely to show this sign as are women [29].

b. A T in V1 taller than the T in V6 in an otherwise normal ECG has been shown by the Framingham heart study to have no prognostic value in terms of the development of coronary disease and is not more prevalent in those with known coronary disease [25]. It is a normal finding in subjects with an inferior frontal axis and a transition zone shifted to the right in the horizontal plane [16].

c. A QRS-T angle of less than 90° suggests a normal relation between depolarization and repolarization. Most normal QRS-T angles are 45° or less, but minor metabolic changes, e.g., those caused by a meal or anxiety, could extend the normal QRS-T angle to 90°.

AGE OF INFARCT

1. Old: Only necrosis vectors present, i.e., Q waves of infarction.
2. Acute: Injury current present, i.e., S-T vectors of infarction.
3. Hyperacute: T wave going in same direction as S-T vectors, i.e., T not yet pointing away from infarction site.
4. Age indeterminate: Only T wave abnormalities of infarction present.
5. Acute or aneurysm: Injury current present for longer than a week.

T NEGATIVITY IN PERICARDITIS

1. Where in the myocardium is the ischemia in acute pericarditis?
   ANS.: It is usually a pansubepicardial ischemia.
2. What is the T direction in pericarditis?
   ANS.: Away from the mean QRS; i.e., the T waves become negative in the leads with the predominantly positive QRS complexes.
3. What is peculiar about the timing of the occurrence of T negativity in the subepicarditis of acute pericarditis?
   ANS.: It often appears only after the S-T injury current has returned to the baseline, occasionally even a few days afterward, leaving an intermediate stage during which the ECG is transiently normal. This intermediate stage is sometimes helpful in ruling out coronary disease as a cause of abnormal T waves.

POSTEXTRASYSTOLIC, POST-TACHYCARDIA, AND POSTPULMONARY EDEMA T ABNORMALITIES

1. Why may the T of the QRS that follows a premature ventricular contraction be different from the usual T wave and so serve as a kind of test for coronary insufficiency?

   ANS.: A premature depolarization has a positive inotropic effect on the heart, increasing its contractility because of changes in calcium flux. Any increase in contractility requires more oxygen consumption and so could exaggerate the effects of poor coronary filling. It has been shown that the more depressed the contractile state of the myocardium, the greater is the postextrasystolic contractile potentiation [23] and the greater is the postextrasystolic T change [8]. Also, the longer the compensatory pause after a premature ventricular depolarization, the greater is the postextrasystolic T change presumably because of the greater Starling effect and afterload reduction causing a greater increase in contractility [10].

2. When does a postextrasystolic T change not necessarily mean coronary insufficiency?

   ANS.: If the T change is of only minor degree [9] (see ECG 66). It is because any change in the duration of diastole can alter contractility [24] and any alteration in contractility, whether an increase or a decrease, can cause a change in repolarization [8]. The earlier the premature beat, the greater the postextrasystolic T change and therefore the less does it signify coronary insufficiency [10]. Thus a postextrasystolic T change signifies an abnormality only if it is disproportionately marked, i.e., disproportionate to the degree of prematurity. A relatively late premature beat should not normally produce much postextrasystolic T change. A marked inversion of a positive T wave is probably also a sign of ischemia unless the previous premature ventricular contraction is interpolated. (See p. 519 for an explanation of interpolation and p. 522 for T changes with interpolation).

   Note: A long pause following a short cycle in atrial fibrillation can also produce a T change in the cycle after the long pause. The T change may be marked if the patient has myocardial damage.

3. When is cessation of a paroxysm of tachycardia likely to be followed by inverted T waves?

   ANS.: If the attack is prolonged.

   Note: a. The T inversion may persist for a few hours or for a few days and rarely for a few months.

   b. Some causes of nonischemic pulmonary edema T negativity are: valvular disease, idiopathic dilated cardiomyopathy, hypertension, chronic renal insufficiency, and acute volume overload [19A].

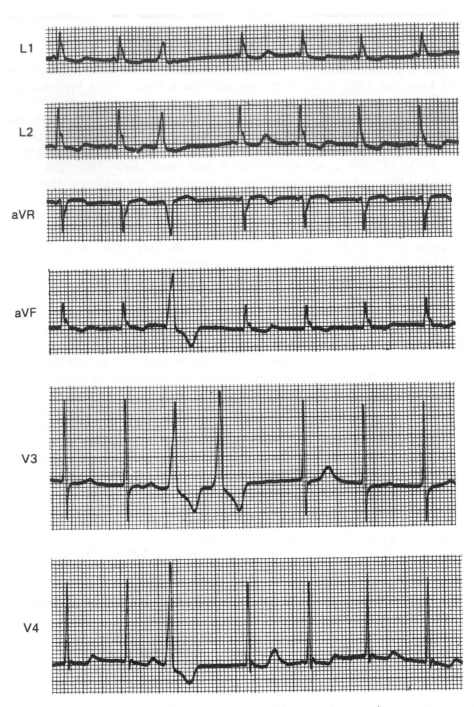

ECG 66. *Postextrasystolic T changes in an 87-year-old man with no cardiac symptoms or signs and a normal chest x-ray. The T in the normal beat following every premature ventricular contraction is moderately changed. The changes are not marked enough and do not have the S-T depressions to denote coronary insufficiency. (The very short P-R interval, seen best in leads 1 and 2, indicates atrio–His preexcitation.)*

REFERENCES

1. Abildskov, J. A. The sequence of normal recovery of excitability in the dog heart. *Circulation* 52:442, 1975.
2. Arkin, B. M., Hueter, D. C., and Ryan, T. J. Predictive values of ECG patterns in localizing left ventricular asynergy. *Am. Heart J.* 97:453, 1979.
3. Ashman, R., and Byer, E. The normal human ventricular gradient. *Am. Heart J.* 25:36, 1943.
4. Ashman, R., and Byer, E. The normal ventricular gradient. *Am. Heart J.* 25:16, 1943.
5. Bayley, R. H., and LaDue, J. S. Electrocardiographic changes of impending infarction, and the ischemia-injury pattern produced in the dog by total and subtotal occlusion of a coronary artery. *Am. Heart J.* 28:54, 1944.
6. Chamberlain, D. A., and Edmonds-Seal, J. Effects of surgery under general anesthesia on the electrocardiogram in ischemic heart disease and hypertension. *Br. Med. J.* 2:784, 1964.
7. Denes, P., et al. A characteristic precordial repolarization abnormality with intermittent left bundle-branch block. *Ann. Intern. Med.* 89:55, 1978.
8. Edmands, R. E., and Bailey, J. C. The postextrasystolic T wave change. *Am. J. Cardiol.* 28:536, 1971.
8A. Eisenstein, I., et al. ECG and VCG diagnosis of posterior infarction. *Chest* 88:409, 1985.
9. Engle, T. R., Meister, S. G., and Frankl, W.S. Postextrasystolic T wave change and angiographic coronary disease. *Br. Heart J.* 39:371, 1977.
10. Fisch, C., Edmands, R. E., and Greenspan, K. The post-extrasystolic T wave change: A correlate of the inotropic state. *Isr. J. Med. Sci.* 5:491, 1969.
11. Frick, M. H., Virtanen, K., and Savela, J. Modification of digitalis-induced ECG changes by propranolol and potassium. *Ann. Clin. Res.* 4:213, 1972.
12. Fritz, W. F., and Sjoerdsma, A. The possible significance of a T wave variant as determined from its age distribution and prevalence prior to myocardial infarction. *Am. Heart J.* 50:203. 1955.
13. Haiat, R., et al. Pseudo normalization of the repolarization during transient episodes of myocardial ischemia. *Am. Heart J.* 94:390, 1977.
14. Hammer, W. J., Luessenhop, A. J., and Weintraub, A. M. Observations on the ECG changes in subarachnoid hemorrhage. *Am. J. Med.* 59:427, 1975.
15. Hartman, R. B., Clark, P. I., and Schulman, P. Pronounced and prolonged ST segment elevation. *Arch. Intern. Med.* 142:1917, 1982.
16. Hirsch, S. T1 less than T111 and TV1 greater than TV6 in the electrocardiograms of normal subjects. *Kardiol. Pol.* 8:31, 1965.
17. Kaufman, J. M., and Lubera, R. Preoperative use of atropine and electrocardiographic changes. *J.A.M.A.* 200:109, 1967.
18. Kereiakes, D., et al. Apical hypertrophic cardiomyopathy. *Am. Heart J.* 105:855, 1983.
19. Lamb, L. E. Electrocardiographic changes noted at the onset of coronary occlusion and myocardial infarction. *Am. J. Cardiol.* 8:521, 1961.
19A. Littmann, L. Large T wave inversion and QT prolongation associated with pulmonary edema. *J. Am. Coll. Cardiol.* 34:1106–1110, 1999.
20. Nissen-Druey, C. 'Infarction T wave' in effort ECG. *Schweiz. Med. Wochenschr.* 105:48, 1975.
21. Noble, R. J., et al. Normalization of abnormal T waves in ischemia. *Arch. Intern. Med.* 136:391, 1976.
22. Pantridge, J. F. Observations on the electrocardiogram and ventricular gradient in complete left bundle branch block. *Circulation* 3:589, 1951.
23. Ranganathan, N., Sivaciyan, V., and Chisholm, R. Effects of postextrasystolic potentiation on systolic time intervals. *Am. J. Cardiol.* 41:14, 1978.
24. Robitaille, G. A., and Phillips, J. H. A study of the postextrasystolic T wave changes associated with interpolated premature ventricular beats. *Am. J. Med. Sci.* 250:107, 1965.
25. Schneider, J. F., Thomas, H. E., Jr., and Kannel, W. B. Precordial T wave vectors in the detection of coronary heart disease: The Framingham study. *Am. Heart J.* 94:568, 1977.
26. Sharpey-Schafer, E. P. Potassium effect on T wave inversion in myocardial infarction and preponderance of a ventricle. *Br. Heart J.* 5:80, 1943.
27. Steingo, L., et al. Apical hypertrophic nonobstructive cardiomyopathy. *Am. Heart J.* 105:635, 1982.

28. Tei, C., et al. Asymmetrical apical hypertrophy: Relationship to the giant T wave inversion. *J. Cardiogr.* 7:121, 1977.
29. Teicholz, L. E., Young, E., and Gorlin, R. T wave in V1 greater than T wave in V6 in coronary artery disease. *Am. J. Cardiol.* 31:161, 1973.
30. Weyn, A. A., and Marriott, H. J. L. The TV1 taller than TV6 pattern. *Am. J. Cardiol.* 10:764, 1962.
31. Zakopoulos, K. S., Herrlich, H. C., and Lepeschkin, E. Effects of subendocardial injury on the electrocardiogram of intact dogs. *Am. J. Physiol.* 213:143, 1967.

2. Nonischemic T Abnormalities

TALL T WAVE DIFFERENTIAL DIAGNOSIS

1. What is meant by an abnormally tall T wave?

   ANS.: The T height must be related to QRS amplitude, i.e., the larger the QRS, the greater may be the T. In general, a T is seldom normally as tall as a left ventricular QRS.

   Note: A tall T in the mid-precordial leads may mean only that the electrode was close to the heart. There is no upper limit of normal for a tall T in the mid-precordial leads.

2. List the three causes of tall, upright precordial T waves that are most likely to imitate the transmural ischemia of posterior myocardial infarction.

   ANS.: a. Hyperkalemia.

   b. Early repolarization, i.e., normal variant [12].

   c. Cerebrovascular accidents [12].

   Note: Anything that can produce the effect of stimulation to the left stellate ganglion or depression of the right stellate ganglion can cause tall, upright precordial T waves (see p. 349 for details). Cerebral hemorrhage and carotid occlusion are the usual causes.

3. What can help to differentiate the tall, peaked hyperkalemic T from the posterior ischemic T?

   ANS.: a. The base of the T may differ. In hyperkalemia the T is more likely to have a narrow base even if the Q-T is prolonged. This is because a prolonged Q-T with hyperkalemia is almost always due to a long S-T segment from hypocalcemia associated with uremia. The Q-T of myocardial infarction is often prolonged and produces a wide T base.

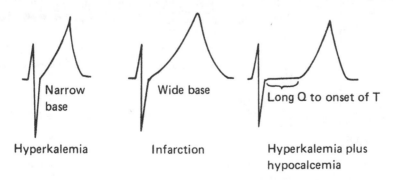

Narrow base	Wide base	Long Q to onset of T
Hyperkalemia	Infarction	Hyperkalemia plus hypocalcemia

   b. The presence of U waves tends to rule out hyperkalemia.

   c. The S-T segment differs. Although in both infarction and hyperkalemia there may be precordial J point (RS-T) depression, in infarction there is more likely to be sagging with the depression.

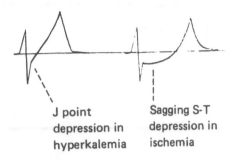

J point
depression in
hyperkalemia

Sagging S-T
depression in
ischemia

In posterior infarcts, the S-T depression and sagging in the precordial leads is the reciprocal of the S-T elevation and upward coving that would be found on the posterior chest. Therefore it is found in the right side of the chest. In hyperkalemia the S-T depression changes may be only over the left precordium.

*d. The P and QRS may differ. As hyperkalemia progresses, the P waves become lower and the QRS duration becomes prolonged. The P-R interval also becomes prolonged owing to both increased atrioventricular (AV) nodal conduction time and slow conduction along the bundle of His and bundle branches [27].

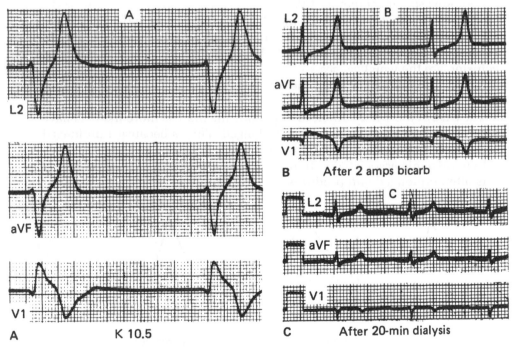

A. Wide QRS, wide Q wave, absent P wave, and S-T elevation in V1 when the potassium is very high. There is a marked left axis deviation. B. Antihyperkalemic effect of sodium bicarbonate. P waves are still absent. The left axis deviation has disappeared. Note the narrow-based T waves due to the flat and slightly prolonged S-T segments. C. Return of the P waves and narrow QRS when only moderate hyperkalemia is present after dialysis. Note that C is taken at half-standard. The P-R is prolonged.

* Material marked with an asterisk is included for reference and for advanced students in cardiology.

4.   What is meant by a spinous T wave?
     ANS.: A T that is peaked with a narrow base.
          Note: About one-third of alcoholics have a peaked T wave in V2–V4 [22A].
*5. List the causes of tall, peaked upright T waves that do not usually mimic posterior infarction.
     ANS.: a.   Iron deficiency anemia within 2 weeks of treatment with iron [26].
           b.   Vagotonia, as in athletes [41].
           c.   Volume or pressure overloads of the left ventricle.
           d.   Severe mitral stenosis.
                Note: About 15 percent of male patients with severe mitral stenosis in one series had tall, peaked mid-precordial T waves thought to be an early sign of right ventricular hypertrophy (RVH). It has been called 'T mitrale' [72].
           e.   Alcoholism.
                Note: In one study alcoholic patients were found to have taller T waves than normal. This finding is surprising because it was discovered during efforts to confirm earlier reports that in alcoholic cardiomyopathies there are notched T waves, and notched T waves are usually low [33]. It is even more surprising to find tall T waves in view of the discovery that most hospitalized alcoholic patients have hypokalemia. Because prolonged alcohol intake can cause magnesium deficiency and T wave peaking has been found to be an early manifestation of magnesium depletion, perhaps these tall T waves are a manifestation of magnesium imbalance [59, 68]. Magnesium deficiency may first cause loss of intracellular potassium, resulting in a relative extracellular hyperkalemia. When, however, magnesium and potassium deficiency occur together in dog experiments, terminal T negativity is seen [59].
           f.   Metabolic acidosis.
6.   In what situation is vagotonia seen as a cause of tall T waves?
     ANS.: In young athletes. It is usually associated with an elevated S-T segment and is then called 'early repolarization' (see ECG 54, p. 260).
          Note: The tall T of young people can usually be distinguished from a hyperkalemia T wave by
           a.   The heart rate. Patients with hyperkalemia rarely have heart rates of less than 70, whereas such heart rates are common in normal subjects with tall T waves [10].
           b.   The presence of a U wave. A U wave is not expected with elevated potassium levels.
           c.   Symmetry. Compared to the vagotonic T, the tall T of hyperkalemia is more symmetrical ('church steeple T'). The reason is that the base of the T is narrowed by a shift of the proximal limb of the T (which is normally longer than the terminal limb) to the right (pushed away from the QRS) by a prolonged S-T segment.
*7. What happens to the S-T, T *direction* from either the hyperkalemia of renal disease or the ingestion of a large dose of potassium chloride?
     ANS.: Nothing. Only their magnitude is changed.
          Note: The S-T magnitude can be so exaggerated by hyperkalemia that it may mimic the injury current of acute pericarditis.

8. What are the two most common causes of hyperkalemia? Why is it usually easy to diagnose by ECG?

   ANS.: a. Uremia. The hypocalcemia plus the hyperkalemia gives a characteristic picture in at least one lead. The hypocalcemia flattens and prolongs the S-T, whereas the T is sharp and peaked (see ECG 68A, p. 318).

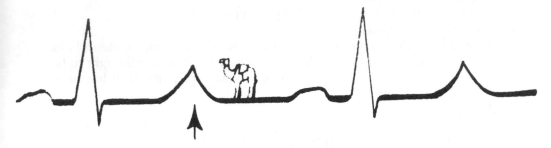

Tent on the desert

The sharp, upright T is like a tent on the desert of a long, flat S-T segment. This pattern is characteristic of uremia.

   b. Potassium administration for hypokalemia problems.

   Note: a. Hypocalcemia, as seen with uremia, exaggerates the T wave abnormalities [63].

   b. Elevation of serum potassium is a more reliable indication for hemodialysis in acute renal failure than is the ECG evidence of hyperkalemia [48].

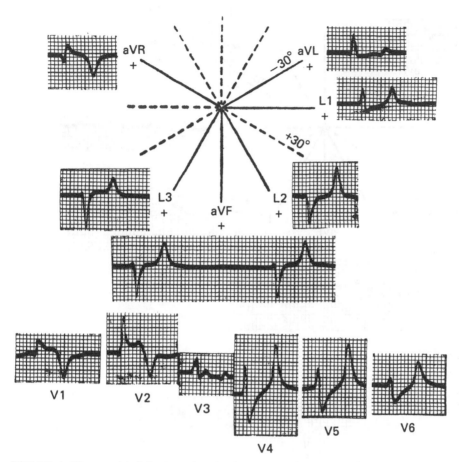

ECG 67. A 60-year-old diabetic patient had uremia and a serum calcium of 7.5 mg per dl
(low normal is 9 mg/dl). Despite a blood urea nitrogen of 87 mg per dl, he had been receiving
60 mEq of potassium chloride per day intravenously. He died before the serum potassium was
determined.
Note the narrow base of the tall, peaked T waves in V4 and V5. Because the S-T depression and
tall T waves are seen only in the left precordium, they are not due to posterior ischemia but must
be due to a high serum potassium. (The flat S-T of hypocalcemia is seen well only in L3. It is not a
long enough S-T, however, to be typical for hypocalcemia.)

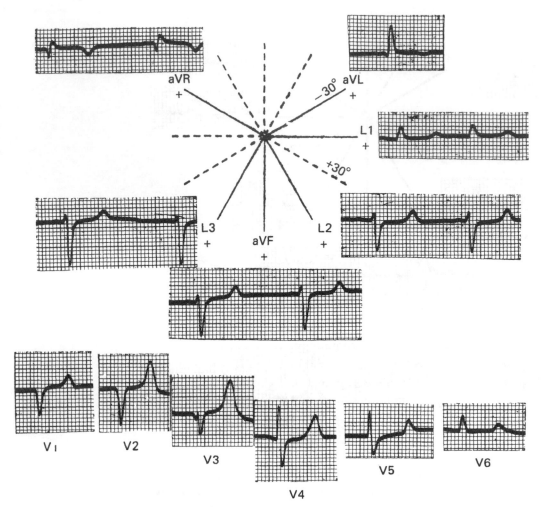

ECG 68A. A patient with chronic glomerulonephritis; blood urea nitrogen 131; potassium 9 mEq; calcium 8.5 mg. The long, flat S-T segment with the sharp, peaked T is almost diagnostic of uremic hypocalcemia and hyperkalemia. Note also the extremely low P waves characteristic of advanced hyperkalemia in leads 2, 3, and aVF. The P waves tend to disappear with potassium levels of 9 to 10 mEq.

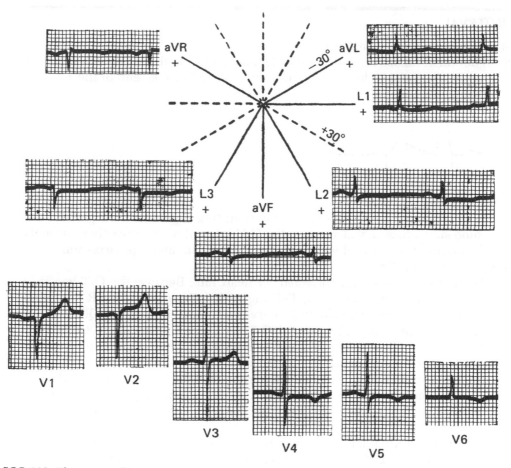

ECG 68B. The same subject as in ECG 68A but after dialysis. The negative T waves in V4, V5, and V6 suggest an underlying cardiomyopathy.

*9. List the causes of T wave alternans reported in the literature.

ANS.: a. Hypomagnesemia with severe alcoholism [43, 53].

b. Severe pancreatic disease with shock, renal failure, and low calcium and potassium.

c. Rapid blood transfusion during surgical hypothermia [49].

d. Renal failure with hypertension and hypocalcemia.

e. Prolonged supraventricular tachycardia and heart failure in a patient on quinidine [70].

f. Parathyroid deficiency with severe hypocalcemia [49].

g. After either a cardiac syncopal episode or exercise in the congenital long Q-T interval syndromes [49, 56].

Note: The alternans may be either in voltage or in axis.

Q-T INTERVAL

1. What is meant by the Q-T interval?

    ANS.: The time taken by ventricular depolarization and the major forces of repolarization, i.e., from the beginning of the QRS to the end of the T.

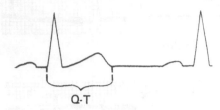

Q-T

Note: Because the U wave also occurs during repolarization, probably of some subendocardial structures, the Q-U interval more correctly represents the *complete* process of ventricular depolarization and repolarization.

*2. What is meant by a Q-Tc?

    ANS.: The corrected Q-T, i.e., corrected for heart rate. Because the Q-T becomes longer with slower heart rates, dividing by the square root of the R-R interval corrects for heart rate. (The R-R interval is the cycle length or QRS-to-QRS interval in seconds.) The normal Q-Tc is 390 ± 40 msec (0.39 ± 0.04 sec). The upper limit of 430 msec is for women. For men and for patients under age 50, it is about 10 msec shorter [61].

3. Without using square root tables, how can one tell that the Q-T is prolonged?

    ANS.: a. By inspection alone; if the T ends at more than 50 percent of the R-R interval, the Q-T is prolonged. This method works only up to a heart rate of 80.

    *b. The top normal for a heart rate of 70 is 400 msec (0.40 sec), or two large divisions on ECG paper. For every 10 beats per minute over 70, it shortens by 2 msec (0.02 sec). For every 10 beats per minute under 70, it lengthens by 30 msec (0.03 sec). (To aid your memory: it lengthens by a larger number than it shortens.) This method of judging the Q-T works for rates from 50 to 110 beats per minute. The Q-T tends to be 10 msec longer for women. For example, a man with a heart rate of 80 should have an upper normal Q-T of 400 − 20 = 380 msec. For a woman the Q-T should be no longer than 390 msec.

4. What happens to the Q-T if the patient is on digitalis?

    ANS.: It shortens.

5. What commonly used drugs can lengthen the Q-T, i.e., the Q-Tc?

    ANS.: a. The antiarrhythmic agents quinidine, procainamide, and lidocaine.

    b. The phenothiazines [6].

*6. What happens to the Q-T with left ventricular hypertrophy?

    ANS.: Even enough left ventricular hypertrophy (LVH) to produce a strain pattern and cardiac enlargement as seen on a chest x-ray film does not cause much Q-T prolongation [18].

*7. How can the Q-T help to distinguish myocarditis alone from myocarditis associated with acute pericarditis?

    ANS.: Carditis prolongs the Q-T and pericarditis shortens or does not change it. Therefore the presence of a long Q-T tells you that pericarditis is probably not present, at least not as the only problem [65, 67].

Note: A long Q-T interval and an increased risk of sudden death occurs in about one-third of adult celiac disease patients. It is inversely related to serum potassium [14A].

*8. How is the Q-T affected by acute myocardial infarction? What is the cause?

ANS.: The Q-T reaches a maximum by about the second day and returns to normal by about the fifth day. The prolongation is thought to be due to focal extracellular hypocalcemia with intracellular calcium accumulation. Injured cells take up large amounts of calcium into their mitochondria [17].

Note: Patients with acute infarction who developed ventricular fibrillation in hospital usually had a prolonged Q-Tc of 0.46 sec or more [2]. If repeated early postinfarction and Q-Tc intervals are prolonged to 0.44 second or more, there is a markedly increased incidence of either reinfarction or sudden death over the next year, especially if the patient is under age 66 and without bundle branch block [3].

*9. What syndromes are associated with a congenital prolongation of the Q-T interval?

ANS.: a. The surdocardiac or cardioauditory syndrome, which is an autosomal recessive abnormality with nerve deafness and cardiac syncopal attacks, the latter precipitated by fright, anger, or exertion. Sudden death during childhood occurs in about one-half of these patients [51]. The Q-T is strikingly prolonged, mostly due to a long Q to onset of T (S-T segment), and the T may appear to be ischemic. These ECG changes may be due to sympathetic nervous system imbalance and may be seen only after exercise [52].

Note: This rare situation is sometimes called the Jervell and Lange-Nielsen syndrome, after the authors of the first description [32].

b. The Romano-Ward syndrome, an autosomal dominant abnormality in which syncopal attacks and sudden death occur due to ventricular arrhythmias that are precipitated by exercise or emotional stress, is associated with a prolonged Q-T interval but no deafness [23, 34, 52]. In a family some members may have only the prolonged Q-T, whereas others may also have deafness [44].

Note: a. The Q-T may vary on different occasions and even from one cycle to the next.

b. With exercise these patients often have lower than normal heart rates, which suggests decreased right stellate sympathetic stimulation [57].

c. The Q-T may be shortened by right stellate ganglion stimulation and left stellate ganglion block [15].

d. These ventricular arrhythmias are occasionally suppressed by phenobarbital [45].

e. Abnormally large after-depolarizations or after-potentials (see p. 529) were found in a patient with the long Q-T syndrome [60]. They are enhanced by beta-adrenergic stimulation and may attain firing threshold. They may be blocked by propranolol.

f. All four cases of Romano-Ward syndrome in one autopsy study had a chronically inflamed ventricular myocardium [8].

10. How does the measured Q-T interval change during a 20-second Valsalva maneuver in (a) normal subjects, (b) familial long Q-T syndrome subjects?

ANS.: a. The Q-T shortens.

    b. The Q-T lengthens.

    Note: In relatives the Q-T may also lengthen, thus helping to detect latent cases.

11. What T abnormalities can occur with the long Q-T syndrome?

  ANS.: a. Alternation of the T wave often follows the same stimuli that trigger the syncopal attacks [57].

    b. Markedly notched T waves resulting from humps or bulges or protruberances just beyond the apex or on the descending limb of an upright wave can occur in patients and in blood relatives [37A]. After the pause of a PVC these bulges may become more prominent. They have sometimes been thought to be U waves [68A].

    Note: Postextrasystolic U wave or T hump augmentation may identify patients at risk for VT/VF even when the baseline Q-T is normal [68B].

12. How can gender be suggested by the S-T, T and Q-T interval?

  ANS.: In males (a) the J point tends to be higher as in early repolarization which is much more common in males (b) the upstroke and downslope of the T wave are steeper. These changes are dependent on testosterone levels and are best seen in the leads with the greatest T amplitude—usually V1 to V4 [8A]. This explains the longer Q-T in women.

Q-T and Hypercalcemia

1. How does hypercalcemia affect the Q-T?

  ANS.: It shortens it.

    Note: It is easy to remember that elevated serum calcium shortens the Q-T because calcium acts like digitalis on the myocardium. Indeed, digitalis is thought to work through calcium. Therefore if digitalis can shorten the Q-T, so should calcium. The short S-T of hypercalcemia, however, is not associated with a sagging S-T, as it is with digitalis (see ECG 69).

2. Which part of the Q-T is shortened by calcium?

  ANS.: The Q to onset of the T; i.e., the S-T segment is shortened [11].

Q to onset of T is normal here

Q to onset of T here has been shortened by hypercalcemia

Note: a. When the serum calcium is at very high levels (more than 18 mg/100 ml), it has been noted that the T may be prolonged and the slope of the downstroke is shallower than normal [9]. This picture suggests that the Q to peak of T might be more reliable than the Q-T. In actual practice, because it is difficult to find the onset of T accurately, it is not surprising that the Q to apex of T shows a better correlation with serum calcium than does either Q to onset of T or Q-T. The Q to apex of T corrected for heart rate by dividing by the square root of the R-R interval is the Q-aTc [50].

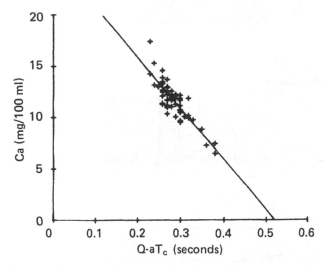

Serum calcium as a function of Q-aTc. Calcium = 25.7 – 49.5 (Q-aTc); standard deviation ± 0.92; p value < 0.001. (Modified from D. W. Nierenberg and B. J. Ransil. Am. J. Cardiol. 44:243, 1979.)

    b. The Q-T interval does not correlate well with the sudden hypercalcemia produced by intravenous calcium chloride or the acute hypocalcemia produced by blood transfusions [54].

    c. Hyperkalemia can also shorten the S-T segment.

    d. One study found that shortening of the Q-T is an unreliable sign of chronic hypercalcemia, e.g., only five of 15 instances of hypercalcemia had a Q to peak of T shorter than normal [73].

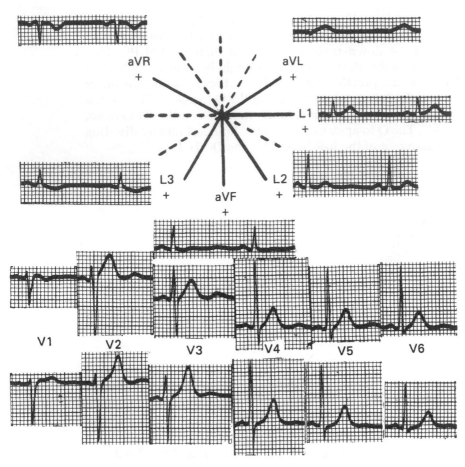

ECG 69. A 49-year-old man has metastatic cancer to bone, primary site unknown. He has marked muscle weakness. His serum calcium is 15.2 mg per 100 ml. The bottom line was taken 3 months earlier when he had normal serum calcium. Compare the short S-T segments of hypercalcemia with the normal S-T segments when his calcium was normal.

Q-T and T in Hypocalcemia

*1. How is the T direction affected by hypocalcemia?

ANS.: Although most subjects have posterior turning (often with terminally negative T waves in most of the precordial leads), some have anterior turning with tall, peaked precordial T waves; on the other hand, the T may not be affected at all.

Note: a. Intravenous calcium has almost no effect on any abnormal T direction produced by hypocalcemia.

b. The serum calcium must be less than 8 mg per 100 ml before it can be recognized on an ECG.

2. How is the Q-T affected by hypocalcemia such as that in hypoparathyroidism?

ANS.: It is lengthened. The T duration, however, is rarely affected [11].

Note: The P-R also is often prolonged in hypocalcemia [11].

3. How, then, does hypocalcemia prolong the Q-T if it rarely affects the T?
   ANS.: It prolongs the Q to onset of the T; i.e., the S-T segment is prolonged [11]. (This situation is best seen in the precordial leads.)

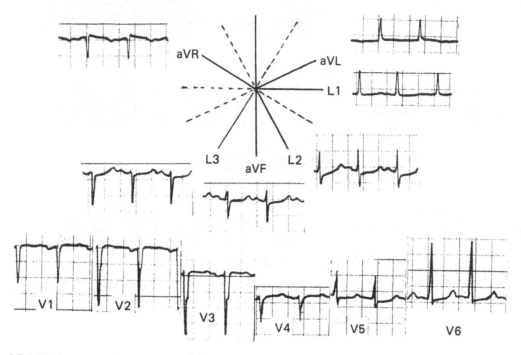

ECG 70. A normotensive 57-year-old woman had paresthesias 20 years after a partial thyroidectomy. Her calcium level was 5.4 mg/dl due to hypoparathyroidism.

U WAVE

1. What is meant by a U wave?
   ANS.: It is any wave that occurs just after the T and before the next P.
2. What is the direction of the normal U wave?
   ANS.: The same direction as the normal T, i.e., anterior and slightly leftward.
3. In which precordial leads are normal U waves best seen? Why?
   ANS.: In the mid-precordial leads V2 and V3, probably because these electrodes are closest to the heart and can pick up the tiny potentials of the normal U wave, which averages 0.3 mm in height; rarely, it rises to 2 mm.
4. When does T-U fusion occur?
   ANS.: Whenever the Q-T interval is prolonged, as with quinidine, hypocalcemia, or central nervous system disease (i.e., when the end of the T wave is late), the U wave does not move away from the T but stays relatively close to the QRS and so fuses with the T wave [40].
5. What is the commonest cause of a normal high U wave?
   ANS.: Bradycardia (see ECG 71).

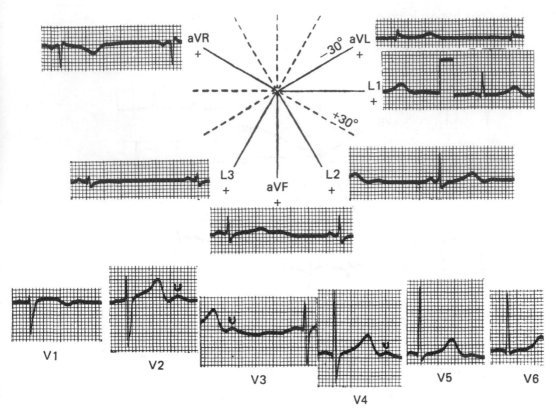

ECG 71. A high U wave in a 46-year-old normal black man with bradycardia. It is normal because the T is much higher in the leads with the highest U waves. Although the patient has been drinking heavily for the previous 6 months, his electrolytes were normal. (The short P-R interval and absent P-R segment suggest atrio-His preexcitation.)

6. What is the cause of the U wave?

    ANS.: It is unknown. Because it begins with isovolumic relaxation, a useful concept is to consider it as a residual repolarization potential 'left over' after repolarization has made a T wave during systole. Assume that because of the high pressure generated in the ventricular muscle during systole all of repolarization is not possible until ventricular relaxation begins. It must be understood that the T wave is inscribed during systole.

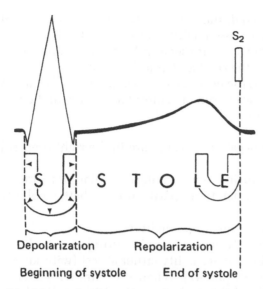

Depolarization   Repolarization

Beginning of systole   End of systole

The U wave begins at about the time of the second sound and occurs with ventricular expansion or diastole. Some think it is due to repolarization of the papillary muscles [21]; others believe it is due to late repolarization of the septum because only the septum has high pressure on both sides during systole.

7. Why is the foregoing concept (of the U as a 'leftover' repolarization after the T is finished) useful?

    ANS.: It may explain why relatively high U waves are so commonly seen with low T waves in abnormal states; i.e., the less the T, the more the U. For example, when epinephrine is given and the T wave amplitude decreases, the U wave increases [40].

        Note: a. In normal hearts the higher the T, the higher the U.

          *b. U wave alternans has been found in some patients with pulsus alternans, suggesting that the height of the U wave may be associated with the degree of contraction or contractility [19].

          c. The magnesium deficiency of prolonged alcoholism has produced both T wave alternans and U wave alternans [7, 53].

ABNORMAL U WAVES

*Negative U Waves

*1. When is a negative U wave most likely to be seen?

    ANS.: a. With myocardial infarction, subendocardial fibrosis, or subendocardial ischemia, as in angina pectoris patients [39].

        Note: In one study, patients with a history of ischemic heart disease and negative U waves had a high incidence of anterior descending coronary artery obstruction [4, 25].

      b. In severe LVH, especially the LVH of pure aortic regurgitation [39].

        Note: The negative U waves in hypertensive patients are usually of short duration because the final part of the U is isoelectric [22]. When blood pressure is lowered, the U waves become upright, usually with a concomitant decrease in QRS amplitude [24, 64].

Note: a. In LVH the negative U waves are seen in leads 1, V5, and V6; i.e., the U tends to point to the right and anteriorly [39].

b. If the infarct is anterior, the negative U waves are in leads 1 and V4 to V6; i.e., they point away from the anterolateral area of the heart. If the infarct is inferior, the negative U waves are in the inferior leads L3 and aVF [21].

c. In mitral stenosis the negative U waves are in the right precordial leads [22].

d. Negative U waves during acute anterior infarction identify patients with smaller infarctions partly due to better collateral circulation [66A].

*2. How may negative U waves help in the diagnosis of angina?

ANS.: A negative U in V5, although usually occurring only during an actual attack of chest pain, may be the only ECG abnormality either at rest (without pain) or during and after an exercise test [35, 47]. When it occurs with exercise, it is usually associated with a simultaneous increase in QRS amplitude [64]. A negative U appearing with normalization of a negative T during exercise is highly specific for critical anterior descending stenosis [34A].

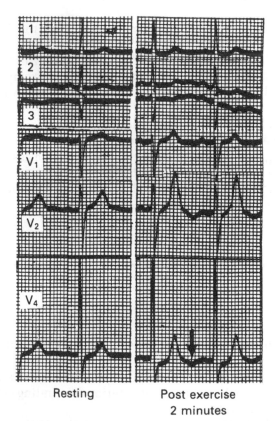

Resting   Post exercise
2 minutes

ECG 71A. Negative U waves developed after exercise in this patient with angina pectoris. The QRS amplitude increased slightly in V4. Negative or biphasic U waves after exercise have been reported in about two-thirds of patients with angina pectoris [39].

3. What is the significance of initial versus terminal U wave inversion?
    ANS.: Initial inversion is related to elevated blood pressure; terminal inversion is associated with regional ischemia [46A].

Relatively High U Wave

1. What is meant by a relatively high U wave?
    ANS.: If the U is almost as high as the T, even a small U should be considered relatively tall. High U waves may be normal with bradycardia but then they are associated with a normal T that is much taller than the U (see ECG 71).

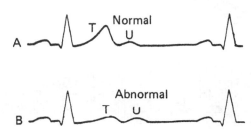

A. The U wave is normal because the T is tall and there is a bradycardia, which can exaggerate a U wave. B. The U is abnormal because it is associated with a low T wave; i.e., it is a relatively high U wave even though it is the same absolute height as the normal U in A.

2. List some causes of relatively high U waves.
    ANS.: a. Hypokalemia.
        b. Digitalis.
        c. Any cardiomyopathy.
        d. LVH.
        e. Quinidine.
        f. Phenothiazines, especially thioridazine.
        g. Diabetes.
        h. Central nervous system disease, e.g., subarachnoid hemorrhage.
        i. Tricyclic antidepressants.
    Note: a. All the preceding conditions and drugs are associated with abnormally notched T waves except hypokalemia, digitalis, and diabetes.
        b. The high U waves (and tall P waves) seen in some patients with subarachnoid hemorrhage can be abolished by propranolol [16].

Hypokalemia and U Waves

1. List the classic ECG changes seen in hypokalemia.
    ANS.: A depressed and sagging S-T, with a low T wave and a relatively high U.
        Note: When the S-T segment is not depressed, consider causes of relatively high U waves other than low potassium [20].

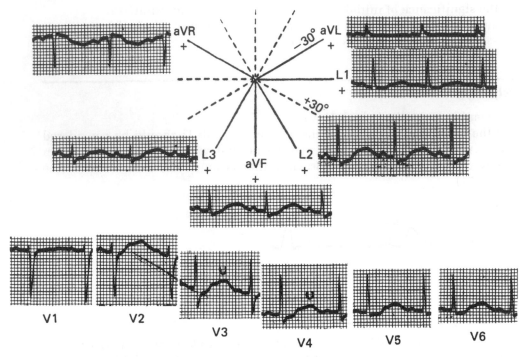

ECG 72. This 24-year-old woman with a normal heart received 80 to 120 mg of furosemide per day for months as treatment for idiopathic edema of the hands and legs. Her serum potassium was 1.2 mEq. Note that the leads showing the relatively high U waves have depressed or sagging S-Ts. This pattern is characteristic of the classic ECG of hypokalemia.

2. How can a U wave imitate a prolonged Q-T?
   ANS.: A Q-T that blends with a tall U wave merging with its peak is really a Q-U interval.
   Note: a. Of all the causes of a relatively high U, hypokalemia is the commonest cause of a Q-U masquerading as the Q-T.

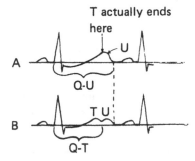

A. A long Q-T due to a Q-U, with the U imperceptibly attached to the T, as in servere hypokalemia. B. From the same patient as in A, but with slightly less hypokalemia. The relatively high U wave has separated from the T.

  b. The Q-U interval masquerading as a Q-T interval has led to the mistaken notion that hypokalemia significantly prolongs the Q-T interval.

  c. Marked magnesium deficiency, as after a prolonged alcoholic bout, may also cause an apparently prolonged Q-T, which is more likely to be a Q-T blending with a relatively high U wave [42, 67].

3. How can a U wave help to distinguish hyperkalemia from other causes of high-peaked T waves?

  ANS.: In hyperkalemia U waves are rarely present.

*4. List the differences between hypokalemia and hypocalcemia on an ECG.

  ANS.: a. Hypocalcemia prolongs the Q-T interval. Hypokalemia causes very little if any prolongation of the Q-T. The Q-T, however, may appear to be prolonged because a giant U wave may attach itself imperceptibly to the end of the T.

  b. Hypocalcemia prolongs the Q to onset of T. Hypokalemia does not [71].

  c. Hypocalcemia rarely lowers T wave amplitude. Hypokalemia does.

5. Are the ECG changes of hypokalemia related to intracellular or to serum potassium?

  ANS.: This question is controversial. The changes are thought by some to be more related to intracellular potassium because hypokalemic ECG changes have been found with low, normal, or even high serum potassium, but they are always seen when the red blood cell potassium levels are low [62]. On the other hand, the infusion of potassium results in prompt disappearance of hypokalemic ECG changes. These changes depend more on the rate of potassium infusion than on the quantity of potassium infused [36].

  Note: a. Repletion studies suggest that the T and U changes in the ECG reflect intracellular potassium depletion, and the S-T depression may be related to the reduced potassium perfusing the heart [66].

  b. Some diabetic patients have Q-Tc prolongation exceeding 0.46 second and a U/T amplitude of 0.50 or more in a V lead despite the absence of hypokalemia. This prolongation is thought due to decreased cellular potassium and has been called the 'hypokalcellic ECG' [1].

T WAVES OF CARDIOMYOPATHIES (MYOCARDIAL INFILTRATION, FIBROSIS, INFLAMMATION)

1. Can you usually tell the difference between an ischemic T and a fibrotic or infiltrative T?

  ANS.: No. Any kind of fibrosis or any infiltrate such as amyloid or carcinoma can cause T waves that imitate the T of ischemia.

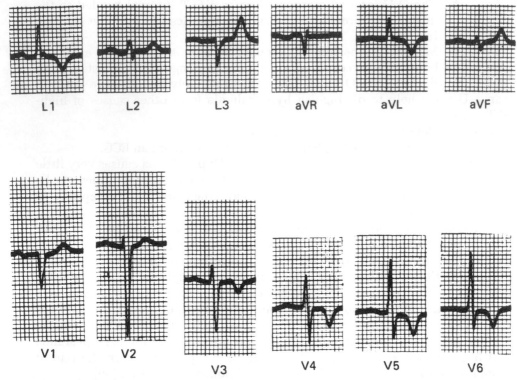

ECG 73. *A 36-year-old man died 1 month after this ECG with a lymphosarcomatous tumor mass involving the full thickness of the left ventricle. The leftward axis (0 degrees) with terminal positivity in aVR qualifies this ECG for a diagnosis of a minor degree of anterior divisional block. The T negativity in V3 to V6 and in lead 1 is due to the infiltrate.*

2. What is a clue that the T negativity is due to fibrosis or inflammation and not to the ischemia of an acute infarct or coronary insufficiency?
   ANS.: a. If it is only shallow T negativity, i.e., less than 5 mm deep [14].
        b. If it is only an exaggerated notch; i.e., there are slight 'shoulders' at or above the baseline that are still part of the T (see ECG 74).

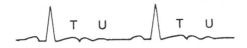

Notched T Waves

1. In which lead is the T normally notched?
   ANS.: It is normal to have notching of the T at the transition T zone between a negative T and a positive T in the precordial leads (see ECG 75).

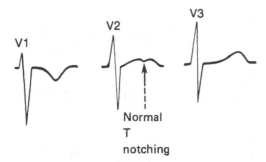

2. List the usual cardiomyopathies[1] that can cause an abnormally notched T wave.
   ANS.: a. Coronary disease causing fibrosis (see ECG 74).
   b. LVH causing fibrosis [14] (see ECG 78).
   c. Myocarditis or inflammation in or around the heart such as that produced by thoracic radiation [68], pericarditis, or infectious diseases, e.g., infectious mononucleosis.
   d. Metabolic diseases affecting the heart, e.g., thyrotoxicosis.
   e. Any infiltrate, e.g., amyloid.
   Note: A long P-R interval and a notched T are the only characteristic findings seen in a small proportion of subjects with hyperthyroidism. The Q-T interval may shorten in some [5, 29].

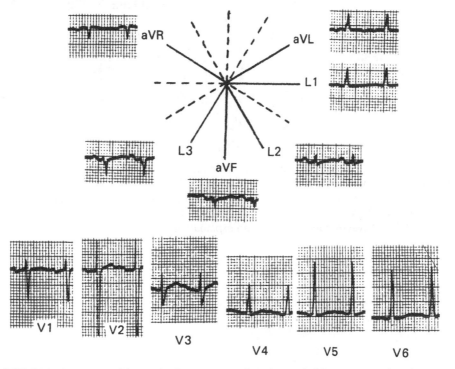

ECG 74A. A 60-year-old man had a necropsy that showed old anteroseptal and posterolateral myocardial infarction. The notched Ts in V3, V4, and V5 are the only signs of cardiac damage. The sum of SV2 and RV6 was the only voltage criterion for the LVH that he had (necropsy revealed biventricular hypertrophy).

[1] The term *cardiomyopathy* is being used in the nonspecific sense of the word. It should be qualified by an adjective to indicate the cause, e.g., 'coronary' or 'idiopathic' cardiomyopathy.

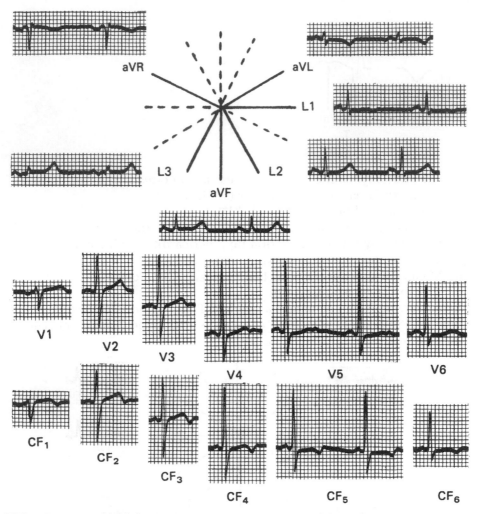

ECG 74B. A 53-year-old man had angina only on first morning effort and during sleep. The notched T waves, well seen in V4 and V5, are due to the fibrosis of coronary disease. The CF leads show that the notch is really a minor degree of T negativity. There are still 'shoulders' belonging to the T wave above the baseline in CF3 to CF5. Therefore these are really only deeply notched T waves. (See p. 339 for an explanation of CF leads.)

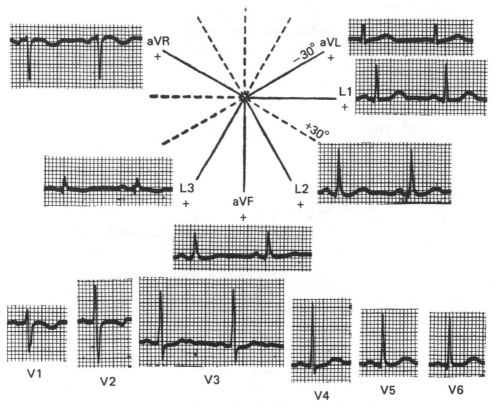

ECG 75. The notched T in V3 is transitional between the negative T in V2 and the positive T in V4. Therefore this notch is normal in this 33-year-old normal black woman. Note the relatively high U that almost always follows a notched T, regardless of whether the notch is normal. The flat-topped T in V4 probably represents a minor degree of notching. Therefore the transition zone for the T is actually spread over two leads.

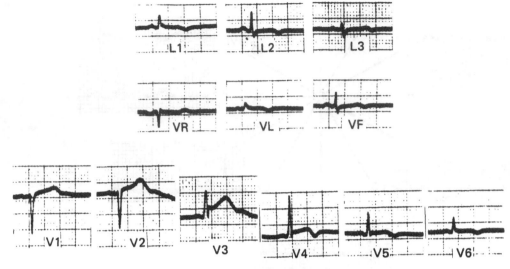

ECG 76. This patient had biopsy-proved amyloidosis of the heart. The S-T elevation in V1 to V6 had been present for years despite normal coronary arteries. Note that only the limb leads show low voltage (less than 10 mm). The negative T waves in many leads have shoulders above the baseline and are therefore really deeply notched T waves.

*3. What noncardiac conditions can produce notched T waves?
ANS.: a. Increased intracranial pressure and cerebral damage, which results in an autonomic imbalance effect on repolarization [31]. These notched T waves may, however, sometimes be due to minor myocardial damage secondary to an autonomic storm, as suggested by the focal myocardial necrosis produced in mice with experimental cerebral hemorrhage [46].
b. The effect of such drugs as alcohol, quinidine, procainamide, or some psychotropic drugs, e.g., lithium or tranquilizers such as phenothiazines, especially thioridazine [6, 55]. The notching occurs at therapeutic doses and with or without Q-T prolongation [30].
c. Marked hypomagnesemia [69].

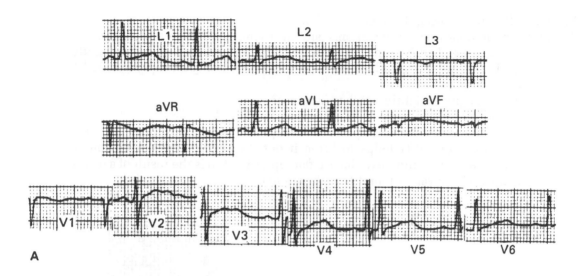

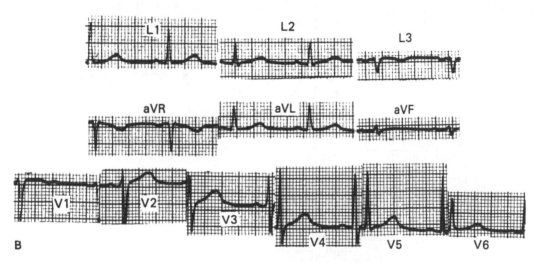

ECG 77. A. Quinidine toxicity in a 65-year-old man with vomiting and diarrhea. He was also receiving digoxin and furosemide. The quinidine level was 8.5 mg per liter. Note the notched T waves and a prolonged Q-T. The Q-Tc is 510 msec (upper limit of normal is 430 msec). B. Two days after quinidine was stopped the Q-Tc was 460 msec, and the notched T waves were gone.

Note: a. About 20 percent of alcoholic patients have various degrees of T notching or inversion in left precordial leads if an ECG is taken on the same day as the last drink [58].

b. The abnormal notch caused by phenothiazines can be reversed by an overnight fast, 10 g of potassium chloride, or 40 mg of propranolol [3]. It is often seen only after a meal [13].

c. A rare cause of T notching is an allergic reaction to penicillin [28].

d. Muscular dystrophies such as Friedreich's ataxia can produce any degree of T abnormalities from notching to deep negativity.

4. Why is it difficult to recognize a notched T wave?

    ANS.: With the poor frequency response and overdamping of many direct writers, a slightly notched T often appears only flat-topped [14]. Also, a slightly negative T with its shoulders above the baseline is really a deeply notched T (see CF4 in ECG 74).

5. How can you recognize slightly notched T waves?

    ANS.: Any low or flat-topped T followed by a relatively high U wave should be looked at closely for notching. A double-sensitivity (double-standardization) ECG helps to bring it out, especially if taken at double speed. T waves should never have a flat top. A flat top is the result of a direct writing stylus's vain attempt to make a notch.

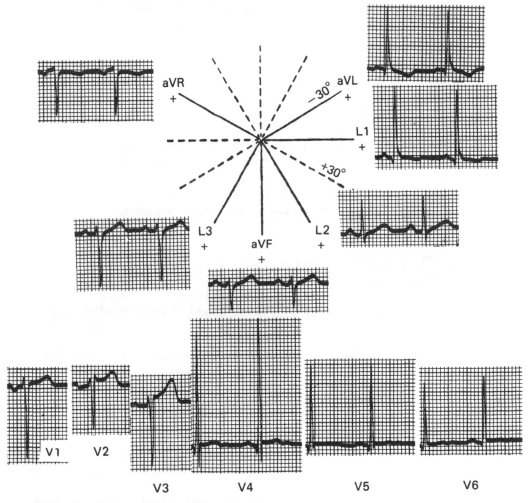

ECG 78. This ECG is from a hypertensive woman age 47 years. Note the notched T in V4, V5, and V6. This pattern is one of the common secondary changes found in the ECGs of subjects with LVH. (The T in V1 is larger than the T in V6. Therefore it is turned more anteriorly than usual. Also, the T in V5 and V6 is less than 10 percent of the QRS. Therefore these Ts are abnormally low. These changes are all secondary signs of LVH.)

*6. What proof is there that an abnormally notched T is really a minor degree of T inversion?

ANS.: If one uses a CF chest lead (see Note at end of answer), it often converts a precordial notched T into an inverted T (see ECG 74).

Note: A CF chest lead is a bipolar lead with a negative electrode as the foot electrode and a positive electrode as the chest exploring electrode. (It is no longer used as a routine chest lead.) If the machine has no built-in CF lead system, you can perform a CF type of precordial exploration by using any bipolar lead, e.g., lead 1. If you use lead 1, put the right arm negative electrode on a leg and use the positive left arm electrode for the chest leads. Then switch to lead 1 on the machine.

DIGITALIS EFFECT ON THE T WAVE

1. Does digitalis affect the direction of a T wave?

ANS.: Not in the basal state. In response to minor autonomic or hypertrophic metabolic changes, the T may change direction. It may bring out an LVH strain pattern that was not present before digitalis. Also it can turn the T posteriorly away from the right ventricle in patients with RVH [38].

2. What does digitalis do to the T wave even in the basal state?

ANS.: a. It decreases its magnitude (see ECG 57, p. 265).

b. It shortens its duration; i.e., the Q-T interval is shortened.

c. It causes the S-T segment to sag, usually below the baseline.

T WAVE IN HYPOTHYROIDISM

How can hypothyroidism affect the T?

ANS.: It tends to turn the T away from the QRS to make a wide QRS-T angle in all planes. The T amplitude usually remains low, often in all 12 leads (see ECG 93, p. 382).

REFERENCES

1. Abarquez, R. F., Jr. Hypokalcellic electrocardiograms and diabetes mellitus. *Far East Med. J.* 2:272, 1966.

2. Ahnve, S., Lundman, T., and Shoaleh-var, M. The relationship between QT interval and ventricular arrhythmias in acute myocardial infarction. *Acta Med. Scand.* 204:17, 1978.

3. Alvarez-Mean, S. C., and Frank, M. J. Phenothiazine-induced T-wave abnormalities. *J.A.M.A.* 224:1730, 1973.

4. Ameur-Hedrich, et al. Onde U négative a valeur diagnostique et prognostique: Apropos de 100 cas. *Ann. Cardiol. Angeiol.* (*Paris*) 25:103, 1976.

5. Baker, S. P., Landowne, M., and Gaffney, G. W. Electrocardiographic changes following the administration of thyroid stimulating hormone (thyrotropin). *Am. J. Cardiol.* 6:905, 1960.

6. Ban, T. A., and St. Jean, A. Electrocardiographic changes induced by phenothiazine drugs. *Am. J. Cardiol.* 16:575, 1965.
7. Bashour, T., Rios, J. C., and Gorman, P. A. U wave alternans and increased ventricular irritability. *Chest* 64:377, 1973.
8. Bharati, S. and Lev, M. Cardiac disease in sudden death. *Arch. Intern. Med.* 144:1811, 1984.
8A. Bidoggia, H., Maciel, J. P., Capalozza, N., Mosca, S., et al. Sex-dependent electrocardiographic pattern of cardiac repolarization. *Am. Heart J.* 140:430–436, 2000.
9. Bradlow, B. A., and Segel, N. Acute hyperparathyroidism with electrocardiographic changes. *Br. Heart J.* 2:197, 1956.
10. Braun, H. A., Surawicz, B., and Bellet, S. T waves in hyperpotassemia: Their differentiation from simulating T waves in other conditions. *Am. J. Med. Sci.* 230:147, 1955.
11. Bronsky, D., et al. Calcium and electrocardiogram. *Am. J. Cardiol.* 7:840, 1961.
12. Burch, G. E., and Phillips, J. H. The large upright T wave as an electrocardiographic manifestation of intracranial disease. *South. Med. J.* 61:331, 1968.
13. Chouinard, G., and Anable, L. Phenothiazine-induced ECG abnormalities. *Arch. Gen. Psychiatry* 34:951, 1977.
14. Constant, J., and Carlisle, R. The notched T in LVH and in alcoholism. *Chest* 57:540, 1970.
14A. Corazza, G. R., et al. Investigation of Q-T interval in celiac disease. *Br. Med. J.* 304:1285, 1992.
15. Crampton, R. Preeminence of the left stellate ganglion in the long Q-T syndrome. *Circulation* 59:769, 1979.
16. Cruickshank, J. M. Effect of oral propranolol on ECG changes in subarachnoid hemorrhage. *Cardiovasc. Res.* 9:236, 1975.
17. Doroghazi, R. M., and Childers, R. Time-related changes in the Q-T interval in acute myocardial infarction: Possible relation to local hypocalcemia. *Am. J. Cardiol.* 41:684, 1978.
17A. Dreyfuss, D., et al. Tall T waves during metabolic acidosis. *Crit. Care Med.* 17:404, 1989.
18. Elek, S. R., et al. The Q-T interval in myocardial infarction and left ventricular hypertrophy. *Am. Heart J.* 45:80, 1953.
19. Eyer, K. M. U wave alternans: An electrocardiographic sign of left ventricular failure. *Am. Heart J.* 87:41, 1974.
20. Fisch, C., et al. Potassium and the monophasic action potential, electrocardiogram, conduction and arrhythmias. *Cardiovasc. Comp.* 1:52, 1966.
21. Furbetta, D., et al. Abnormality of the U wave of the T-U segment of the electrocardiogram: The syndrome of the papillary muscles. *Circulation* 14:1129, 1956.
22. Furbetta, D., et al. Morphologic aspects of the negativity of the U wave and their corresponding electrocardiographic and clinical data. *Circulation* 14:859, 1956.
22A. Gardner, K., et al. The spinous T wave. *Am. J. Cardiol.* 48:201, 1981.
23. Garza, L. A., et al. Hereditable Q-T prolongation without deafness. *Circulation* 41:39, 1970.
24. Georgopoulos, A. J., Proudfit, W. L., and Page, I. H. Relationship between arterial pressure and negative U waves. *Circulation* 23:675, 1961.
25. Gerson, M. D., and McHenry, P. L. Resting U wave inversion as a marker of stenosis of anterior descending. *Am. J. Med.* 69:545, 1980.
26. Gonzalez-de-Cossio, A., Sanchez-Medal, L., and Smyth, J. F. Electrocardiographic modifications in anemia. *Am. Heart J.* 67:166, 1964.
27. Gould, L., Reddy, C. V. R., and Gomprecht, R. F. His bundle electrograms in a patient with hyperkalemia. *J.A.M.A.* 230:87, 1974.
28. Haden, R. F., and Langsjoen, P. H. Manifestations of myocardial involvement in acute reactions to penicillin. *Am. J. Cardiol.* 8:420, 1961.
29. Hoffman, I., and Lowrey, R. D. The electrocardiogram in thyrotoxicosis. *Am. J. Cardiol.* 6:893, 1960.
30. Huston, J. R., and Bell, G. E. The effect of thioridazine and chlorpromazine on the ECG. *J.A.M.A.* 198:134, 1966.
31. Jachuck, S. J. Electrocardiographic abnormalities with increased intracranial pressure. *Br. Med. J.* 1:242, 1975.

32. Jervell, A., and Lange-Nielsen, F. Congenital deaf-mutism, functional heart disease with prolongation of the Q-T interval and sudden death. *Am. Heart J.* 54:59, 1957.
33. Jorgensen, F. S., and Hedebo, S. Elektrokardiografiske undersogelser hos kroniske alkoholikers. *Nord. Med.* 80:1441, 1968.
34. Harhunen, P., et al. Syncope and Q-T prolongation without deafness: The Romano-Ward syndrome. *Am. Heart J.* 80:820, 1970.
34A. Hasegawa, K., Sawayama, T., Nezuo, S., Mitani, K. Exercise-induced T wave normalization associated with U wave inversion in detection of critical left anterior descending artery stenosis.
35. Kast, G., and Klepzig, H. The clinical significance of a negative U-wave in the electrocardiographic exercise test. *Z. Kreislaufforsch.* 54:1156, 1965.
36. Klutsch, K. Extracellular and intracellular potassium, blood pressure and electrocardiogram in potassium depletion by hemodialysis. *Arch. Kreislaufforsch.* 47:246, 1966.
37. Leachman, D. R., Dekmer, G. J., and Hills, L. D. Evaluation of postextrasystolic T alterations. *Am. Heart J.* 102:658, 1981.
37A. Lehmannm, M. H., Suzukim, F., Fromm, B. S., Frankovich, D. A., et al. T wave 'humps' as a potential electrocardiographic marker of the long QT syndrome. *J. Am. Coll. Cardiol.* 24:746–754, 1994.
38. Lemberg, L., Boucek, R. J., and Castellanos, A. Digitalis as an indicant of ventricular disease. *Dis. Chest* 52:490, 1967.
39. Lepeschkin, E. The U wave of the electrocardiogram. *Mod. Concepts Cardiovasc. Dis.* 38:39, 1969.
40. Lepeschkin, E. et al. Effect of epinephrine and norepinephrine on the electrocardiogram of 100 normal subjects. *Am. J. Cardiol.* 5:594, 1960.
41. Lichtman, J. et al. Electrocardiogram of the athlete. *Arch. Intern. Med.* 132:763, 1973.
42. Loeb, H. S. et al. Paroxysmal ventricular fibrillation in two patients with hypomagnesemia: Treatment by transvenous pacing. *Circulation* 38:210, 1968.
43. Luomanmaki, K., Heikkila, J., and Hartikainen, M. T-wave alternans associated with heart failure and hypomagnesemia in alcoholic cardiomyopathy. *Eur. J. Cardiol.* 3/3:167, 1975.
44. Mathews, E. C., Jr., Blount, A. W., Jr., and Townsend, J. I. Q-T prolongation and ventricular arrhythmias, with and without deafness in the same family. *Am. J. Cardiol.* 29:702, 1972.
45. McVay, M. R., et al. Idiopathic long Q-T syndrome. *J. Electrocardiol.* 15:189, 1982.
46. Millar, K., and Abildskov, J. A. Notched T waves in young persons with central nervous system lesions. *Circulation* 37:597, 1968.
46A. Miwa, K., Miyagi, Y., Fujita, M., Fujiki, A., Sasayama, S. Transient terminal U wave inversion as a more specific marker for myocardial ischemia. *Am. Heart J.* 125:981–987, 1998.
47. Morris, S. N., and McHenry, P. L. Role of exercise stress testing in healthy subjects and patients with coronary disease. *Am. J. Cardiol.* 42:659, 1978.
48. Narasimahan, P. Electrocardiography and hyperkalemia. *Lancet* 2:317, 1960.
49. Navarro-Lopez, F., et al. Isolated T wave alternans. *Am. Heart J.* 95:369, 1978.
50. Nierberg, D. W., and Ransil, B. J. QaT$_c$ interval as a clinical indicator of hypercalcemia. *Am. J. Cardiol.* 44:243, 1979.
51. Olley, P. M., and Fowler, R. S. The surdo-cardiac syndrome and therapeutic observations. *Br. Heart J.* 32:467, 1970.
52. Phillips, J., and Ichinose, H. Clinical and pathologic studies in hereditary syndrome of long QT interval, syncopal spells, and sudden death. *Chest* 58:236, 1970.
53. Ricketts, H. H., Denison, E. K., and Haywood, L. J. Unusual T-wave abnormality: Repolarization alternans associated with hypomagnesemia, acute alcoholism, and cardiomyopathy. *J.A.M.A.* 207:365, 1969.
54. Rumancik, W. M., et al. The QT interval and serum ionized calcium. *J.A.M.A.* 240:366, 1978.
55. Saint-Jean, A., and Desautels, S. Changements électrocardiographiques avec un neuroleptique: la thioridazine. *Union Med. Can.* 95:554, 1966.
56. Schwartz, P. J. and Malliani, A. Electrical alternation of the T-wave: Clinical and experimental evidence of its relationship with the sympathetic nervous system and with the long Q-T syndrome. *Am. Heart J.* 89:45, 1975.
57. Schwartz, P. J., Periti, M., and Malliani, A. The long Q-T syndrome. *Am. Heart J.* 89:378, 1975.

58. Sereny, G. Effects of alcohol on the electrocardiogram. *Circulation* 44:558, 1971.
59. Seta, K., et al. Effect of potassium and magnesium deficiency on the electrocardiogram and plasma electrolytes of pure-bred beagles. *Am. J. Cardiol.* 17:516, 1966.
60. Shechter, E., Freeman, C. C., and Lazarra, R. Afterdepolarizations as a mechanism for the long Q-T syndrome. *J. Am. Coll. Cardiol.* 3:1556, 1984.
61. Simonson, E. The effect of age on the electrocardiogram. *Am. J. Cardiol.* 29:64, 1972.
62. Soloff, L. A., Kanosky, S. A., and Boutwell, J. H. The relationship of the electrocardiographic pattern of potassium depletion to the concentration of potassium in red blood cells. *Am. J. Med. Sci.* 240:280, 1960.
63. Surawicz, B. Electrolytes and the electrocardiogram. *Am. J. Cardiol.* 12:656, 1963.
64. Surawicz, B. U wave–the controversial genesis and the clinical significance. *Jpn. Heart. J.* (Suppl.) 23:17, 1982.
65. Surawicz, B., and Lasseter, K. C. Electrocardiogram in pericarditis. *Am. J. Cardiol.* 26:471, 1970.
66. Swales, J. D. Hypokalemia and the electrocardiogram. *Lancet* 2:1365, 1964.
66A. Tamura, A., Watanabe, T., Nagose, K., Mikuriya, Y., Nasu, M. Significance of negative U waves in the precordial leads during anterior wall acute myocardial infarction. *Am. J. Cardiol.* 79:897–900, 1997.
67. Taran, L. M., and Ordorico, D. Electrical systole (Q-T intervals in acute rheumatic pericarditis in children). *Pediatrics* 5:947, 1950.
68. VanderArk, C. R., Ballantyne, F., III, and Reynolds, E. W., Jr. Electrolytes and the electrocardiogram. *Cardiovasc. Clin.* 5:270, 1973.
68A. Viskin, S., Heller, K., Barron, H. V., Kitzis, I., Hamdan, M., et al. Post-extrasystolic U wave augmentation, a new marker of increased arrhythmic risk in patients without the long QT syndrome. *J. Am. Coll. Cardiol.* 28:1745–1752, 1996.
68B. Viskin, S., Kitzis, I., Heller, K., Olgin, J., et al. Postextrasystolic U-wave augmentation: A potential new risk marker for sudden arrhythmic events in patients with normal QT. *Circulation* (Suppl.), 92:1–681, 1995.
69. Wan-Chun, C., and Xin-Xiang, F. Electrocardiographic changes of magnesium deficiency. *Am. Heart J.* 104:1115, 1982.
70. Wellens, H. J. J. Isolated alternans of the T wave. *Chest* 64:319, 1972.
71. Whitfield, A. G. W., and Kunkler, P. B. Radiation reactions in the heart. *Br. Heart J.* 19:53, 1957.
72. Williams, J. A., Littmann, D., and Warren, R. Experiences with the surgical treatment of mitral stenosis. *N. Engl. J. Med.* 258:623, 1958.
73. Wortsman, J., and Frank, S. The Q-T interval in clinical hypercalcemia. *Clin. Cardiol.* 4:87, 1981.

23. Benign T Abnormalities and Syndromes

List the types of T abnormalities and syndromes associated with a normal myocardium.

ANS.: a. Juvenile T pattern.
b. Neurotic heart T syndrome.
c. Hyperventilation T abnormalities.
d. Isolated T negativity syndrome.
e. Benign T negativity of athletes.
f. Cerebral autonomic T abnormalities.
g. Prolapsed mitral valve syndrome.
h. Suspended heart syndrome.
i. T inversion of schizophrenia.
j. T changes after artificial pacing.
k. Post-tachycardia T abnormalities.
l. T changes in intermittent left bundle branch block [1].

JUVENILE T PATTERN

1. What is meant by the 'juvenile T pattern'?
ANS.: As used in the literature, there are three possible meanings.
a. Any T negativity in the right precordium, even if only in V1 and V2.
b. T negativity from V1 to V3 or V4.
*c. T negativity from V1 to V3 or V4 with the T slightly posterior to the QRS; i.e., if the QRS is positive or equiphasic in V3, the T is negative in V3 (see ECG 79).
Note: a. A T that is negative in the right precordium should always have a negative QRS. If the negative T has an equiphasic QRS, it means that the T is posterior to the QRS.
b. The juvenile T may show as negativity from only V1 to V2, but the T may be notched as far as V5 [44].

---

* Material marked with an asterisk is included for reference and for advanced students in cardiology.

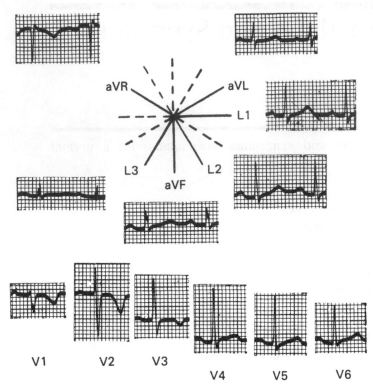

ECG 79. A juvenile T pattern in a normal 34-year-old black woman in the hospital for a
hysterectomy because of fibroids. The QRS is positive in V3, yet the T is still negative.
Note: Even the QRS is 'juvenile' because the patient has an atypical right bundle branch block
pattern, common in children; i.e., there is an S in L1, L2, and L3 and a shallow S in V1.

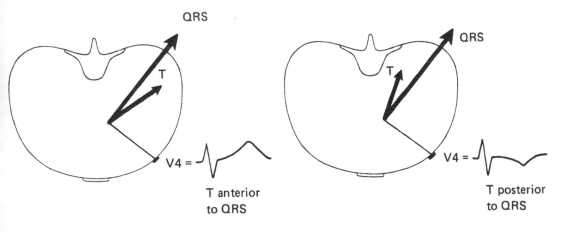

T anterior
to QRS

T posterior
to QRS

2. Why is it called the *juvenile* T pattern?
    ANS.: Because the T is normally negative in the right precordium in children, but
           by adolescence the T is rarely negative beyond V1.
           Note: The usual adult age group in which the juvenile T pattern is seen is
           between 20 and 40. Although it is said to be common in young black men, it
           was seen in only 1 percent in a study in a northern state in the United States,

and even then the T negativity did not go beyond V3 [42]. In another study on black college students in a southern state, about 10 percent showed it [44].

*3. What is the importance of recognizing the juvenile T pattern?

ANS.: It is the only time that a T is normally posterior to a QRS.

*4. Which maneuvers can change the juvenile pattern into the adult pattern?

ANS.: a. A deep inspiration.

b. Atropine-like drugs (suggesting that it is a manifestation of hypervagotonia [46]).

c. Repeating the ECG with the patient in a fasting state [40].

d. A large dose of oral potassium chloride. (This method is dangerous in patients with myocardial damage [44].) You should probably not use more than 45 mEq of liquid potassium chloride [15, 38]. The T negativity due to organic heart disease either becomes more negative or remains unchanged after potassium chloride [8].

e. Hyperventilation for 3 minutes.

Note: Hyperventilation for 10 to 15 seconds can produce a juvenile T pattern in about 10 percent of normal subjects, although less often in whites than in blacks [45]. In view of the fact that a short period of hyperventilation can produce S-T, T abnormalities, it is surprising that prolonged hyperventilation often normalizes them. This phenomenon may be explained by the finding that a short period of hyperventilation initiates a vagal reflex [46].

---

*NEUROTIC HEART T SYNDROME

*1. What is the neurotic heart T syndrome?

ANS.: Some nervous persons with symptoms of palpitations, weakness, and chest pains of a nonanginal type have ECGs showing T waves that are low or negative in the inferior leads and left precordium. The T negativity may be exaggerated or seen only on standing. This condition is often referred to as neurocirculatory asthenia.

Note: a. The neurotic heart T negativity is usually due to sympathetic overactivity but occasionally to sympathetic underactivity. This finding is suggested by the fact that it can be reversed by beta blockade (propranolol) [5] or by the atropine-like drug propantheline bromide (Pro-Banthine) [45]. Persons with sympathetic overactivity often have episodes of sinus tachycardia of 150 per minute or more documented during their daily routine without undue effort [43].

b. A short period of hyperventilation is vagotonic and can sometimes make the neurotic T negativity worse. This situation can be prevented by atropine. (Hyperventilation has the same effect on the juvenile T pattern and the lowered or diphasic T of a standing athlete.)

c. Ingestion of 100 g of glucose can worsen benign T abnormalities in young people in about 25 minutes [33, 39].

*2. Which kind of patient other than neurotic subjects may show orthostatic T lowering or negativity?

ANS.: Not only may subjects with ischemic heart disease have this pattern, but the left ventricular T waves of 25 to 50 percent of the normal population are lowered on standing, even if they are athletes [26]. However, these T wave changes are, at most, biphasic and not inversions.

Note: The lowered T on standing in many normal subjects is not due to changes in heart position because

a. The T wave can be seen to revert from upright to diphasic in a gradual manner as the subject stands [26].

b. Amyl nitrite or fever can reproduce the T changes in the recumbent position.

c. Some orthostatic T changes in normal people can be produced only with hyperventilation as the subject stands [26].

d. The T changes can be prevented by propranolol or potassium chloride administration [15, 32].

*3. What metabolic abnormality has been blamed for producing minor T abnormalities in subjects with such neurotic symptoms as palpitations, fatigue, and anxiety?

ANS.: A possible hypoovarian state was suggested by reversal of both symptoms and T abnormalities with the administration of estrogens in women who had menstrual irregularities or pelvic surgery prior to the development of symptoms [37]. There are reports of women with fibroids who have T wave abnormalities. One such patient had normal T waves only during heavy periods and after an oophorectomy and hysterectomy [17].

Note: Palpitations, fatigue, and anxiety are also seen in some patients with prolapsed mitral valves. These patients also have minor T abnormalities (see p. 354).

HYPERVENTILATION SYNDROME T ABNORMALITIES

1. What is the hyperventilation syndrome?

ANS.: It is a syndrome that usually occurs in young and middle-aged adults and consists in tension-induced chest discomfort (sharp pain, dull ache, or heaviness) without a definite relation to exertion but often with dyspnea, fatigue, nervousness, and palpitations. These patients tend to hyperventilate under tension. The syndrome is seen most often in women.

2. What effect does 3 minutes of voluntary hyperventilation have on the T in V5 or V6 of (a) normal subjects, (b) subjects with the hyperventilation syndrome?

ANS.: Various degrees of T negativity, from slight notching up to 4 mm of inversion.

Note: a. The vagotonic effect of a short period of hyperventilation (30–60 sec) can cause T negativity even in athletes [26].

b. The T changes of hyperventilation can be reversed by intravenous potassium chloride (20–30 mEq), intravenous phentolamine, or oral propranolol [7]. They can be prevented by eliminating the respiratory alkalosis (breathing 6% CO_2) [50].

c. Several theories are postulated to account for the T changes of hyperventilation.

According to one theory, since prolonged hyperventilation causes a combined effect of respiratory alkalosis and catecholamine excess, there is a migration of potassium from inside to outside the cell. (The coronary sinus potassium level increases during hyperventilation, and serum potassium levels also rise with epinephrine injection [50].)

*S-T, T ABNORMALITIES AND THE VALSALVA MANEUVER

*1. What happens during a Valsalva maneuver to the S-T, T abnormalities due to hyperventilation and to organic heart disease?
ANS.: Hyperventilation abnormalities are often rectified, but the T wave abnormalities due to organic disease are not affected by a Valsalva test unless the subject also has an autonomic imbalance [27].

*2. How can a Valsalva maneuver help diagnose the false-positive functional T abnormalities of an exercise test?
ANS.: A Valsalva maneuver exaggerates the autonomic imbalance and always magnifies the T abnormality of the control tracing.
Note: To exaggerate an autonomic imbalance, the subject should strain as long as possible and strongly enough to produce a tachycardia and peaking of the P waves in leads 2 and aVF.

ISOLATED T NEGATIVITY SYNDROME

1. What is the isolated T negativity syndrome?
ANS.: A negative T (often only terminal negativity) in only one or two mid-precordial leads.

*2. What has suggested that an isolated T negativity is due to picking up some vectors that depend entirely on proximity for their recording?
ANS.: A deep inspiration can make them disappear.
Note: It does not mean, however, that an area of localized T negativity is surrounded by an area of positivity. When the null zone for the T is drawn, it merely takes a tortuous S-shaped course down the chest. Deep inspiration merely rotates the heart so that the null zone is shifted slightly to the right, shifting the chest electrode into the positive side of the null zone [4]. (See p. 66 for an explanation of 'null zone.')

*3. What is the danger when neurotic heart T negativity or isolated T negativity occurs together with the S-T elevation of early repolarization?
ANS.: The combination of these two benign changes resembles acute myocardial infarction. This normal variant is most commonly seen in black patients (see ECG 56, p. 262).

Early repolarization   Isolated T negativity   Both together

BENIGN T NEGATIVITY OF ATHLETES

1. In which leads is the benign T negativity of athletes seen?

   ANS.: In the inferior and left precordial leads, i.e., in the same leads as in the neurotic T abnormalities.

   Note: Athletes of championship caliber tend to show these changes [21].

*2. What can correct this T abnormality of athletes?

   ANS.: a. Maximal or near-maximal exercise. (A Master two-step has no effect on these T inversions [31].)

         b. Isoproterenol infusion [51].

         c. Interruption of training [21].

*3. What theory has been proposed to account for these T changes?

   ANS.: Excess sympathetic inhibition in top-ranking athletes somehow causes an uneven repolarization process in the left ventricle. Excess vagotonia cannot be inferred because there is supposedly little direct parasympathetic influence on ventricular repolarization.

   Note: These T abnormalities are seen in some nonathletes who have an excess sympathetic inhibition of unknown etiology [16]. This situation is suspected from their bradycardia and proved by seeing the T waves disappear with atropine or exercise. (See pp. 262 and 379 for other ECG changes seen in athletes.)

*4. What surgical procedure can produce an autonomic abnormality that can affect the T waves?

   ANS.: Following truncal vagotomy, about 10 percent of patients have marked T wave abnormalities that mimic acute infarction [19].

CEREBRAL AUTONOMIC T ABNORMALITIES

*1. Which parts of the left ventricle do the right and left sympathetic pathways supply?

ANS.: The right sympathetic pathways supply the anterior left ventricle, and the left pathways supply the posterior wall.

*2. Why do cerebral hemorrhage, unilateral carotid occlusion, and intracranial lesions cause T wave abnormalities?

ANS.: Experiments in animals have shown that unbalancing the sympathetic nerve supply to the myocardium by ablation or stimulation of one stellate ganglion causes the T waves to move markedly anteriorly or posteriorly, depending on which stellate ganglion was made dominant. Stimulation of the right ganglion or left stellate ganglionectomy produces negative T waves, whereas reversing the sides that are stimulated and ablated produces upright T waves [49].

Note: a. Either excess sympatheticotonia or sympathetic inhibition can cause or correct T wave abnormalities. It is not surprising that an imbalance of sympathetic input to different parts of the heart can be corrected by either beta-adrenergic stimulation or beta blockade by allowing more homogeneous repolarization of the myocardium. Isoproterenol can completely correct the abnormal T waves seen in intracranial lesions but not the T waves of ischemia, bundle branch block, or LVH [14].

b. Hearts of patients dying of subarachnoid hemorrhage usually have focal necrotic lesions, probably catecholamine-induced because they can be prevented by propranolol [30].

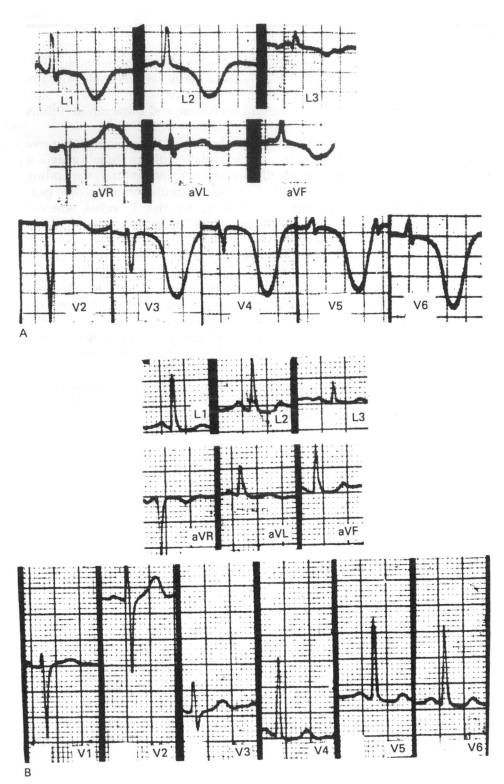

ECG 80. A. A 32-year-old woman was admitted with a diagnosis of sudden left carotid occlusion. B. This ECG was taken 2 days after cerebral angiography had confirmed the diagnosis. It has returned almost to normal.

*3. How severely can an ECG be affected by cerebral hemorrhage?

ANS.: a. The T waves in the precordium can become either deeply negative or very tall and peaked [3, 22]. (*Giant negative T waves* and *giant peaked upright T waves* are commonly used terms [25, 36].) The Q-T is usually prolonged, and the T may fuse with a large U wave.

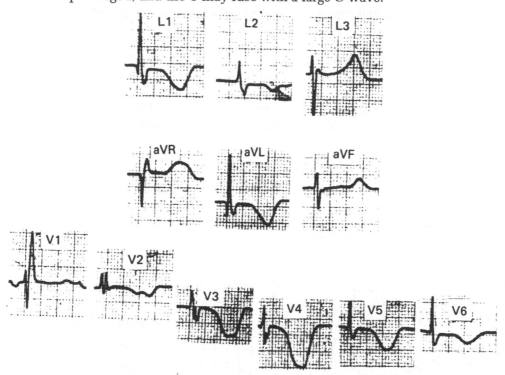

ECG 81. *This ECG with giant negative T waves in the precordium is from a young woman who had had a cerebral hemorrhage 1 week before, when the T waves in V4 and V5 were even deeper. The notched T in V2 is easily confused with a T + U. The sharp second peak of the T in V1 is a P wave. (She had intermittent atrioventricular block with junctional escape beats.) There is also a right bundle branch block and left axis deviation due to anterior divisional block.*

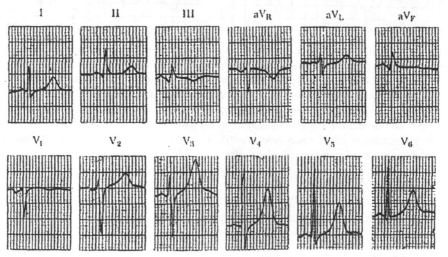

Tall, positive T waves in a 58-year-old man with subarachnoid hemorrhage.

      b. Necrosis vectors and subendocardial injury currents may occur owing to myocardial necrosis, probably of neurohumoral origin [9, 20].

    Note: a. Actual myocardial damage has been documented histologically in many reports of patients dying from intracranial lesions, either after neurosurgery or spontaneously [12, 34].

        b. Transmural injury currents may also occur, and at least three subjects with such an injury current were found at autopsy to have had normal hearts [13, 23].

4. What is the slightest T abnormality that can be caused by cerebral damage?

    ANS.: a. An abnormal notch on the T wave. (See p. 332 for definition of normal notch.)

        b. An inferior turning of the T axis (negative in aVL) [24].

5. List some of the causes of giant T inversions other than cerebral damage or carotid occlusion.

    ANS.: a. Acute myocardial infarction.

        b. Right ventricular hypertrophy [25].

        c. Injection of contrast material for coronary angiography [25].

        d. Pheochromocytoma.

        e. Steroid therapy for complete antrioventricular block or following a Stokes-Adams attack [25].

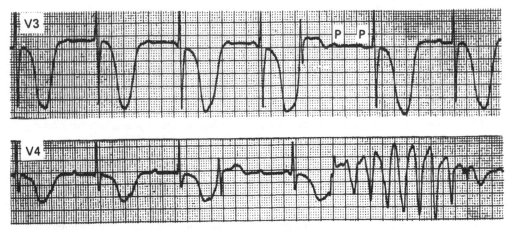

ECG 82. Giant T negativity in a 35-year-old woman with aortic stenosis and syncopal attacks due to complete atrioventricular block and paroxysms of ventricular flutter. The Q-T is prolonged (more than 50 percent of the R-R). Giant T inversion with complete atrioventricular block and a prolonged Q-T tells you that the patient has syncopal (Stokes-Adams) attacks. The atria are manifesting sinus tachycardia, and the lower pacemaker is in the junctional area (only slightly widened QRS). The premature complexes may be either junctional premature beats or capture beats due to 'supernormal' conduction (see p. 490). A rapid ventricular tachycardia at a rate of 220 is generally considered to be ventricular flutter.

f. Truncal vagotomy [19].
g. Hypertensive encephalopathy [41].
h. After electronic pacing of the ventricle.
i. LV apical hypertrophy.

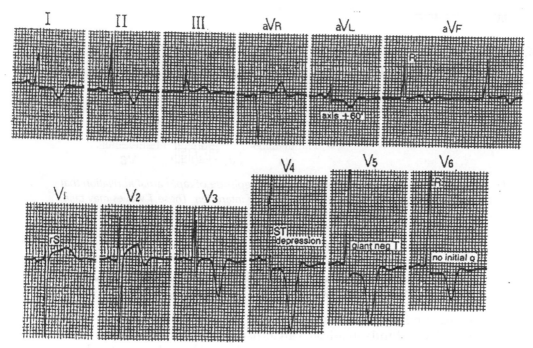

This ECG is from a 46-year-old female with hypertrophy confined to her left ventricular apex.

j. Large muscular false tendons within the LV and anomalously placed papillary muscles.
k. During active upper intestinal bleeding usually with alcoholism and hypertension and low potassium but no apparent coronary disease. The T waves normalize with transfusions of packed red blood cells [11A].
l. Effect of a long period of tachycardia or the post-tachycardia ECG.

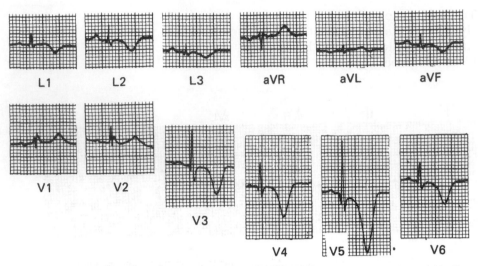

| L1 | L2 | L3 | aVR | aVL | aVF |

| V1 | V2 | V3 | V4 | V5 | V6 |

ECG 83. This ECG is from an elderly woman 6 days after an episode of rapid atrial fibrillation that lasted about 1 day, without symptoms or enzyme changes of infarction. These T waves may take several weeks to return to the normal appearance of the patient's pretachycardia ECG.

---

*PROLAPSED MITRAL VALVE SYNDROME

*1. What is the prolapsed mitral valve syndrome?

ANS.: A congenitally redundant mitral valve, usually with myxomatous transformation, part of which protrudes into the left atrium abnormally during systole, often producing a nonejection click with or without a mitral regurgitant murmur and nonspecific chest pain. The syndrome includes

a. A tendency toward ventricular or atrial arrhythmias.

b. T notching or frank negativity in left ventricular leads, sometimes spreading to mid-precordial leads.

c. A superior turning of the T wave, so that in aVF it becomes negative.

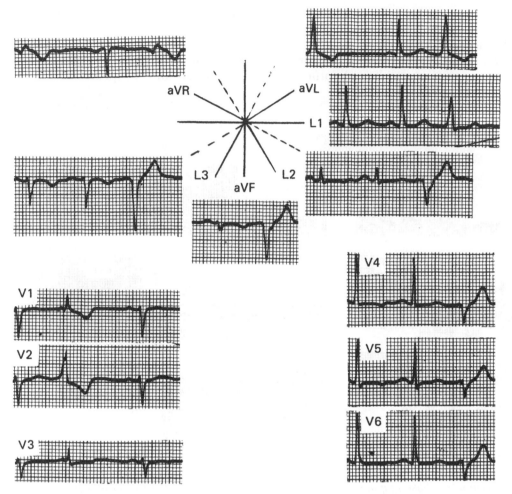

ECG 83A. T abnormality and frequent premature ventricular complexes in a 30-year-old woman with an apical click and faint late systolic murmur due to a prolapsed mitral valve, confirmed angiographically. The T is superiorly directed (negative in aVF). The first negative T in V4, V5, and V6 is the result of a preceding long diastole, which is not shown here. The second T follows a normal diastole and has a positive T. The aVF strip shows the cycle after a long diastole. After a normal cycle, which is not shown here, the T in aVF (and in lead 3) is not quite so deep but is still negative.

*Note: a. If a patient with Marfan's syndrome has a negative T in aVF, a myxomatous mitral valve is probable.

b. An occasional patient has a necrosis Q wave abnormality despite normal coronary arteries and normal myocardial motion on angiography [28].

c. In one study of patients with mitral valve prolapse, most had a prolonged Q-T interval, possibly accounting for the occasional ventricular arrhythmias and sudden death in these patients [6].

d. About 25 percent usually have inferolateral S-T depression, T wave inversions, or Q-T prolongation. These changes are as common in asymptomatic as in symptomatic patients [29A].

*2. What is the cause of the T abnormalities and arrhythmias of the prolapsed valve syndrome?

ANS.: The cause is unknown.

> *Note:* a. Dangerous ventricular arrhythmias are to be expected only in patients with T abnormalities in the inferior and left precordial leads [10].
>
> b. In many subjects the T abnormalities are largely on an autonomic basis, as they may be normalized by a beta blocker [2].

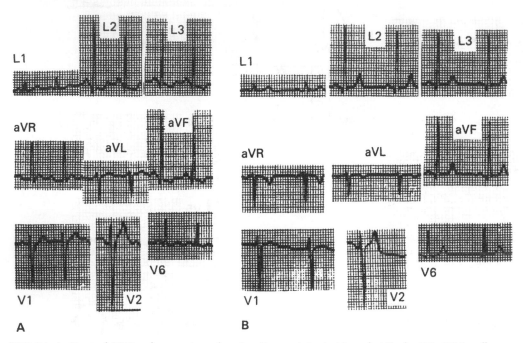

ECG 84. A. Control ECG, taken supine, showing T negativity in L3 and aVF; the T in V1 is taller than the T in V6. There is a slight tachycardia. B. One hour after oral propranolol, the heart rate is slower and the T wave is normal.

---

*SUSPENDED HEART SYNDROME

*1. What is the suspended heart syndrome?

ANS.: Nonspecific chest pains with

> a. Leftward and posterior axis of the T wave even with deep inspiration (negative T in the inferior limb leads and left chest leads) and often with S-T depression in the leads with the negative T waves. The QRS axis is often inferior.
>
> b. The heart moving an unusual distance from the diaphragm on deep inspiration, especially in the oblique views [18].
>
> *Note:* This syndrome has not yet been generally accepted as a real entity by cardiologists.

*2. In which direction does the normal T vector tend to turn on deep inspiration? What is the effect on leads 3 and aVF?

ANS.: Inferiorly. Therefore the T should become taller in leads 3 and aVF. (It is why the suspended heart syndrome is so unusual; i.e., despite no pathologic findings, the T becomes even more negative or stays the same in lead 3 on deep inspiration.)

*T INVERSION OF SCHIZOPHRENIA

*1. Where is the T inverted in some schizophrenic patients?
   ANS.: In lead 1 or lead 2 [47].
      Note: These T inversions sometimes look markedly ischemic.
*2. How can one tell if the T inversion in some schizophrenic patients is really due to myocardial ischemia?
   ANS.: It has been shown that having the patient stand up and giving him nitroglycerin or potassium chloride produces no change if the T inversion is ischemic, but it does produce an upright T if the patient is schizophrenic [47].
*3. What proof is there that this nitroglycerin test is valid?
   ANS.: It has been used to test the effect of nitrates, with very consistent results [48].
      Note: The nitrates that give the greatest effect according to the tests on the ability to normalize T waves on standing in the schizophrenic patient are nitroglycerin, isosorbide dinitrate (oral or sublingual), and erythrityl tetranitrate (only if sublingual).

Summary of Maneuvers to Identify Physiologic T Abnormalities

1. Report the ECG in the fasting state.
   a. During a deep inspiration.
   b. Standing.
   c. After 1 to 3 minutes of hyperventilation.
   d. During a Valsalva maneuver.
   e. During exercise [40].
   f. During beta-adrenergic stimulation with isoproterenol.
   g. During beta-adrenergic blockade. (Propranolol can be used intravenously in a dose of 0.15 mg per kilogram given at a rate of 1 mg per minute.)
2. If the results of the foregoing are equivocal, then try
   a. Administration of 45 mEq of oral potassium chloride.
   b. Administration of 2 mg of atropine subcutaneously or 30 mg of propantheline bromide intravenously [45].

*T WAVES AFTER ARTIFICIAL PACING

*1. What ECG changes occur after implanted pacemakers have been disconnected? What causes these changes?

ANS.: Deeply negative T waves, often with depressed S-T segments [11]. The cause is unknown. It is not produced by atrial pacing [11].

Note: The T waves in about one-third of patients tend to turn superiorly and show negative T waves only in leads 2, 3, and aVF. In others the T turns inferiorly, and in still others it also turns posteriorly, with giant T negativity in all the chest leads.

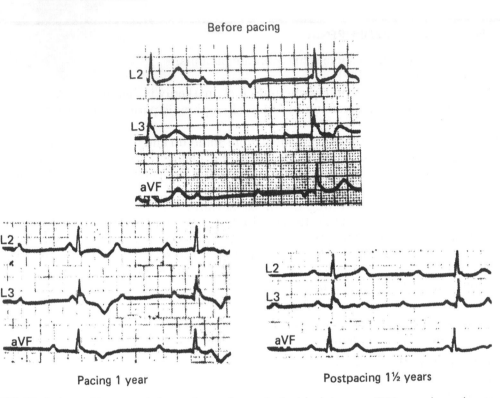

ECG 85. *Patient with congenital complete atrioventricular block (narrow QRS complexes denote a junctional pacemaker). The negative P waves seen before pacing in leads 2 and aVF are blocked premature atrial complexes. Note the superiorly turned T waves after 1 year of pacing.*

*2. In what proportion of patients with electronic pacemakers do T wave changes develop?

ANS.: In one study it occurred in almost three of every four patients in whom a prepacing and postpacing ECG was available [35].

Note: a. Only the pacemaker power and not its rate influences the severity of the changes. However, with high rates as well as high voltage, the changes begin within only 10 minutes of pacing and may be marked after only 1 day of pacing [29].

b. The T changes may last from hours to years, depending on how long the pacing had been going on before it was discontinued [35].

c. Patients with intermittent left bundle branch block often show precordial T inversions during normal conduction that are similar to those following right ventricular pacing. These inversions can revert to normal during prolonged periods of normal conduction and are not correlated with the presence of coronary disease [1].

REFERENCES

1. Abben, R., Rosen, K. M., and Denes, P. Intermittent left bundle branch block: anatomic substrate as reflected in the electrocardiogram during normal conduction. *Circulation* 59:1040, 1979.
2. Abinander, E. G. Adrenergic beta blockade and ECG changes in the systolic click murmur syndrome. *Am. Heart J.* 91:297, 1976.
3. Ashby, D. W., and Chadha, J. S. Electrocardiographic abnormalities simulating myocardial infarction in intracerebral haemorrhage and cerebral thrombosis. *Br. Heart J.* 30:732, 1968.
4. Awa, S., et al. Isolated T-wave inversion in the electrocardiograms of children. *Am. Heart J.* 81:158, 1971.
5. Behar, S., and Kariv, I. Effect of propranolol on 'nonspecific' S-T segment and T-wave changes: differentiation of coronary from noncoronary ECG changes. *Chest* 63:376, 1973.
6. Bekheit, S., and Ali, A. Q-T interval in idiopathic prolapsed mitral valve. *Am. J. Cardiol.* 41:374, 1978.
7. Biberman, L., Sarma, R. N., and Surawicz, B. T-wave abnormalities during hyperventilation and isoproterenol infusion. *Am. Heart J.* 81:166, 1971.
8. Boyadjian, N., Eechamps. G., and VanDooren, F. Ingestion of massive doses of potassium in the etiologic diagnosis of negative T-waves. *Acta Cardiol. (Brux.)* 13:607, 1958.
9. Burch, G. E., et al. Acute myocardial lesions. *Arch. Pathol.* 84:517, 1967.
10. Campbell, R. W. F., et al. Ventricular arrhythmias in syndrome of balloon deformity of mitral valve: definition of possible high risk group. *Br. Heart J.* 38:1053, 1976.
11. Chatterjee, K., et al. T-wave changes after artificial pacing. *Lancet* 1:759, 1969.
11A. Colleran, J. A., Papademetriou, V., and Narayan, P. Electrocardiographic abnormalities suggestive of myocardial ischemia during upper gastrointestinal bleeding. *Am. J. Cardiol.* 75:312–314, 1995.
12. Connor, R. C. R. Heart damage associated with intracranial lesions. *Br. Med. J.* 3:29, 1968.
13. Cropp, G. J., and Manning, G. W. Electrocardiographic changes simulating myocardial ischemia and infarction associated with spontaneous intracranial hemorrhage. *Circulation* 22:25, 1960.
14. Daoud, F. S., and Surawicz, B. The effect of isoproterenol (ISP) on the electrocardiogram in patients with intracranial lesions. *Am. J. Cardiol.* 26:629, 1970.
15. Dodge, H. T., Grant, R. P., and Seavey, P. W. The effect of induced hyperkalemia on the normal and abnormal electrocardiogram. *Am. Heart J.* 45:725, 1953.
16. Echenique, R. I. R., and Gonzalez, G.T wave inversion of the electrocardiogram of healthy individuals with vagotonia. *Aerospace Med.* 40:318, 1969.
17. Edeiken, J. Cyclic changes in T waves. *J.A.M.A.* 180:460, 1962.
18. Evans, W., and Lloyd-Thomas, H. C. The syndrome of the suspended heart. *Br. Heart J.* 19:153, 1957.
19. Gallivan, G. L., Levine, H., and Canzonetti, A. J. Ischemic electrocardiographic changes after truncal vagotomy. *J.A.M.A.* 211:798, 1970.
20. Hammermeister, K. E., and Reichenbach, D. D. QRS changes, pulmonary edema, and myocardial necrosis associated with subarachnoid hemorrhage. *Am. Heart J.* 78:94, 1969.
21. Hanne-Paparo, N., Wendkos, M. H., and Brunner, D. T wave abnormalities in the electrocardiograms of top-ranking athletes without demonstrable organic heart disease. *Am. Heart J.* 81:743, 1971.
22. Harrison, M. T., and Gibb, B. H. Electrocardiogram in stroke. *Lancet* 2:429, 1964.
23. Hugenholtz, H. Electrocardiographic abnormalities in cerebral disorders: report of six cases and review of the literature. *Am. Heart J.* 63:451, 1962.
24. Hunt, D., McRae, C., and Zepf, P. Electrocardiographic and serum enzyme changes in subarachnoid hemorrhage. *Am. Heart J.* 77:479, 1969.
25. Jacobson, D., and Schrire, V. Giant T wave inversion. *Br. Heart J.* 28:768, 1966.
26. Kemp, G. L., and Ellestad, M. H. The significance of hyperventilative and orthostatic T-wave changes on the electrocardiogram. *Arch. Intern. Med.* 121:518, 1968.
27. Leon-Sotomayor, L. The use of the Valsalva EKG test for differentiation of functional from organic T-wave abnormalities. *Angiology* 19:511, 1968.

28. Lobstein, H. P., et al. Electrocardiographic abnormalities and coronary arteriograms in the mitral click-murmur syndrome. *N. Engl. J. Med.* 289:127, 1973.

29. Lyon, L. J. T-wave inversions. *Arch. Intern. Med.* 135:745, 1975.

29A. Meyers, D. G., et al. Repolarization abnormalities in mitral valve prolapse. *Am. Heart J.* 113:1414, 1987.

30. Neil-Dwyer, C., and Walter, P. Effect of propranolol on stress-induced myocardial necrosis. In *World Congress of Cardiology Abstracts*, 1978, P. 297.

31. Nevins, M. A., Levy, A., and Lyon, L. J. When professional athlete's electrocardiogram mimics heart disease. *Physician Sportsmed.* 2:27, 1974.

32. Nordenfelt, O. Orthostatic electrocardiographic changes and the adrenergic beta receptor blocking agent, propranolol (Inderal). *Acta Med. Scand.* 173:393, 1965.

33. Ostrander, L. D., Jr. Effect of glucose ingestion upon electrocardiograms. *Am. J. Med. Sci.* 251:399, 1966.

34. Rajs, J. Relation between craniocerebral injury and subsequent myocardial fibrosis and heart failure: report of 3 cases. *Br. Heart J.* 38:396, 1976.

35. Reddy, R., Swamy, M., and Gould, L. Electrocardiographic changes: pacemaker induced. *N.Y. State J. Med.* 77:1080, 1977.

36. Runge, P. J., and Bousvaros, G. Giant peaked upright T waves in cerebrovascular accidents. *Br. Heart J.* 32:717, 1970.

37. Scherf, D., and McGavack, T. H. The estrogen-like action of desoxycorticosterone acetate upon the altered ECG in various hypo-ovarian states. *Am. J. Med. Sci.* 204:41, 1942.

38. Schneider, R. G., and Lyon, A. F. Use of oral potassium salts in the assessment of T wave abnormalities in the ECG: a clinical test. *Am. Heart J.* 77:721, 1969.

39. Simonson, E., and McKinlay, C. A. The meal test in clinical electrocardiography. *Circulation* 1:1000, 1950.

40. Sleeper, J. C., and Orgain, E. S. Differentiation of bening from pathologic T waves in the electro-cardiogram. *Am. J. Cardiol.* 11:338, 1963.

41. Surawicz, G. ECG pattern of cerebrovascular accident. *J.A.M.A.* 197:191, 1966.

42. Thomas, J., Harris, E., and Lassiter, G. Observations on the T wave and S-T segment changes in the precordial electrocardiogram of 320 young Negro adults. *Am. J. Cardiol.* 5:468, 1960.

43. Tzivone, D., et al. ECG characteristics of neurocirculatory asthenia. *Br. Heart J.* 44:426, 1980.

44. Wasserburger, R. H. Observations on the 'juvenile pattern' of adult Negro males. *Am. J. Med.* 18:428, 1955.

45. Wasserburger, R. H., and Lorenz, T. H. The effect of hyperventilation and Pro-Banthine on isolated RS-T segment and T-wave abnormalities. *Am. Heart J.* 51:666, 1956.

46. Wasserburger, R. H., Siebecker, K. L., Jr., and Lewis, W. C. The effect of hyperventilation on the normal adult electrocardiogram. *Circulation* 13:850, 1956.

47. Wendkos, M. H. The effects of potassium mixture on abnormal cardiac repolarization in hospital-ized psychiatric patients. *Am. J. Med. Sci.* 249:412, 1965.

48. Wendkos, M. H., and Logue, R. B. Unstable T waves in leads II and III in persons with neuro-circulatory asthenia. *Am. Heart J.* 31:711, 1946.

49. Yanowitz, F., Preston, J. B., and Abildskov, J. A. Functional distribution of right and left stellate innervation to the ventricles. *Circ. Res.* 18:416, 1966.

50. Yu, P. N., Yim, J. B. B., and Stanfield, A. C. Hyperventilation syndrome. *Arch. Intern. Med.* 103:902, 1959.

51. Zeppilli, P., Pirrami, M. M., and Fenici, R. T wave abnormalities in top ranking athletes: effect of isoproterenol. *Am. Heart J.* 100:213, 1980.

24. Left Ventricular Hypertrophy

PROBLEM OF INCREASED VOLTAGE

1. Why does QRS voltage increase in patients with left ventricular hypertrophy (LVH)?

    ANS.: An increased muscle mass produces more electrical potential. There is no evidence of any increase in the magnitude of single-cell voltage generated by a hypertrophied heart [80].

    Note: a. A dilated left ventricle (LV) from any cause, even with only a slightly thickened wall, can cause increased QRS voltage if total muscle mass is increased [79].

    b. When an acute increase in volume occurs, as when a subject with ischemic heart disease and myocardial dysfunction exercises, there may be an increase in voltage. This effect is known as the Brody effect, because during the mid-1950s Brody postulated that R wave amplitude would vary directly with left ventricular volume because of the radial orientation of the electromotive forces of the LV [7]. In normal subjects, however, both volume and QRS voltage decrease during exercise.

    c. In one study of normal subjects at rest there was a tendency for a decrease in voltage with an increase in volume [77]. It may have been due to an increase in chest wall circumference and thickness in normal subjects with increased heart volumes.

    If hyperosmolar contrast medium is injected into normal male volunteers, the ECG voltage decreases as the end-diastolic volume increases [88A].

    d. Anemia can also cause increased voltage. Low resistivity of the intracavitary blood has been demonstrated to cause this increase in voltage [5].

*2. What is the effect of an acute change in ventricular systolic pressure on QRS voltage?

    ANS.: Very little. Exercise testing can raise systolic pressure to more than 200 mm Hg with very little effect on a normal subject's QRS voltage.

*3. Are there more muscle fibers in a hypertrophied heart?

    ANS.: It depends on whether the hypertrophy is moderate or severe. With moderate hypertrophy the fibers are merely thicker, not greater in number. Because voltage from a thick cell is not increased, the greater ECG voltage from moderate hypertrophy must be due to some changed spatial relation that enhances current density. With severe hypertrophy there are more fibers [42], i.e., there is hyperplasia.

---

* Material marked with an asterisk is included for reference and for advanced students in cardiology.

Note: A heart weight of 400 g is considered the upper limit of normal in pathologists' reports that try to correlate ECG and necropsy findings [1]. A heart weighing more than 400 g has usually been considered hypertrophied without reference to height, weight, age, or sex. It has been shown, however, that if heart weight is related to height and sex alone, the normal heart weight in men 66 inches tall is 317 ± 40 g and in women of the same height 277 ± 30 g. Therefore in many studies some women with a heart weight less than 400 g (e.g., as low as 350 g) could have had LVH but nonetheless were considered normal [90].

4. How do you determine the height (in millimeters) of a positive or negative wave if the baseline is thick (chisel point stylus)?

    ANS.: Count from top to top for positive waves and from bottom to bottom for negative waves.

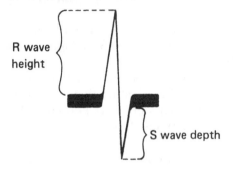

FRONTAL PLANE LVH CRITERIA

1. What are the frontal plane voltage criteria for LVH?

    ANS.: a. The most useful and common is the index of Lewis: net positivity in lead 1 plus net negativity in lead 3 of 17 mm or more. Net positivity is calculated as follows:

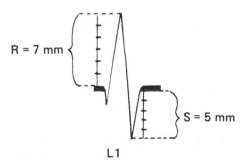

If the R is 7 mm and the S is 5 mm, the net positivity is 2 mm.

    b. Index of Ungerleider: R in lead 1 + S in lead 3 = 25 mm [29]. It is not necessary to subtract opposite deflections; i.e., this index does *not* refer to net positivity or negativity. It is not a sensitive index.

  *c. R in aVL more than 11 mm [47, 74].

d. R in aVF more than 20 mm.

*e. In infants up to 3 months of age, an axis of + 30° or less (lead 3 equiphasic or negative); or up to age 1 year, 0° or less (aVF equiphasic or negative [13]).

Note: Sir Thomas Lewis did the earliest ECG research reported in the British literature, wrote the first books on electrocardiography in English, and was the editor of the first heart journal in English. In Lewis's time, only bipolar limb leads and one chest lead were used. This fact makes it easier to remember that the index of Lewis utilizes bipolar leads, i.e., leads 1 and 3 (see ECG 86).

Ungerleider proposed his frontal plane voltage criteria of 25 mm for LVH in 1943 when bipolar limb leads were still the only ones in general use.

2. Why is the LVH criterion of an R of 11 mm in aVL usually redundant for those who use the index of Lewis?

ANS.: The R of 11 mm in aVL is rarely found without a positive index of Lewis, but the latter is often present without the aVL criterion (see ECG 86).

On rare occasions, when the subtraction of an S wave in lead 1 prevents a positive index of Lewis, the voltage in aVL alone may be positive for LVH.

Note: a. When dilatation occurs in patients with hypertension or coronary disease, the aVL or index of Lewis criteria are more likely to be met than are horizontal plane criteria [76]. (For other ECG signs of left ventricular dilatation, see p. 383.)

b. A 25-mm Ungerleider voltage index is very specific; i.e., it gives few false positives. It is, however, very insensitive in that only rarely is it present in a patient with LVH especially as subjects grow older because in the older age groups the QRS tends to swing out of the frontal plane and into the horizontal plane.

c. In 1917 White and Bock [86] proposed 20 mm as the upper limit of normal for R1 + S3. However, because they used net voltage (i.e., they subtracted opposites: S in lead 1 and R in lead 3), their 20-mm index is probably not much different from Ungerleider's 25-mm index, as he did *not* subtract opposites. Because White and Bock noted that in some normal subjects the voltage could be 20 mm, we can assume that Ungerleider's index of 25 mm must also include some normal subjects. Only if White and Bock used 30 mm could they eliminate normal subjects.

d. It has also been proposed that 7.5 mm in aVL increases the sensitivity of aVL for LVH. However, the incidence of false positives is double that found for the 11-mm criterion [47, 63]. The 7.5-mm criterion can be useful if there are no other voltage criteria, but instead there are many of the secondary criteria discussed under Secondary LVH Criteria.

Note: Of 31 patients with aVL over 11, 6 had increased left ventricular mass by echocardiogram when corrected for age and/or body surface area [35A].

3. How does the index of Lewis or Ungerleider relate to the axis?

ANS.: It usually implies at least a leftward axis; i.e., in order to have a tall R in lead 1 and a deep S in lead 3, the axis must be at least less than + 30°.

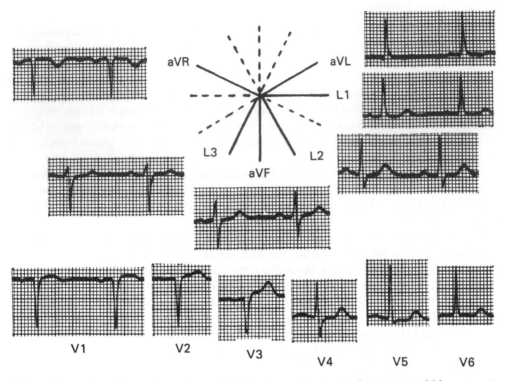

ECG 86. *The index of Lewis is not the only LVH voltage criterion in this 76-year-old hypertensive woman (blood pressure 160/115 mm Hg) with a slightly enlarged heart on x-ray. The R in L1 plus the S in L3 is about 20 mm. Subtracting the R in L3 still leaves 17 mm. The secondary criteria are incomplete LBBB pattern (no septal q in V5, V6, or L1, no septal r in V1 or V2) and the slightly flat and depressed S-T in V4, V5, and V6. Note that aVL has an R with an amplitude of more than 11 mm. When this voltage index is positive, usually the index of Lewis is also positive. The reverse occasionally occurs; i.e., aVL is occasionally 11 mm or more with a negative index of Lewis.*

4. What can cause a false-positive index of Lewis of 17 mm?
    ANS.: a. Obesity.
        b. Youth, i.e., age under 30.
      *c. Congenital corrected transposition (inversion of the ventricles) [22].
        Note: a. Anterior divisional block causes limb lead voltage to increase and therefore is said to cause a false-positive index of Lewis. However, because the index of Lewis was noted to be valid before divisional blocks were defined, it included patients with divisional blocks. Divisional blocks probably uncover LVH rather than produce false LVH [64]. An anterior divisional block can even bring out an LVH strain pattern that was not present without the block [55]. (Rosenbaum and Elizari [64] required the S in lead 3 to be at least 15 mm deep, the axis to be at least – 60°, and the Q in lead 1 to be small or absent before they allowed a reading of LVH in the presence of anterior divisional block.)
        b. In a study of U.S. Air Force personnel in 1964, the index of either Lewis or Ungerleider appeared to be valid for both young and middle-age persons [44]. For example, the upper limit of normal

for R in lead 1 plus S in lead 3 was found to be 16 for the younger age groups and 17 for the middle-age groups. This finding gives the index of Lewis (which subtracts opposites to make 17) even greater validity, especially for women, as they tend to have lower voltages than men.

5. Why is a positive index of Lewis present with obesity?

ANS.: Obese subjects have physiologic LVH [1]. Therefore this result is a false positive only in that there is no pathologic LVH. Remember that an index of Lewis requires at least a leftward axis in order to give a reasonably tall R in lead 1 and a deep S in lead 3. Obese subjects tend to have a leftward axis (because of their high diaphragms), which is the first stage toward a positive index of Lewis [33].

When obese patients have pathological LVH they are more likely to show the increased voltage in the frontal than in the horizontal plane [47A].

*6. What kind of transposition of the great vessels produces a positive index of Lewis without LVH actually being present?

ANS.: Isolated corrected transposition, i.e., with no other intracardiac abnormality [22]. When the systemic posterior right ventricle (RV) hypertrophies to do the work of an LV, it affects the ECG as though LVH were present.

7. How can you overcome the false positives of the index of Lewis or Ungerleider?

ANS.: By not accepting voltage criteria alone if the subject is either under age 30 or is obese unless there are secondary changes that help confirm the presence of LVH. A point-score system has been devised to assist in diagnosing LVH by utilizing secondary criteria [62].

HORIZONTAL PLANE LVH CRITERIA

1. List the horizontal plane voltage criteria for LVH.

ANS.: 1. S in V1 + R in V5 or V6 = 35 mm or more (index of Sokolow) [74].

Note: a. For ease of remembering, this index is about twice the index of Lewis, which is 17 mm.

b. V6 is rarely used because it is seldom larger than V5.

2. S in V2 + R in V6 = 35 mm or more (modified index of Sokolow) (see ECG 8, p. 97, and ECG 74A, p. 333).

3. Any R + any S in the precordium = 45 mm or more (index of McPhie [48]).

*4. R in V5 or V6 more than 26 mm [73]. However, this degree of voltage in V5 and V6 is rarely present without the Sokolow SV1 + RV5 or V6 criterion's being positive; and in 5 percent of normal subjects between the ages of 20 and 60, the amplitude is between 26 and 30 mm.

Note: a. You are more likely to be correct when you read a positive Sokolow index in women because, on the basis of the 97.5 percentile upper limit, SV1 + RV5 is 35 mm for men (over age 30) but only 33 mm for women [73]. Horizontal plane vector magnitudes have been found to be 30 percent lower in women than in men [54].

     b. You are also more likely to be correct when you read a positive Sokolow (or Lewis) index in the elderly because QRS voltage decreases with age [2].

     c. For the probability that an infant or child has LVH to be high, 40 mm in V5 or V6 alone is necessary [58].

2. How is aVL used in the Cornell index for LVH voltage?

  ANS.: If the amplitude of the R in aVL plus the S in V3 is equal to or is greater than 28 mm for men and 20 mm for women [10A].

    Note: a. For sedentary students age 20–30 index of Sokolow maximum should be 40 mm for males and 36 mm for females. For athletic students maximum is 50.3 mm for males and 36 mm for females [6A].

       b. The index of Sokolow has been found to vary from 33 mm to 40 mm during serial studies as a normal day-to-day variability [21A].

3. How does proximity affect precordial voltage?

  ANS.: The closer the chest electrode is to the heart, the greater is the voltage. With the electrode placed directly on the heart, the voltage is about five times that recorded from the surface. A mastectomy increases precordial voltage [39]. The largest adult voltage I have ever seen was in a patient with LVH due to aortic regurgitation who had had a left mastectomy. The unexpected finding is that for unknown reasons the voltage in V1 increases even after a left mastectomy [39].

4. Why should an S in V2 plus an R in V6 of 35 mm be as reliable a voltage criterion for LVH as an S in V1 plus an R in V5?

  ANS.: V2 is relatively more of a proximity lead than V1, and V6 is relatively less of a proximity lead than V5. Also V1 to V5 is separated by the same distance as is V2 to V6.

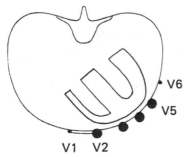

The large spots indicate electrodes that are relatively proximal to the heart. The index of Sokolow uses V1 and V5, i.e., one distant and one close electrode. The modified index of Sokolow, using V2 and V6, also adds one distant to one close lead. Also V1 to V5 equals the distance of V2 to V6. Thus both criteria should have equal validity.

5. Why does an S on the right precordium plus an R on the left precordium logically reflect LVH voltage?

  ANS.: Because the S on the right precordium represents the same vector as the R seen on the left precordium; i.e., the S on the right precordium is produced by the LV, as is the R on the left precordium.

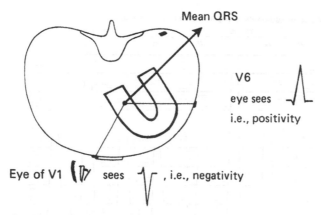

If you imagine that a right precordial electrode is like an eye watching the QRS vector moving away from the electrical center, it sees predominant negativity for the QRS in the diagram; i.e., V1 produces a dominant S wave. Similarly, V6, seeing the same vector, produces a dominant R wave.

6. What are the commonest causes of falsely high precordial voltage?

    ANS.: Youth and race [72]. In 1957 Grubschmidt and Sokolow [28] raised the upper limit for the younger age groups to 40 mm. In 1964 the findings of a U.S. Air Force study indicated that in subjects under 30 years of age the index should be raised to 53 mm [44]. Young black male subjects, both children and adults, are especially prone to excessively high voltage in the absence of LVH [46]. They have been found in one study to have a thicker left ventricular posterior wall in diastole and the heart is located closer to the chest wall [61A].

    Note: a. The physiologic LVH of athletes can cause precordial voltage that satisfies the criteria for LVH [82].

    b. It is so hazardous to diagnose LVH on the basis of voltage alone in subjects under age 30 that if no secondary criteria are present (see p. 369), you should simply report 'within normal limits' [50]. If the patient is over age 30, you should report 'nonspecific voltage increase in limb or precordial leads.'

    c. Pediatric precordial voltage varies with age. The diagram below gives upper normal amplitudes from the first year of life to 16 years.

NORMAL AMPLITUDE MEASUREMENTS IN CHILDREN AT VARIOUS AGES

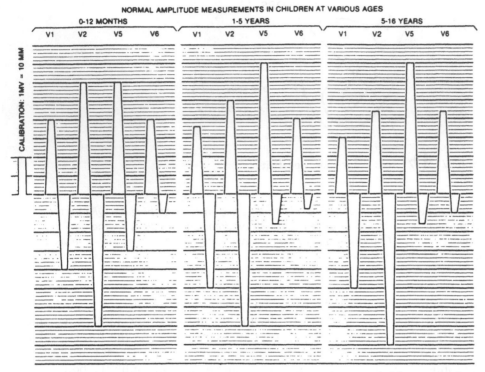

Images of the QRS complex in V1, V2, V5, and V6 in children at various ages.

Images of the QRS complex in V1, V2, V5, and V6 in children at various ages.

*7. When a hypertensive patient is successfully treated, which is more likely to change: the frontal or horizontal plane QRS vectors? In what direction does the change occur?

ANS.: The horizontal plane QRS vector is much more likely to change, moving more anteriorly [18]. This fact suggests that the frontal plane QRS direction is not so much affected by the LVH of hypertension as is the horizontal plane QRS.

Note: When congenital aortic valvular stenosis is successfully treated surgically, the ECG voltage is decreased. Provided aortic regurgitation has not been induced, voltage changes can be used to tell you whether the gradient is diminished [53].

8. When is voltage alone likely to mean LVH in the absence of any clinical information?

ANS.: When there are positive voltage criteria in both frontal and horizontal planes [17].

9. In what percentage of subjects found at autopsy to have LVH were no voltage criteria observed in any plane, when as many as 33 of the criteria available in the literature were used?

ANS.: In 15 percent [63].

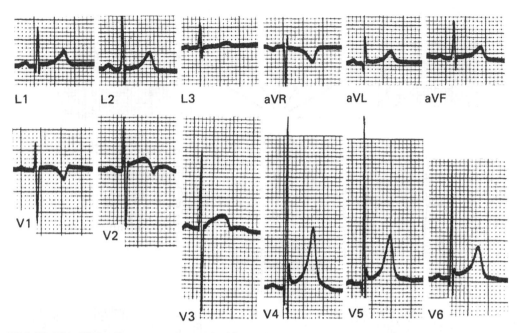

ECG 87. This ECG is from a 25-year-old athlete. The tall T waves assure you that the elevated S-Ts that begin with a 'hook' are due to normal 'early repolarization' rather than to pericarditis. The extremely high voltage in the precordium is due partly to youth and partly to physiologic LVH.

10. How is precordial lead voltage affected by albumin?
    ANS.: The lower the albumin, the lower the voltage, and LVH may be under-diagnosed [29B].

SECONDARY LVH CRITERIA

1. Which secondary changes are helpful in confirming the presence of LVH when voltage criteria are present?
   ANS.: a. Almost any nonspecific QRS, S-T, or T abnormalities.
   b. Voltage criteria in both limb leads and chest leads, i.e., in both frontal and horizontal planes.
   c. ECG evidence of left atrial overload.
2. Which frontal plane QRS changes suggest LVH when found with voltage criteria?
   ANS.: a. A deep Q in lead 3, especially if the amplitude of the Q is greater than that of the R.
   Note: The R in lead 1 plus the Q in lead 3 may be used as the index of Lewis, which confirms the fact that the Q in lead 3 can become deep simply due to LVH (see ECG 88; see also ECG 34, p. 175).

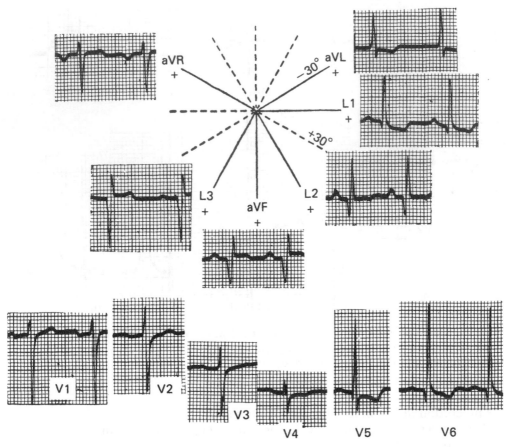

ECG 88. A 60-year-old hypertensive man had an old inferior infarction and cardiomegaly. The Q in L3 and aVF is 40 msec (0.04 sec) wide. The extreme depth of the Q is secondary to LVH. The R in L1 plus the Q in L3 is 26 mm. After subtracting the Q in L1 plus the R in L3 (7 mm), a net sum of 19 remains. Therefore the index of Lewis is positive. Note that V6 is larger in amplitude than V5. This finding is very unusual and suggests cardiac dilatation.

    b. Mid-conduction or terminal conduction defects producing leftward axes or marked left axis deviation.

    c. A delayed intrinsicoid deflection, i.e., a ventricular activation time of 50 msec (0.05 sec) or more in leads with a left ventricular complex; 60 msec is highly specific for LVH (in the absence of complete left bundle branch block [LBBB] or preexcitation) [65].

  *d. A prolonged QRS due to a delayed intrinsicoid deflection is much more likely to be found in dilated hearts (due to heart failure, aortic regurgitation, or mitral regurgitation) than in pure LVH, as in aortic stenosis or hypertension [4].

    e. Initial right-to-left conduction (i.e., no q in aVL and lead 1), with no r or a very small r in V1. This finding suggests some degree of LBBB (see ECG 86, p. 364). If the QRS is not widened, however, the term incomplete LBBB *pattern* is preferable to *incomplete LBBB*.

  *f. Initial right-to-left conduction in LVH does not necessarily mean that the septum is depolarized only from right to left. Electrodes placed on each side of the septum have shown that septal activation is often still from left to right. Therefore the right-to-left conduction seen in the ECG (no q in lead 1, V5, or V6), may be the result of subendocardial hypertrophy or septal scarring unbalancing the initial forces, presumably slowing conduction along the septal fascicle [1].

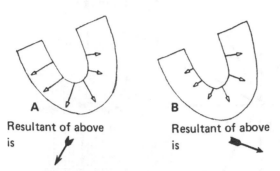

A. The septal vectors dominate. An increase in septal forces or a decrease in free wall subendocardial forces causes the initial vector to move from left to right. B. Septal scarring has decreased or slowed septal forces.

*3. Which of the preceding conduction defects are the most specific for LVH?

ANS.: a. A delayed intrinsicoid deflection in left ventricular leads, i.e., aVL, V5, or V6, in the absence of complete LBBB or preexcitation [65].

b. A left axis (0° or more leftward) (see ECG 86).

Note: The left axis seen in many subjects with LVH is not due to any change in the gross anatomic relation of the LV to the chest cavity [4]. An exception to this leftward axis shift may be seen in congenital aortic stenosis. Many subjects with severe congenital aortic stenosis have inferior axes with no right ventricular overload to account for them [61] (see ECG 89). This axis does not change with age, and the higher the left ventricular pressure, the more inferior the QRS [35].

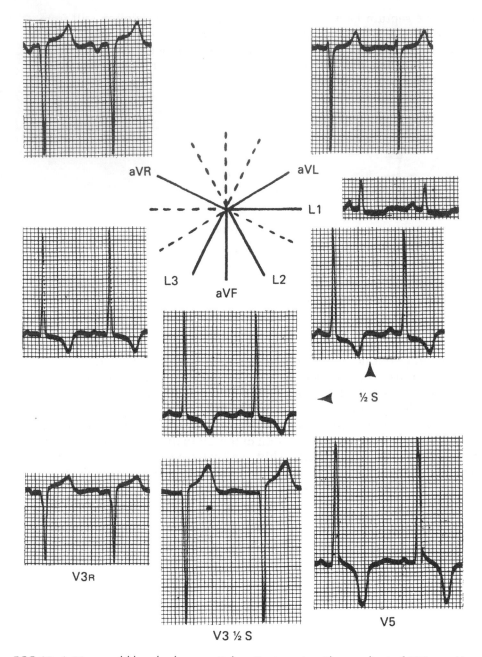

ECG 89. A 16-year-old boy had congenital aortic stenosis with a gradient of 200 mm Hg across the valve. Note the inferior axis of about 70° (aVL markedly negative). The fantastic voltage seen with hypertrophy in this age group is shown here where leads 2, aVF, and V3 are taken at one-half standard (½ S). Seven years after aortic valvotomy this patient's ECG was normal, even in voltage.

SECONDARY HORIZONTAL PLANE LVH CRITERIA

*1. How can LVH affect the septal vector or Q wave in left ventricular leads other than making it disappear?

ANS.: It can mimic the Q waves of infarction because it can cause a deep and slightly wide Q in left ventricular leads.

Note: a. It may be due to thickening of the septum or to the myocardial fiber disarray in the septum seen in asymmetrical septal hypertrophy.

b. In about 10 percent of patients with hypertrophic subaortic stenosis and asymmetrical septal hypertrophy, the Q may be exceptionally deep in the left precordium, with reciprocally tall R waves in V3R and V1 [87]. There may even be a Q with greater voltage in V4 than in V5 or V6.

c. A tall 'septal' R wave in V1 is also seen in patients with pseudo-hypertrophic muscular dystrophy [43].

d. Apical hypertrophy with or without upper septal or diffuse hypertrophy usually orients the initial forces from right to left, and the QRS tends to be posterior [36]. Asymmetric septal hypertrophy differs in that initial conduction is usually from left to right and the QRS tends to be more anterior than with pure apical hypertrophy [56].

2. What is the commonest QRS conduction change seen in patients with LVH?

ANS.: Incomplete LBBB or an incomplete LBBB pattern without a block, i.e., initial right-to-left conduction with at least a slight delay in intrinsicoid deflection, seen best in left precordial leads. In V1, of course, the 'septal r' is either absent or reduced in amplitude (see ECG 86).

Note: LVH is suggested by a delayed intrinsicoid deflection beyond 40 msec (0.04 sec) in the first chest lead with a septal Q [75]. If no Q is present in the left precordium, a delayed intrinsicoid deflection of 60 msec (0.06 sec) in V5 or V6 is highly specific for LVH but rarely occurs [65, 71].

3. What happens to the QRS-T angle in the horizontal plane when LVH changes develop?

ANS.: The QRS-T angle widens; i.e., the QRS turns posteriorly, and the T turns anteriorly.

4. What happens to the T voltage in the right and left precordium as the T turns more and more anteriorly?

ANS.: The T grows taller in the right precordium and lower in the left precordium (see ECG 15, p. 129; see also ECG 89).

5. What is the lowest normal T in left precordial leads?

ANS.: The absolute voltage of the T depends too much on the proximity of the electrodes to the heart to be of any use; i.e., even a very low T may be normal if the total voltage is reduced. You can, however, recognize an abnormally low T in the left precordium despite the effects of proximity by using the rules that (a) the lowest normal T in a left ventricular lead is one-tenth of the R wave, and (b) the T in V1 is rarely ever taller than the T in V6.

Note: A left ventricular lead is one with a left ventricular complex, i.e., an R wave with a Q or S that is either small or absent.

6. What is the final stage of a T abnormality that can develop secondary to LVH alone?

ANS.: The LVH strain pattern.

LVH STRAIN PATTERN

1. Which S-T and T abnormalities are especially specific for LVH?

   ANS.: The LVH strain pattern, i.e., a predominantly positive or left ventricular QRS, with a depressed J point, a straight or upward convex, downward sloping, long S-T leading to a negative T wave with a short terminal limb.

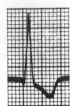

V6 or aVL (left ventricular leads)

2. What is the advantage of the expression 'LVH strain pattern'?

   ANS.: It can take the place of the 37-word description used in question 1.

   Note: a. All degrees of flattening or depression of the S-T segment can be changes secondary to LVH, i.e., there may be minor degrees of strain pattern before its full development (see ECG 86). However, only the full-blown strain pattern has specificity.

   *b. The original 'left ventricular strain' ECG—when the expression was first used in 1929—consisted only of negative T waves in leads 1 and 2. No mention was made of the S-T segment or the shape of the T [3].

3. What is wrong with the term *left ventricular strain*?

   ANS.: It implies that the S-T, T changes always have a volume or pressure overload etiology and cannot occur simply from the LVH alone, as, for example, in idiopathic hypertrophy. That is why the word *pattern* should always accompany the expression. When the abbreviation LVH is used, it is convenient to say 'LVH strain pattern.'

4. What is the commonest stimulus to the LV that causes the LVH strain pattern to develop?

   ANS.: Any condition that causes a higher-than-normal systolic pressure in the LV. It is known as systolic or pressure overloading of the LV. In the absence of idiopathic hypertrophy or aortic stenosis, however, the full-blown strain pattern is rare without cardiac dilatation as well as hypertrophy [46, 78] (see ECG 88).

5. What are the two most common causes of systolic overloading of the LV?

   ANS.: a. Systemic hypertension.

   b. Aortic stenosis (see ECG 90).

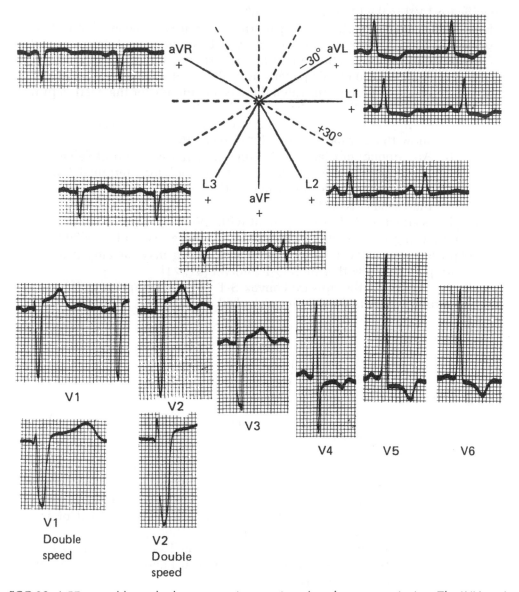

ECG 90. A 57-year-old man had severe aortic stenosis and moderate regurgitation. The LVH strain pattern is fully developed in the left ventricular leads (L1, aVL, V5, and V6). Note the reciprocal of the S-T, T strain pattern in the right ventricular leads V1 and V2. The small q in front of the septal r in V1 and V2 is invisible to the beginner but obvious to the experienced ECG reader. A strip run at double speed demonstrates this tiny q, which is due to myocardial necrosis. The patient's myocardial function was markedly depressed owing to myocardial damage.

*6. How reversible is the LVH strain pattern after successful surgery for severe aortic stenosis? What is the significance?

ANS.: About 50 percent still show the LVH strain pattern after surgery, even with the gradient abolished. The pattern is therefore probably often fixed by fibrosis [51].

Note: The LVH strain pattern of severe hypertension is also often reversible with successful treatment [20].

7. How specific for LVH is the LVH strain pattern?

   ANS.: Even without voltage criteria this pattern almost always means that LVH is present [27, 71]. However, the secondary S-T, T changes of any widened QRS, as in LBBB, imitate the LVH strain pattern.

   Note: a. A rare cause of this pattern in leads 3 and aVF is the 'suspended heart syndrome,' in which there is a tendency for the heart to pull away from the diaphragm on deep inspiration (see on fluoroscopy). Leads V5 and V6 may reflect the inferior leads and also show this normal variation [21] (see p. 356).

   b. Autonomic imbalance as in some patients with mitral valve prolapse may simulate the strain pattern. Look for a terminal T wave positivity or overshoot which with the strain pattern denotes an increased mass [71A].

8. How does digitalis affect the S-T, T of a patient with LVH?

   ANS.: a. It may bring out the strain pattern; i.e., if there was only a slight S-T depression and low T before digitalis, the drug may develop it into a strain pattern but with a short Q-T interval [41, 71].

   b. It may straighten the upward convex S-T or even completely eliminate the strain pattern and substitute a marked digitalis S-T, T pattern.

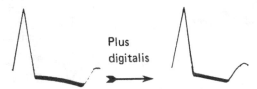

Plus
digitalis

Note how digitalis not only shortens the Q-T interval but also straightens out the upward convex S-T of the LVH strain pattern.

9. How does the LVH strain pattern differ from the injury and ischemic S-T, T pattern of acute transmural infarction?

   ANS.: a. In the LVH strain pattern the S-T is depressed in leads with the negative T, but with myocardial infarction the S-T is usually elevated or isoelectric in the leads with the inverted T.

   b. With LVH, the proximal downward limb of the T is usually longer than the distal limb, but with ischemia the downward and distal limbs of the T are often almost symmetrical.

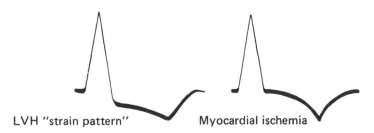

LVH "strain pattern"   Myocardial ischemia

*10. How does the precordial ECG pattern of anterior subendocardial infarction or fibrosis differ from the LVH strain pattern?

ANS.: a. The subendocardial infarction or fibrosis S-T depression occurs not only in left ventricular leads but also in the mid-precordial leads, i.e., those with an S wave. The LVH strain pattern occurs only in the left ventricular leads (leads with almost entirely positive QRS, such as the usual appearance of leads 1, aVL, V5, and V6). If the S wave in the mid-precordium and left precordium is due to an anterior divisional block, however, the S-T, T part of the strain pattern in these leads may signify LVH just as if the S-T, T abnormality were with a pure left ventricular complex [55].

b. The subendocardial infarction T waves are often upright in the mid-precordium and left precordium. Also, when subendocardial infarction causes negative T waves in those leads, the negativity is usually deep, i.e., 5 mm or more.

Note: The LVH strain pattern can occur with or without coronary obstruction.

OTHER SECONDARY T CRITERIA FOR LVH

1. List some T abnormalities, other than some stage of strain pattern development, that can be used with voltage criteria to provide minor secondary criteria to help diagnose LVH.

ANS.: a. A negative T in a critical lead, i.e., in lead 1, 2, or aVF.

b. A notched T wave [14] (see ECG 74, p. 333).

c. An anterior T wave, i.e., the T in V1 taller than the T in V6.

d. A T less than 10% of the R in a left ventricular complex.

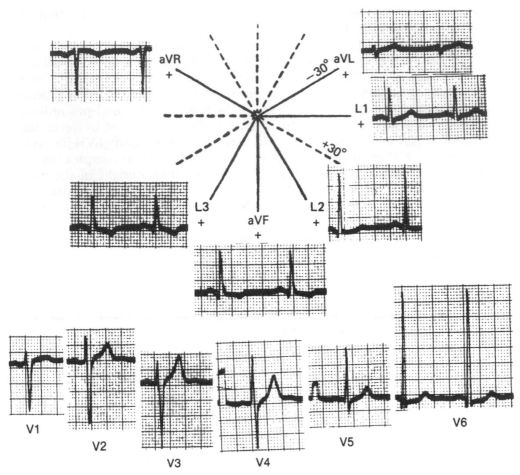

ECG 90A. From a 45-year-old man with moderate cardiomegaly due to moderately severe mitral regurgitation. He has voltage criteria by the modified index of Sokolow (SV2 + RV6 is more than 35 mm). Note that the T is negative in aVF and is less than 10 percent of the R in V6.

2. Is the wide QRS-T angle seen in the horizontal plane of patients with LVH due to rotation of the QRS or rotation of the T?

　　ANS.: Both. The T turns anteriorly, but the QRS turns posteriorly; i.e., the wide QRS-T angle of LVH is due to both a posterior QRS and an anterior T.

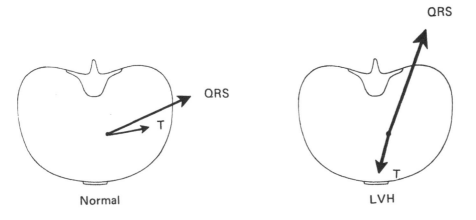

3. Why does the anterior T wave of LVH imitate myocardial infarction?

    ANS.: The anterior T may turn so rightward that it is negative from V3 to V6. Because of a proximity effect, V4 may have a deeper T than V5 or V6 and be so symmetrical and deep that the myocardial ischemia of acute infarction is suggested [52]. If we do not know the clinical story, we should teach such T waves in the presence of LVH criteria as 'myocardial ischemia or fibrosis.' By 'ischemia' we suggest the possibility of acute infarction.

*4. How does the height of the T in V1 relate to the height of the T in V6 in normal adults?

    ANS.: Normally, the T is the same height or is taller in V6 than in V1. (In about one-fifth of men and one-twentieth of women, the reverse is true [57].)

    Note: LVH tends to make the T in V1 greater than the T in V6 [32]. This finding can be used, especially in women, as a minor sign of LVH when combined with voltage criteria.

*5. What T wave change may be the only sign of LVH in infants and children?

    ANS.: T negativity in left ventricular leads [37].

*6. When is a taller-than-normal T seen in LVH?

    ANS.: In the physiologic LVH of athletes the frontal T is taller and more leftward than in matched controls.

    Note: a. In athletes the P-R interval, the rate-corrected Q-T interval, and the cycle length may all be prolonged, and the QRS may be more anterior than usual [6]. This fact helps you to recognize the athlete's ECG [35, 82]. Because P-R prolongation is not found in all studies of athletes, it may be present only in selected types of athletes or it may depend on the degree of the athlete's training [6].

    b. The anterior QRS may be due to the concomitant right ventricular hypertrophy that is said to occur in athletes.

CAUSES OF REDUCED VOLTAGE

1. What is meant by a low-voltage ECG?

    ANS.: You should not use the expression 'low voltage' to describe an entire ECG unless every lead has a QRS amplitude of less than 10 mm.

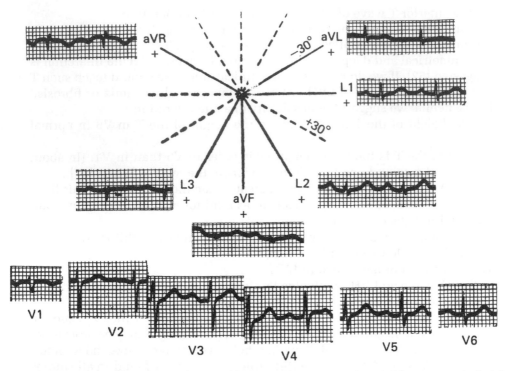

ECG 91. A 63-year-old woman with normal heart and lungs was in hospital for a cosmetic facial operation. The low voltage in only the limb leads is a normal variant and is never worth noting unless emphysema, mitral stenosis, or amyloidosis is being considered. Because V3 has a voltage of 13 mm, the low limb lead voltage alone should not be read as 'low voltage' because all leads are not less than 10 mm. Note the indeterminate axis caused by the atypical right bundle branch block pattern. A right bundle branch block pattern is probably a variation of normal in all age groups.

2. What are the causes of reduced voltage only in the frontal plane?
   ANS.: Most of the time it is a normal variant. The commonest abnormal causes are chronic obstructive pulmonary disease and mitral stenosis. Rare causes are constrictive pericarditis, amyloid disease, myxedema, and cachexia. Low voltage (5 mm or less) in lead 1 alone has the same possible causes. In cachectic patients not only is the voltage of both QRS and T decreased but the duration of the QRS is decreased as well [9].
   Note: The voltage in lead 1 in mitral stenosis may be low for the same reason that it is low in chronic obstructive pulmonary disease because mitral stenosis patients have been found to have increased residual lung volume due to a loss of the elastic properties of the lung [24].
3. How can myocardial disease reduce precordial voltage in the absence of edema or effusions?
   ANS.: By replacing voltage-producing myocardium with fibrous tissue or other infiltrates such as amyloid. Patients with amyloid disease, however, usually show significant low voltage only in the frontal plane [8].

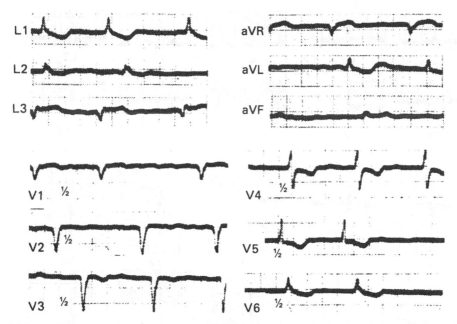

ECG 92. *Skin and liver biopsy revealed amyloidosis in this 48-year-old white man with macroglossia, intermittent fevers, aching muscles and joints, purpuric spots on the lower extremities, hepatomegaly, and congestive heart failure. Although the limb leads show low voltage, the chest leads (taken at one-half standard) have normal voltage.*

4. How can cardiomegaly and congestive heart failure lower voltage despite the large volume and LVH?

ANS.: The reason is unknown. If it is not due to occult pericardial effusion, perhaps in some patients peripheral edema creates a skin resistance that results in lower voltage. (The lower voltage is seen in both the frontal and horizontal planes.)

Note: a. A large heart volume alone does not produce low voltage because bleeding an animal and making the heart smaller makes the voltage lower [45]. Because anemia can increase voltage and polycythemia can decrease it, it is not the anemia caused by the hemorrhage that decreases the voltage [66].

b. Anasarca can reduce voltage because as the resistance of the conducting medium around the heart decreases the ECG potentials are attenuated by being shortened [42A]. Plasma has lower resistivity than lung or fat [24A].

*5. How can voltage be used to follow a patient with congestive heart failure?

ANS.: As the failure improves and the heart decreases in size, the voltage increases [32]. Because these voltage changes are best seen in the horizontal plane, scrupulous lead placement is necessary to record the changes accurately. This voltage increase is presumably secondary to a change in skin resistance due to the reduction of edema.

Note: Voltage can also be used to follow a patient with pericardial effusion. In one study, with each 100 ml of fluid removed, the voltage increased by about 0.5 mm in limb leads and by almost 1 mm in precordial leads [81].

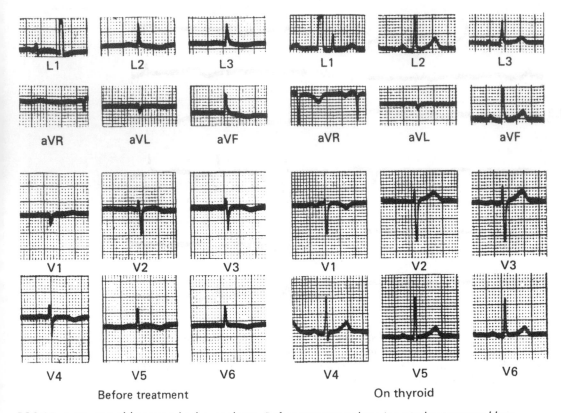

Before treatment   On thyroid

ECG 93. A 40-year-old woman had myxedema. Before treatment there is a tendency toward low voltage (V2 barely makes more than 10 mm), and the T waves are negative in L1, L2, and V3 to V6. After 4 months of desiccated thyroid treatment, the patient's ECG is completely normal. Even the P waves have more voltage, and the slight atypical right bundle branch block pattern (S in L1) has disappeared.

*6. How can myxedema cause reduced voltage?

ANS.: By producing either pericardial effusion, increased skin resistance, myocardial edema, or nonspecific infiltration [49, 69].

7. What is the commonest cause of reduced voltage in precordial leads in the absence of emphysema, cardiomyopathy, or pericardial disease?

ANS.: Obesity.

Note: a. Precordial voltages tend to vary inversely with the square of the distance of the recording electrode from the center of the left ventricular mass [31]. Obesity not only does not diminish limb lead voltage but actually tends to produce a false-positive index of Lewis [33].

b. A left-sided pleural effusion or left pneumothorax can also insulate the heart from the chest electrode and so produce low voltage. Other ECG signs of a large left-sided pneumothorax are a shift of frontal axis interiorly and inversion of precordial T waves [19].

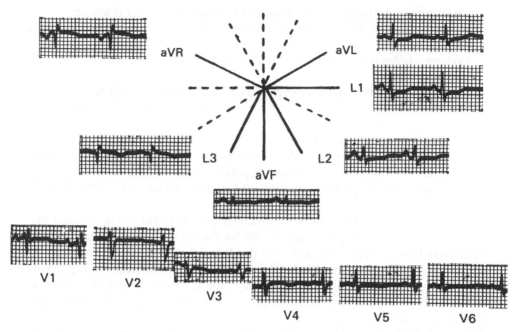

ECG 94. Because every lead has less than 10 mm amplitude, this pattern should be read as a low voltage ECG. It is from a 62-year-old woman with a pericardial effusion secondary to carcinoma of the lung. She is thin and cachectic, so the low voltage in the chest leads is even more signifi-cant. Note that the right bundle branch block pattern has produced an indeterminate axis.

8. How can the ECG technician produce an ECG that is false negative or false positive for LVH?

    ANS.: By overstandardizing or understandardizing.

*9. Which conduction defects, other than complete right or left bundle branch block, can mask LVH precordial voltage?

    ANS.: a. A right bundle branch block (RBBB) *pattern* alone because if the terminal QRS is controlled by the part of the RV responsible for the RBBB pattern, voltage for LVH may be reduced.

    b. An anterior divisional block, because the terminal superior and leftward forces are often not picked up in the left precordial leads, which are usually slightly inferior to the electrical center [26, 31].

ACQUIRED VENTRICULAR DILATATION

1. How does diagnosing left ventricular dilatation help you to diagnose LVH?

    ANS.: A dilated LV is almost always accompanied by some LVH unless the dilata-tion is acute, which is rare [4].

2. Which chest leads are closer to the heart, V5 or V6? How does this positioning affect voltage?

    ANS.: Usually V5 is either closer to or equally as far from the heart as V6. Therefore the *total voltage* in V5 is almost always larger than or equal to that of V6 [30].

*3. How can you recognize left ventricular dilatation in acquired heart disease?

ANS.: Dilatation is suggested by the presence of voltage criteria for LVH plus one of the following:

   a. V6 larger in total voltage than V5 [15] (see ECG 24, p. 157; ECG 32, p. 173; and ECG 88).

   b. *A sudden transition* from a deep S in one chest lead to a tall R in the next lead to the left [38]. A tiny transition lead at V4 or V5 has the same meaning (see ECG 88). If the sudden transition zone is between V5 and V6, dilatation is even more likely.

   c. A completely developed LVH strain pattern in the absence of aortic stenosis or hypertrophic cardiomyopathy. (It is rare for a strain pattern to be caused by hypertension without some dilatation [78].) (See ECG 15, p. 129.)

4. Why does a V6 voltage larger than the V5 voltage suggest left ventricular dilatation?

ANS.: If the heart is closer than normal to V6 by dilatation, V6 may be larger in amplitude than V5 [15]. Even if only the R in V6 is taller than the R in V5 (i.e., not considering total voltage [R + S]), about 75 percent of such patients have cardiac dilatation as shown by x-ray [30]. Cardiac shifts to the left due to thoracic abnormalities such as pectus excavatum or high diaphragm nullify this sign.

Note: A T in V6 taller than the T in V5 has also been found to be highly suggestive of left ventricular dilatation, but only when anterior myocardial infarction was excluded [27].

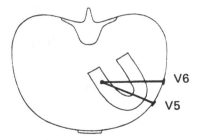

Normally, V6 is farther or the same distance from the heart as in V5.

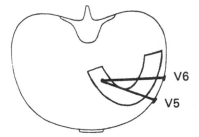

If the heart is dilated, V6 may be closer to the heart than is V5.

*5. What does it imply about the QRS vector to say that a sudden transition zone or small transitional lead at V5 rather than at V3 or V4 is highly suggestive of left ventricular dilatation?

ANS.: A transition zone that is shifted to the left implies that the QRS turns more posteriorly when LVH and dilatation develop.

Note: When vector loops are understood, it will be seen that a small transitional lead at V5 means a narrow, posterior loop. When it occurs as a result of the LVH, the stage of congestive heart failure with right ventricular enlargement has usually been reached [89].

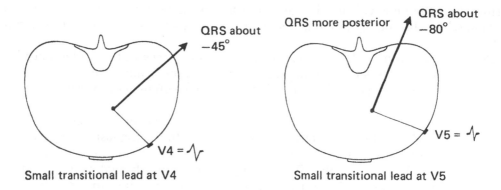

QRS about −45°

QRS more posterior

QRS about −80°

V4 =

Small transitional lead at V4

V5 =

Small transitional lead at V5

*6. What is the older term for a shift of the transition zone to the left as a result of posterior turning of the QRS?

ANS.: *Clockwise rotation of the heart,* meaning around its longitudinal axis as viewed from below, i.e., from the apex. It was thought that there was clockwise rotation of the heart when the transition zone was shifted to the left, i.e., toward V5 or V6, because the transition zone (equiphasic precordial lead) was considered to represent the site of the septum and interventricular sulcus, with the RV on its right and the LV on its left.

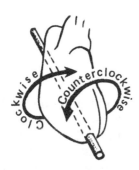

*7. What is wrong with the term *clockwise rotation of the heart?*

ANS.: a. There is no evidence that posterior turning of the QRS vector is necessarily associated with any displacement of the interventricular sulcus. Also, the term *clockwise* in relation to heart rotation on its longitudinal axis has no vector concept associated with it and so must be considered outdated. Vector concepts require that vector rotations be related to body axes and planes, e.g., the frontal X and Y axes and the horizontal X and Z axes.

b. Looked at from above, a posterior rotation of the QRS is actually a counterclockwise rotation of the vector (see diagram for question 5). There may, however, be horizontal plane QRS axis changes due to anatomic clockwise rotation in patients with right ventricular hypertrophy and to counterclockwise rotation with tortuous or elongated aortas.

Counterclockwise anatomic rotation of the heart may actually occur if aortic atherosclerosis causes elongation and tortuosity. This finding may account for the shift of the transition zone (and septal Q) to the right (at about V2) in some elderly patients with such aortas [88].

*8. How does the QRS voltage change in the frontal plane relative to the horizontal plane when chronic dilatation is due to (a) coronary disease, (b) idiopathic cardiomyopathy?

ANS.: a. In coronary disease the voltage often decreases in the horizontal plane but changes little or may also decrease in the frontal plane.

b. In idiopathic cardiomyopathies the voltage often decreases in the frontal plane but tends to increase in the horizontal plane. One study found that if frontal plane voltage is computed as the sum of the peak-to-trough QRS amplitudes in any two limb leads with the highest voltage, and the horizontal plane voltage is taken as the sum of the maximum voltage in (V1 or V2) plus (V5 or V6), a horizontal/frontal voltage ratio of more than 3.5 strongly suggests dilatation due to an idiopathic cardiomyopathy [25].

BUNDLE BRANCH BLOCK AND LVH

1. How can you best diagnose LVH in the presence of LBBB?

ANS.: In the frontal plane [32A]:
   a. aVL 11 with axis – 40°.
   b. Index of Ungerleider.
   In the horizontal plane [32A]:
   a. RV5 or 6 ≥ 25.
   b. 5V1 + RV5 or 6 ≥ 45 [34].
   c. Left atrial overload.
   d. QRS duration > 155 msec [29A].
   Note: a. A tall, slender R with no mid-QRS notch is probably due to LVH rather than LBBB, despite a QRS width of 120 msec (0.12 sec).
   *b. Of patients with complete LBBB, 80 percent have LVH at autopsy as determined by left ventricular thickness, and 96 percent have a heart weight greater than 0.43 percent of body weight in men or greater than 0.40 percent in women [59, 91].
   c. If necropsy studies are done on patients who had LBBB and hypertension or clinical coronary disease, 100 percent of such patients have LVH when the weight of the LV (plus the septum) and Zeek's upper normal values by body height are used [70, 90].

2. Is the index of Lewis valid in RBBB? Why?

ANS.: Probably yes, because RBBB tends to decrease QRS voltage. Some left ventricular forces are eliminated because the change of direction to the right and anteriorly caused by the block begins in the *middle* of the QRS *even before the terminal slowing.*

3. Is the index of Sokolow valid in RBBB?

ANS.: Yes, because RBBB tends to decrease both the S voltage in the right precordium and the R voltage in the left precordium.

Note: Even an RBBB pattern can mask the voltage of LVH.

*SIGNIFICANCE OF LVH ON THE ECG IN SYSTOLIC OVERLOADS

1. Which horizontal plane index for LVH is most sensitive for calcific aortic stenosis in the elderly?

   ANS.: The index of McPhie [22A].

*2. Can severe aortic stenosis be present with a normal ECG?

   ANS.: Yes. In children the ECG can be normal on repeated examinations until a severe LVH strain pattern is seen, when 6 months before there were no abnormalities. It is especially true with discrete subvalvular stenosis (see ECGs 95A and 95B).

   Note: a. Although voltage criteria are of no help in judging gradients across an aortic valve in congenital aortic stenosis, severe stenosis is indicated by
   - (1) A frontal T axis superior to + 15°, i.e., a T axis leftward enough at least to make the T in lead 3 negative.
   - (2) A sum of frontal and horizontal QRS-T angles of more than 100°.
   - (3) An R/T ratio in V5 or V6 greater than 10, i.e., an abnormally low T in V5 or V6 [23]. If the V6 R peak is later than the V2 S peak, the ejection fraction is less than 55 percent with a specificity of about 90 percent [61B].
   b. In hypertrophic subaortic stenosis (hypertrophic obstructive cardiomyopathy), LVH is absent on an ECG usually only in subjects with no resting gradient and no mitral regurgitation, even if abnormal Q waves suggestive of myocardial infarction are present [84].
   c. In hypertrophic cardiomyopathies without obstruction, the QRS tends to be anterior (transition at V2 or V3), the R wave tallest in V4, and the T waves markedly negative in the mid-precordium [11]. If the hypertrophic cardiomyopathy is of the type with asymmetric septal hypertrophy and no obstruction to outflow, the voltage is often markedly high in V4 or V5, i.e., 40 mm or more. This picture is not usual with hypertrophic subaortic stenosis (hypertrophic obstructive cardiomyopathy) [36].

*3. Is there a correlation between the degree of systemic hypertension and ECG criteria for LVH?

   ANS.: Yes, the higher the peripheral resistance, the more ECG changes due to LVH are found [67].

   Note: a. The presence of S-T or T changes is more related to systolic than to diastolic blood pressure in patients with both pressures elevated [60].
   b. Successful blood pressure treatment can significantly reverse T wave abnormalities [60].
   c. A normal ECG in a hypertensive patient suggests labile hypertension or the type with an increased cardiac output and heart rate with normal peripheral resistance [67]. (In these patients, diastolic hypertension is presumably due to lack of time for peripheral runoff because of the tachycardia and a lack of a compensatory drop in peripheral resistance.)

d. The degree of frontal leftward axis and horizontal posterior axis
correlates best with systolic pressure.

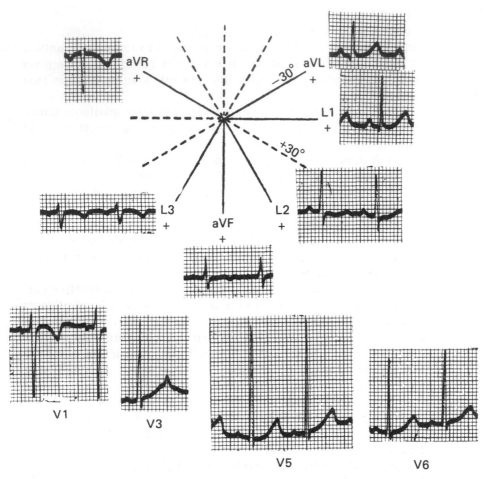

ECG 95A. An 8-year-old girl had discrete subvalvular aortic stenosis (a subvalvular membrane).
The index of Sokolow is positive for LVH, but this criterion is unreliable in this age group. There
are no secondary signs of LVH. Therefore if there were no clinical data, LVH could not be read
here. The gradient across the obstruction was 200 mm Hg.

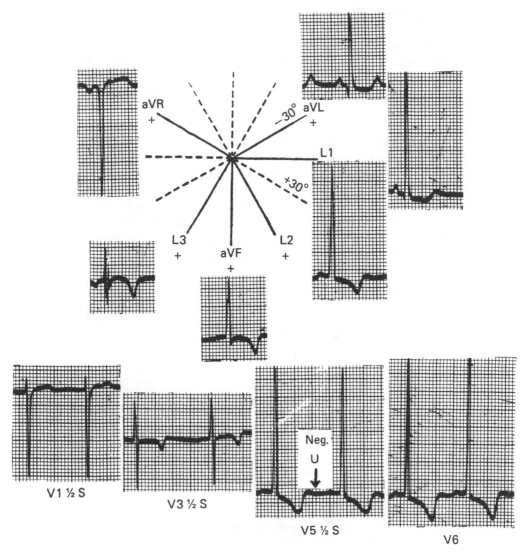

ECG 95B. This ECG is from the same girl as in ECG 95A but was obtained 10 months later. There is now a fully developed LVH strain pattern and a great increase in voltage. The transition zone has shifted to V3; i.e., the QRS is more posterior. Secondary muscular hypertrophic stenosis was found at surgery.

*4. What suggests in some patients with LVH secondary to hypertension that the S-T, T changes are secondary as much to coronary disease as to a hypertrophied myocardium?
    ANS.: In some hypertensive patients, disproportionate and often abrupt S-T, T changes develop when compared with voltage increases over the years [16].

VOLUME OVERLOADING OF THE LEFT VENTRICLE

1. What is the opposite of systolic overloading of the LV?
    ANS.: Diastolic or volume overloading, as in aortic or mitral regurgitation, ventricular septal defect (VSD), and persistent ductus arteriosus.

2. What is the generally accepted characteristic ECG pattern of volume overloading of the LV?

ANS.: The left ventricular leads are just like normal ones but with deep Q waves, tall R waves, and tall, peaked T waves; i.e., *it is as if a normal V5 and V6 were taken at double standard or double sensitivity* [10]. (A slightly delayed intrinsicoid deflection is also usual.) Another way to remember is to consider that, so long as hypertrophy is secondary and proportionate to the dilatation, both the QRS and the T increase their voltage proportionately. Pressure loads cause a disproportionate hypertrophy, which causes a disproportionate increase in QRS voltage relative to the T wave.

Note: This volume overload picture is not reliable for predicting the clinical situation when there is associated myocardial damage, as in any acquired heart disease, because then all degrees of LVH strain pattern can develop [40]. Therefore only in congenital heart disease, in which a relatively normal myocardium is expected, is the left ventricular diastolic overload pattern reliable, e.g., in VSD and persistent ductus arteriosus (see ECG 96).

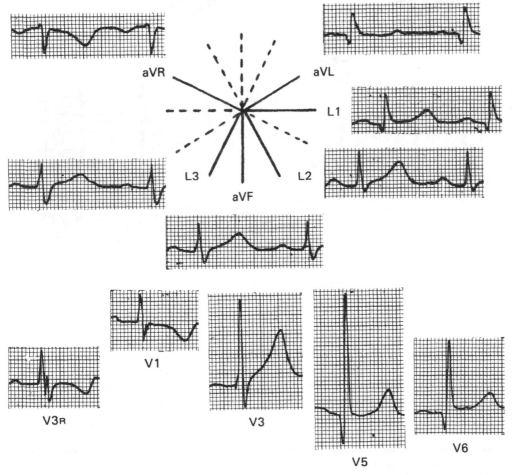

ECG 96. This double-speed ECG is from a 3-year-old child with a moderately large VSD. Pediatric ECGs are commonly run at double paper speed (50 mm/second). The large QRS and deep Q in V5 are characteristic of the left ventricular volume overload pattern as seen in congenital heart disease. The absence of a deep left ventricular S in V3r and V1 suggests combined ventricular overload.

3. How does chest lead voltage differentiate the left ventricular dilatation of aortic regurgitation from that of mitral regurgitation?

ANS.: Although both conditions produce high voltage R waves in the left precordium, only aortic regurgitation produces equally deep or deeper S waves over the right precordium. In one study of mitral regurgitation the R wave in V6 was always larger than the S wave in V1 [68]. (See ECG 90A.)

4. How can the QRS amplitudes help to show severe depression of ejection fraction in patients with aortic regurgitation?

ANS.: When the total 12-lead QRS amplitudes are less than 215 mm, together with an LVH strain pattern.

Note: The greatest voltage in one study of AR occurred in V2 and V3 [61C].

5. What does the isolated diastolic overload ECG pattern tell you about VSD hemodynamics?

ANS.: There is no important elevation of pulmonary artery pressure, i.e., not more than 30 mm Hg [26].

Note: A normal ECG in VSD does not necessarily mean a small shunt, and an isolated diastolic overload pattern does not always mean a large shunt [26].

*6. What is the most reliable sign of diastolic overloading in V5 and V6 in congenital heart disease: the deep Q, the tall R, or the tall T?

ANS.: The deep Q. The tall R and T are more often absent than are deep Q waves [49].

Note: a. A deep Q in V6 (2 mm or more) in the presence of an atrial septal defect suggests an endocardial cushion defect with a left ventricular volume overload due to mitral regurgitation [85].

b. In general, the larger the pulmonary/systemic flow ratios, the deeper is the Q in V6 [85].

c. In the presence of RBBB, a deep Q in left ventricular leads has been shown to mean a left ventricular overload, especially after a shunt operation for tetralogy of Fallot.

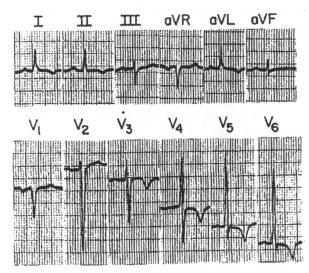

From a patient with severe AR who had his aortic valve replaced after the ECG was taken. Note that the S V2 is deeper than the RV5 or 6.

REFERENCES

1. Amad, K. H., Brennan, J. C., and Alexander, J. K. The cardiac pathology of chronic exogenous obesity. *Circulation* 32:740, 1965.
2. Bachman, S., Sparrow, D., and Smith, L. K. Effect of aging on the electrocardiogram. *Am. J. Cardiol.* 48:513, 1981.
3. Barnes, A. R., and Whitten, M. B. Study of T-wave negativity in predominant ventricular strain. *Am. Heart J.* 5:14, 1929.
4. Baxley, W. A., Dodge, H. T., and Sandler, H. A quantitative angiocardiographic study of left ventricular hypertrophy and the electrocardiogram. *Circulation* 37:509, 1968.
5. Bayley, R. H., Kalbfleisch, J. M., and Berry, P. M. Changes in the body's QRS surface potentials. *Am. Heart J.* 77:517, 1969.
6. Beswick, F. W., and Jordan, R. C. Cardiological observations at the sixth British Empire and Commonwealth Games. *Br. Heart J.* 23:113, 1961.
6A. Bjornstad, L., Storstein, L. Electrocardiographic findings of left, right and septal hypertrophy in athletic students and sedentary controls. *A.C.C. Curr. J. Rev.* 67, 1993.
7. Brody, D. A. A theoretical analysis of intracavitary blood mass influence on the heart-lead relationship. *Circ. Res.* 4:731, 1956.
8. Buja, L. M., Khoi, N. B., and Roberts, W. C. Clinically significant cardiac amyloidosis: Clinicopathologic findings in 15 patients. *Am. J. Cardiol.* 26:394, 1970.
9. Burch, G. E., Phillips, J. H., and Ansari, A. The cachectic heart. *Chest* 54:5, 1968.
10. Cabrera, E., and Gaxiola, A. A critical re-evaluation of systolic and diastolic overloading patterns. *Cardiovasc. Dis.* 2:219, 1959.
10A. Cassale, P. N., et al. Improved sex-specific criteria of LVH, validation by autopsy. *Circulation* 75:565; 1987.
11. Chen, C., Nobuyoshi, M., and Kawai, C. ECG pattern in nonobstructive hypertrophic cardiomyopathy. *Am. Heart J.* 97:687, 1979.
12. Cokkinos, D. V., Demopoulos, J. N., and Vorides, E. M. ECG criteria for left ventricular hypertrophy in left bundle branch block. *Br. Heart J.* 40:320, 1978.
13. Coleman, E. N. Ventricular hypertrophy and the electrical axis of the QRS complex in infancy. *Br. Heart J.* 24:139, 1962.
14. Constant, J., and Carlisle, R. The notched T in left ventricular hypertrophy and in alcoholism. *Chest* 57:540, 1970.
15. Constant, J., Schiller, N. B., and Lippschutz, E. J. Ventricular dilatation or volume overload diagnosed by QRS relationships of V4, V5, and V6. *Am. J. Med. Sci.* 253:61, 1967.
16. Cosby, R. S., and Herman, L. M. Sequential changes in the development of the electrocardiographic pattern of left ventricular hypertrophy in hypertensive heart disease. *Am. Heart J.* 63:180, 1962.
17. Cumming, G. R., and Proudfit, W. F. High-voltage QRS complexes in the absence of left ventricular hypertrophy. *Circulation* 19:406, 1959.
18. Dern, P. L., et al. Serial electrocardiographic changes in treated hypertensive patients with reference to voltage criteria, mean QRS vectors, and the QRS-T angle. *Circulation* 36:823, 1967.
19. Diamond, J. R., and Estes, M. M. ECG changes associated with left pneumothorax simulating anterior infarction. *Am. Heart J.* 103:303, 1982.
20. Doyle, A. E. Electrocardiographic changes in hypertension treated by methonium compounds. *Am. Heart J.* 45:363, 1953.
21. Evans, W. The syndrome of the suspended heart. *Br. Heart J.* 19:153, 1957.
21A. Farb, A., Devereux, R. B., Klingfield P. Day-to-day variability of voltage measurements used in electrocardiographic criteria for left ventricular hypertrophy. *Am. Coll. Cardiol.* 15:618–623, 1990.
22. Fernandez, F., et al. Electrocardiogram in corrected transposition of the great vessels of the bulbo-ventricular inversion type. *Br. Heart J.* 32:165, 1970.
22A. Forker, A. D., et al. Atypical presentations of patients with calcific aortic stenosis. *J.A.M.A.* 212:774, 1970.
23. Fowler, R. S. Ventricular repolarization in congenital aortic stenosis. *Am. Heart J.* 70:603, 1965.
24. Garbagni, R., et al. Residual lung volume in mitral disease. *Br. Heart J.* 20:479, 1958.

24A. Geddes, L. A., Baker, L. E. The specific resistance of biological material. *Med. Biol. Eng.* 5:271–2793, 1967.

25. Goldberger, A., Dresselhaus, T., and Bhargava, W. Dilated cardiomyopathy: Utility of the transverse: frontal plane QRS voltage ratio. *J. Electrocardiol.* 18:35, 1985.

26. Grayzel, J., and Neyshaboori, M. Left axis deviation: Etiologic factors in one-hundred patients. *Am. Heart J.* 89:419, 1975.

27. Griep, A. H. Pitfalls in the electrocardiographic diagnosis of left ventricular hypertrophy. A correlative study of 200 autopsied patients. *Circulation* 20:30, 1959.

28. Grubschmidt, H. A., and Sokolow, M. The reliability of high voltage of the QRS complex as a diagnostic sign of left ventricular hypertrophy in adults. *Am. Heart J.* 54:689, 1957.

29. Gubner, R. S., and Ungerleider, H. E. Electrocardiographic criteria of left ventricular hypertrophy. *Arch. Intern. Med.* 72:196, 1943.

29A. Haskell, R. J., Ginzton, L. E., and Laks, M. M. Electrocardiographic diagnosis of left ventricular hypertrophy in the presence of left bundle branch block. *J. Electrocardiogr.* 20(3): 227–232, 1987.

29B. Heaf, J. G. Albumin-induced changes in the QRS complex. *Am. J. Cardiol.* 55:1530, 1985.

30. Holt, D. D., and Spodick, D. H. The RV6:RV5 voltage ratio in left ventricular hypertrophy. *Am. Heart J.* 63:65, 1962.

31. Horton, J. D., Sherber, H. S., and Lakatta, E. G. Distance correction for precordial electrocardiographic voltage in estimating left ventricular mass. An echocardiographic study. *Circulation* 55:509, 1977.

31A. Huwez, F. U. Variable patterns of S-T, T abnormalities in patients with LVH and normal coronary arteries. *Br. Heart J.* 67:304, 1992.

32. Ishikawa, K., Berson, A. S., and Pipberger, H. V. Electrocardiographic changes due to cardiac enlargement. *Am. Heart J.* 81:635, 1971.

32A. Kafka, H., Burggraf, G. W., Milliken, J. A. Electrocardiographic diagnosis of left ventricular hypertrophy in the presence of left bundle branch block: an echocardiographic study. *Am. J. Cardiol.* 55:103–106, 1985.

33. Kilty, S. E., and Lepeschkin, E. Effect of body build on the QRS voltage of the electrocardiogram in normal men. *Circulation* 31:77, 1965.

34. Klein, R. C., et al. Electrocardiographic diagnosis of left ventricular hypertrophy in left bundle branch block (abstract). *Circulation* 57/58:II-198, 1978.

35. Klemola, E. Electrocardiographic observations on 650 Finnish athletes. *Ann. Med. Intern. Fenn.* 40:121, 1951.

35A. Knopf, W. D. Increased aVL voltage lack of correlation with echocardiographic LVH. *J. Am. Coll. Cardiol.* 3:597, 1984 (Abstract).

36. Kondo, T., Hisida, H., and Mizuno, Y. Electrocardiographic manifestations of hypertrophic cardiomyopathy. *J. Cardiogr.* 9:1, 1979.

37. Kossmann, C. E., et al. The electrocardiogram in ventricular hypertrophy and bundle branch block. *Circulation* 26:1337, 1962.

38. Kuramoto, K., et al. Correlative study of electrocardiographic criteria of left ventricular hypertrophy in the aged. *Ronnenbyo (Jpn. J. Geriatr.)* 4:631, 1960.

39. LaMonte, C. S., and Freiman, A. H. The electrocardiogram after mastectomy. *Circulation* 32:746, 1965.

40. Lasser, J. J., and Lasser, R. P. Hemodynamic correlations of the electrocardiographic pattern of left ventricular hypertrophy, 'diastolic overloading.' *Dis. Chest* 41:180, 1962.

41. Lemberg, L., et al. Digitalis as an indicator of ventricular disease. *Chest* 52:490, 1967.

42. Linzbach, A. J. Heart failure from the point of view of quantitative anatomy. *Am. J. Cardiol.* 5:370, 1960.

43. Manning, G. W., and Cropp, G. J. The electrocardiogram in progressive muscular dystrophy. *Br. Heart J.* 20:416, 1958.

44. Manning, G. W., and Smiley, J. R. QRS voltage criteria for left ventricular hypertrophy in a normal male population. *Circulation* 29:224, 1964.

45. Manoach, M., et al. Influences of hemorrhage on the QRS complex of the electrocardiogram. *Am. Heart J.* 82:55, 1971.

46. Masica, D. N., Maron, B. J., and Krovetz, L. J. Racial variations in the childhood electrocardiogram: Preliminary observations. *Am. Heart J.* 84:153, 1972.

47. Massoleni, A., et al. Correlation between component cardiac weights and electrocardiographic patterns in 185 cases. *Circulation* 30:808, 1964.

47A. McLenachan, J. M., Henderson, E., Morris, K. I., Dargie, H. J. Electrocardiographic diagnosis of left ventricular hypertrophy: influence of body build. *Clin. Sci.* 75:589–592, 1988.

48. McPhie, J. Left ventricular hypertrophy: Electrocardiographic diagnosis. *Aust. Ann. Med.* 7:317, 1958.

49. Means, J. H. *The Thyroid and Its Diseases* (2nd ed.). Philadelphia: Lippincott, 1948.

50. Morganroth, J., et al. Electrocardiographic evidence of left ventricular hypertrophy in otherwise normal children. *Am. J. Cardiol.* 35:278, 1975.

51. Morrow, G. M., Goldblatt, A., and Braunwald, E. Congenital aortic stenosis. *Circulation* 27:450, 1963.

52. Myers, G. B. QRS-T patterns in multiple precordial leads that may be mistaken for myocardial infarction. *Circulation* 1:844, 1950.

53. Nadas, A. S., and Fyler, D. C. *Pediatric Cardiology* (3rd ed.). Philadelphia: Saunders, 1972. P. 485.

54. Namati, M., et al. The orthogonal electrocardiogram in normal women. Implications of sex differences in diagnostic electrocardiography. *Am. Heart J.* 95:12, 1978.

55. Neuman, A. Intermittent regional delay of left ventricular activation: The influence of such a delay on the standard electrocardiogram. Report of 33 cases. *Chest* 61:633, 1972.

56. Numa, T., et al. Vectorcardiogram in various types of non-uniform ventricular hypertrophy. *J. Cardiogr.* 8:305, 1978.

57. Okamoto, N., Simonson, E., and Blackburn, H. The T-V1 T-V6 for electrocardiographic diagnosis of left ventricular hypertrophy and ischemia. *Circulation* 31:719, 1965.

58. Okuni, M. A proposal of new pediatric electrocardiographic criteria for ventricular hypertrophy. *Jpn. Heart J.* 16:189, 1975.

59. Petersen, G. V., and Tikoff, G. Left bundle branch block and left ventricular hypertrophy: Electrocardiographic pathologic correlations. *Chest* 59:174, 1971.

60. Poblete, P. F., et al. Effect of treatment on morbidity in hypertension. Veterans Administration cooperative study on antihypertensive agents. Effect on the electrocardiogram. *Circulation* 58:481, 1973.

61. Postell, W. N., et al. Vectorcardiographic and electrocardiographic manifestations of increasing left ventricular pressure overload. *Am. Heart J.* 77:33, 1969.

61A. Rao, P. S., Thapar, M. K., Harp, K. J. Racial variations in electrocardiograms and vectorcardiograms between black and white children and their genesis. *J. Electrocardiogr.* 17(3):239–52, 1984.

61B. Recke, S. H., et al. ECG markers of impaired ejection performance in aortic stenosis. *J. Electrocardiol.* 22:45, 1989.

61C. Roberts, W. C. Electrocardiographic observations in clinically isolated, pure, chronic, severe aortic regurgitation: Analysis of 30 necropsy patients aged 19 to 65 years. *Am. J. Cardiol.* 55:431–438, 1985.

62. Romhilt, D. W., and Estes, E. H. Point-score system for the electrocardiographic diagnosis of left ventricular hypertrophy. *Am. Heart J.* 75:752, 1968.

63. Romhilt, D. W., et al. A critical appraisal of the electrocardiographic criteria for the diagnosis of left ventricular hypertrophy. *Circulation* 40:185, 1969.

64. Rosenbaum, M. B., and Elizari, M. V. Left anterior and left posterior hemiblocks. Electrocardiographic manifestations. *Postgrad. Med.* 53:61, 1973.

65. Rosenfeld, I., et al. The electrocardiographic recognition of left ventricular hypertrophy. *Am. Heart J.* 63:731, 1962.

66. Rosenthal, A. Influence of acute variations in hematocrit on QRS complex of Frank electrocardiogram. *J.A.M.A.* 218:908, 1971.

67. Sannerstadt, R., Bjure, J., and Varnauskas, E. Correlation between electrocardiographic changes and systemic hemodynamics in human arterial hypertension. *Am. J. Cardiol.* 28:117, 1970.

68. Schamroth, L., et al. Electrocardiographic differentiation of the causes of left ventricular diastolic overload. *Chest* 89:95, 1966.

69. Schultz, A. Uber einen Fall von Athyreosis congenita (Myxodem) mit besonderer Berucksichtigung der dabei beobachteten Muskelveranderungen. *Virchows Arch.* 232:302, 1921.

69A. Scognamiglio, R., et al. Detection of left ventricular function in aortic regurgitation. *Eur. Heart J.* 9:54, 1988.

70. Scott, R. C., and Norris, R. J. ECG-pathologic correlation study of LVH and LBBB. *Circulation* 20:766, 1959.

71. Selzer, A., et al. Electrocardiographic findings in concentric and eccentric left ventricular hypertrophy. *Am. Heart J.* 63:320, 1962.

72. Simonson, E., and Keys, A. The effect of age on mean spatial QRS and T vectors. *Circulation* 14:100, 1956.

73. Simonson, E., et al. Sex differences in the electrocardiogram. *Circulation* 22:598, 1960.

74. Sokolow, M., and Lyon, T. P. The ventricular complex in left ventricular hypertrophy as obtained by unipolar precordial and limb leads. *Am. Heart J.* 37:161, 1949.

75. Soloff, L. A., and Lawrence, J. W. The electrocardiographic findings in left ventricular hypertrophy and dilatation. *Circulation* 26:553, 1962.

76. Talbot, S. Electrical axis and voltage criteria of left ventricular hypertrophy. *Am. Heart J.* 90:420, 1975.

77. Talbot, S., et al. QRS voltage of the electrocardiogram and Frank vectorcardiogram in relation to ventricular volume. *Br. Heart J.* 39:1109, 1977.

78. Toshima, H., and Mori, F. Studies on the abnormal T waves: Left ventricular dilatation and T changes. *Jpn. Circ. J.* 25:307, 1961.

79. Toshima, H., Koga, Y., and Kimura, N. Correlations between electrocardiographic vectorcardiographic, and echocardiographic findings in patients with left ventricular overload. *Am. Heart J.* 94:547, 1977.

80. Uhley, H. N., and Proctor, J. Study of the transmembrane action potential, electrogram, electrocardiogram and vectorcardiogram of rats with left ventricular hypertrophy. *Am. J. Cardiol.* 7:211, 1961.

81. Unverferth, D. V., Williams, T. E., and Fulkerson, P. K. Electrocardiographic voltage in pericardial effusion. *Chest* 75:157, 1979.

82. VanGansa, W., et al. The electrocardiogram of athletes. *Br. Heart J.* 32:160, 1970.

83. Wada, T. Left ventricular activation time in left ventricular hypertrophy and in left bundle-branch block. *Circulation* 19:873, 1959.

84. Walston, A., II, et al. Electrocardiographic and hemodynamic correlations in patients with idiopathic hypertrophic subaortic stenosis. *Am. Heart J.* 91:11, 1976.

85. Watson, D. G., and Keith, J. D. The Q waves in lead V6 in heart disease of infancy and childhood with special references to diastolic loading. *Am. Heart J.* 65:629, 1962.

86. White, P. D., and Bock, A. V. Electrocardiographic evidence of abnormal ventricular preponderance and of auricular hypertrophy. *Am. J. Med. Sci.* 156:17, 1918.

87. Wigle, E. D., and Baron, R. H. Effects of left and right ventricular conduction defects on the electrocardiogram in muscular subaortic stenosis. *Circulation* [Suppl. 11] 31–32:219, 1965.

88. Yanagisawa, N. Counterclockwise rotation of the heart. *J. Electrocardiol.*, 14:233, 1981.

88A. Yanagisawa, A., Kanemitsu, H., Shirato, C., Ishikawa, M., et al. Influence of acute intracardiac volume expansion upon the QRS complexes in normal men. *Jpn. Heart J.* 23:531–533, 1982.

89. Yano, K., and Pipberger, H. V. Correlations between radiologic heart size and orthogonal electrocardiograms in patients with left ventricular hypertrophy. *Am. Heart J.* 67:44, 1964.

90. Zeek, P. M. Heart weight. *Arch. Pathol.* 34:820, 1942.

91. Zmyslinski, R. W., Richeson, J. F., and Akiyama, T. Left ventricular hypertrophy in the presence of complete left bundle branch block. *Br. Heart J.* 43:170, 1980.

25. Right Ventricular Hypertrophy

FRONTAL PLANE CRITERIA

1. What would you expect to happen to the frontal plane QRS axis in right ventricular hypertrophy (RVH)?
   ANS.: The axis ought to turn inferiorly and to the right, because the right ventricle (RV) is slightly rightward in relation to the left ventricle (LV).

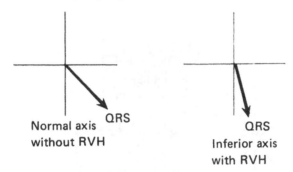

Normal axis without RVH

Inferior axis with RVH

2. How rightward a QRS should you consider suggestive of RVH?
   ANS.: It depends on the age and chest shape of the subject. The younger the patient and the longer the chest, the more inferior and to the right is the axis normally. Therefore among subjects with short, squat, stocky chests in whom the axes tend to be leftward, even a young patient should not normally show a very inferior axis.
   Note: A right bundle branch block (RBBB) can cause a slight right axis deviation.

3. In the patient over age 40, what is the maximum limit of an inferior or rightward QRS?
   ANS.: About 90°. Beyond 90° probably means RVH or posterior divisional block.
   Note: In a patient under age 40, the axis should be beyond 110° before strongly suggesting RVH.

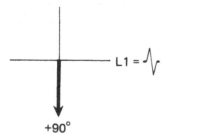

Normal inferior QRS axis in an adult with a long chest.

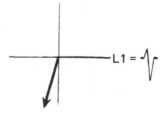

Normal rightward QRS axis in a child without RVH.

*4. What can cause a right axis deviation of more than 90° without RVH or RBBB?

ANS.: A terminal conduction defect of the posterior divisional block type.

Note: a. Because an anterior divisional block produces a left axis deviation, RVH is obscured by such a conduction defect [47].

b. A Q in lead 1 deep enough to cause a right axis deviation can be caused by infarction.

5. How can you tell at a glance that the QRS suggests RVH in the frontal plane, i.e., that there is a rightward axis in the frontal plane?

ANS.: If lead 1 is predominantly negative (its S is deeper than the R is tall), and the inferior leads are positive. (The 'inferior leads' are leads 2, 3, and aVF.)

6. Are there voltage indexes in the frontal plane for RVH just as there are left ventricular hypertrophy (LVH) voltage indexes such as the index of Lewis?

ANS.: Yes. If the S in lead 1 + the R in lead 3 = at least 14 mm (after subtracting opposite deflections).

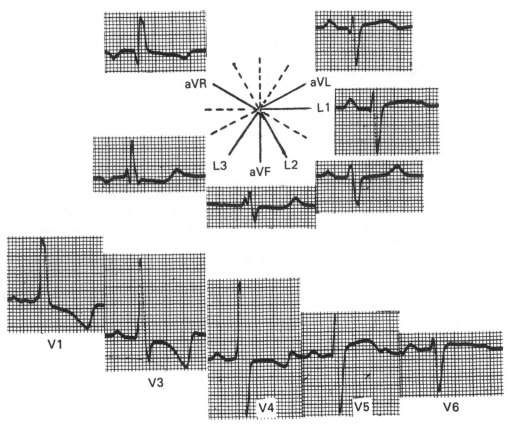

ECG 97. A 50 mm per second (double-speed) pediatric ECG of severe pulmonary valvular stenosis from a 10-year-old girl with a right ventricular pressure of 140 mm Hg, which was greater than her aortic pressure of 120 mm Hg. The R in L3 plus the S in L1 (after subtracting the R in L1 and the S in L3) is 19. The marked right axis deviation of about + 170° is another frontal plane characteristic of RVH.

---

* Material marked with an asterisk is included for reference and for advanced students in cardiology.

*7. Because the axis in normal infants may normally be more than 90°, how much right axis deviation is suggestive of RVH in an infant?

ANS.: It depends on the child's age. At birth the RV is about 15 percent heavier than the LV, so that all normal infants are born with RVH, and under age 1 month even 180° may be normal. The ECG signs of RVH begin to regress at about the end of the first month, when the LV becomes heavier than the RV. If the infant is over 3 months of age, a right axis deviation of more than 120° suggests RVH. Therefore aVR should not be predominantly positive over age 3 months.

Note: In premature infants the LV is heavier than the RV [25].

*8. Does the axis turn more rightward in RBBB when there is RVH?

ANS.: Yes. Therefore a marked right axis deviation, even in the presence of RBBB, suggests RVH or a block in the posterior division of the left bundle, i.e., a bifascicular block.

*9. Does the axis in the frontal plane turn either inferiorly or rightward if RVH is present with left bundle branch block (LBBB)?

ANS.: Yes.

Note: The presence in LBBB of a change in axis due to RVH seems surprising as in LBBB the RV presumably is completely depolarized long before the LV has even begun to be activated. However, according to one theory, the inferior one-third of the right part of the septum belongs to the RV; i.e., it is a right ventricular septal mass [58]. If RVH hypertrophies both the RV and this septal mass, the initial part of the activation in LBBB, which is entirely due to right ventricular depolarization, could point rightward, inferiorly, and anteriorly, i.e., toward the hypertrophied septal mass. This situation could also cause a large initial positivity in V1, which would be unexpected in uncomplicated LBBB.

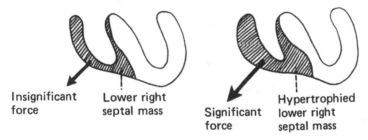

Insignificant force — Lower right septal mass

Significant force — Hypertrophied lower right septal mass

10. Why is the axis range of −90° to 180° the 'no man's land' of the axis world?

ANS.: A QRS axis in this area could be due to a very marked left or very marked right axis deviation.

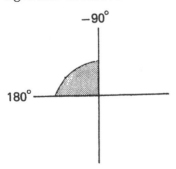

Note: This range of axes is characteristic of some patients with transposition of the great vessels and is probably due to a combination of the marked right axis deviation caused by the RVH and the marked left axis deviation that the LV produces in transposition. This situation produces a resultant in the upper right quadrant [29]. This range of axes is very rarely caused by any other congenital abnormality.

ECG IN EMPHYSEMA, OR CHRONIC OBSTRUCTIVE PULMONARY DISEASE

Frontal Plane

1. Can an inferior axis be due to chronic obstructive pulmonary disease (COPD) alone *without significant RVH?*
   ANS.: Yes.
2. How could COPD cause an inferior axis without the patient's necessarily having RVH?
   ANS.: One theory is that in COPD the lungs are such poor conductors of electricity that all X axis forces are diminished, leaving Y axis vectors dominant.
   Note: It also produces a voltage of less than 10 mm in lead 1. The differential diagnosis of low voltage in lead 1 is most commonly a normal variant in a long chest, COPD, or mitral stenosis. Rarely, it is chronic constrictive pericarditis, cachexia, amyloid disease, or myxedema. Voltage of 5 mm or less in lead 1 is even more likely to be one of the above diagnoses.
   Note: The low voltage in lead 1 in mitral stenosis occurs for the same reason as in COPD; i.e., there is an attenuation of X axis vectors by the lung, and the QRS tends to turn posteriorly into the horizontal plane.

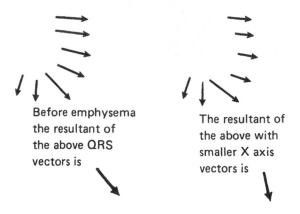

Before emphysema the resultant of the above QRS vectors is

The resultant of the above with smaller X axis vectors is

3. How could a dilated RV with an elevated pressure in it cause delayed conduction along the right bundle?
   ANS.: The right bundle is a thick thread that travels so close to the right side of the ventricular septum that a catheter pressing on the ventricular septum during cardiac catheterization can produce various degrees of RBBB, depending on the amount of pressure applied. A dilated RV can stretch the right bundle. Stretching the right bundle has been said to delay conduction along it, thereby producing the ECG picture of RBBB.

Note: The right bundle is a relatively thick, distinct, easily dissectible cord that pursues a well defined course to the apex of the RV before ramifying. In contrast, the left bundle branch divides almost immediately into thin radicles or rootlets. According to the neuropraxic principle, large-diameter nerves are more susceptible to compression than are small-diameter nerves [7]. Hypertrophy of a wall protects the conduction fibers from compression. Therefore

a. The RV with a sudden high pressure, as with an acute pulmonary embolism, is likely to cause a compression delay in right bundle branch conduction.

b. The filamentous left bundle branches are not so likely to suffer from significant compression delays, so that LBBB does not usually result from increased pressure in the LV.

c. When COPD results in RVH, it protects against RBBB.

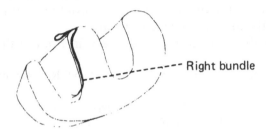

4. What other surprising QRS axis is common in COPD?

 ANS.: Marked left axis deviation of even as much as − 80°.

 Note: The 'axis illusion' theory has been given as a cause of marked left axis deviation in COPD. It utilizes the fact that the QRS commonly points almost straight backward and slightly inferiorly. It appears to be markedly inferior in the frontal plane.

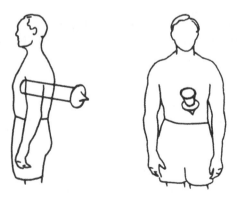

Now note that a slight tilt of the axis inferiorly can produce a marked inferior axis.

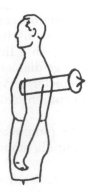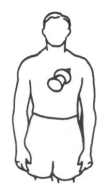

Also a slightly superior tilt of the QRS takes on the appearance of a marked left axis deviation. One theory of the cause of the almost straight-backward tilt of the QRS vector is that there is a backward tilt of the apex of the heart in COPD as the low diaphragm pulls down on the pericardium.

Another theory is that a relative increase of lung space in front of the heart attenuates anterior forces.

5. What does the posterior turning of the QRS in COPD tend to do to the QRS voltage in the limb leads?

ANS.: a. It tends to make the voltage low in all limb leads but *especially in lead 1* because of the simultaneous verticalization of the QRS, so that it tends to become perpendicular to the lead line of lead 1 [14].

b. Because the P waves do not turn posteriorly, as does the QRS, it tends to make the P waves relatively tall in comparison to the QRS in the frontal plane.

Note: In chronic constrictive pericarditis there also tends to be an inferior axis or frank right axis deviation with low voltage in all the limb leads, especially in the presence of atrial fibrillation [2].

6. What happens to the P wave in COPD other than becoming relatively tall?

ANS.: It becomes more inferior than + 60°, so that the P in aVL is usually negative. See pages 434–6 for explanation of P axis in COPD.

7. How does the P axis for COPD differ from restrictive lung disease? Why?

ANS.: In COPD the P axis is between 70° and 90°. In purely restrictive lung disease the P axis is usually between 40° and 60° [54A].

8. What P axis is virtually diagnostic of COPD?

ANS.: About + 90°; i.e., the P in lead 1 is almost flat (see ECG 98).

Note: a. The Ta wave may be exaggerated if the P wave is relatively tall in leads 2, 3, and aVF [65]. (See p. 443 for explanation of the Ta wave.)

b. An acute pulmonary embolism causing acute cor pulmonale can also turn the P wave inferiorly up to + 90° [12].

9. What percent of patients have a negative P in aVL if they have (a) COPD, (b) interstitial fibrosis?

ANS.: a. 80 percent.

b. 25 percent.

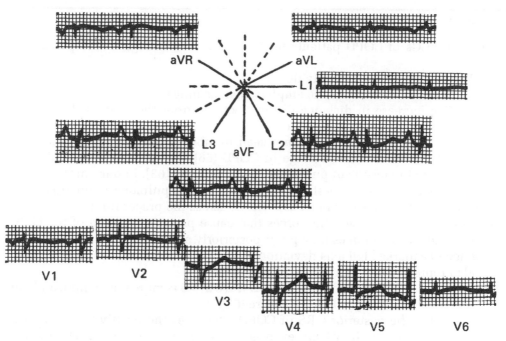

ECG 98. An 83-year-old man had COPD but normal CO_2 and vital capacity. His PO_2 in room air was 65 mm Hg. His 1-second vital capacity was 60 percent of predicted capacity. Note the low voltage L1, relatively tall P wave in aVF, negative P in aVL, and almost flat P in L1; i.e., the P is about + 85°. (*The negative P in both V1 and V2 is also a feature of COPD.)

*10. What can be seen in the frontal ECG of COPD patients with chronic cor pulmonale when a bout of hypoxia occurs?

   ANS.: When a bout of hypoxia, acidosis, and pulmonary hypertension occurs, only those with chronic cor pulmonale show various degrees of temporary
   a. Inferior axis shift of more than 30°.
   b. S-T depression in the inferior leads.
   c. T negativity in the right chest leads, i.e., V1 and V2 [37].
   d. RBBB of various degrees.

   Note: About 5 percent of patients with COPD show biventricular hypertrophy on the ECG with no obvious cause for the LVH. This finding has been explained on the basis of bronchopulmonary shunts and hypoxia, as well as the heart functioning as a single unit in hypertrophy [49]. The latter is suggested by the finding of LVH in patients with pure pulmonary stenosis at necropsy [31].

*11. What frontal plane pattern has been associated with the worst degree of COPD?

   ANS.: The S1, S2, S3 pattern. (It is usually a pattern without a definite axis; i.e., it often produces an interdeterminate axis.) Hypertrophy of the outflow tract of the RV probably causes the terminal vector to take this form of RBBB pattern. The initial and terminal forces then usually go in opposite directions.

   Note: a. A P axis of more than + 80° correlates with the next most severe degree of COPD. In general, the P turns more rightward (inferiorly) with increasing obstructive lung disease [61].
   b. Those with the worst pulmonary impairment tend to have the fastest heart rates [13].

Horizontal Plane

1. Why do the ECGs of COPD patients tend to show low voltage in the precordial leads?

   ANS.: The low voltage is probably due to
   a. Poor conductivity of the emphysematous lungs.
   b. The increase in distance of the electrode from the heart if the antero-posterior diameter is increased.

   Note: Even if low voltage is not seen in most of the precordial leads, V6 almost always has low voltage in COPD [66]. The lower the R in V6, the worse are the results of pulmonary function tests [63]. In one study an R in V6 of 6 mm or less suggested a severe decrease in pulmonary function [55].

2. Why does COPD tend to show itself as S waves across the precordium?

   ANS.: The S waves represent the forces that cause posterior turning of the QRS; i.e., the terminal forces may point posteriorly and to the right. (In the presence of a marked left axis deviation, the S waves in the left precordium may also represent the inferior lead S waves.)

   Note: a. COPD is very likely if the S wave in V6 is more than 5 mm, and the COPD is likely to be severe [63].
   b. The posterior QRS of COPD attenuates the positivity in V1, and r waves in V1 are even absent in 20 percent of COPD patients. A terminal positivity, or R', is also rare.
   c. Some mitral stenosis patients also have a posterior QRS as with COPD. Together with the low voltage in lead 1, the imitation of COPD is marked. Vectorcardiographic loops have shown that some mitral stenosis patients imitate the QRS loops of COPD almost exactly [27].

3. Why may poor precordial R wave progress not be a valid sign of COPD, although in most books and articles it is mentioned as typical of the ECG of COPD?

   ANS.: a. The R/S progression may be normal, i.e., the R may not become larger but the S does become smaller.
   b. In the occasional reports of patients with COPD and a poor R wave progression as well as poor R/S progression there was often no angiographic or necropsy confirmation of the absence of infarction.
   c. If the electrodes are placed one interspace lower, good R wave progression and R/S ratio progression may be seen.

*4. If the QRS is posterior and to the right, is the transition zone shifted to the right or to the left?

   ANS.: It may be shifted either way, e.g.,

These QRS vectors are posterior and rightward

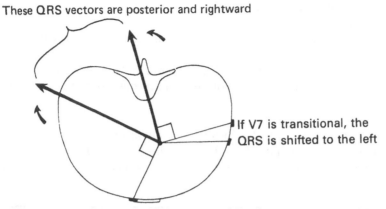

If V7 is transitional, the QRS is shifted to the left

If V1 is transitional, the QRS is shifted to the right

Note: The posterior QRS of COPD shifts the transition zone to the left [9]. This move tends to make the R/S ratio in V6 less than 1. If the QRS is posterior and rightward enough, only lead V3R may show the RVH sign of Rs or qR.

5. How does bronchospasm affect QRS voltage?

   ANS.: It may cause marked fluctuation in QRS voltage with respiration, especially in low-voltage equiphasic leads. It may occur because there are exaggerated axis shifts, which are best seen in transitional leads.

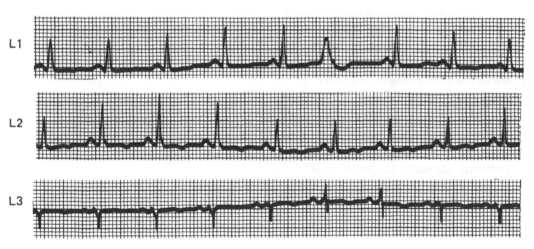

ECG 99. This ECG is from a man with marked bronchospasm. Note the marked variation in amplitude and axis. The changes are best seen in the lead that is lowest in voltage and closest to being equiphasic. Even in normal subjects, a low-voltage equiphasic lead commonly shows respiratory variations in amplitude.

---

*Pectus Excavatum Versus Emphysema

*1. In which way is the heart in pectus excavatum like that of a patient with COPD?

   ANS.: The apex is posteriorly displaced in both.

*2. How does the posterior apex in subjects with pectus excavatum affect the ECG?

ANS.: a. Both P and T are predominantly negative in V1 [20].
   b. V1 has a qR.

*3. How does the posterior apex in subjects with a pectus excavatum produce a qR in V1?

ANS.: An electrode directly on the right atrium in a normal subject records a qR. A posterior apex plus the concave chest depression may force the right atrium to be adjacent enough to the V1 electrode for it to pick up direct right atrial complexes.

4. When does the P become negative in V1 in pectus excavatum?

ANS.: When the pectus is deep enough to displace the heart to the left.

Note: The P negativity has a large enough area to suggest left atrial overload.

Cachectic Heart Versus COPD

1. What is meant by the cachectic heart?

ANS.: The heart in a patient dying from malignancy or another debilitating disease. At autopsy a soft, flabby heart with minimal atherosclerosis and epicardial fat is observed. The x-ray shows a small heart [10].

2. How is the ECG of the cachectic heart similar to the ECG in COPD?

ANS.: a. Leads 1 and V6 have low voltage.
   b. The P waves are inferior, i.e., more than + 60°.

3. How does the ECG of the cachectic heart differ from the ECG of COPD?

ANS.: a. The P waves, even though inferior, are low or normal in amplitude [10].
   b. The QRS axis tends to be normal.
   c. The S waves do not tend to go to V6.

Summary of the ECG Features of COPD

One or More QRS Signs

1. Low voltage in all limb leads but lowest in lead 1.
2. Low voltage in chest leads but especially in V6.
3. Inferior axis or marked left axis deviation.
4. RBBB patterns, atypical, i.e., no R′ in V1.
5. S waves across the precordium and small RV6 with the S in V6 more than 5 mm (posterior and rightward QRS).
6. Occasionally, QS through the right precordium and mid-precordium.

P Signs

1. Inferior P axis, i.e., negative in aVL and especially diagnostic if more than + 80°, so that the P is low or flat in lead 1.
2. Relatively tall and peaked P in aVF.
3. Tall P waves when atrial tachycardias occur. (Atrial tachycardias tend to have low P waves.)
4. An exaggerated Ta wave in leads 2, 3, and aVF. (See p. 443 for an explanation of the Ta wave.)

Note: a. The preceding signs are not necessarily those of RVH. The pattern of classic RVH should not be expected with COPD. The ECG signs of COPD are due to the effects of the lungs on electrical conduction. RVH occurs rarely, as does significant pulmonary hypertension, i.e., in only 8 percent or less of COPD patients [41]. In general, it has been shown that the more severe the COPD (i.e., the lower the FEV_1/VC), the more likely are the signs of RVH to show, i.e., P waves of more than 2.5 mm, deep Ta waves, QRS axes more than 75°, and an S in V5 and V6 more than 5 mm [63].

   b. All the preceding findings except the P axis of more than 80° may be found in normal young people.

HORIZONTAL PLANE CRITERIA FOR RVH

Anterior QRS in RVH

1. If the RV is an anterior and slightly rightward structure, in what direction would you expect the mean QRS to point in the presence of RVH?
   ANS.: The QRS should be shifted anteriorly and rightward.

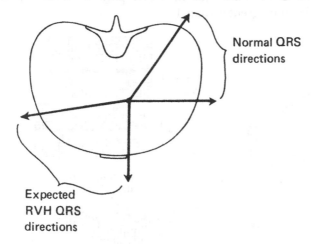

Normal QRS directions

Expected RVH QRS directions

2. How does the anterior and rightward direction of a QRS show on the ECG?
   ANS.: The right chest leads have increased positivity (see ECGs 100 and 108).
3. In LVH we add the S in the right precordium to the R in the left precordium because they represent left ventricular forces. What part of the precordial complexes represents right ventricular forces?
   ANS.: The R in the right precordium and the S in the left precordium.
4. What is the index of Sokolow for RVH?
   ANS.: If the R in V1 plus the S in V5 or V6 is 11 mm or more, RVH is likely [59]. (The only other voltage criterion that uses the number 11 is the aVL maximum voltage for LVH.) This chest lead criterion would be of use in the presence of an anterior divisional block, which can also produce deep S waves in the left precordium.
   Note: The physiologic RVH seen in athletes may show the anterior QRS type of RVH index of Sokolow. It is found in at least 10 percent of endurance athletes [40].
5. What is the normal R/S ratio in V1?
   ANS.: In adults it is usually less than 1; i.e., the R is usually smaller than the S. (In infants the R/S ratio in V1 can normally reach 4.) In adults V1 usually =

although it may occasionally be exactly 1, i.e.,

6. What can happen to the R/S ratio in V1 if RVH develops in the adult?
   ANS.: It can become greater than 1. This ratio is the result of the mean QRS vector's turning anteriorly and to the right.

   *It is rarely seen in RVH due to COPD, in which the R/S ratio in V1 is usually normal because in COPD the QRS turns posteriorly. Only if the pulmonary vascular resistance increases markedly (as in a few patients with COPD) does the R/S ratio in V1 become greater than 1.

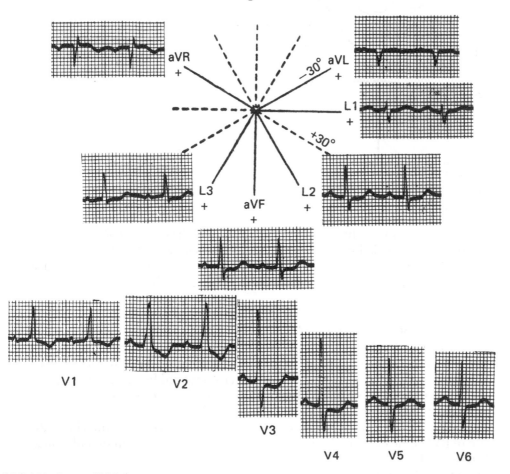

ECG 100. Severe RVH due to systemic levels of pulmonary hypertension secondary to mitral stenosis in a 55-year-old woman. Note the anterior QRS (perpendicular to a lead in about the V7 position). The frontal axis is at about 110°.

7. What cardiac abnormalities may produce a QRS anterior enough to increase the R/S ratio in V1 and thus imitate RVH?

ANS.: a. A posterior myocardial infarction can cause the R/S ratio in V1 to be greater than 1.

b. An RBBB or RBBB pattern can cause the R/S in V1 to be greater than 1 because the S may be very shallow.

Note: You can separate RVH from the preceding by observing that in RVH not only is the R/S ratio in V1 greater than 1 but also the R/S ratio in V6 is less than 1; i.e., the S is greater than the R [51].

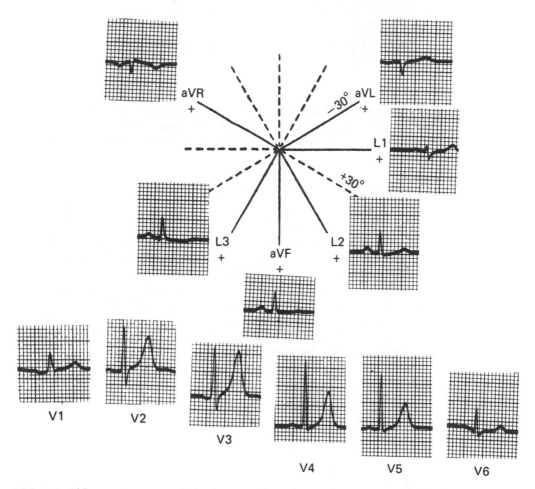

ECG 101. Old posterior myocardial infarction. The right axis deviation is probably due to a posterior divisional block. The tall, peaked precordial T waves are due to posterior fibrosis or ischemia. The markedly anterior QRS (positive QRS across the precordium) is due to loss of posterior forces.

8. What is the upper limit of normal for an R in V1 in the adult?

ANS.: 7 mm [20].

*9. At what age is a 7-mm upper normal R in V1 invalid?

ANS.: A V1 of more than 7 mm is present in about 25 percent of subjects under age 10 and in about 10 percent of those between the ages of 10 and 15.

Note: a. An R of more than 7 mm in V1 is likely to mean RVH even in a child if the upstroke is slurred. About 50 percent of patients with

RVH have a slurred upstroke of the R in V1 [6]. In the presence of RVH, a notched R or small rsR' can almost invariably be found if additional exploratory right chest leads are taken slightly higher, lower, or to the right [66]. A rapid paper speed of 50 mm per second can yield a higher percentage of slurred upstrokes than the usual 25 mm per second (see ECG 97).

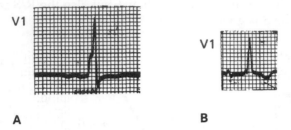

A

B

A is from a 4-year-old boy with a pulmonary artery pressure of 80 mm Hg due to a ventricular septal defect and a pulmonary artery band. B is from a 50-year-old woman with severe pulmonary hypertension secondary to mitral stenosis.

b. You should expect that the maximum normal septal R in aVR would be less than the maximal normal septal R in V1 because, although they both represent the rightward and anterior forces of the normal septal vector, the anterior component ought to dominate because of the proximity effect of the V1 electrode. In fact it does, the maximum being 7 mm in V1 versus 5 mm in aVR.

c. The adult ventricular activation time in V1 and RVH may become prolonged beyond the upper normal of 30 msec (0.03 sec) in the absence of any degree of RBBB. In infants with RVH, however, there is rarely such a prolongation. (An RsR' in V1 can be due to either RVH or some degree of RBBB.)

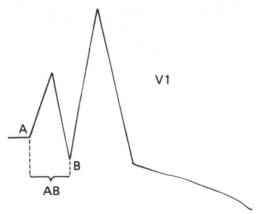

A marks the onset of left ventricular depolarization. B marks the onset of right ventricular depolarization. If AB is 30 msec or longer, there is some degree of RBBB [66].

Posterior QRS in RVH

*1. What can explain a QRS to the right and posterior in RVH?
ANS.: The reasons for the posterior QRS in COPD have already been given (see
p. 402).

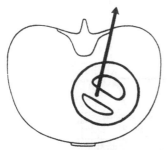

Posterior but still leftward QRS   Posterior and slightly rightward QRS

Another theory is that some forms of RVH produce a dominant hypertrophy
of the posterior part of the RV. Therefore the mean force of the QRS vector
points in this posterior and rightward direction.

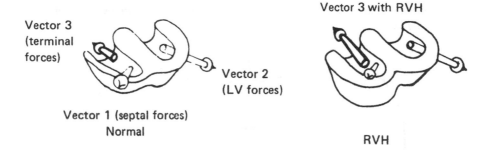

Vector 3
(terminal
forces)

Vector 2
(LV forces)

Vector 1 (septal forces)
Normal

Vector 3 with RVH

RVH

*2. What do the chest leads look like if the QRS is posterior and to the right?
ANS.: There are deep S waves across the precordium, with or without a tall R in
V1.

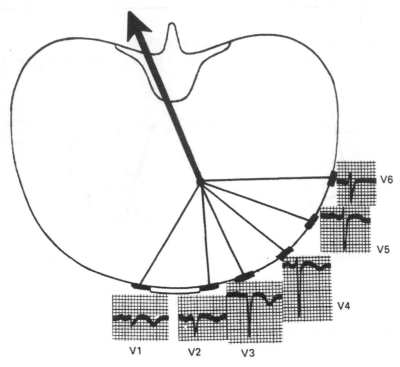

This rightward and markedly posterior QRS produces predominant negativity in every precordial lead.

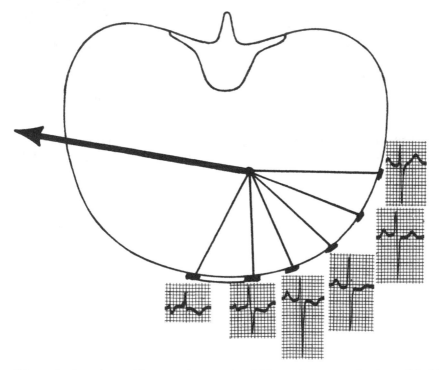

This markedly rightward but slightly posterior QRS produces a predominant R in V1 and predominant S waves across the rest of the precordium.

*3. If the QRS is posterior and to the right, is the transition zone shifted to the right or to the left?

ANS.: It may be shifted either way. In the first vector diagram in question 2, a posterior axillary lead V7 would be transitional, and the transition may be considered shifted to the left. In the second vector diagram, the transition is between V1 and V2 and may be considered shifted to the right (see p. 405).

4. List the other causes of a very posterior QRS with the transition zone at V5 or V6 other than RVH.

ANS.: a. LVH and dilatation in the late stages of failure, when right ventricular dilatation is present (see p. 384).

b. Anterior infarction.

c. LBBB.

Note: In RVH a portion of the QRS is more likely to be also *rightward*; i.e., there is likely to be a right axis deviation in the frontal plane.

*5. What does a posterior QRS do to the R/S ratio in V6?

ANS.: It decreases it; i.e., the S grows at the expense of the R.

Note: The normal minimal R/S ratio in V6 is 1, i.e., the same as the maximal R/S ratio in V1.

*6. What other than right ventricular overloads and RBBB patterns imitates the low R/S ratio in V6?

ANS.: Anterior divisional block. A marked left axis deviation causes terminal negativity in all inferior leads. The left precordium is usually below the electrical center of the chest and so often reflects the same vectors as do the inferior leads.

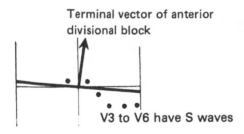

Terminal vector of anterior divisional block

V3 to V6 have S waves

Note: The maximum normal S in V5 or V6 is said to be 7 mm. (This fact is convenient to remember because 7 mm is the maximum normal R in V1, and both are RVH criteria.)

*7. Why is lead V3R or V4R often recommended as a means of diagnosing RVH?

ANS.: Deep S waves across the precordium, as in some anterior divisional blocks, could be mistaken for the posterior QRS of RVH. If the precordial pannegativity is due to RVH, V3R and V4R are often the only precordial leads to show a predominantly positive QRS [46]. Very occasionally it is necessary to take a V6R to show predominant positivity [19].

Note: a. One explanation for the positive QRS coming from an anterior electrode on the right chest despite a predominantly posterior mean QRS is that we are picking up multiple dipolar forces. Here is where the single dipole theory for production of the total QRS can be shown to be of no use. It is generally accepted that the heart does not function as a single dipole.

b. A V4R R/S ratio greater than 1 is usually diagnostic of severe RVH, provided no posterolateral myocardial infarction is present. In one study it was more sensitive than V1 [14]. If the abnormal V4R is due to myocardial infarction, V1 almost invariably also has an R/S ratio greater than 1.

R/S Ratio Regression Sign of RVH

1. What is characteristic of the R/S ratio across the precordium in patients with RVH and either a normal or a posterior QRS axis?

ANS.: The R/S ratio tends to diminish from V1 to the transition lead; i.e., there is a regression of the R/S ratio between at least two successive precordial leads [56].

Note: With the R/S ratio sign there is often a shallow, slurred S in V1. It is the first stage of RBBB [56].

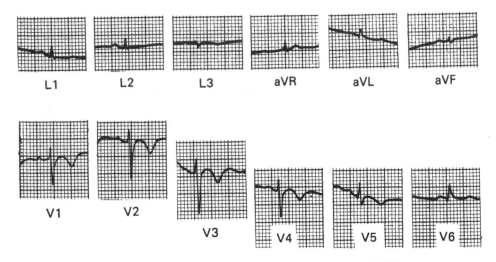

ECG 102. This ECG is from an elderly woman whose autopsy showed diffuse pulmonary carcinomatosis, RVH, and dilatation. The lack of R/S ratio progression between V1 and V3 and the T negativity from V1 to V5 are signs of the RVH. Note the absence of an inferior P wave (the P in aVL is not negative), tending to rule out COPD as a cause of the RVH.

2. Is the R/S ratio regression an early or late sign of right ventricular overload?

ANS.: An early sign. It can even occur in acute pulmonary embolism [56, 57].

Note: Mitral stenosis and COPD are the two acquired conditions causing RVH in which the QRS often tends to be posterior. The R/S poor progression sign is important when patients with COPD or mitral stenosis show a posterior QRS because they rarely show other signs of RVH unless the RVH is severe.

3. With what is the R/S ratio poor progression sign of RVH easily confused?
   ANS.: Because the R/S ratio may regress in anterior infarction, the latter must always be considered in the differential diagnosis.
   Note: a. When the r wave diminishes from V1 to V3, so that in V3 it is 2 mm or less, an anterior infarct is not present if there is either a right axis deviation or an S in lead 1 of more than 1 mm to warn that RVH is probably present.
   b. An anterior divisional block may also produce a poor R/S progression. The reason is that the initial and terminal forces are, as in RBBB patterns, relatively independent of one another.

*INITIAL NEGATIVITY IN V1 WITH RVH

*1. With RVH, what happens to the anatomic relation between the RV and the LV? How does it affect the septum?
   ANS.: The RV rotates clockwise (as viewed from the apex). Therefore the plane of the ventricular septum becomes more parallel to the frontal plane of the body [45]. It is especially true when the RV is volume overloaded as with an atrial septal defect [35].

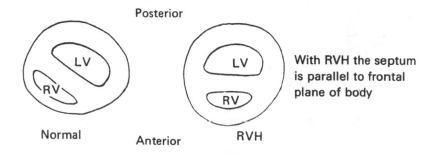

*2. If the 'initial septal vector' is normally from left to right, what may happen to its direction with RVH and a rotated septum?
   ANS.: The septal vector may move directly anteriorly or even from right to left [35].

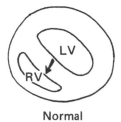

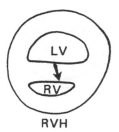

Normal

RVH

In normal subjects the septal vector is from left to right.

With RVH the septal vector may turn from right to left.

*3. How can RVH with a rotated septum affect the appearance of the QRS in both V1 and lead 1?

ANS.: A qR can be produced in V1. Initial negativity is due to initial right-to-left conduction. This situation also produces an absent q in lead 1; i.e., lead 1 looks like

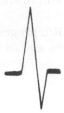

with an initial R due to initial right-to-left conduction.

Note: The preceding rotation would not produce negativity in V1 unless it actually turned the initial vector even more to the left. This situation could be explained if the inferior right septal mass were hypertrophied and rotated the vector to the left. It has been shown that hypertrophy of the right side of the septum causes an increase in the velocity of right-to-left conduction proportional to the degree of hypertrophy [39].

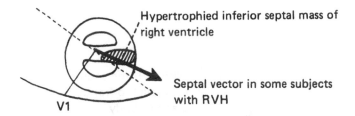

Hypertrophied inferior septal mass of right ventricle

Septal vector in some subjects with RVH

V1

*4. How can the right atrial dilatation seen in many patients with RVH account for a qR in V1?

ANS.: The V1 electrode may be able to pick up proximity effects as if the electrode were directly on the right atrium. A direct right atrial electrode depicts a qR [57].

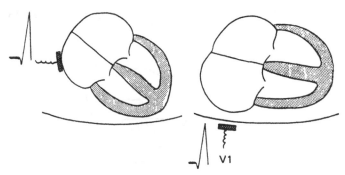

V1

In patients with RVH, an electrode directly on the atrium shows a qR. With dilatation of the right atrium plus rotation of the heart, the V1 electrode may reflect events as if the electrode were on the right atrium. Therefore a qR in V1 should mean not only RVH but also right atrial dilatation.

Note: a. It has been shown that in many patients with a qR in V1, an rsR′ can be picked up by exploring the right chest. It has also been shown that the q of qR is often really the s following an isoelectric initial r [66] (see ECG 103).
   b. A q in V1 is never normally seen in a child at any age [1].

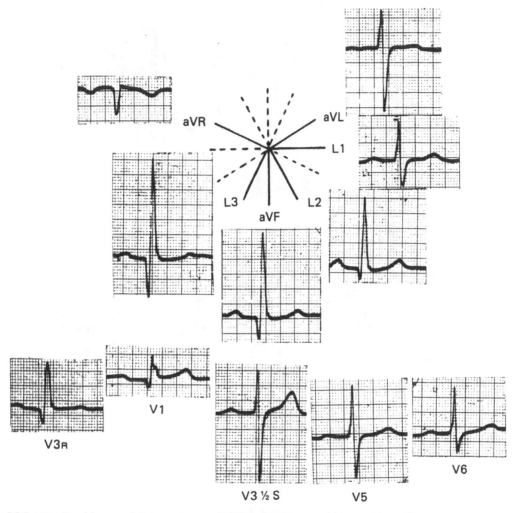

ECG 103. Double-speed (50 mm/second) ECG of a 15-year-old boy with an Eisenmenger reaction secondary to transposition of the great vessels and a single ventricle.

S-T, T IN THE RIGHT PRECORDIUM WITH RVH

1. What happens to the S-T, T with RVH?
   ANS.: As with LVH, they move in a direction opposite to the QRS and can make a pattern similar to the LVH strain pattern in those leads with a positive QRS. In other words, the QRS-T angle widens.
2. Where on the precordium does the right ventricular strain pattern appear?
   ANS.: In the right precordial leads, i.e., in the V1 area (see ECGs 100 and 104).

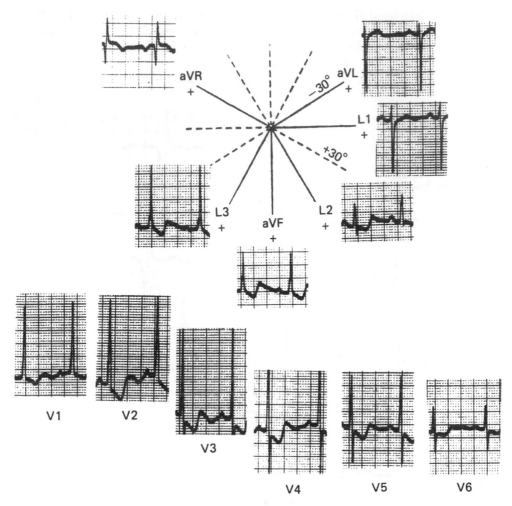

ECG 104. RVH in a 20-year-old girl with severe primary pulmonary hypertension. Note the RVH strain pattern in the inferior leads and in the right precordial leads.

    Note: With acute pulmonary embolism the S-T may become depressed in the mid-precordium and left precordium. This finding may be due to a subendocardial injury current secondary to the coronary insufficiency that may be caused by severe obstruction to flow into the LV.

3. What does a right ventricular strain pattern tell you about the RVH?
   ANS.: The right ventricular pressure is at systemic levels or higher.
4. How may acquired RVH affect the precordial T waves?
   ANS.: It may produce T negativity in the right precordium. A sudden right ventricular overload, as with an acute pulmonary embolism, can produce T negativity in the right precordium as its only ECG sign [44].
   Note: Chronic overloads, as with severe pulmonary hypertension, have produced giant T inversions in all the precordial leads, but this occurrence is rare.

RIGHT VENTRICULAR SYSTOLIC AND DIASTOLIC OVERLOADING

ECG with Systolic or Pressure Overloading

1. How does ventricular enlargement in response to a chronic pressure load differ from the ventricle's response to a chronic volume load; i.e., which type of load stimulates hypertrophy, and which causes dilatation?

   ANS.: The ventricle responds to a chronic pressure load by hypertrophy and to a chronic volume load by dilatation, with proportionate hypertrophy.

   Note: The kind of heart problems other than pulmonary stenosis that can produce a hypertrophied RV without dilatation are those that result in pulmonary hypertension.

2. Describe the systolic overload pattern of RVH.

   ANS.: V1 has an R wave with either a small s after it or a tiny q preceding it. The T is negative, except during the first few years of life.

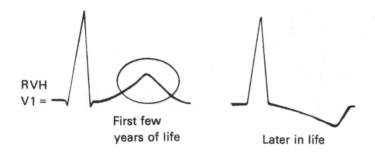

3. For how long after birth is the T normally upright in the right precordium?

   ANS.: It gradually turns posteriorly, so that by 7 days the T is negative in the right precordium.

   Note: a. If the T is upright in the right precordium after the first week of life, right ventricular overload is likely. After age 5 the normal T may again become upright in V1 [48]. However, it usually remains negative in the right precordium until adolescence or early adulthood and is called the juvenile T pattern.

   b. A positive T in V1 in an infant is not a sign of RVH even after the first week unless V6 is also positive. If the T is negative in V6, the positive T in V1 may be due to LVH [48].

   c. The R/S in V1 must be at least 1 or more before an upright T in the right precordium is definitely a sign of RVH (see ECG 105A).

   d. In the frontal plane the T should be between 0° and 60° by the seventh day.

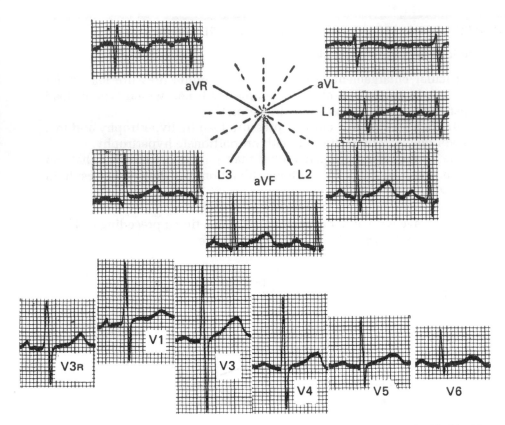

ECG 105A. A double-speed (50 mm/second) ECG showing RVH in a 7-month-old girl with tetralogy of Fallot. Both left and right ventricular systolic pressures were 100 mm Hg. Her pulmonary artery pressure was 22/10 mm Hg. Her systemic oxygen saturation was 90 percent. Note that the right precordial leads V3R and V1 have upright T waves. Together with an R/S ratio greater than 1, these T waves are the only sign of RVH in this infant. The T in V6 is also positive. If it were negative, RVH could not be assumed.

*4. Draw all characteristic V1 QRS and T patterns seen in RVH with pressure loads on the RV.
ANS.:

Not diagnostic

Diagnostic only in children (after 24 hours)

Diagnostic in adults

All these QRS-T patterns have been seen in RVH pressure loads.

*5. What is the direction of T in a ventricular septal defect (VSD) with pulmonary hypertension due to high resistance, i.e., the type that is generally inoperable?
ANS.: The T points anteriorly and to the left, as in the newborn, producing upright T waves across the precordium.
Note: a. The degree of pulmonary hypertension in VSD is better correlated with the QRS-T angle than with the T direction alone because the QRS-T angle widens with increasing right ventricular pressure.

b. The absence of significant pulmonary vascular disease in VSD is strongly suggested by the concomitant left ventricular overload signs of a Q deeper than 4 mm in V5 or V6, a leftward axis, or any S in V1. Lone RVH is virtually diagnostic of severe pulmonary vascular disease [32].

c. If R/S is greater than 1 in V1, it tells you that the pulmonary artery pressure is probably more than 45 mm Hg. Whether the pulmonary hypertension is hyperkinetic or due instead to a high resistance is not indicated by this ECG pattern. However, if there is a deep Q in the left precordial leads, the resistance is probably close to normal [67].

6. When can the voltage of an R' in V1 in RBBB be high enough to suggest strongly that RVH is highly likely?

ANS.: If incomplete RBBB is present, it must be at least 18 mm high. If complete RBBB is present, it must be at least 20 mm high [5].

---

*RVH of Pulmonary Stenosis

*1. How does the amplitude of R in V1 correlate with the degree of pulmonary stenosis (in the absence of RBBB)?

ANS.: a. The ECGs of children under age 15 have higher voltage than those of adults for the same gradient, so that there is almost no significant correlation with gradient unless age is considered. After puberty, however, an R of less than 8 mm usually means a mild gradient and an R between 8 and 16 mm suggests a moderate gradient of not more than 60 mm Hg. An R of 20 mm or more suggests a right ventricular pressure of at least 70 mm Hg, but if combined with an S-T, T strain pattern in V1 the pressure is at least 100 mm Hg [15].

b. At all ages the R in V1 correlates moderately well with the pulmonary valve *area*; i.e., it correlates with *systolic flow* through the valve. For example, a high-voltage R in V1 in the absence of RBBB means a small valve area with a low flow, even though the gradient may be small [4].

c. An R' in V1 without bundle branch block in pulmonary stenosis signifies that the stenosis is not more than moderate unless the R' is tall. A tall R' suggests a significant gradient and has the same meaning as a pure R about twice as high [24].

d. An absent S in V1 or V4R tells nothing about the right ventricular pressure in pure pulmonary stenosis.

e. An R' in V1 with a negative T is considered the classic diastolic overload pattern, but it is found in many patients with pure pressure overloads when there is mild to moderate stenosis [4].

f. The duration of the QRS or the ventricular activation time in V1 correlates poorly with pulmonary valve area or gradient (either to the peak of the R or R').

*2. Which correlates better with the pressure gradient in pulmonary stenosis: the QRS axis, the T axis, or the QRS-T angle?

ANS.: The frontal T axis and QRS-T angle correlate well and about equally. The frontal QRS axis correlates poorly [4]. In the horizontal plane the QRS-T angle correlates well with the pressure gradient, whereas the T axis correlates poorly. It is not surprising that the horizontal T axis by itself correlates poorly with right ventricular pressure in pulmonary stenosis because up to about puberty a leftward and anterior T is seen with high pressures in the right ventricle. In the adult, however, a leftward and posterior T is associated with high pressure in the right ventricle.

Note: a. Although the greater the pressure gradient in pulmonary stenosis the more the right axis deviation, there are occasionally marked right axis deviations with mild to moderate gradients. The use of the QRS-T angle can then help because the greater the gradient the wider the QRS-T angle, so that the average mean QRS-T angles for mild, moderate, and severe stenosis is about 5°, 75°, and 170°, respectively. In the horizontal plane, in almost all cases of severe stenosis, the QRS-T angles are greater than 100° [4].

b. With tetralogy, there is no correlation between the hemodynamic severity and the ECG criteria for right ventricular hypertrophy [50].

3. What change does the initial vector in RVH due to severe pulmonary stenosis have in common with the initial vector of LVH due to severe aortic stenosis?
ANS.: The more severe the stenosis, the more likely will the initial force go from right to left.

RBBB Pattern and Right Ventricular Overloading

1. What percentage of normal persons have an RBBB pattern, i.e., an S in lead 1, a terminal positivity in V1, and no widening of the QRS?
ANS.: The incidence varies from 5 to 95 percent. The younger the age group studied, the higher the incidence of RBBB pattern. The more often chest leads are taken in the V3R or V4R position, the higher is the reported incidence [21].
2. What causes the RBBB pattern in normal persons?
ANS.: It is thought to be due to domination of the terminal depolarization by the outflow tract of the RV [21].

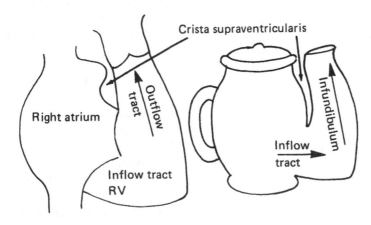

Note: This outflow tract, which is like the spout of a kettle, is separated from the main body or inflow tract of the RV by bands of muscle called the crista supraventricularis. Conduction through the crista may account for the terminal conduction in the RBBB pattern, which is also called the 'cristal pattern' [42].

3. What is meant by an atypical RBBB pattern?

ANS.: A pattern in which, instead of terminal positivity in V1, a shallow S is present; i.e., the terminal vector is not quite so anterior as in the typical pattern.
Note: An atypical pattern is more likely than a typical pattern.

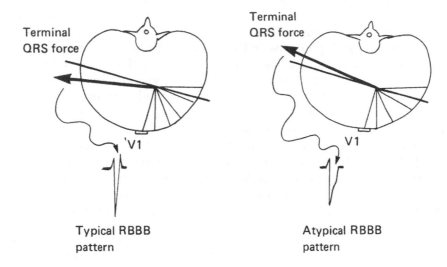

Typical RBBB
pattern

Atypical RBBB
pattern

*4. What is the RBBB pattern called if there is an S not only in lead 1 but also in leads 2 and 3?

ANS.: The S1, S2, S3 syndrome.
Note: There is no more known significance to the S1, S2, S3 syndrome than there is to any other RBBB pattern; i.e., it is either normal or due to RVH.

RVH WITH ACUTE PULMONARY EMBOLISM

1. What is the relation between the appearance of an RBBB pattern and pulmonary embolism?

ANS.: If an RBBB pattern suddenly appears, it suggests a sudden right ventricular overload such as that brought about by acute pulmonary edema or pulmonary embolus (see ECGs 35A, 35B, and 35C, pp. 178–180).
Note: The RV must dilate in order to overcome a sudden elevation in outflow resistance. Its effect may therefore be considered a combination of pressure and volume overload.

2. What are the classic frontal plane QRS changes in acute pulmonary embolism?

ANS.: a. The initial vector may turn superiorly; i.e., a Q is often seen to develop in lead 3 and aVF.

b. The terminal vector may turn inferiorly or rightward (an S develops in aVL or in L1).

Note: A combination of (a) and (b) can produce the S1, Q3 pattern. This combination occurs in about 15 percent of patients with acute pulmonary embolism.

c. All degrees of leftward shift, even to marked left axis deviations. This situation occurs about twice as often as an inferior or rightward shift [33]. The picture of RBBB and anterior divisional block is a characteristic ECG change in massive pulmonary embolism.

d. Posterior rotation of the QRS (transition zone shifts to the left [28]).

e. A slurred upstroke of S in V1.

f. A regression of the R/S ratio across the precordium.

Note: Remarkably slight ECG changes are seen in some patients with massive pulmonary embolism [60].

*3. What kind of divisional block produces an S1, Q3 where there was none before?

ANS.: A posterior divisional block not only produces an S in lead 1 but also produces a Q in lead 3. Perhaps a posterior divisional block occurs in pulmonary embolism if a sudden high right ventricular pressure can selectively stretch the posterior part of the septum and produce a conduction delay along the posterior fibers of the left bundle [53].

Further confirming the postulate that a posterior divisional block is the cause of the S1, Q3 change is the occasional appearance of Q waves in the right precordium exactly simulating an acute anteroseptal (as well as inferior) infarct [16]. Posterior divisional blocks can cause Q waves in the precordium if the chest electrodes are low enough to pick up the initial superior forces as negative deflections.

Note: a. With pulmonary embolism a leftward shift of the axis is actually twice as frequent as a rightward shift. This axis suggests selective stretching of the anterior division [42].

b. Another theory for the S1, Q3 in acute pulmonary embolism is that sudden dilatation of the RV can cause a clockwise anatomic rotation on the heart's longitudinal axis. In dogs it can cause an S1, Q3 pattern [17].

4. Which frontal T changes suggest that the S1, Q3 is due to a pulmonary embolus?

ANS.: The T may turn leftward (away from the RV) and superiorly to produce a negative T in the inferior leads. It then is called 'S1, Q3, T3' for short (see ECG 105B).

Note: a. When patients with chronic cor pulmonale go into acute respiratory failure because of infection, a negative T in leads 3 and aVF rarely develops.

b. The S1, Q3, T3 change is often called the McGinn-White syndrome, but the complete syndrome really requires the following:

(1) Symptoms and signs of massive pulmonary embolus.

(2) A depressed S-T in lead 2 and a depressed J point in lead 1.

(3) A late inversion of the T in lead 3 (toward the end of the T) [43].

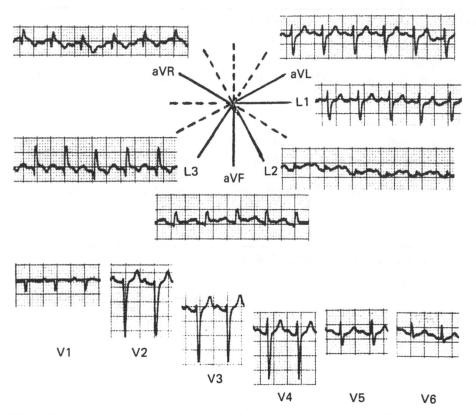

ECG 105B. An elderly man had sudden pleuritic pain and hemoptysis. The marked right axis deviation, the S1, Q3, T3 pattern, and the tachycardia of 150 (perhaps atrial tachycardia in view of the relatively long P-R interval) are characteristic of acute pulmonary embolism.

*5. What frontal S-T changes may occur with an acute pulmonary embolism? Why?
    ANS.: The S-T may become depressed in the left ventricular leads, i.e., usually leads 1 and 2. It may be due to coronary insufficiency when the obstruction to flow is extreme.
*6. What frontal P changes suggest an acute pulmonary embolism?
    ANS.: The P may become taller in inferior leads, suggesting right atrial overload. It usually occurs only in patients with chronic cor pulmonale. Therefore in such a patient this P change should always suggest either acute infectious respiratory failure or embolism. An abnormally tall P wave due to a high pulmonary artery pressure is called 'P pulmonale.'
    Note: A spontaneous pneumothorax can produce ECG changes similar to those of acute pulmonary embolism [52].
*7. How can heart rate and rhythm help determine that the cause for a sudden appearance of RBBB is pulmonary embolism?
    ANS.: With pulmonary embolism there is usually a sinus tachycardia and occasionally a change of rhythm to atrial flutter or fibrillation.

Horizontal ECG Changes in Acute Pulmonary Embolism

1. How does the QRS change in the chest leads in pulmonary embolism?
   ANS.: There may be
   a. Posterior rotation of the QRS posteriorly (transition zone shift to the left) [28].
   b. A slurred upstroke of S in V1.
   c. A regression of R/S ratio across the precordium.
   d. A qs or qr pattern in one or all of V4R to V6 R [18A].
2. What S-T changes may occur in the horizontal plane in acute pulmonary embolism?
   ANS.: There may be S-T elevation in one or all of V4R, V5R, and V6R [18A].
   Note: Remarkably slight ECG changes are seen in some patients with massive pulmonary embolism [60].

Summary of Changes with Acute Pulmonary Embolism

The sudden appearance of
1. S1, Q3, T3.   } This combination
2. T negativity in the right precordium.   } is diagnostic.
3. RBBB pattern or complete RBBB.
4. RBBB in precordial leads, with marked left axis (anterior divisional block).
5. S-T depression in leads 1 and 2, as well as in mid-precordial and left precordial leads.
6. Sinus tachycardia, atrial flutter, or atrial fibrillation.
7. A more inferior and taller P if chronic cor pulmonale is present.
8. A slurred upstroke of S in V1.
9. A regression of the R/S ratio across the precordium.
10. Posterior turning of the QRS (transition shifted to the left).
11. A qs or qr in V4R or V6R.
12. S-T elevations in V4R, V5R, or V6R.

Right Ventricular Diastolic Overload Pattern

1. Give some examples of conditions with a right ventricular diastolic or volume overload.
   ANS.: Atrial septal defect (ASD), tricuspid or pulmonary regurgitation.
2. Describe the right ventricular diastolic or volume overload pattern.
   ANS.: It is an RBBB pattern in V1. The T wave (as in the usual RBBB picture in V1) is negative [11].
   Note: In most patients with moderate to severe tricuspid regurgitation the RBBB pattern in V1 is associated with low voltage (less than 7 mm) [54].
*3. What part of the RV is said to hypertrophy in chronic volume loads?
   ANS.: The crista. It can hypertrophy with no hypertrophy of the free wall. This fact explains why patients with ASDs, with a chronic right ventricular volume load, so characteristically show an RBBB or cristal pattern.
4. Is the right ventricular diastolic or volume overload pattern as reliable or valid as the systolic or pressure overload pattern?

ANS.: No. It is seen in many normal subjects, especially the young. It is even seen with pressure overloads, as in moderate pulmonary stenosis.

*5. What abnormality has been found in the right bundle of hearts with ASDs that could account for the right bundle conduction delay?

ANS.: The right bundle in these hearts has been found to be twice as long as normal.

*6. How can a T wave shape suggest the size of the left-to-right shunt in ASD?

ANS.: Observe the right precordial T transition area. If there is a biphasic T or an S-T, T that shows only a terminal, angular, positive T, the magnitude of the late-phased dart T wave has a close linear correlation with the shunt at the atrial level [3]. The range of the T dart in more than 70 patients with ASDs was from 1 mm for the smallest shunt to 11 mm for the largest.

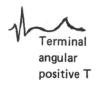

Terminal
angular
positive T

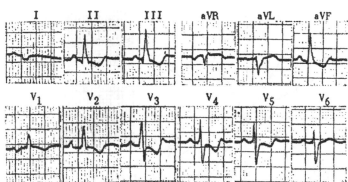

This from a 48-year-old woman with RVH secondary to an ASD.

Note: a. When a notch is seen on the R wave of an inferior lead in a patient with an ASD, the shunt is usually large [26A].

b. Some cardiologists believe that the ventricular septum can be localized from the site of the QRS transition zone on the precordial leads. It has been shown that there is no significant correlation between the location of the septum and the transition zone [30].

Combined Ventricular Overloads

1. If LVH by the index of Sokolow is seen in the chest leads, how can the limb leads suggest that RVH is also present?

ANS.: If the frontal axis is inferior, combined overload of both ventricles is probable (see ECG 106).

*Note: a. An exception to this rule is congenital aortic stenosis, which may produce LVH by the index of Sokolow but also an inferior frontal axis that may persist into middle age. The reason is unknown.

b. If the cause of the combined ventricular overload is a VSD or an aortopulmonary shunt for tetralogy of Fallot, the double overload can be recognized by voltage adequate for an index of Sokolow plus large equiphasic leads in the mid-precordium. It is known as the Katz-Wachtel phenomenon [34]. If you study vector loops, you learn that it means a wide loop in the horizontal plane. The original 1937 article by Katz and Wachtel described only large equiphasic complexes in at least two of the three *bipolar limb leads* as diagnostic of 'congenital heart disease' [34]. The phenomenon has been extended by others to the mid-precordial leads as a criterion for combined ventricular hypertrophy—a weak criterion because it commonly occurs in normal subjects. In the presence of significant pulmonary hypertension, a left ventricular overload (meaning operability still probable) is shown by:

(1)   A Q of 4 mm or more in V6 in patients over age 3.

(2)   A QRS frontal axis of 60° or less in infants under age 3.

(3)   An S greater than 25 mm in V1 or an R greater than 25 mm in V6 [22].

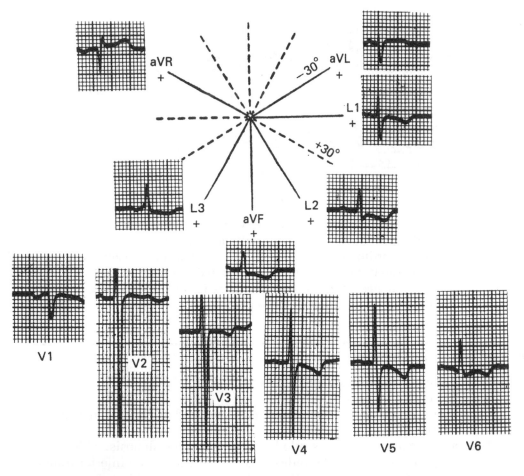

ECG 106. Right and left ventricular overload due to severe congestive failure as a result of hypertension and coronary disease in a 63-year-old woman. Note the right axis deviation and positive modified index of Sokolow (V2 + V6 = more than 35 mm).

*2. How can S waves in the left precordium help to diagnose combined ventricular overloads?

ANS.: If there is LVH by either frontal or chest lead criteria, S waves in the left precordium may represent exaggerated rightward forces from an enlarged or hypertrophied RV (in the absence of RBBB or marked left axis deviation).

*3. How can the T waves suggest RV overload in a suspected VSD with a pattern of diastolic LV overload?

ANS.: a. In the transition zone of the T wave, a 'dome-and-dart' configuration of a bifid, or notched, T wave is often seen. If the second peak, or 'dart,' is taller than the dome, a right ventricular overload is suggested [3].

*4. How can the ECG help determine if a complete transposition of the great vessels has (a) a small communication between the pulmonary and systemic circuit or (b) a large communication?

ANS.: a. Pure RVH is seen.

b. Biventricular overload is seen.

Note: A left axis deviation with complete transposition suggests either aortic arch obstruction or a communication from the LV to the right atrium [23].

Differential Diagnosis of RVH

1. How can you tell the right axis deviation of posterior divisional block from RVH?

ANS.: a. Look for signs of inferior myocardial infarction, which is expected with posterior divisional blocks.

b. Look for the P waves of right atrial overload or COPD (see section on right atrial overloads), which is not expected in posterior divisional blocks.

*2. When can constrictive pericarditis imitate RVH?

ANS.: When the QRS is rightward and anterior (about 5 percent of patients with constriction). In a few it is due to subpulmonic annular constriction. In others, it may be due to some distortion and rotation caused by fibrosis at the base of the heart [18].

3. What can cause right axis deviation besides youth, RVH, and posterior divisional block?

ANS.: Congenital absence of the pericardium. Also the transition zone is shifted to the left in these patients because the heart is shifted markedly into the left axilla.

REFERENCES

1. Alimurung, M. M., et al. The unipolar precordial and extremity electrocardiogram in normal infants and children. *Circulation* 4:420, 1951.
2. Avgoustakis, D., et al. The electrocardiogram in constrictive pericarditis before and after radical pericardectomy. *Chest* 57:460, 1970.

3. Awa, S., et al. The significance of late-phased dart T wave in the electrocardiogram of children. *Am. Heart J.* 80:619, 1970.

4. Bassingthwaighte, J. B., et al. The electrocardiographic and hemodynamic findings in pulmonary stenosis with intact ventricular septum. *Circulation* 28:893, 1963.

5. Booth, R. W., Te-Chuan, C., and Scott, R. C. Electrocardiographic diagnosis of ventricular hypertrophy in the presence of right bundle-branch block. *Circulation* 18:169, 1958.

6. Braunwald, E., et al. A study of the electrocardiogram and vectorcardiogram in congenital heart diseae. *Am. Heart J.* 50:591, 1955.

6A. Broadbent, J. C., et al. Congenital deficiency of the pericardium. *Dis. Chest* 50:237, 1966.

7. Brock, S. *The Basis of Clinical Neurology.* Baltimore: Williams & Wilkins, 1945. P. 11.

8. Brotmacher, L., and Campbell, M. Ventricular septal defect with pulmonary stenosis. *Br. Heart J.* 20:379, 1958.

9. Burch, G. E., and DePasquale, N. P. The electrocardiographic diagnosis of pulmonary heart disease. *Am. J. Cardiol.* 11:622, 1963.

10. Burch, G. E., Phillips, J. H., and Ansari, A. The cachectic heart. *Dis. Chest* 54:5, 1968.

11. Cabrera, E., and Gaxiola, A. A critical re-evaluation of systolic and diastolic overloading patterns. *Prog. Cardiovasc. Dis.* 2:219, 1959.

12. Caird, F. I., and Stanfield, C. A. The electrocardiogram in asphyxial and in embolic acute cor pulmonale. *Br. Heart J.* 24:313, 1962.

12A. Caird, F. L. The ECG in interstitial disease of the lung. *Am. J. Cardiol.* 10:14, 1962.

13. Calatayud, J. B., et al. P-wave changes in chronic obstructive pulmonary disease. *Am. Heart J.* 79:444, 1970.

14. Camerini, F., Goodwin, J. F., and Zoob, M. Lead V4R in right ventricular hypertrophy. *Br. Heart J.* 18:13, 1956.

15. Cauler, G. C., Ongley, P., and Nadas, A. S. Relation of systolic pressure in the right ventricle to the electrocardiogram. *N. Engl. J. Med.* 258:979, 1958.

16. Cernohorsky, J. The electrocardiogram in pulmonary embolism simulating anterior infarction. *Cor Vasa* 5:273, 1963.

17. Cherchi, A., and Liguori, G. Electrocardiogram and position of the heart. *Folia Cardiol.* 14:407, 1955.

18. Chesler, E., Mitha, A. S., and Matisonn, R. E. The ECG of constrictive pericarditis — pattern resembling right ventricular hypertrophy. *Am. Heart J.* 91:420, 1976.

18A. Chia, B. L., Tan, H.-C., Lim, Y. T. Right sided chest lead electrocardiographic abnormalities in acute pulmonary embolism. *Int. J. Cardiol.* 61:43–46, 1997.

19. Coelho, E., et al. Electrocardiographic and vectorcardiographic alterations in chronic cor pulmonale. *Am. J. Cardiol.* 10:20, 1962.

20. DeOliveira, J. M., Sambhi, M. P., and Zimmerman, H. A. The electrocardiogram in pectus excavatum. *Br. Heart J.* 20:495, 1958.

21. DePasquale, N. P., and Burch, G. E. Analysis of the RSR' complex in lead V1. *Circulation* 28:362, 1963.

22. DuShane, J. W., et al. The electrocardiogram in children with ventricular septal defect and severe pulmonary hypertension. *Circulation* 22:49, 1960.

23. Elliott, L. P., et al. Complete transposition of the great vessels: II. An electrocardiographic analysis. *Circulation* 27:1118, 1963.

24. Ellison, R. C., and Miettinen, O. S. Interpretation of RSR' in pulmonic stenosis. *Am. Heart J.* 88:7, 1974.

25. Emergy, J. L., and Mithal, A. Weights of cardiac ventricles at and after birth. *Br. Heart J.* 23:313, 1961.

26. Fisher, J. M., et al. Electrocardiographic sequelae of right ventriculotomy in patients with ventricular septal defects. *Circulation* 22:280, 1960.

26A. Hagege, A. A., Heller, J., Besse, B., Desnos, Guerot, C. 'Crochetage' in the R wave in inferior leads: A new independent ECG hallmark of atrial septal defect (ASD) related to shunt severity. *J.A.C.C. (Abstr.)* 111A, 1995.

27. Graf, W. S., Gunther, L., and Allenstein, B. QRS pattern in mitral stenosis. *Am. J. Cardiol.* 14:266, 1964.
28. Grank, N. Aid for prompt recognition of pulmonary embolism. *J.A.M.A.* 227:203, 1974.
29. Grant, R. P. The morphogenesis of transposition of the great vessels. *Circulation* 26:819, 1962.
30. Guntheroth, W. G., Ovenfors, C. O., and Ikkos, D. Relationship between the electrocardiogram and the position of the heart as determined by biplane angiocardiography. *Circulation* 23:69, 1961.
31. Harick, E., et al. The left ventricle in congenital isolated pulmonary valve stenosis. A morphological study. *Br. Heart J.* 39:429, 1977.
32. Hollman, A., Goodwin, J. F., and Basta, L. Cardiographic assessment of pulmonary vascular disease in ventricular septal defect. *Br. Heart J.* 24:529, 1962.
33. Kamper, D., et al. The reliability of electrocardiographic criteria of chronic obstructive lung disease. *Am. Heart J.* 80:445, 1970.
34. Katz, L. N., and Wachtel, H. The diphasic QRS type of electrocardiogram in congenital heart disease. *Am. Heart J.* 13:202, 1937.
35. Kawai, N., et al. Correlation between direction of the interventricular septum and the initial QRS vectors. *J. Electrocardiol.* 17:401, 1984.
36. Kereiakes, D. J., et al. Apical hypertrophic cardiomyopathy. *Am. Heart J.* 105:856, 1983.
37. Kilcoyne, M. M., Davis, A. L., and Ferber, M. I. A dynamic electrocardiographic concept useful in the diagnosis of cor pulmonale. *Circulation* 42:903, 1970.
38. Kossmann, C. E., et al. Intracardiac and intravascular potentials resulting from electrical activity of the normal human heart. *Circulation* 2:10, 1950.
39. Kyriacopoulos, J. D., et al. Activation of the free wall of the right ventricle in experimental right ventricular hypertrophy with and without right bundle branch block. *Am. Heart J.* 67:81, 1964.
40. Lichtman, J., et al. Electrocardiogram of the athlete: Alterations simulating those of organic heart disease. *Arch. Intern. Med.* 132:763, 1973.
40A. Liebman, J. The initial QRS vector in ventricular hypertrophy. *Jpn. Heart J.* 23:480, 1982.
41. Littman, D. The electrocardiographic findings in pulmonary emphysema. *Am. J. Cardiol.* 5:339, 1960.
42. Lynch, R. E., Stein, P. D., and Bruce, T. A. Leftward shift of frontal plane QRS axis as a frequent manifestation of acute pulmonary embolism. *Chest* 61:443, 1972.
43. McGinn, S., and White, P. D. Acute cor pulmonale resulting from pulmonary embolism. *J.A.M.A.* 104:1473, 1935.
44. McIntyre, K. M., Sashahara, A. S., and Littman, D. Relation of the electrocardiogram to hemodynamic alterations in pulmonary embolism. *Am. J. Cardiol.* 30:205, 1972.
45. Munoz-Armas, S., et al. Symposium on electrocardiography in congenital heart disease. Part II. Tetralogy of Fallot and pulmonary stenosis with intact interventricular septum. *Am. J. Cardiol.* 21:773, 1968.
46. Myers, G. B., Klein, H. A., and Stofer, B. E. The electrocardiographic diagnosis of right ventricular hypertrophy. *Am. Heart J.* 35:1, 1948.
47. Neuman, A., Intermittent regional delay of left ventricular activation: The influence of such a delay on the standard electrocardiogram; Report of 33 cases. *Chest* 61:633, 1972.
48. Okuni, M. Report of Expert Committee of Pediatric Electrocardiogram. A proposal of new pediatric electrocardiographic criteria for ventricular hypertrophy. *Jpn. Heart J.* 16:189, 1975.
49. Padmavati, S., and Ralzada, V. Electrocardiogram in chronic cor pulmonale. *Br. Heart J.* 34:658, 1972.
50. Roberts, D. L., Wagner, H. R., and Lambert, E. C. The electrocardiogram in tetralogy of Fallot. *J. Electrocardiol.* 5:155, 1972.
50A. Rodman, D. M., et al. The electrocardiogram in COPD. *J. Emergency Med.* 8:607, 1990.
51. Roman, G. T., Walsh, T. J., and Massie, E. Right ventricular hypertrophy: Correlation of electrocardiographic and anatomic findings. *Am. J. Cardiol.* 7:481, 1961.
52. Rulliere, R., and Capronnier, C. Acute cor pulmonale due to spontaneous pneumothorax. *Coeur Med. Interne* 5:149, 1966.
53. Scott, R. C. The S Q pattern in acute cor pulmonale: A form of left posterior hemiblock. *Am. Heart J.* 82:135, 1971.

54. Sepulveda, G., and Lukas, D. S. The diagnosis of tricuspid insufficiency. *Circulation* 11:552, 1955.

54A. Shah, N. S., Koller, S. M., Janower, M. L., Spodick, D.H. Diaphragm levels as determinants of P axis in restrictive vs obstructive pulmonary disease. *Chest* 107:697–700, 1995.

55. Silver, H. M., and Calatayud, J. B. Evaluation of QRS criteria in patients with chronic obstructive pulmonary disease. *Chest* 59:153, 1971.

56. Smith, McK., and Ray, C. T. Electrocardiographic signs of early right ventricular enlargement in acute pulmonary embolism. *Chest* 58:205, 1970.

57. Sodi-Pallares, D., Bisteni, A., and Hermann, G. R. Some views on the significance of qR and QR type complexes in right precordial leads in the absence of myocardial infarction. *Am. Heart J.* 43:716, 1952.

58. Sodi-Pallares, D., et al. *Deductive and Polyparametric Electrocardiography*. Mexico City: Instituto Nacional de Cardiologia, 1970.

59. Sokolow, M., and Lyon, T. P. The ventricular complex in right ventricular hypertrophy as obtained by unipolar precordial and limb leads. *Am. Heart J.* 38:272, 1949.

60. Spodick, D. H. Electrocardiographic responses to pulmonary embolism: Mechanisms and sources of variability. *Am. J. Cardiol.* 30:695, 1972.

61. Spodick, D. H., et al. The electrocardiogram in pulmonary emphysema. *Am. Rev. Respir. Dis.* 88:14, 1963.

62. Surawicz, B., and Lasseter, K. C. Effect of drugs on the electrocardiogram. *Prog. Cardiovasc. Dis.* 13:26, 1970.

63. Tandon, M. D. Correlations of electrocardiographic features with airway obstruction in chronic bronchitis. *Chest* 63:146, 1973.

64. Toscano-Barboza, E., and DuShane, J. W. Ventricular septal defect: Correlation of electrocardiographic and hemodynamic findings in 60 proved cases. *Am. J. Cardiol.* 3:721, 1959.

65. Wasserburger, R. H., et al. The electrocardiographic pentalogy of pulmonary emphysema: A correlation of roentgenographic findings and pulmonary function studies. *Circulation* 20:831, 1959.

66. Wasserburger, R. H., et al. Further electrocardiographic observations on direct epicardial potentials in congenital heart lesions. *Circulation* 26:561, 1962.

67. Witham, A. C., and McDaniel, J. S. Electrocardiogram, vectorcardiogram, and hemodynamics in ventricular septal defect. *Am. Heart J.* 79:335, 1970.

6. Atrial Overloads

GENERAL PRINCIPLES

1. Why is the term left or right atrial *overload* preferable to left or right atrial *hypertrophy*?
   ANS.: The ECG cannot distinguish between an enlarged atrium and one that is hypertrophied [53].
2. Which parts of the P wave represent the right and left atrium?
   ANS.: The first part of the P wave is due to depolarization of the right atrium (the sinoatrial [SA] node is in the right atrium), and the second part reflects left atrial depolarization.
3. How does right and left atrial overload usually affect the height and width of the P wave in the limb leads?
   ANS.: Right atrial overload tends to increase the height of the P wave, and left atrial overload increases its width.

RIGHT ATRIAL OVERLOAD

P Axis in Right Atrial Overload

1. What is the normal direction of the frontal plane axis of the right atrial portion of the P wave?
   ANS.: Downward and slightly leftward.

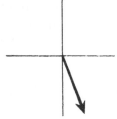

2. What is the normal direction of the frontal axis of the left atrial portion of the P wave?
   ANS.: Leftward and slightly inferior.

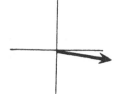

3. What is the normal direction of the frontal axis of the total P?
   ANS.: Leftward and inferior, but between the right and left atrial vectors.

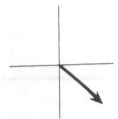

*4. If the right atrial portion of the P predominates because of right atrial overload, would you expect the frontal direction of the total P to be inferior, or would you expect it to be leftward?
   ANS.: Although you would expect it to be inferior, in fact the total P axis remains 'neutral'; i.e., it is neither inferior nor leftward with right atrial overloads. Only if chronic obstructive pulmonary disease (COPD) is present is the P direction inferior, and even here it is not due to right atrial overload.
   Note: With atrial septal defects with a leftward P (negative P in lead 3), it has been found in some series that such a P suggests either a sinus venosus type or the presence of a left superior vena cava [28]. In other series such a correlation has not been found [58]. With a left axis deviation of the QRS, a leftward P suggests an endocardial cushion defect with a common atrium [30].

P Axis in COPD

1. How are the P wave direction and height affected by COPD?
   ANS.: COPD causes an inferior turning of the P and a *relatively* tall P in inferior leads such as aVF. In COPD the P becomes more inferior than + 60°; i.e., the P is negative in aVL [54].
   Note: There is no correlation between the amount of cor pulmonale, or right ventricular hypertrophy (RVH), in COPD and the degree of inferior direction of the P wave axis. The inferior turning of the P should be thought of as due to the effect of the attenuation of X axis vectors by poorly conducting lung tissue and to lowering of the diaphragm. There is some correlation, however, with pulmonary function in COPD and the degree of inferior turning of the P wave.
   Note: There is no correlation with right ventricular pressure, right atrial pressure, or their wall thickness. Therefore, it is probably due mainly to the vertical anatomical position of the heart and an exaggeration of the vertical forces which is known to occur in COPD patients [40A].
2. When is a negative P in aVL most likely to mean COPD?
   ANS.: a. When the patient is over age 50.
      b. When the patient is stocky and with a short chest, so that a leftward P would have been expected. A long chest can produce a negative P in aVL in a normal subject.

* Material marked with an asterisk is included for reference and for advanced students in cardiology.

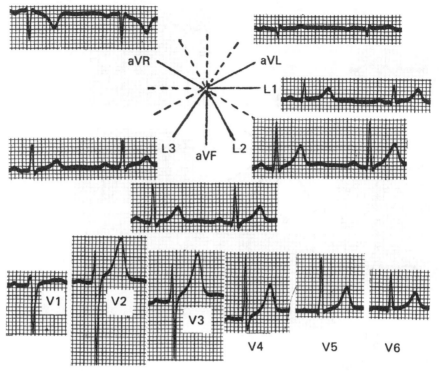

ECG 107. An inferior P wave in a tall, slender, normal physician, age 26. Note the negative P in aVL; i.e., its vector is about + 70°.

    c. When the P is inferior enough to be almost + 90°, i.e., when it is almost isoelectric in lead 1 (see ECG 98, p. 403).

    d. When the P is relatively tall in the Y axis, i.e., when in aVF it is 30 percent or more of the R (in absence of an S).

    e. When it is associated with the QRS signs of COPD (see ECG 98, p. 403).

3. Which of the foregoing is the most reliable P vector sign of COPD?

    ANS.: A P of almost + 90°.

        Note: a. A P wave of more than + 90° (negative in lead 1) is probably an ectopic P.

              b. The right atrial overload due to right ventricular hypertrophy (RVH) secondary to congenital heart disease, e.g., pulmonary stenosis, is not associated with an inferior P wave. In these cases the P wave has even been seen to be leftward for some unknown reason (see ECG 97, p. 398).

              c. The right atrial overload due to pulmonary fibrosis without COPD is also not necessarily associated with an inferior P wave (see ECG 108).

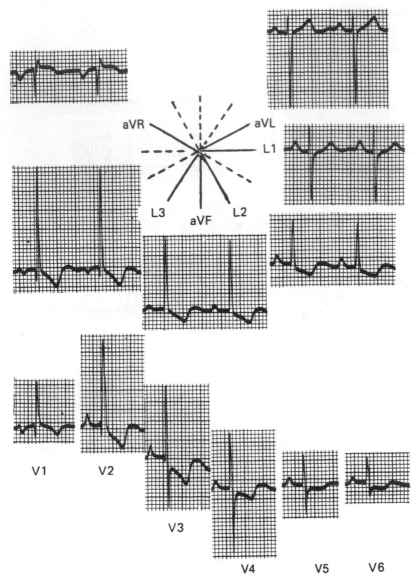

ECG 108. This ECG is from a 69-year-old woman with dyspnea at rest and a PO$_2$ of 49 mm Hg due to severe idiopathic pulmonary fibrosis. The P is peaked in L2 and V2 to V6, but there is a leftward P axis of about + 15°, unlike the inferior P seen in COPD.

Right Atrial Overload

P Pulmonale

1. What happens to the frontal plane P wave when right atrial overload occurs?
   ANS.: The P wave becomes taller.
2. What are the upper normal limits of P wave height and width?
   ANS.: The P wave's upper normal limits are 2.5 mm in height and 100 msec (0.10 sec) in duration. Thus in terms of small divisions a normal P wave may be 2.5 × 2.5 mm.

Note: a. Actually, in only about 3 percent of normal subjects is the P wave taller than 2 mm [38].

b. Both increased body weight and vital capacity correlate with increased P wave height [5].

c. The duration of the P decreases with increasing heart rate [1].

3. What is meant by P pulmonale?

ANS.: A frontal plane P wave that is more than 2.5 mm tall owing to right atrial overload.

4. How other than becoming tall does the P pulmonale of right atrial overload tend to show itself in the frontal plane P wave contour?

ANS.: The P wave becomes symmetrical and peaked (see ECG 109A).

5. What other than right atrial overload and increased body weight can cause an increased P height?

ANS.: a. Sympathetic stimulation, as with sinus tachycardia due to emotion, exercise, or acute myocardial infarction [31].

*b. Hypokalemia [17].

*c. Hypoxia, as in congestive heart failure or severe asthma [44].

*d. Subarachnoid hemorrhage [20]. The tall P waves with subarachnoid hemorrhage are usually associated with a sinus tachycardia and nonspecific T abnormalities [56].

*e. Tall P waves have also been reported with meningitis and intracranial tumors [56].

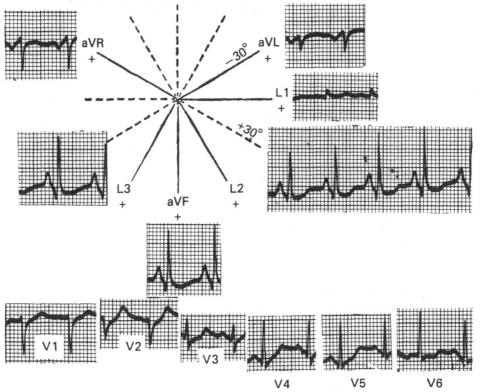

ECG 109A. *P pulmonale due to a severe asthmatic attack in a 43-year-old woman with a normal heart. The hypoxia, sympathetic stimulation, and right atrial overload due to acute pulmonary hypertension combined to produce a 3-mm P wave in L2, L3, and aVF. See ECG 109B taken 2 days later.*

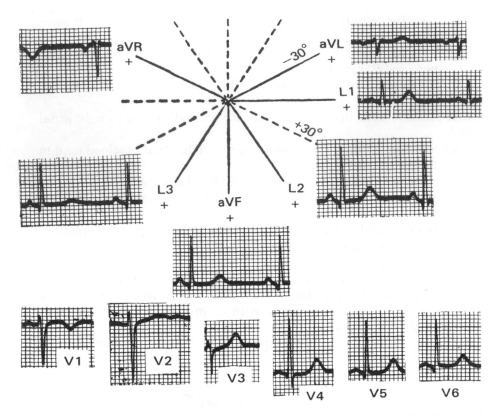

ECG 109B. Same patient as in ECG 109A, showing normal P waves 2 days after the acute attack subsided.

Note: a. The desaturation of cyanotic congenital heart disease shows no correlation with the height of the P wave [3].

b. A volume overload of the right atrium that is not associated with a high right atrial pressure, as in most atrial septal defects (ASDs), often does not cause the cells of the right atrium to hypertrophy. This fact probably accounts for the rarity of right atrial overload signs in the P waves of patients with ASDs and normal pulmonary artery pressures [21].

c. The only congenital lesion in which the P wave height in lead 2 is known to correlate significantly with right ventricular systolic pressure is the ostium primum type of ASD in which the P waves may rise from 1.5 mm for pressures between normal and 50 mm Hg to 3 mm at 100 mm Hg [37].

6. What is the probable cause of the taller P wave that occurs with the sympathetic stimulation of exercise or when epinephrine is administered?

ANS.: Because the normal P notch (see p. 439) that separates right from left atrial depolarization tends to disappear with exercise or epinephrine, it may be due to almost synchronous excitation of the right and left atrium [31]. Another possibility is that because the site of the SA node cells that cause severe tachycardias is known to be different from that for slower rates, the impulse may enter the atrium at a different site, use different internodal pathways preferentially, and so produce a different P wave contour.

Lead 2 P wave

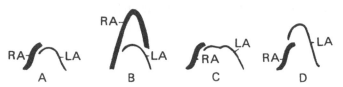

The heavy lines represent the right atrium (RA); the thin lines, the left atrium (LA). A = normal;
B = tall P wave due to right atrial overload; C = wide, notched P wave due either to left atrial
overload, or to intraatrial conduction delay or block; D = tall P wave due to epinephrine or
exercise, caused by nearly simultaneous right and left atrial depolarization.

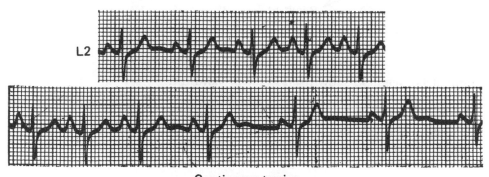

Continuous tracing

The changing rate here is due to the effect of respiration (sinus arrhythmia). Note how the P wave
height changes vary directly with the heart rate.

Pseudo P Pulmonale

1. What are the causes of tall, inferior P waves in normal subjects with normal heart
   rates?
   ANS.: Both the amplitude and the inferiorness of P axes are correlated positively
   with vital capacity in normal subjects [25]. Because vital capacity correlates
   positively with height, it follows that the taller the subject, the taller and
   more inferior is the P (see ECG 107).
   Note: The taller-than-normal P waves seen in some athletes may be due to
   physiologic RVH and true right atrial overload.
*2. What abnormal conditions are most commonly associated with an imitation of the
   tall P wave of P pulmonale with normal heart rate?
   ANS.: a. Systemic hypertension is the commonest cause of a pseudo P pulmonale
            [15].
         b. Some patients with coronary disease, either chronic or due to acute myo-
            cardial infarction, have pseudo P pulmonale [27].
         c. Subarachnoid hemorrhage [20].

Horizontal Plane Signs of Right Atrial Overload

1. What are the horizontal plane mean vectors for the right and left atrial portions of the P wave?
   ANS.:

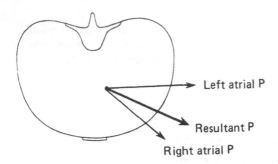

2. How does right atrial overload show itself in the precordium?
   ANS.: a. Tall upright P waves in the right precordium and often even extending over toward the left precordium [51] (see ECG 111, p. 442).
   b. A sharply peaked, upright P wave (not necessarily tall) in the right precordial leads (see ECGs 100, 108, and 110).

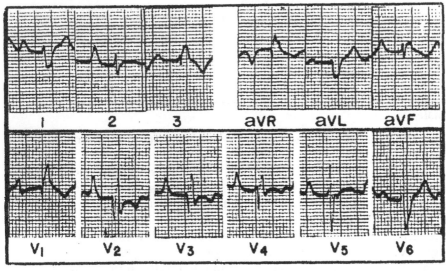

This is from a 17-year-old boy with Ebstein's anomaly. Note the tall P waves, the long P-R, the complete RBBB, and the qR in V1.

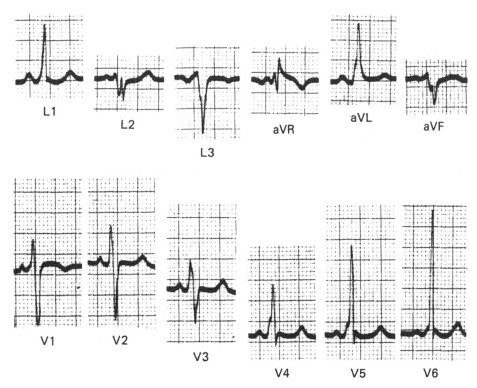

ECG 110. *Atrioventricular preexcitation in a 16-year-old boy with Ebstein's anomaly. The sharply peaked P waves in V1 and V2 are the only clues to the presence of right atrial overload. Although the delta wave (best seen in V4, V5, and V6) points anteriorly and inferiorly, the QRS points posteriorly and superiorly and so makes it a type B. Because there was no history of tachycardia, this boy did not have Wolff-Parkinson-White syndrome.*

   c. A qR in the right precordium [48] (see p. 415 for explanation). It is highly correlated with a markedly dilated right atrium (see ECG 103, p. 417).

*d. A total QRS amplitude ratio of V2 to V1 of 4 or more [48].

*e. A large terminal P negativity force, as in left atrial overload. It is seen in marked right atrial enlargement problems, e.g., large ASDs [13].

Note: It is usually possible to tell whether the large area of terminal P negativity in V1 is due to a very marked right atrial overload or to a left atrial overload. If it is due to the former, aVR shows a large area of P negativity because V1 can reflect large frontal plane forces when it is above the electrical center.

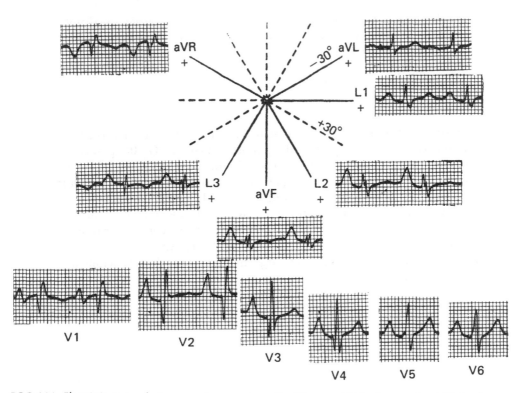

Note that the large frontal P force of right atrial overload goes away from both aVR and V1.

3. Which congenital lesions may have the largest right atrial P waves?
   ANS.: a. Ebstein's anomaly. (In addition to the large P waves, these patients usually have a right bundle branch block [RBBB] with lower voltage than expected for such a wide QRS.) (See ECG 111.)
   b. Vying with the P waves of Ebstein's anomaly are the tall P waves associated with total anomalous pulmonary venous connection, severe pulmonary stenosis, and tricuspid atresia with P waves occasionally as high as 6 mm [3].

ECG 111. Ebstein's anomaly in a nearly asymptomatic 25-year-old black man. An ASD is also present. The P is not only high but prolonged to 120 msec.

*4. Why does right atrial overload sometimes increase the width of the P wave, even though usually it does not?

ANS.: It can take such a long time to conduct through a very large right atrium, as in Ebstein's anomaly, that left atrial depolarization is completed before right atrial depolarization is completed (see ECG 111).

Note: Even though the P wave is prolonged in Ebstein's anomaly, the P-R segment is not short because there is often a block or delayed conduction either in or below the atrioventricular (AV) node [35].

Ta WAVE AND P-R SEGMENT

1. What is a Ta wave?

ANS.: The wave due to repolarization of the atrium, i.e., the T wave of the atrium.

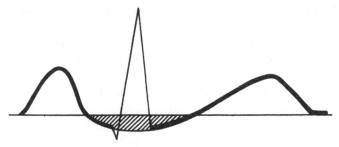

The striped area is the Ta wave.

2. How does the direction of the atrial repolarization vector relate to the P vector?

ANS.: It is opposite in direction to the P vector. This relation is supposedly due to the thinness of the atrial wall and the low pressure it generates. It allows repolarization to occur in the same direction as depolarization, but with an opposite leading edge charge.

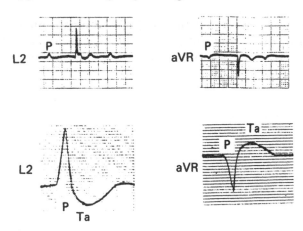

The lower panels show an electronic magnification of the P and Ta wave from the ECG of a 26-year-old woman with a normal heart except for congenital complete AV block, so that the P waves are separated from the QRSs. The top panel shows the patient's usual P waves with almost invisible Ta waves.

Note: In dogs an imbalance of vagal or sympathetic stimulation to each side of the heart can cause the Ta wave to move in the same direction as the P wave [32].

3. When should you expect a large Ta wave?
   ANS.: When there is a large P wave.

4. How long is a Ta wave in relation to the P wave, P-R segment, and QRS?
   ANS.: The Ta wave encompasses the P-R segment and the entire QRS. Although it is normally about three times the duration of the P wave, with atrial damage it may be longer. Also, the longer the P-P interval, the longer is the Ta wave [29].
   Note: It is important to be aware of a Ta wave in exercise tests because a J point depression due to a Ta wave may be misinterpreted as an S-T segment depression.

*5. How can a Ta wave help to diagnose an infarction?
   ANS.: An atrial injury current can be recognized by noting a P-R segment vector that is not opposite in direction to the P wave or that is becoming progressively more depressed or elevated simultaneously with S-T segment changes.

   A major criterion of atrial infarction is PR segments (Ta wave) elevation greater than 0.5 mm in V5 and 6 with reciprocal depressions in V1 and V2 [40B].

   Note: a. Suspect atrial infarction if an intraatrial block or atrial arrhythmias develop during the course of acute infarction [24, 39].

   b. Occasionally atrial infarction can be diagnosed by ECG when the diagnosis of ventricular infarction is questionable. Thus atrial infarction may be the only clue to ventricular infarction. Chronic atrial fibrosis can also manifest as a Ta wave that in at least some leads is in the same direction as the P wave [29].

   c. Atrial infarction is exceedingly rare with anteroseptal infarction. If, however, the right coronary artery is occluded to produce an inferior or posterior infarction, or the circumflex is occluded to produce a lateral or anterolateral infarction, atrial infarction is common [22].

   d. If with clinical acute infarction the ECG shows atrial infarction, suspect an aortic dissection with a hematoma compressing the ostium of the coronary artery and/or direct compression of the atrial myocardium.

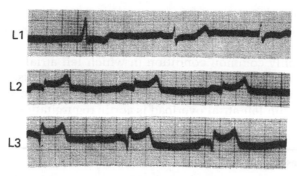

ECG 111A. A 69-year-old man had necropsy proof of an acute postero-inferior infarction with involvement of the right atrium and septum. The circumflex artery was thrombosed 2 cm from its origin. Note the P-R segment elevations in leads 2 and 3.

*6. How can a Ta wave help in the diagnosis of right atrial overload in COPD?

ANS.: Even if the P is not absolutely tall, a relatively tall P can be suspected if the Ta wave is deep in lead 3 or aVF. Also, as pulmonary disease progresses, the Ta wave becomes deeper [11].

Note: The Ta wave is normally about one-third the height of the P wave. The Ta amplitude may be increased not only by atrial hypertrophy but also by atrial damage [29].

*7. What should you suspect if an ECG shows a tachycardia and marked Ta wave?

ANS.: Alkalosis, commonly the hyperventilation-induced type but also the alkalosis of vomiting [7].

Note: Acute alkalosis or acidosis has been found to produce no significant QRS or T alterations [49].

LEFT ATRIAL OVERLOAD

Physiology and Etiologies

1. Why is the left atrium almost always affected by left ventricular hypertrophy?

ANS.: During diastole the left ventricle (LV) and atrium are in communication through an open mitral valve. Therefore their pressures are almost equal. Left ventricular hypertrophy (LVH) reduces the compliance (increases the stiffness) of the LV, so that at the end of diastole, with the mitral valve still open, the left atrium becomes part of a stiff 'atrioventricle.' A normal volume of blood entering the stiff atrioventricle from the pulmonary veins raises the pressure in the atrium to a higher level than normal. The Starling effect of this high pressure on the walls of the left atrium stimulates the atrium to contract more forcefully, which in turn results in left atrial hypertrophy. This effect, then, is the mechanism for left atrial pressure overload. If, on the other hand, the LV is dilated and hypertrophied because of mitral regurgitation, the left atrium is overloaded with a volume load and, depending on the left ventricular pressure at the end of diastole, may even have an additional left atrial pressure load.

2. How does left atrial overload help in diagnosing LVH?

   ANS.: Left atrial overload on the ECG can be used as a secondary criterion for LVH even if no other secondary criteria are present.

   Note: a. The only common condition in which left atrial overload occurs without left ventricular overload is mitral stenosis.

   b. The only volume overload of the LV that is not necessarily associated with left atrial overload is aortic regurgitation.

Wide, Notched P Waves in Left Atrial Overload (Intraatrial Block)

1. What is the upper normal width (duration) of a P wave?

   ANS.: Although you should commit to memory that a P wave is normally 2.5 small divisions high and 2.5 mm small divisions wide (i.e., 2.5 mm high and 100 msec long), some studies have shown that a normal P wave can be 110 msec (0.11 sec) in duration. Therefore you should feel safe only in considering a P wave of 120 msec (0.12 sec) as definitely abnormal [10].

2. What is meant by *P mitrale*? What is wrong with using this term for the P wave in left atrial overload?

   ANS.: It means the wide, notched P wave that is commonly found in the left atrial overload of mitral stenosis. It was first called P mitrale by Winternitz in 1935 [6]. Wide, notched P waves can also result from an interatrial conduction defect between the right and left atrium or from conditions other than mitral disease that cause left atrial overload [33] (see ECG 112). Therefore although the term should be specific for the left atrial overload of mitral disease, the wide, notched P wave is not [62]. It occurs in only about 30 percent of patients with mitral stenosis [24] and should be attributed to the rheumatic damage of the atrial muscle rather than to left atrial overload.

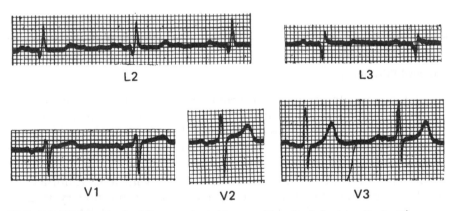

L2   L3

V1   V2   V3

ECG 112. Widely notched P waves in a 66-year-old male diabetic patient with intermittent claudication and no cardiac symptoms or signs. X-ray showed a normal cardiac size and no left atrial enlargement. The notch on the P waves separates peaks by about 60 msec (0.06 sec). Therefore this abnormality is an intraatrial conduction defect or block.

Note: a. A widely notched P wave is best called an intraatrial block.

b. Some electrocardiographs have a dampened frequency response, and the notch may not be as apparent as with other machines. With a high-enough frequency response, all P waves are notched because of asynchrony of right and left atrial depolarization; i.e., left atrial depolarization follows the beginning of right atrial depolarization by 20 to 30 msec.

c. An interatrial block can be produced experimentally by cutting Bachmann's bundle (a tract that runs horizontally from the SA node to the left atrium). The P wave will be notched if the left portion of the bundle is damaged [40C].

3. Which lead is usually the best one to examine for the widest P wave?

ANS.: The P wave in lead 2, because the frontal plane P vector is commonly between 45° and 65°.

4. Why does left atrial overload widen a P wave?

ANS.: Because the SA node is in the right atrium and the right atrium is depolarized first, the end of the P normally represents the left atrium. If the left atrium is enlarged, the terminal part is late in depolarization and so widens the P wave. P widths of at least 0.11 second are found in almost all patients with left atrial enlargement by echocardiogram [14].

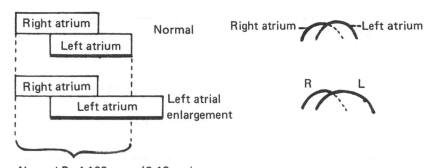

Normal P of 100 msec (0.10 sec)

5. If all P waves are slightly notched, how can you tell that a P wave is abnormally notched?

ANS.: a. If the peaks of the notch are 40 msec (0.04 sec) or more apart (i.e., one small division apart), the P wave is probably abnormally notched [8]. To be certain, however, it is safer to read an abnormal notch if the peaks are *more than* 40 msec apart.

b. If the duration of the P wave is 120 msec (0.12 sec) or more [10].

*6. What is the Macruz index for left atrial overload?

ANS.: Because a wide P due to left atrial overload must encroach on the P-R segment (the part between the end of the P and the beginning of the QRS), the wider the P wave the shorter is the P-R segment. It has been found that a ratio of the P to the P-R segment of 1.16 or more suggests a left atrial overload [40].

Note: The Macruz index cannot be trusted because

a. The P-R segments can be short owing to preexcitation by nodal bypass fibers, and the P-R segments may be prolonged owing to AV block. (The P-R segment represents conduction time through the AV node and through the bundle of His and bundle branches.)

b. A P wave can be prolonged and encroach on the P-R segment if there is a right intraatrial block or a very large right atrium, so that the right atrial depolarization is delayed and thus completed late.

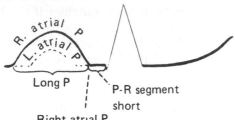

P Axis in Left Atrial Overloads

1. How does the left atrial portion of the P wave change direction in left atrial overloads?
   ANS.: It shifts the terminal portion of the P leftward or superiorly [12].
2. How can you recognize the terminal P leftward shift?
   ANS.: The terminal portion of the P in lead 3 or aVF is negative.

Horizontal Plane Signs of Left Atrial Overload

1. Which part of the P wave represents left atrial depolarization?
   ANS.: The terminal part.
2. What should happen to the terminal P force in left atrial overloads?
   ANS.: It should become larger and should turn slightly more posteriorly. (The left atrium is a central and posterior structure; it is not on the left side of the chest.)

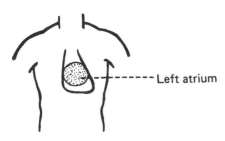

3. How can you detect the presence of a larger-than-normal terminal P force in the precordial leads?

ANS.: If an area of P terminal negativity in V1 is at least one small square in area, i.e., a square 1 mm by 1 mm (1 mm down and 40 msec across) in area [43] (see ECG 113). This area is known as an Ashman unit.

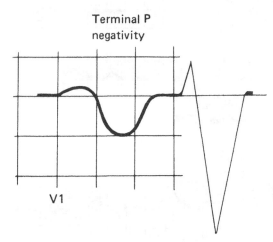

Terminal P negativity

V1

The area of negativity is 1 mm by 1 mm = 1 sq mm = left atrial overload.

Note: a. In children, if the negative portion of the P wave in V1 exceeds one-half of a small square, it is probably abnormal [50].

b. If the terminal P negativity in V1 is 60 msec (0.06 sec) across, even if the depth is only 0.5 mm, an Ashman unit of area is not achieved, but left atrial overload is likely [5, 9].

c. If Morris's original abnormal P terminal area of 0.03 (he used millimeter-seconds) is used, it includes about 5 percent of normal subjects [23]. Presumably, it is because an increased P duration can be caused by an intraatrial block. Therefore depth is more specific than duration for diagnosing left atrial overload accurately. Using at least 0.04 mm in depth as abnormal eliminates most normal subjects.

4. How can the terminal P negativity in V1 be used to tell the ejection fraction in patients with aortic stenosis?

ANS.: A Morris index (duration in seconds times amplitude in mm of the terminal negative P in V1) of 0.06 has a specificity of about 90 percent for an ejection fraction of less than 55 percent.

5. How can you detect abnormal posterior turning of the terminal P force?

ANS.: When the terminal P negativity is seen not only in V1 but also farther toward the left precordium, i.e., also in V2 or V3 [57] (see ECG 113).

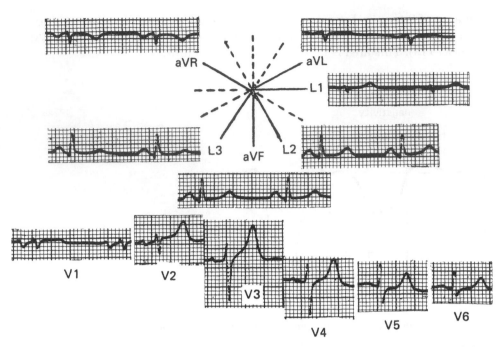

ECG 113. Moderate mitral stenosis in a 52-year-old man. The low-voltage QRS in L1 and the large-area terminal P negativity of left atrial overload in V1 are both characteristic of mitral stenosis. The presence of terminal P negativity in V2 also suggests left atrial overload.

6. What is the direction of left atrial depolarization in the horizontal plane?
   ANS.: It goes directly to the left; i.e., it is usually perpendicular, or slightly less than perpendicular, to V2.

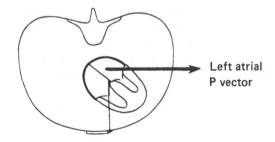

Left atrial P vector

7. Why does posterior turning of the terminal P vector cause the P to become progressively negative across the precordium, i.e., negative not only in V1 but also in V2 or even V3?
   ANS.: Because the farther across the left precordium that negativity is seen, the more posterior is the vector.

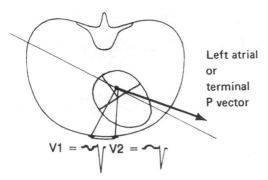

This terminal P is more than 90° from V1 but still positive in V2. It is the usual terminal P vector; i.e., V1 is commonly biphasic.

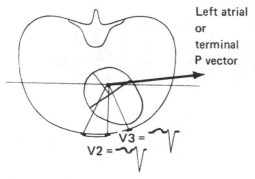

This terminal P is now more than 90° from V2 but less than 90° to V3. Therefore it is negative in V2 but positive in V3 and is now suggestive of left atrial overload.

Note how the vector turns more posteriorly as it shows progressive negativity from the right to the left precordium.

*8. In which conditions without left atrial overload can there be P negativity of one small square in V1? Why?

ANS.: a. Emphysema, or COPD. Here the electrical center may be too low for the normal electrode placement of V leads; i.e., the electrodes are placed relatively too high, so that all P forces tend to point away from the electrodes.

b. Pectus excavatum. Here the posterior tilt of the apex may place the superior aspect of the right atrium more anteriorly and tilt its vector posteriorly [18].

c. A large right atrium in a patient with a low electrical center, i.e., with V1 similar to aVR. See p. 441 for explanation of this problem.

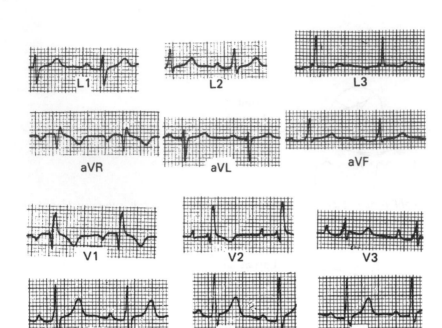

ECG 114. A 20-year-old woman with an ASD. Note the large area of P negativity in V1, which is similar to the P area in aVR. It is a pseudo left atrial overload P wave due to a large right atrium with the V1 electrode placed high relative to the electrical center. The sharply peaked P waves in V2 and V3 also are due to right atrial overload.

*9. How can you exaggerate the large-area terminal P negativity in a patient with mitral stenosis?

ANS.: Repeat V1 after exercise. A normal subject shows no change in the V1 terminal P force [60].

*10. Why may constrictive pericarditis commonly cause left atrial overload?

ANS.: The left ventricle may be constricted early in the course of the disease before the left atrium becomes constricted [52].

---

*Left Atrial Overload in Coronary Disease

*1. What does left atrial overload signify in patients with acute myocardial infarction?

ANS.: A large terminal P force in V1 usually means a high mean left atrial pressure. A return toward normal of the P force means that the left atrial pressure is either more normal or stabilizing [13]. If the abnormal terminal P force remained at the time of discharge, the 5-year mortality rate in one study was about 50 percent [47].

Note: Atrial pressure (acute or chronic) is probably a stronger determinant of the terminal P force than is atrial size [19].

*2. With which clinical aspects of acute infarction do ECG signs of left atrial overload correlate best?

ANS.: a. With papillary muscle dysfunction associated with mitral regurgitation [36].

b. With pulmonary edema; i.e., ECG signs of left atrial overload correlate with the degree of left ventricular failure [36].

Note: a. Because a widely notched P may merely denote an intraatrial block, it is not surprising that V1 terminal P negativity is more reliable than wide notching for predicting elevation of left atrial pressure [34].

b. In one study of patients with coronary, hypertensive, or primary myocardial disease, the P terminal force was always abnormal if the left atrial pressure was more than 24 mm Hg. The P terminal force was never abnormal if the left atrial pressure was less than 14 mm Hg [19].

c. The P terminal force in V1 can help to differentiate an acute pulmonary embolus from its two most important imitators, which are acute pulmonary edema or acute infarction. This is because with pulmonary edema due to left ventricular failure as well as in patients with acute myocardial infarction, the P terminal force is often abnormal. Acute pulmonary embolism, on the other hand, does not as a rule cause an abnormal P terminal force [2].

3. What is the normal shape of the P wave in lead 2?

ANS.: Almost symmetrical or with a slightly longer ascent than descent (see ECG 2, p. 46).

*4. How is the rise (ascent) time of a P wave affected by age?

ANS.: The ascending limb of the P takes longer to reach its peak with increasing age, so that under age 50 it occupies only 50 percent of the P, i.e., the P is symmetrical. In subjects over age 50, the ascending limb occupies 60 percent of the duration of the P.

Note: a. An abnormal ascent usually occupies more than two-thirds of the P wave [26]. (See lead 1 in ECG 19, p. 150; see also lead 1 in ECG 63A, p. 301.)

b. The response of the P wave to impairment of blood supply due to coronary atherosclerosis is
(1) Prolongation of the P beyond the upper normal of 100 msec (0.10 sec) [26].
(2) Delayed rise time to reach its peak [26].
(3) Wide notching (intraatrial block) [8].

*5. What suggests biatrial overload (a) in the precordial leads? (b) in the frontal plane?

ANS.: a. In the horizontal plane, a large area of terminal negativity of left atrial overload in V1 plus a few millimeters of peaked initial positivity.

b. In the frontal plane, a double-peaked P wave, with the first peak taller than the second. This pattern has been characteristically seen in tricuspid atresia and has been called 'P tricuspidale.'

*6. How can an exercise ECG help to diagnose a high left atrial pressure in a patient with old myocardial infarction or angina with a normal resting cardiogram?

ANS.: If it results in a left atrial overload terminal P force in V1 that was not present at rest, the end-diastolic pressure is more than 18 mm Hg with a sensitivity of 90 percent and a specificity of 85 percent.

*ATRIAL OVERLOADS IN ATRIAL ARRHYTHMIAS

*1. How can right atrial overload be recognized in the presence of such arrhythmias as atrial tachycardia or atrial fibrillation?

ANS.: The ectopic P waves of atrial tachycardia are taller than expected. The f waves of atrial fibrillation in V1 may be very coarse, i.e., increased in amplitude.

Note: a. Because atrial flutter is usually caused by right atrial overload, it is not surprising that the amplitude of the f waves of atrial flutter do not correlate with left atrial size on echocardiograms [61].

b. In one study coarse fibrillation waves in ischemic heart disease were found only with paroxysmal fibrillation [41].

c. With idiopathic atrial fibrillation the f waves are usually fine [46].

d. When the dilated atria of heart failure are normalized with treatment, the f waves may become smaller [55].

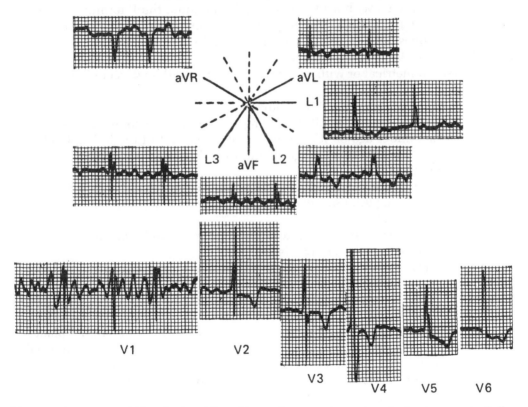

ECG 115. An 18-year-old boy had an idiopathic cardiomyopathy and marked enlargement of all chambers. The giant waves in V1 probably reflect biatrial overload.

*2. When can small f waves be present in V1 despite atrial overload?

ANS.: When the fibrillation has been present for many years, or there is much atrial fibrosis [4].

Note: a. Because much fibrosis can reduce the size of the f wave of atrial fibrillation and because large f waves cannot tell you whether it is the right or the left atrium that is the enlarged chamber, it is not surprising that f wave amplitude cannot be correlated with left atrial size by echocardiography [42, 59].

b. After cardioversion, most patients with coarse f waves show an abnormal P terminal force in V1, and those with fine f waves show a normal P terminal force [45].

*3. When can a premature contraction cause a change in the postectopic P wave?

ANS.: A premature atrial contraction can cause aberrant atrial conduction in the postextrasystolic beat if organic heart disease is present [16].

REFERENCES

1. Abildskov, J. A. The atrial complex of the electrocardiogram. *Am. Heart J.* 57:930, 1959.
2. Abrahams, C., and Furman, K. I. Analgesic abuse and microvascular changes. *Am. Heart J.* 95:268, 1978.
3. Anselmi, G., et al. Electrocardiographic patterns of right atrial overloading in some congenital heart conditions. *Am. J. Cardiol.* 21:628, 1968.
4. Aravanis, C., Toutouzas, P., and Michaelides, G. Diagnostic significance of atrial fibrillatory waves. *Cardiovasc. Comm.* 1:19, 1966.
5. Arevalo, A. C., Spagnuolo, M., and Feinstein, A. R. A simple electrocardiographic indication of left atrial enlargement. A study of young patients with rheumatic heart disease. *J.A.M.A.* 185:358, 1963.
6. Bekheit, S., et al. His bundle electrogram in P mitrale. *Br. Heart J.* 34:1057, 1972.
7. Bernreiter, M. Prominent auricular T waves (Ta) as an important guide to the diagnosis of alkalosis. *Angiology* 18:191, 1967.
8. Bethell, H. J. N., and Nixon, P. G. F. Electrical and mechanical aspects of left atrial activity. *Br. Heart J.* 35:507, 1974.
9. Bethell, H. J. N., and Nixon, P. G. F.P waves of electrocardiogram in early ischaemic heart disease. *Br. Heart J.* 34:1170, 1972.
10. Bradley, S. M., and Marriott, H. J. L. Intra-atrial block. *Circulation* 14:1073, 1956.
11. Calatayud, J. B. Analysis of atrial T wave in patients with COPD. *Dis. Chest* 56:5, 1969.
12. Calatayud, J. B. Leftward shift of the terminal P forces with left atrial enlargement. *Am. Heart J.* 71:727, 1966.
13. Chandraratna, P. A. N., and Hodges, M., Electrocardiographic evidence of left atrial hypertension in acute myocardial infarction. *Circulation* 47:493, 1973.
14. Chirife, R., Freitosa, G. S., and Frankl, W. S. Electrocardiographic detection of left atrial enlargement. *Br. Heart J.* 37:1281, 1975.
15. Chou, T. C., and Helm, R. A. The pseudo P-pulmonale. *Circulation* 32:96, 1965.
16. Chung, E. K. Aberrant atrial conduction: Unrecognized electrocardiographic entity. *Br. Heart J.* 34:341, 1972.
17. Chung, E. K. Electrocardiographic findings in hypokalemia. *Postgrad. Med.* 51:285, 1972.
18. DeOliveira, J. M., Sambhi, M. P., and Zimmerman, H. A. The ECG in pectus excavatum. *Br. Heart J.* 20:495, 1958.
19. DiBianco, R., et al. Left atrial overload – a hemodynamic echocardiographic, electrocardiographic and vectorcardiographic study. *Am. Heart J.* 98:478, 1979.
20. Eisalo, A., Perasalo, J., and Halonen, P. I. Electrocardiographic abnormalities in patients with subarachnoid hemorrhage. *Br. Heart J.* 34:217, 1972.
21. Fenoglio, J. J., Jr., et al. Right atrial ultrastructure in congenital heart disease. II. Atrial septal defect: Effects of volume overload. *Am. J. Cardiol.* 48:820, 1979.
22. Ferrer, M. I. The sick sinus syndrome. *Circulation* 47:635, 1973.

23. Forfang, K., and Erikssen, J. Significance of P wave terminal force in presumably healthy middle-aged men. *Am. Heart J.* 96:739, 1978.
24. Gilbert-Queralto, J., and Tornar-Soler, M. The electrocardiogram in mitral stenosis: Before and after commissurotomy. *Am. Heart J.* 49:548, 1955.
25. Gross, D. Electrocardiographic characteristics of P pulmonale waves of coronary origin. *Am. Heart J.* 73:453, 1967.
26. Gross, D. The clinical significance of P waves with delayed ascent. *Am. Heart J.* 63:496, 1962.
27. Grossman, J. I., and Delman, A. J. Serial P wave changes in acute myocardial infarction. *Am. Heart J.* 77:336, 1969.
28. Hancock, E. W. Coronary sinus rhythm in sinus venosus defect and persistent left superior vena cava. *Am. J. Cardiol.* 14:608, 1964.
29. Hayashi, H., Okajima, M., and Yamada, K. Atrial T (Ta) wave and atrial gradient with A-V block. *Am. Heart J.* 91:689, 1976.
30. Hung, J.-S., et al. Electrocardiographic and angiographic features of common atrium. *Chest* 63:970, 1973.
31. Irisawa, H., and Seyama, I. The configuration of the P wave during mild exercise. *Am. Heart J.* 71:467, 1966.
31A. Ishida, T., et al. Exercise induced T wave changes. *Jpn. Heart J.* 23:630, 1982.
32. James, T. N., Urthaler, F., and Isobe, J. H. Neurogenic influence on the atrial repolarization (P-Tp) segment. *Am. J. Cardiol.* 32:799, 1973.
33. Josephson, M. E., Kastor, J. A., and Morganroth, J. Electrocardiographic left atrial enlargement. *Am. J. Cardiol.* 39:967, 1977.
34. Kasser, I., and Kennedy, J. W. The relationship of increased left atrial volume and pressure to abnormal P waves and the electrocardiogram. *Circulation* 39:339, 1969.
35. Kastor, J. A., et al. Electrophysiologic characteristics of Ebstein's anomaly of the tricuspid valve. *Circulation* 52:987, 1975.
36. Keikkila, J., and Luomanmaki, K. Value of serial P wave changes in indicating left heart failure in myocardial infarction. *Br. Heart J.* 32:510, 1970.
37. Kulbertus, H. E., Coyne, J. J., and Hallidie-Smith, K. A. Electrocardiographic correlation of ana-tomical and haemodynamic data in ostium primum atrial septal defects. *Br. Heart J.* 30:464, 1968.
38. Lamb, L. E. *Electrocardiography and Vectorcardiography.* Philadelphia: Saunders, 1965.
39. Liu, C. K., Greenspan, G., and Piccirillo, R. T. Atrial infarction of the heart. *Circulation* 23:331, 1961.
40. Macruz, R., Perloff, J. K., and Cass, R. B. A method for the electrocardiographic recognition of atrial enlargement. *Circulation* 17:882, 1958.
40A. Maeda, S., et al. Lack of coorelation between P pulmonale and right atrial overload in COPD. *Br. Heart J.* 65:132, 1991.
40B. Mayuga, R., Jr., Singer, D. H. Atrial infarction: clinical significance and diagnostic criteria: An update. *Pract. Cardiol.* 11(12):1–10, Nov. 1985.
40C. Medrano, G. A. Interatrial conduction in experimental atrial damage. *J. Electrocardiol.* 20:357, 1987.
41. Mihulova, L. Diagnostic importance of nature of fibrillation wave. *Unitrni Lek. Vnitrni.* 11:562, 1965.
42. Morganroth, J., et al. Relationship of atrial fibrillatory wave amplitude to left atrial size and etiology of heart disease. *Am. Heart J.* 97:184, 1979.
43. Morris, J. J., et al. P-wave analysis in valvular heart disease. *Circulation* 29:242, 1964.
44. Penneys, R., and Thomas, C. B. The relationship between the arterial oxygen saturation and the cardiovascular response to induced anoxemia in normal young adults. *Circulation* 1:415, 1950.
45. Peter, R. H. Relationship of fibrillatory waves and P waves in the electrocardiogram. *Circulation* 33:599, 1966.
46. Peter, R. H. Significance of fibrillatory waves in idiopathic atrial fibrillation. *Ann. Intern. Med.* 68:1296, 1968.
47. Pohjola, S., Siltanen, P., and Romo, M. The prognostic value of the P wave morphology in the discharge electrocardiogram. *Am. Heart J.* 98:32, 1979.

47A. Recke, S. H., et al. ECG markers of impaired ejection performance in aortic stenosis. *J. Electrocardiol.* 22:45, 1989.

47B. Reeves, W. C., et al. 2-D Echocardiographic assessment of electrocardiographic criteria for right atrial enlargement. *Circulation* 64:387, 1981.

47C. Reeves, W. C. ECG in right atrial enlargement. *J. Am. Coll. Cardiol.* 9:469, 1987.

48. Reeves, W. C., et al. 2-D Echocardiographic assessment of electrocardiographic criteria for right atrial enlargement. *Circulation* 64:387, 1979.

49. Reid, J. A., et al. The effect of variations in blood pH on the electrocardiogram in man. *Circulation* 31:369, 1965.

50. Reynolds, J. L. The electrocardiographic recognition of left atrial enlargement in childhood. *Am. Heart J.* 81:748, 1971.

51. Reynolds, J. L. The electrocardiographic recognition of right atrial abnormality in children. *Am. Heart J.* 81:748, 1971.

52. Samad, A., Rekman, M., and Shafgat, S. H. Left atrial enlargement in chronic constrictive pericarditis. In Abstracts World Congress of Cardiology, Tokyo, 1978, p. 289.

53. Saunders, J. L., et al. Evaluation of ECG criteria for P-wave abnormalities. *Am. Heart J.* 74:757, 1967.

54. Silver, H. M., and Calatayud, J. B. Evaluation of QRS criteria in patients with chronic lung disease. *Chest* 59:153, 1971.

55. Skoulas, A., and Horlick, L. The atrial F wave in various types of heart disease and its response to treatment. *Am. J. Cardiol.* 14:174, 1964.

56. Stolar, I., et al. P wave changes in intracerebral hemorrhage. *Am. Heart J.* 107:784, 1984.

57. Sutnick, A. J., and Soloff, L. A. Posterior rotation of the atrial vector. *Circulation* 26:913, 1962.

58. Thomas, H. M., Jr., Spicer, M. J., and Nelson, W. P. Evaluation of P wave axis in distinguishing anatomical site of atrial septal defect. *Br. Heart J.* 35:738, 1973.

59. Thurmann, M., and Janney, J. G., Jr. The diagnostic importance of fibrillatory wave size. *Circulation* 25:991, 1962.

59A. Waldo, A. L., et al. Effects on the canine P wave of lesions in the atrial tracts. *Circulation Res.* 29:452, 1971.

60. Yokoyama, M., et al. P wave changes on exercise in patients with isolated mitral stenosis. *Am. Heart J.* 87:15, 1974.

61. Zoneraich, O., et al. Atrial flutter. Electrocardiographic, vectorcardiographic and echocardiographic correlation. *Am. Heart J.* 96:286, 1978.

62. Zoneraich, S., et al. Electrocardiographic findings in diabetic patients without clinical evidence of heart involvement. *N.Y. State J. Med.* 77:1254, 1977.

27. Arrhythmia Diagnosis: Part 1. Nodal Abnormalities, Escape Beats, and Premature Atrial Contractions[1]

READING HEART RATES

1. How do you tell heart rate by inspection?

    ANS.: Count the number of large divisions (five small divisions, or 200 msec [0.20 sec]) between R waves and divide into 300. For example, if there are five large divisions between R waves, the rate is 60 beats per minute.

    Because rates vary from minute to minute, report the rate to the nearest 5 or 10; e.g., 98 is reported as 100, and 97 is reported as 95.

2. How do you count heart rate if it is so fast that there are fewer than two large divisions between R waves; i.e., the rate is more than 150?

    ANS.: Divide the number of 40-msec (0.04 sec) small divisions between complexes into 1500; e.g., if there are eight small divisions between R waves, the rate is 188 beats per minute (reported as a rate of 190). This method is useful for counting rapid rates.

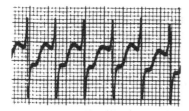

There are 7½ small divisions between R waves. Therefore the rate is 1500 divided by 7.5, which is 200 per minute.

3. How can you tell the heart rate from marks on the edges of most ECG paper?

    ANS.: Vertical marks 3 seconds apart are usually printed on the margins. Count the number of R waves in 6 seconds and multiply by 10. If there are no 3-second markers, count the number of complexes in 30 large divisions (6 seconds long) and multiply by 10.

4. When must you use the 3-second marks on the paper's edge or count the number of R waves in 6 seconds to count the heart rate?

    ANS.: When the rhythm is irregular, as with atrial fibrillation. Do not report a range; report the average rate per minute.

---

[1] A systematic approach to the interpretation of an arrhythmia is outlined on page 586 and to reading an electrocardiogram on page 609.

ARRHYTHMIAS FROM THE SINOATRIAL NODE

Sinus Tachycardia and Bradycardia

1. What is the anatomic location of the sinoatrial (SA) node?
   ANS.: High in the lateral right atrium, where the right atrium joins the superior vena cava. The 'head' is anterosuperior. The 'tail' is inferior and may be posterior as well [3].

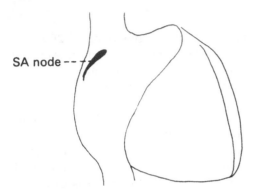

SA node

The SA node is about 1.5 cm long and 5 mm wide.

2. Above how many beats per minute is the rate considered a sinus tachycardia?
   ANS.: Although a rate of more than 90 is faster than a normal resting rate, by electrocardiographic (ECG) convention a sinus tachycardia is a rate of 100 or more.
   Note: a. In the newborn infant the rate is about 95 to 155, which can last about 2 weeks.
   b. At age 1 month the range is between 110 and 200. The maximum rate then falls by about 10 beats per month so that by 1 year it is 140. The adult range is reached at about age 6.
   c. Diabetic patients have faster resting heart rates than do age-matched normal subjects [107].

3. Below how many beats per minute is the rate considered a sinus bradycardia?
   ANS.: Because a rate of 55 or less in a subject age 55 or older is associated with a higher risk of coronary disease than normal, we should probably call 55 or less a bradycardia even though most physicians call 60 or less a bradycardia.
   Note: a. Bradycardia is a recognized feature of the trained athlete. The degree of bradycardia is greatest in endurance athletes. The average rate for runners is 55 and for wrestlers 65.
   *b. A pure form of sinus bradycardia is inherited as an autosomal dominant. Although the prognosis in terms of mortality is relatively benign, the Wolff-Parkinson-White (WPW) syndrome tends to develop in these patients [128]. An impure form of familial sinus bradycardia exists in which complete atrioventricular (AV) block with a high mortality develops in many members of these families [128].

---

* Material marked with an asterisk is included for reference and for advanced students in cardiology.

*4. What are the maximal heart rates attained by healthy subjects under the tension of (a) driving in heavy traffic? (b) driving in a professional auto race?
ANS.: a. About 150 per minute.
b. About 200 per minute.
Note: Resting rates of more than 150 in adults are usually ectopic tachycardias. However, sinus rates may be more than 150 in severe respiratory failure, massive pulmonary embolism, and severe pulmonary edema [92].

*Autonomic Control of the SA Node

*1. What drug test can tell you whether a sinus bradycardia is due to sinus node disease or merely to excess vagal tone?
ANS.: Atropine should produce at least a 20 percent increase in heart rate if excess vagotonia is present.
*2. What influences the resting heart rate more in normal subjects, sympathetic or parasympathetic tone?
ANS.: Parasympathetic influences predominate [113]. This fact is shown by the finding that after vagal blockade the resting heart rate increases by about 50 percent [113]. If, however, sympathetic blockade by spinal anesthesia is produced, the heart rate slows by only about 10 percent [113].
Note: Digitalis slows the sinus rate entirely through its vagal stimulating effects. In an isolated atrium, digitalis actually speeds up the sinus pacemaker [10].
*3. List the metabolic causes of chronic sinus bradycardia.
ANS.: a. Obstructive jaundice (probably the effect of bile salts on the SA node).
b. Myxedema.
c. Hypothermia.

Sinus Arrhythmia

1. How is the heart rate affected by respiration; i.e., what is the effect of respiration on the SA node?
ANS.: The heart rate speeds up with inspiration (owing to inhibition of the vagus) and slows with expiration.
2. What is this change of rate by respiration called?
ANS.: Sinus arrhythmia.
Note: An easy way to remember this terminology is *in*spiration causes an *in*crease in rate. Therefore '*in causes in.*'
3. How is sinus arrhythmia recognized on an ECG?
ANS.: By gradual shortening and then gradual lengthening of the R-R intervals (accordion or concertina effect).

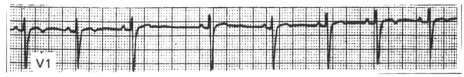

This ECG is from a healthy 18-year-old boy. The progressive changes in R-R intervals indicate sinus arrhythmia. The faster rates occur during inspiration.

4. What common physiologic states can exaggerate a sinus arrhythmia?
   ANS.: a. The relative vagotonia of the athlete.
   b. The vagotonia of sleep (as shown by ECG monitoring in coronary care units).
5. When is sinus arrhythmia not dependent on respiration? What is this type called?
   ANS.: In some elderly patients it appears to depend on spontaneous autonomic fluctuations. Thus it is termed *nonphasic*, or *nonrespiratory*, sinus arrhythmia. *Phasic*, or *respiratory*, sinus arrhythmia is dependent on the phases of respiration. *Respiratory* and *nonrespiratory* sinus arrhythmias are probably better terms.

Natural Pacemakers and the Transmembrane Action Potential

1. What part of the heart other than the SA node may become a pacemaker?
   ANS.: Almost any part of the conduction system of the heart, because automatic pacemaker cells are normally found only in the conduction system.
   a. In parts of the atrium (Purkinje-like cells in the internodal and interatrial tracts).
   b. Around the distal part of the AV node or node-His area.
   c. In the His-Purkinje system of the ventricles.
   Note: There are no pacemaker cells in the center of the AV node, where the major work of slowing is done. (The reason some investigators have been misled by artifacts into thinking that there are automatic cells in the center of the AV node has been explained by Hoffman [26, 61]. We therefore avoid the term *nodal rhythm* or *nodal premature contractions* and use the term *junctional* for this area.
2. Why is the SA node the usual pacemaker in the heart if many sites in the heart can become pacemakers?
   ANS.: Because the SA node normally contains the most rapidly firing group of automatic cells in the heart. (This statement is explained in the discussion of action potentials that follows.)
3. How is an action potential recorded?
   ANS.: By piercing the cell with a needle microelectrode and connecting it to a distant 'indifferent' electrode through a galvanometer.

4. Draw the action potential pattern of a nonautomatic cardiac cell. Label the phases.
   ANS.:

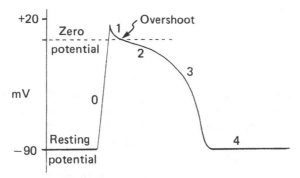

A diagram of an action potential that occurs whenever a cell is depolarized. The phases are labeled 0, 1, 2, 3, and 4. The reasoning behind calling the initial rapid depolarization wave (due to sodium influx into the cell) phase 0 rather than phase 1 is that it is often so fast the writing arm of an ECG machine frequently shows nothing on paper during this rapid upstroke. Phase 0 takes about 1 msec. During phase 3, potassium diffuses out. In phases 0, 1, 2, and 3, calcium also diffuses into the cell. (See question 5, p. 472, for details of calcium flux.)

5. Show how the action potential of a single cell relates to an ECG of the entire heart recorded simultaneously.
   ANS.:

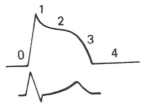

The QRS corresponds to phases 0 and 1. The S-T segment corresponds to phase 2. Because the QRS represents the resultant of the entire heart's billions of cardiac action potentials, it is likely to begin earlier than the action potential of a single cell in the middle of the heart.

6. What is the significance of different amplitudes or different slopes of phase 0?
   ANS.: The lower the amplitude of phase 0 and the shallower its slope, the slower is conduction from cell to cell (the propagation rate is decreased).
7. How does an automatic pacemaker cell action potential such as from the SA node differ most from that of the nonautomatic muscle cell?
   ANS.: Phase 4 of all automatic cells has a visible upward slope. Nonautomatic or 'working' cells have a flat phase 4.

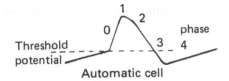

Automatic cell

Note: Phase 4 is often considered the resting phase, but it is really a very active phase because at this time adenosine triphosphatase (ATP) is hydrolyzed to adenosine diphosphatase by ATPase, sodium is pumped out, and potassium reenters the cell. The SA node's action potential phase 0 is slower than in a nonautomatic cell, and the phase 2 plateau is absent. However, this fact is not as important to remember as the fact that in the SA node each cell's phase 4 rises, and when it reaches a certain level (threshold potential) the cell spontaneously depolarizes. The rise in phase 4 of about − 60 to − 70 mv is due to leakage of potassium out of the cell and a slow sodium current into the cell [11]. The phase 4 rise is called diastolic depolarization.

8. What is meant by the threshold potential of an automatic cell?

   ANS.: It is the level to which the phase 4 slope has to rise before the cell fires (depolarizes) spontaneously. (See the foregoing diagram.)

   Note: A working muscle in the atrium or ventricle may become an abnormal automatic cell, i.e., with a rise of phase 4, if physical or metabolic abnormalities reduce their resting membrane potential to − 60 mv [157].

Phase 4 and Heart Rate

1. What alterations in the action potential can increase the firing rate of an automatic cell?

   ANS.: Anything that causes the slope of phase 4 to reach threshold faster. It can be done by:

   a. Increasing the steepness of the slope of phase 4, as by epinephrine.

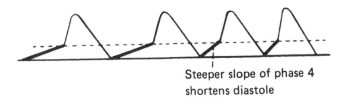

Steeper slope of phase 4
shortens diastole

   *b. Lowering of the threshold potential level (making it more negative), so that it is closer to the resting potential.

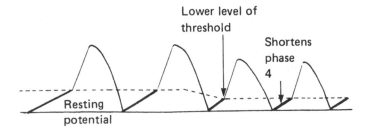

c. Raising the resting potential level closer to threshold potential, as by an increase in serum potassium.

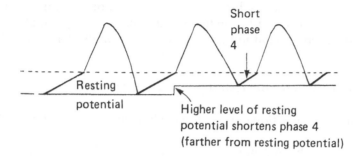

Short
phase
4

Resting
potential

Higher level of resting
potential shortens phase 4
(farther from resting potential)

Note: Raising or lowering the vertical level of the threshold or resting potential is the opposite of raising or lowering the *actual* threshold or resting potential; e.g., if the actual resting potential is given an increased quantity of millivolts, its quantity is raised, but its vertical level is lowered. Do not describe changes in resting potential as higher or lower. It is clearer to describe them as 'increased' or 'decreased' or as 'more' or 'less.' Changes in threshold potential should be related to zero or resting potential. It is better to say 'closer to' or 'farther from' zero potential or resting potential.

2. By which of the previous three mechanisms are sinus pacemaker cells usually changed to produce sinus bradycardia and tachycardia?

ANS.: By a change in the steepness of their phase 4 slope, due to a change in autonomic (vagal and sympathetic) discharge.

Note: Major changes in sinus rates are thought to result from suppression of one pacemaker site within the SA node and dominance of another; i.e., there are said to be many pacemaker cells with different intrinsic rhythmicity in the SA node.

3. How is phase 4 of the action potential of automatic cells, and thus the heart rate, affected by (a) epinephrine? (b) acetylcholine?

ANS.: a. Epinephrine makes the slope steeper and so causes tachycardia.

b. Acetylcholine (the chemical released from vagal nerve endings) does the opposite; i.e., it makes the slope of phase 4 shallower [61]. Vagal stimulation can also delay phase 4 reaching firing threshold by shifting the resting potential downward, away from the threshold potential. This action is called 'hyperpolarization' [88].

Note: Acetylcholine is said to have no effect on the phase 4 slope of automatic cells in the *ventricular* conduction system (His-Purkinje system). It affects only the automatic cells in the atrium [61].

Phase 4 and Dominant Pacemakers

1. How do automatic cells from different sites in the heart differ in their action potential?

ANS.: Phase 4 has different rates of rise at different sites.

2. What usually determines which automatic cells control the heart rate?

ANS.: The area of the heart where automatic cells have the fastest rates of rise in phase 4 becomes the pacemaker of the heart. This is because of the important basic rule of depolarization, which is that if one cell of the conduction system is depolarized, every cell in the heart is depolarized sequentially in all directions unless there is a pathologic or physiologic block. Therefore all the cells that reach threshold first extinguish the phase 4 of all cells that would have reached threshold later.

3. Which automatic cells normally have the fastest phase 4 rate of rise?

ANS.: The SA node.

4. Which automatic cells have the next slower rate of rise when compared with the SA node?

ANS.: The cells just distal to the AV node (i.e., the bundle of His area) have a slightly slower rise of phase 4 than do the sinus node cells. The ventricular automatic cells are still slower.

5. What is another name for the area around the AV node and bundle of His?

ANS.: The junctional area.

6. What is the usual rate of (a) a junctional pacemaker? (b) a ventricular pacemaker?

ANS.: a. Junctional: about 40 to 60 per minute.

   b. Ventricular: about 20 to 40 per minute.

SA Block and Sinus Arrest

1. What does SA node depolarization contribute to the P wave?

ANS.: Nothing. The P wave is due to depolarization of the right and left atrium. SA node depolarization is too small to be seen on an ECG.

2. If the SA node fires regularly, but the impulse occasionally does not leave the SA node, what happens to the P wave?

ANS.: No P wave is produced on the ECG.

3. What term is used to describe blockage of the SA impulse as it tries unsuccessfully to leave the SA node?

ANS.: *SA block.* A concept of a physiologic 'membrane' around the SA node is necessary to explain how an SA node can fire without reaching the atrium, i.e., with an 'exit block.' Nor can variable delays between the SA node firing and reaching the atrium be understood without the 'membrane' concept.

Note: There are cells surrounding the SA node that possess the histologic characteristics of both nodal and ordinary atrial cells. These transitional cells represent a buffer zone and are probably the site of SA blocks [97].

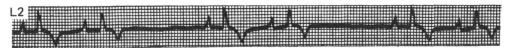

Bigeminy due to SA block every third beat (3:2 block) in a 50-year-old man with angina taking digitalis. The pauses are exactly twice the regular P-P intervals. Atropine eliminated the SA block.

4. How is SA block recognized if there is (a) persistent 2:1 block (i.e., every second firing does not produce a P wave)? or (b) occasional block?

   ANS.: a. Persistent 2:1 SA block with regular firing of the SA node can be diagnosed only if there is at least an occasional *sudden doubling* of the heart rate, either spontaneously or with exercise or atropine. (2:1 SA block is a rare cause of bradycardia.)

   b. Occasional SA block is diagnosed if the occasional long P-P intervals are almost exactly twice—or some other multiple of—the short ones, as in the following strip.

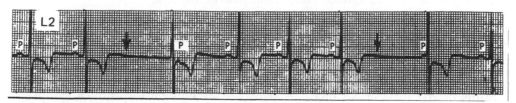

Intermittent SA block as shown by the timing of the absent P waves (indicated by arrows). The arrows show there is almost exactly a place for a P wave that should have appeared if the SA nodal impulse had reached the atrium. Thus the SA node fired but did not get through the paranodal cells; i.e., there was an intermittent exit block from the SA node. The QRS ending the pause is not preceded by a P wave, and the P at the end of the second pause is not producing the QRS that follows it. They are therefore produced by a junctional focus; i.e., they are junctional escape beats. They came at an interval that would have produced a rate of about 40 per minute. Junctional cells generally fire at rates of 40 to 60 per minute. This escape pacemaker, then, is healthier than the one in the illustration for question 5, where the junction escapes at an interval that would have given a pacemaker rate of about 25 per minute.

5. What terms are used when the SA node does not fire at all, either intermittently or permanently?

   ANS.: *Sinus arrest, sinus pause,* or *sinus standstill.*

   Note: A sinus arrest is likely to be temporary following a cardiac operation in which the SA node or its blood supply has been traumatized.

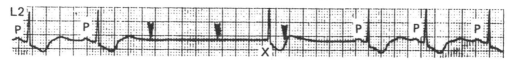

SA block in a man with acute anterior infarction. This pattern is not sinus arrest or standstill because the long interval is an almost perfect multiple of the regular P-P interval. At X is a junctional escape beat that did not penetrate the atrium retrogradely to produce its own P wave.

*6. What are some etiologies of atrial standstill, i.e., the absence of any atrial activity whatever?

   ANS.: Persistent atrial standstill has been described with muscular dystrophy, amyloidosis, and idiopathic or coronary cardiomyopathy.

   Note: If atrial electrical stimulation cannot produce a P wave, it has been called 'persistent atrial quiescence' [161].

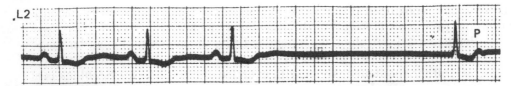

Sinus arrest following surgery for mitral stenosis. This ECG was taken during one of a 40-year-old woman's frequent syncopal attacks, which disappeared within a few weeks. The long P-P interval of the sinus pause is not a multiple of her normal P-P interval; therefore the SA node has probably not fired during the pause. If it had fired but not produced P waves, it would be called SA block, not sinus arrest. The last QRS is a markedly delayed junctional escape beat.

Sinus Node Dysfunction and the Sick Sinus Syndrome

1. What is meant by the sick sinus syndrome (SSS)?

    ANS.: Sinus bradycardia or SA block or arrest severe enough to produce symptoms. The term *sinus node dysfunction* is preferred if no symptoms are present [12]. (A syndrome usually implies the presence of symptoms.)

    Note: The symptoms may be any kind of cerebral disorder, including psychiatric disorders, or any kind of cardiac symptoms, such as pulmonary edema [130]. Angina is not uncommon when there is an inability to increase output with exercise [82].

2. What other than the slow heart rate may produce the symptoms in SSS? What is it called?

    ANS.: Symptoms may result from palpitations, angina, or failure due to intermittent tachycardias. It is then called the 'tachycardia-bradycardia syndrome.'

    Note: a. These patients are greatly at risk for embolism [130].

    b. The arrhythmias are generally supraventricular. Ventricular tachycardias are not a feature of SSS [130].

*3. Why does syncope occur with the tachycardia-bradycardia syndrome?

    ANS.: The tachycardia exaggerates the SA block by overdrive suppression of all pacemaker cells. By suppressing the junctional cells as well, junctional escape is delayed and syncope occurs. The junctional escape mechanism is probably further depressed by the damage to the junctional area that is so common with SSS (see also question 10 for further explanation).

    Note: The production of exit block from a pacemaker cell by an early depolarization is usually much more pronounced for ectopic than for sinus pacemakers unless SA nodal dysfunction is present.

4. What is usually found in the rest of the conduction system in SSS?

    ANS.: About two-thirds of the patients have other conduction abnormalities. They may have intraatrial delays, AV blocks, or His bundle delays. Some even have bundle branch delays.

    Note: a. AV block is commonly associated with SA block presumably because the right coronary artery frequently supplies both SA and AV nodes.

    b. In the presence of an established atrial fibrillation, the AV junctional conduction abnormalities may manifest by a slow ventricular response despite no digitalis or beta blocker [12].

5. How does the coronary artery supply to the SA node explain why coronary disease should not be the commonest cause of sinus node dysfunction?

   ANS.: The artery to the SA node is from the proximal parts of the right coronary artery in 65 percent of subjects and from the proximal few millimeters of the circumflex artery in the rest. However, right coronary and left circumflex obstructions are usually distal to where the sinus node artery takes off.

   Note: The SA nodal artery at autopsy has usually been normal in subjects with SSS. Sinus node artery narrowing has been reported only in patients who died suddenly and fibromuscular dysplasia of unknown etiology has been seen in these patients [65].

*6. What suggests that pathologic sinus bradycardia (persistent P wave rates of 55 or less, with a poor response to exercise or atropine) is a disease of the entire atrium and not just of the SA node?

   ANS.: a. The P waves of patients with pathologic sinus bradycardia tend to have low voltage (almost imperceptible in lead 1).

   b. The frequent episodes of atrial tachycardia or fibrillation in these patients suggest atrial disease [46].

   c. When the tachycardia-bradycardia syndrome occurs, fibrotic lesions of both SA node and atrial myocardium have been noted [144].

   Note: You can distinguish the slow rates of SA block from the slow rates of a persistent, pathologic sinus bradycardia by knowing that

   a. The P waves of SA block are usually of normal amplitude.

   b. Sympathetic stimulation, e.g., exercise or atropine, often suddenly doubles the rate if SA block is present. (A small dose of atropine, i.e., less than 0.4 mg, may paradoxically cause slowing of SA nodal impulses by a vagotonic effect and therefore cannot always be expected to eliminate an SA block [28].)

*7. What drugs can cause SA block?

   ANS.: a. Lithium [40].

   b. Thioridazine [154].

   Note: Digitalis has usually been thought capable of causing SA block. This idea is controversial in view of some studies showing that in SSS patients digitalis appears to improve resting heart rate and sinus node recovery time [15, 160], whereas others show that digitalis can prolong sinus node conduction time [71, 9A]. The effect on the SA node may depend on the baseline autonomic activity in the patient [36]. This effect is shown by the finding that after vagal blockade with atropine digoxin lengthens sinus cycle length and SA conduction and recovery times [119].

8. List the causes of SSS other than trauma to the SA node during surgery and some drugs.

   ANS.: Although in many studies ischemic heart disease (coronary disease) was commonly found, it was not proved to be the cause unless the patients had either a left bundle branch block or a history of infarction [48]. Coronary angiography does not usually reveal significant coronary disease in patients with SSS [55]. Cardiomyopathies such as amyloidosis are the next commonest associated abnormality, although in one study thyrotoxicosis was the commonest cause [154]. An idiopathic familial form with marked sinus bradycardia has also been found [14].

Note: a. The commonest trauma that causes SSS is that due to surgical correction of atrial septal defects.

b. During the acute stage of infarction, sinus node dysfunction may appear within the first few days, often intermittently for an hour or so. The patient may recover, but several months or years later chronic fibrosis may cause permanent changes [48].

c. With advancing age sick sinus syndrome can be produced because:

(1) Fat disposition around the AV node may partially or completely separate the node from the atrial muscle.

(2) The number of pacemaker cells in the SA node begins to decrease by age 60, and by age 75, only about 10 percent of the numbers in a young adult remain [48A].

*9. Which reflex tests can strongly suggest sinus node dysfunction?

ANS.: a. A Valsalva maneuver. No tachycardia during, or bradycardia after, the maneuver suggests SSS.

b. Carotid sinus stimulation.

Note: The SSS patient is excessively sensitive to vagotonic influences. Therefore, whereas 10 seconds of gentle carotid compression in a normal subject with a sinus bradycardia due to vagal effects increases the P-P interval by about only 0.5 second, carotid compression in a subject with SSS may increase the P-P interval by 3 to 5 seconds [87]. (Longer than 450 msec is probably abnormal for a 'corrected carotid sinus recovery time,' which is defined as the prolonged P-P interval minus the usual P-P interval.)

Note: Sinus node dysfunction is present if after 2 mg of intravenous atropine the atrial rate does not go over 90 because although in SSS the sinus node is very sensitive to vagal effects, it is insensitive to antivagal effects [36].

*10. How can an atrial tachycardia or rapid atrial pacing tell you if a patient has sinus node dysfunction?

ANS.: If the atrium is paced rapidly with an electronic pacemaker and the pacemaker is turned off abruptly, there is a delay in the postpacing P wave, presumably because rapid depolarizations of the SA node either cause a depression of phase 4 of the nodal cells' action potential or produce an exit block. This depression of the SA node by a series of rapid depolarizations is called 'overdrive suppression.' The delay in the post-tachycardia P wave due to overdrive suppression is called the *sinus node recovery time*, which should not be longer than 155 percent of the basic cycle length or more than 1700 msec, unless there is sinus node dysfunction [34, 158].

*11. How can a premature atrial contraction (PAC) tell you if a patient has sinus node dysfunction?

ANS.: The PAC has to penetrate the sinus node barrier (probably through transitional cells) to depolarize the SA node. After the SA node fires again, the impulse must pass out through the sinoatrial barrier to produce the next P wave. The interval between the early (ectopic) P to the next sinus P is usually longer than the regular P-P cycle because some degree of SA block is produced by the transitional cells when the SA node is depolarized prematurely. The conduction into and out of the SA node through the surrounding transitional cells is called the *sinus node conduction time*. If the atrium is depolarized by only one early beat, a prolonged sinus node conduction time also is an indication of sinus node dysfunction. If the patient has a spontaneous PAC, a simple calculation can tell if the sinus node conduction time is abnormal. If you call the ectopic P wave the P prime (P′), you can subtract the regular P-P interval from the longer P′-P interval and thus calculate a difference that represents time going both into and out of the SA node. Divide this difference by 2 to get the average time in and out. If the average delay exceeds 115 msec (105 msec in children), sinus node dysfunction is likely [120, 158].

12. What is the cause of a persistent sinus bradycardia in patients over age 60?
ANS.: Increased vagal tone. This situation is suggested by the finding that elderly patients with bradycardia have a much greater heart rate response to atropine than do matched controls. Their normal heart rate and blood pressure response to a Valsalva maneuver shows that they have no autonomic deficit [5].

AV BLOCK

AV Nodal Conduction Properties

1. By about how much is AV nodal conduction slower than atrial conduction?
ANS.: By about one-fifth (200 versus 1,000 mm per second).
2. Into how many parts has the AV node been divided by action potential characteristics? What are these areas called?
ANS.: Into three parts.
a. Upper nodal area or atrionodal region, termed the *AN region.*
b. Mid-nodal region, termed the *N region.*
c. Lower node region, termed the *NH region* (node-His region).
3. How does the action potential of the N region differ from that of the AN and NH regions?
ANS.: The N region has less resting potential, a slower rate of rise in phase 0, and a lower peak than do the AN and NH regions.

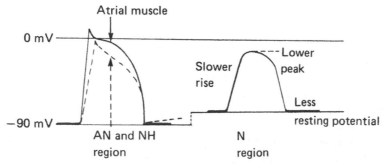

Note that the action potential of the N region is characteristic of a curve produced by calcium flux. (See the illustration for question 5.)

Note: a. The NH region action potentials look much like those in the AN regions in that slight phase 4 depolarization is seen; i.e., some automaticity is apparent in this lower nodal area where it makes its transition into the bundle of His fibers.

b. The major functions of the AV node should be considered to reside in the area called the compact node, or N region, where the major slowing of impulses occurs. Therefore by the 'AV node' we really mean 'N region.'

4. What is meant by decremental conduction in the AV node?

ANS.: As an action potential is being propagated along the AV transmission system, it may gradually become a less and less effective stimulus in the conduction system until complete AV block occurs.

*5. How does the ionic flux that causes the slow response differ from the flux that causes the fast response seen in the usual Purkinje fiber?

ANS.: The fast-channel response is due to a rapid influx of sodium into the cell and efflux of potassium during phase 0. Rapid repolarization begins at phase 1. Phase 2, or the plateau phase (corresponding to the S-T segment of the ECG), and phase 3 are dominated by an influx of calcium via a slow-channel pathway.

Note: a. The sodium channel is not used in the sinus or AV nodes, which are instead depolarized by the inward calcium current.

b. The action potential of the usual Purkinje fiber is best considered a summation of fast and slow channels due to both sodium and calcium influx.

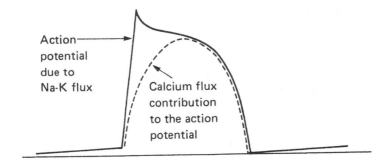

6. What properties of the N region enable it to be the major cause of slowing of the impulse through the AV node? Why?

ANS.: The cells in the AV node N region have

a. A slow rate of rise in phase 0.

b. A decrease in millivolts of resting potential resulting in a lower amplitude of total deflection.

Note: a. The lower the rate of rise in phase 0 and the lower the amplitude of the action potential, the poorer is the propagation of an impulse.

b. The earlier the next action potential occurs during phase 4, the slower is its rate of rise during phase 0 and the lower is the amplitude of that early action potential. This situation is the reverse of what happens in atrial, His, or ventricular tissue, where the earlier in phase 4 that another excitation occurs, the steeper and higher is the next phase 0.

*7. What property of the N region would tend to decrease the great number of impulses getting through in atrial fibrillation (400 ± 50 impulses per second) by not allowing the weak impulses to propagate?

ANS.: It takes a greater stimulus to excite the N region cells than to excite any other cardiac cells.

*8. What property of the N region would slow impulse propagation with vagal stimulation?

ANS.: Acetylcholine decreases both the rate of rise and the height of phase 0 *only in the N region*. In atrial muscle it does the opposite (by changing potassium permeability).

*9. What is meant by first-degree, second-degree, and third-degree AV block?

ANS.: First-degree AV block means a longer-than-normal P-R interval. Second-degree block means an occasional dropped QRS; i.e., occasionally the P wave does not conduct through the AV node. Third-degree block means complete AV block; i.e., the AV node and bundle branches do not allow any supraventricular impulses to pass through them. The term *complete AV block* is preferred.

Note: AV block may be only anterograde, only retrograde, or a different degree of each.

First-Degree AV Block

1. What conduction pathways are represented by the P-R interval; i.e., where in the conduction system can delays prolong the P-R interval?

ANS.: The P-R interval depends on conduction through the atrium, the AV node, the bundle of His, and the bundle branches. Therefore slow conduction through any of these tissues can prolong the P-R interval.

Note: The P-R interval measures the total duration of preventricular depolarization, i.e., from the beginning of the P wave to the beginning of the QRS. The time for intraatrial transmission from the SA node to the AV node is usually about 40 msec (0.04 sec). The sinus impulse thus reaches the AV node about the time that the peak of the P wave is recorded. Therefore during at least the last half of the P wave, while the left atrium is being depolarized, conduction through the AV node is occurring. The P-R segment (between the end of the P and the beginning of the QRS) thus consists of conduction through the last part of the AV node and then conduction through the bundle of His and bundle branches.

2. How does the P-R interval vary with fast heart rates due to (a) emotion or exercise? (b) atrial pacing?

ANS.: a. The P-R interval shortens slightly with fast rates due to emotion or exercise.

b. Atrial pacing at faster and faster rates produces a progressively longer P-R interval because of the properties of the N region described in the previous section; i.e., the earlier an impulse reaches the N cells, the more it is delayed. Sympathetic stimulation, which is the usual cause of fast rates with emotion or exercise, accelerates AV nodal conduction and counterbalances the slowing effect of the short cycles on the N region [80].

3. How does the P-R interval vary with age?

ANS.: It lengthens with age until about puberty, when it stabilizes [93]. By puberty the upper normal is 180 msec (0.18 sec) [2]. Over the next 10 years (the third decade) it increases to 200 msec (0.2 sec) and changes very little after that.

Note: The lengthening of the P-R interval with age in children has been shown to be due to prolongation of conduction in the atrium, bundle of His, and bundle branches, but not in the AV node; i.e., as the heart grows, it takes longer to traverse the increasing length of the atrium, bundle of His, and bundle branches [121].

4. How can you detect a first-degree AV block without referring to tables for age and heart rate?

ANS.: The upper limit of normal P-R interval for adults with average heart rates is 200 msec (0.20 sec), i.e., one large division on ECG paper. Therefore if the heart rate is rapid, 200 msec would be a first-degree AV block. Also, if the patient is very young, a 200-msec P-R interval is probably a first-degree AV block.

Note: a. Women tend to have slightly shorter P-R intervals than do men [136].

b. Over age 60, and with normal heart rates, a P-R of 220 msec (0.22 sec) or more is significantly correlated with ischemic heart disease or with T abnormalities [115].

c. The longest P-R that I have seen was 680 msec (0.68 sec).

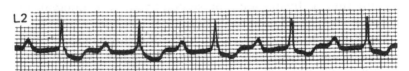

First-degree AV block. The P-R interval is 360 msec (0.36 msec).

Note: a. About 2 percent of the population have first-degree AV block, i.e., P-R intervals of 220 msec or longer. If it is the only abnormality in the young, it probably has no known clinical significance and is usually transient [24]. In the elderly there is a significant correlation with ischemic heart disease [115].

b. A sinus tachycardia with a prolonged P-R interval should make you suspect hyperthyroidism. First-degree AV block has been reported to occur in 2 to 3 percent of hyperthyroid patients. Even second-degree AV block and complete AV block have been reported [45].

*5. Why does a long P-R interval in a child with a fever suggest a diagnosis of rheumatic fever?

ANS.: A long P-R interval is more common in children with the carditis of acute rheumatic fever than with any other of the major features of the disease or with any other kind of streptococcal infection.

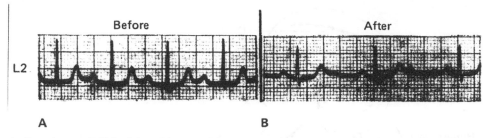

A. First-degree AV block in a 21-year-old woman with migratory polyarthritis, fever, and mitral regurgitation due to acute rheumatic fever. The P-R interval is prolonged to 240 msec (0.24 sec). B. Four days after cortisone was begun. The fever and joint pains had disappeared, and the P-R interval is now normal.

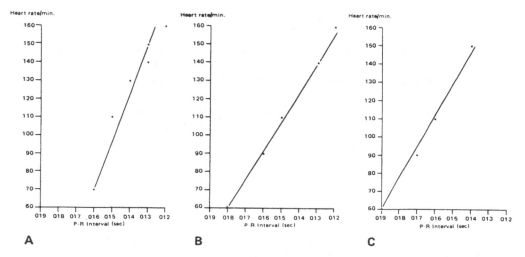

Maximum normal P-R interval according to heart rate and age. A. At 3 to 5 years. B. At 6 to 11 years. C. At 12 to 15 years. (Modified from M. Clark and J. D. Keith, Br. Heart J. 34:472, 1972.)

6. When can a long P-R interval occur in the presence of perfectly normal conduction through the AV node?

ANS.: a. When partial trifascicular block is present, with two fascicles completely blocked and one incompletely blocked, i.e., in incomplete trifascicular block (see ECG 47, p. 228).

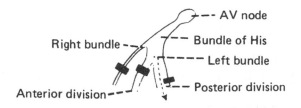

*b. Bundle of His recordings have even shown that prolonged intraatrial conduction can cause a long P-R interval. There are three internodal pathways between the SA and AV nodes. Obstruction of any of these specialized conduction pathways may result in a prolonged P-R interval.

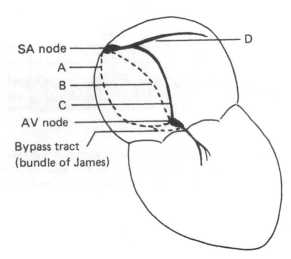

A is the posterior internodal tract, or Thorel's pathway. (It is really posterolateral.) B is the middle internodal tract and C the anterior internodal tract. D is the interatrial tract, or Bachmann's bundle, actually a branch of the anterior tract.

Note: a. Small, discrete lesions in the specialized interatrial tracts can change the direction and duration of P waves. The anterior internodal tract is the most important in causing prolonged atrial conduction if it is damaged [149].

b. The prolonged P-R interval often seen in patients with tricuspid stenosis may be due to compression of either the internodal tracts, the AV node, or the bundle of His by the high pressure in the right atrium.

7. Which drugs can prolong the P-R interval? Where is the prolongation produced?

ANS.: a. Digitalis by prolonging AV nodal conduction.

Note: It is usually impossible to use a prolonged P-R interval as a sign of digitalis effect because with therapeutic doses the effect is entirely vagotonic and the prolongation is rarely by more than 80 msec (0.08 sec) in a subject with a normal AV node [15].

*b. Tricyclic antidepressants, by prolonging both AV nodal conduction and His-bundle branch conduction [129, 148].

Note: Doxepin does not cause delayed conduction.

*c. Clonidine, probably only if with digitalis [68].

*8. Which coronary artery occlusion is likely to produce first-degree AV block due to (a) AV node damage? (b) partial trifascicular block?

ANS.: a. A right coronary occlusion can damage the AV node because this artery supplies the AV node in 90 percent of subjects. In 10 percent of subjects the circumflex artery supplies the posterior descending artery and the AV node.

b. An anterior descending occlusion can cause partial trifascicular block because this artery supplies all three fascicles, to at least some degree [124].

Note: Advanced coronary heart disease only rarely gives rise to a prolonged P-R interval. Surprisingly, the P-R usually shortens with increasingly severe angiographically proved coronary disease [47].

*9. What is the genetic significance of a patient with a secundum atrial septal defect having a first-degree AV block?

ANS.: It usually means that an autosomal dominant hereditary factor is involved, so that there is a 50 percent risk of subsequent siblings or of offspring being affected [9, 66, 114].

   Note: a. A syndrome of secundum ASD, left axis deviation, AV block, and sudden death has been found as a non-sexed-linked autosomal dominant [43].

   b. Most atrial septal defects (ASDs) with large shunts actually result in a slightly longer P-R interval than normal, probably because of the greater distance that the impulse has to travel from SA to AV node through the enlarged right atrium [4].

   c. A first-degree AV block is also common in patients with a common atrium. It should be further suspected if an ASD is clinically apparent and there is a left axis deviation of both the QRS and the P [106]. However, a common atrium is probably a kind of endocardial cushion defect, and in one study it was found that all endocardial cushion defects had longer internodal conduction than did secundum defects [150].

Laddergram

What is a laddergram?

ANS.: It is a method of diagramming impulse formation and conduction from the SA node through the atrium, AV node, and ventricle.

   Note: A laddergram is sometimes called a 'Lewis diagram' or 'AV diagram.'

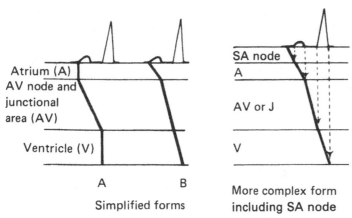

Left. For laddergram A, vertical lines are used for all conduction except through the junctional area. This configuration is the Lewis diagram, the first type of laddergram used. The modern laddergram uses slanted lines, as B, to represent duration through each part of the conduction system. It is more representative of actual events and is used in this book. *Right.* This laddergram is the same as B but adds a bar for the SA node.

Second-Degree AV Block

What is meant by second-degree AV block?

ANS.: The occasional failure of the P wave to get through the AV node.

Type 1

1. What is the commonest type of second-degree AV block?

    ANS.: One in which the P-R gradually lengthens in consecutive cycles until there is a dropped beat; i.e., the P-R becomes longer and longer until for one beat no AV conduction occurs at all.

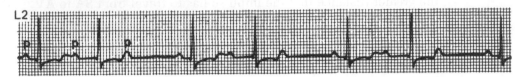

The peaked T wave after every second QRS is due to a superimposed P wave. Because this P did not conduct through the AV node to produce a QRS, it resulted in a dropped beat.

> **Note:* The first P-R interval after any pause may be slightly shorter than the otherwise constant P-R intervals, probably as the result either of improved AV nodal conduction following the rest period afforded by the block or of a junctional escape beat allowed by the long pause. (See p. 492 for discussion of escape beats.)

2. What are the various terms for the P-R pattern of normal, long, longer, and dropped beats?

    ANS.: *Wenckebach phenomenon, Wenckebach periods, type 1 second-degree AV block, Mobitz type 1 AV block.* Another set of terms is based on the ratio of P waves to QRS complexes. Because there must always be one more P wave than there are QRS complexes in each Wenckebach period, the ratio of P waves to QRS complexes is used, so that four P waves to three QRS complexes would be a 4:3 Wenckebach, as shown in the following.

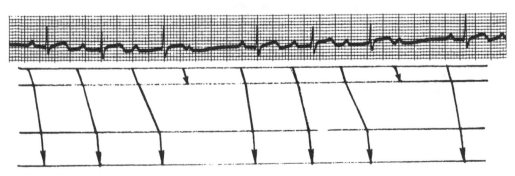

Trigeminy (groups of three) due to 4:3 Wenckebach periods.

*3. What other than 'fatigue' of the AV node could account for type 1 second-degree AV block?

    ANS.: If the P waves arrive at the AV node earlier and earlier in the refractory period of the AV node, the P-R is longer and longer. This progressively early P is initiated by a lengthening of the second P-R over the first.

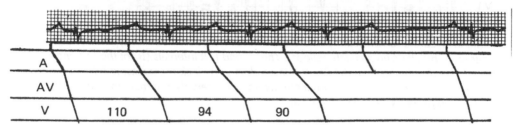

P1   P2   P3

↑   ↑
AV node   AV node first
finally   reached here
traversed here   by P3
after P2

Note that the first long P-R, which is at P2, causes the next P wave, P3, to come closer to the time that the AV node has been finally traversed by P2. Therefore P3 is earlier in the refractory period of the AV node than is P2.

4. What happens to the R-R interval when the P-R interval successively lengthens in type 1 second-degree AV block?

ANS.: The R-R interval successively shortens. The reason is difficult to comprehend but depends on the fact that the P-R lengthens by decreasing increments, e.g.,

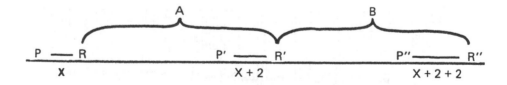

A

AV

V   110   94   90

Wenckebach period. The P-P intervals must be kept constant for a gradually lengthening P-R interval to cause gradual shortening of the R-R interval. Therefore the latter is rarely seen in ECGs because sinus arrhythmias usually vary the P-P intervals too much.

Note: For the mathematically inclined who wish to understand how an R-R can shorten while a P-R lengthens, the following may help.

A   B

P — R   P′ —— R′   P″——— R″

X   X + 2   X + 2 + 2

Let X be the first P-R interval. Let 2 be the increment, and let there be no decreasing increment. To keep the R′-R″ interval B the *same* as the R-R interval A, the P″-R″ must increase the same amount as did the P′-R′; i.e., it must have a P″-R″ interval of X + 2 + 2. However, if the P″-R″ increment is less than the P′-R′ increment, the R′-R″ distance shortens.

5. If P waves are invisible, how can a Wenckebach period be recognized?

ANS.: The pattern of R-R sequence indicates the presence of a Wenckebach period. You usually see a gradually decreasing R-R interval followed by a pause that is less than twice the shortest R-R. (The shortest R-R is usually the R-R before the pause.)

*6. When is the pattern of gradually decreasing R-R intervals not seen in type 1 second-degree AV block?
    ANS.: a. When sinus arrhythmia is present.
          b. When the last cycle of the period has such a long P-R that the impulse can just barely traverse the AV node, thus making the last P-R interval of the period the same or even longer than the preceding one.
          c. When there is nonhomogeneous conduction through the AV node and bundle of His.
          d. When, for unknown reasons, in the middle or end of a Wenckebach period, the P-R occasionally does not lengthen by decreasing increments.
         Note: The type 1 second-degree AV block R-R sequence is most easily seen in atrial tachycardia or flutter because sinus arrhythmias are absent, and the P-P intervals or the flutter wave intervals are usually perfectly constant, thus allowing minor changes in R-R distances to be measured more accurately.

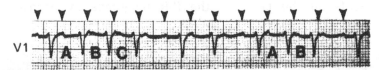

Atrial tachycardia (arrowheads point to P waves) at a rate of 165, with type 1 second-degree AV block (Wenckebach periods). The second R-R intervals (B) of the first and last groups are shorter than the first R-R interval (A). The lack of increasing P-R interval in cycle C is not unusual. It is not uncommon for P-R intervals to remain the same after one or two progressively longer intervals.

*7. How can a sinus Wenckebach, i.e., a type 1 second-degree SA block in the SA node, be recognized?
    ANS.: Here the P waves take the place of the R waves in the Wenckebach sequence. That is, you see a gradually shortening P-P interval until a pause occurs that is less than twice the last or shortest P-P interval. Because there is no AV block, the R-R intervals naturally also have this pattern.

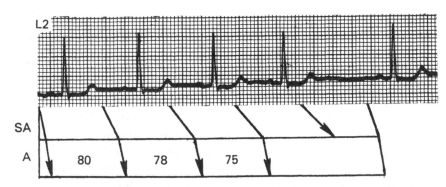

Sinus Wenckebach. The P-R intervals are equal. Therefore the pattern of R-R intervals is not due to type 1 second-degree block at the AV node. The SA node firing in the laddergram is only postulated to fit the P wave sequence.

8. Which cardiac abnormalities may be suggested by a type 1 second-degree AV block?
   ANS.: a. Myocarditis.
   b. Digitalis excess.
   c. A precursor of complete AV block in the setting of acute infarction.
   Note: Some healthy young adults with excessive vagal tone can show type 1 second-degree AV block [79]. It is especially common in highly trained endurance athletes [147].
9. What is the usual anatomic site of type 1 second-degree AV block?
   ANS.: The AV node.
   *Note: Type 1 second-degree AV block, however, occasionally occurs in the bundle of His or bundle branches. This pattern has been shown not only by bundle of His recordings but also by the finding of progressively increasing bundle branch or even divisional blocks with Wenckebach periods [89, 126]. See the following ECGs.

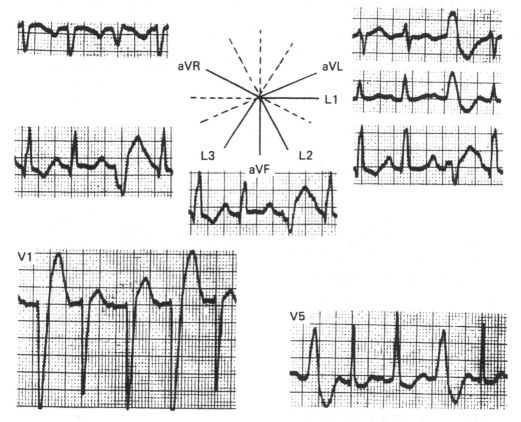

This ECG is from a 45-year-old man with ischemic heart disease. The repeat pattern of gradually increasing QRS width over three beats indicates a type 1 second-degree block in the left bundle. Note that with the incomplete left bundle branch block (third complex in V5) the q wave disappears. The QRS axis changes from about 70° to 60° with the incomplete block and then to about − 30° when the block is complete.

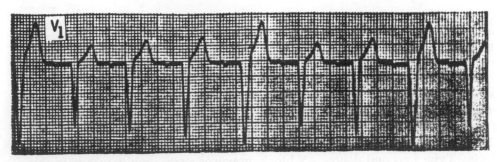

A 60-year-old man had aortic stenosis and regurgitation, first-degree A-V block, and intermittent LBBB. The two patterns of gradually increasing degrees of LBBB are due to a 4:3 Wenckebach period followed by a 3:2 Wenckebach period in the left bundle. There was no divisional block in his 12-lead ECG, only a marked left ventricular hypertrophy (LVH) strain pattern and LVH by index of Sokolow.

*10. What is meant by the 'Wedensky effect' and 'Wedensky facilitation'? What have they been used to explain?

ANS.: The Wedensky effect is the ability of a subthreshold stimulus to reach threshold and induce a response if it is preceded by a suitably strong stimulus. Wedensky facilitation is the enhanced conductivity beyond a blocked zone. These phenomena have been used to explain a bundle branch block that appears only in the first cycle of Wenckebach periods [50]. The Wedensky effect is used to explain the fact that in some patients with artificial pacemakers subthreshold responses can attain threshold if they fall after a strong stimulus.

Note: The existence of a Wedensky effect has not yet been proved in humans [44].

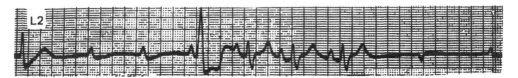

Wedensky facilitation in a 50-year-old man with frequent syncopal attacks. He has intermittent SA and AV block. The P waves do not get through the AV node until the impulse from a ventricular escape beat reaches the area of the AV block retrogradely. This condition presumably lowers the threshold beyond the block and allows conduction of anterograde impulses. After a few sinus beats, SA block occurs, and an atrial escape beat (negative P) is seen.

Type 2

1. What is type 2 second-degree AV block?

ANS.: A sudden AV block producing a sudden absence of the QRS despite no preceding successive P-R lengthening.

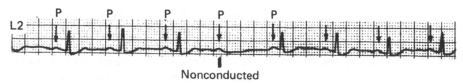

Type 2 second-degree AV block in a 60-year-old man with coronary disease.

2. What name other than Wenckebach is often used to describe type 1 and type 2 block?
   ANS.: Mobitz.
3. Did Wenckebach describe both types of AV block?
   ANS.: Yes [131A].
4. If Wenckebach described both types, why do we use Mobitz's name?
   ANS.: Wenckebach described them but not as types 1 and 2. This addition was by Mobitz [103] 25 years after Wenckebach's description. Wenckebach's name is given only to type 1, but Mobitz's is given to either type 1 or type 2. You can avoid these eponyms altogether by simply saying 'type 1' or 'type 2' second-degree AV block.
5. Where is the anatomic location of the block in type 2 second-degree AV block?
   ANS.: Usually in the bundle of His or in the bundle branches.
   Note: Type 2 second-degree AV block has occasionally been found in the AV node [123]. When a type 2 second-degree AV block is seen with narrow QRS complexes, as in the preceding ECG strip, the block may well be in the AV node. The block, however, may be in the bundle of His [25, 33]. If the block is in the AV node, exercise or atropine decreases it because sympathetic stimulation accelerates AV nodal conduction. If the block is in the bundle of His, exercise or atropine increases it because early impulses to the bundle of His allow less time to recover from its refractory period.
   Note: Type 1 second-degree AV block with bundle branch block, although uncommon, may be in the His-Purkinje system in about 65 percent of cases and has the same poor prognosis as a type 2 block [6A].

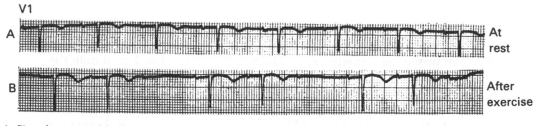

A. First-degree AV block in a 75-year-old woman with congestive failure due to a cardiomyopathy. B. Effect of exercise, producing a second-degree block, characteristic of an intra-His block.

*6. What is meant by a pseudo AV block?
   ANS.: A premature His depolarization that is blocked both ways can partially penetrate the AV node and cause a block at the AV node [16]. This block, of course, can be shown only by His bundle recordings.
7. What is the clinical significance of type 1 and type 2 second-degree AV block?
   ANS.: Type 1, being usually at the AV node, is often due to excess vagotonia. Type 2, being usually below the node, is more likely to mean serious disease in

the bundle of His or bundle branches; i.e., it suggests bilateral bundle branch block and therefore is likely to portend complete AV block [72]. If the QRS is narrow, however, then even with type 2 the prognosis for the development of complete AV block may be benign because the block may be in the AV node and may even be vagotonically induced, as with digitalis [123].

Note: a. Complete AV block developed in almost one-half of eight children and adolescents with type 1 second-degree AV block when they were followed for an average of 11 years. Therefore type 1 second-degree AV block does not always represent just an excessive vagotonic effect on the AV node [159].

b. A type 3 second-degree AV block has been described [18] in which the P-R intervals lengthen and shorten haphazardly, and it is not necessarily the longest P-R interval that is followed by the blocked impulse.

8. What commonly occurs with a type 2 second-degree AV block that confirms that it often means serious disease of the bundle of His or bundle branches?

ANS.: Type 2 second-degree AV block commonly occurs with either concomitant right or left bundle branch block [39].

Note: Type 2 AV block with a normal QRS width may be in the bundle of His or it is really a type 1 block with increments too small to be readily apparent [123]. If the P-R interval is suddenly shorter after the pause it has been called 'pseudo-Mobitz 2' type and is associated with different clinical characteristics than the classic Mobitz 2 in which the P-R does not shorten after the pause [71A].

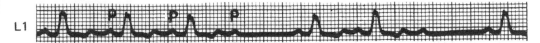

L1

Type 2 second-degree AV block with left bundle branch block. A sudden nonconducted P wave with a wide QRS is more likely to be a type 2 second-degree AV block than if the QRS is narrow. It is because no QRS is produced if a bundle branch block is present and the opposite bundle is intermittently blocked. This pattern, then, represents intermittent bilateral bundle branch block.

9. Is 2:1 AV block type 1 or type 2?

ANS.: It may be a transient phase in either type.

Note: One way to tell whether a 2:1 block is type 1 or type 2 is to note the effect of slowing of the sinus rate, as with very gentle carotid massage. A 1:1 response often develops in the patient with type 2 block, and the rate suddenly doubles [96]. Another maneuver is to exercise the patient (straight leg raising). With exercise a type 1 block decreases so that the QRS rate may suddenly double. A type 2 block may become third-degree.

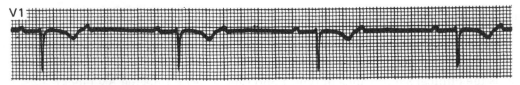

V1

This patient has 2:1 AV block; i.e., every other P wave is blocked. The absence of bundle branch block favors type 1 rather than type 2 second-degree AV block.

Complete AV Block

What is another term for complete AV block? What are the disadvantages to this other term?

ANS.: *Heart block.* There are four disadvantages to this term:

a. SA blocks, bundle branch blocks, and divisional blocks are also 'heart blocks.'

b. The term *heart block* is a very frightening term to the layman.

c. Many physicians use *AV block* for first-degree and second-degree blocks but *heart block* for third-degree block. This terminology implies that there is a difference between third-degree AV block and complete heart block.

d. Finally, when students are learning about AV block for the first time, they know immediately where the block is. If you say 'heart block,' you must teach the site as an additional fact.

Pacemaker Site and Characteristics

1. Where are the pacemakers in complete AV block? What are their usual rates?

ANS.: Anywhere in the conduction system from the bundle of His area (rates approximate 40 to 60) to the most distal Purkinje fibers of the ventricles (rates approximate 20 to 40) [37].

Note: It has been shown in the canine heart that junctional pacemakers can fire at about two-thirds the rate of the sinus pacemaker [145].

2. What are the proximal and distal pacemakers beyond the AV node called?

ANS.: The proximal ones around the bundle of His area are called 'junctional,' or 'bundle of His' pacemakers. The more distal Purkinje pacemakers are called 'idioventricular.'

Note: At one time, when an ECG showed a rhythm with a narrow QRS and a retrograde P wave before, inside, or after each QRS, the pacemaker was called 'nodal.' Bundle of His recordings have shown that pacemakers producing a P inside or after a QRS are in the bundle of His [27]. A retrograde P before a QRS may be from a low atrial focus.

3. How does the ECG showing a bundle of His area pacemaker differ from that of a pacemaker more distal in the ventricle?

ANS.: A bundle of His pacemaker produces an ECG that, compared with that of a more distal pacemaker, usually has

a. A faster intrinsic rate.

b. A narrower QRS.

c. A greater ability to show an increased rate with exercise and catecholamine stimulation [37].

Note: In congenital complete AV block, the interruption may be between the atrium and the AV node, between the AV node and the bundle of His [56] or due to absence of an AV node [78]. Therefore the pacemaker is almost always in the bundle of His and has all the characteristics just listed. Most patients with congenital complete AV block and no other congenital heart disease do well without a pacemaker until they become pregnant or reach the fifth decade. Syncopal attacks during pregnancy may require a temporary pacemaker [95].

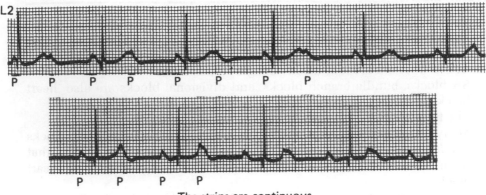

The strips are continuous

Congenital complete AV block in a 4-year-old child. The atrial rate is 125, and the ventricular rate is 55. The narrow QRS and the relatively fast rate tell you that the pacemaker is above the bifurcation of the bundle of His; i.e., it is a junctional pacemaker, probably in the bundle of His.

*4. List the congenital anomalies that are often associated with AV block of some degree.

Note: This material is not for committal to memory but for reference. The common anomalies that should be remembered are in italics.

ANS.: a. Abnormalities of the right atrium (which contains the AV node) ASDs, *usually primum,* but occasionally even secundum [118].

  b. Abnormalities of the aortic root or conal tissue (the bundle branches bifurcate between the right and posterior aortic cusps):

   (1) *Transposition, complete or corrected.* (About 40 percent of all patients with congenital complete AV block have congenitally corrected transposition [62].)

   (2) Hypoplasia of the aortic tract.

  c. Abnormalities of the tricuspid valve (a structure close to the AV node). Tricuspid stenosis atresia or isolated tricuspid regurgitation.

  d. Abnormalities of the membranous ventricular septum (just below which travels the bundle of His with its branches):

   Ventricular septal defects (VSDs), alone or with tetralogy of Fallot (especially after surgical repair), or with aneurysm of the membranous septum.

*5. Can the width of a QRS signify how distal in the Purkinje system the idioventricular focus is in complete AV block? Why?

ANS.: Most of the time yes, because the more distal the focus, the more time it should take for the impulse to reach the opposite branches of the conduction system. If, however, there were a bundle branch block before the AV block developed, even if the pacemaker were in the junctional area the QRS would be wide.

  Note: If the rate of an idioventricular focus is under 40, it tells you that the pacemaker is probably distal to the bundle of His, but how far distal it is cannot be determined by rate alone.

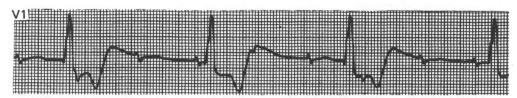

Complete AV block. The atrial rate is about 80; the ventricular rate is 35. Because the P-R interval is varying but the R-R intervals are regular, the P waves are not connected to the QRSs. Therefore it is complete AV block. The wide QRS complexes and slow rate together imply a distal Purkinje idioventricular pacemaker.

> **Note:* When digitalis excess causes complete AV block, the pacemaker is in the bundle of His.

*6. What can cause an idioventricular pacemaker to be slightly irregular with complete AV block?

ANS.: a. There may be varying exit blocks from any pacemaker in the heart.

b. More than one idioventricular pacemaker may be present, with a shift from focus to focus.

> *Note:* a. When two idioventricular pacemakers are vying for control, fusion beats may be seen in complete AV block. This situation is rare [75].
>
> b. A late PVC, i.e., after the T wave, usually delays the postextrasystolic QRS to make a cycle longer than the basic one. An early PVC (on or near the downstroke of the T) is usually followed by an early QRS making the postextrasystolic cycle shorter than the basic one [69].

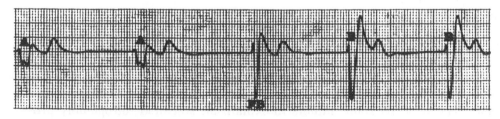

This ECG is from a 75-year-old woman with Stokes-Adams attacks. There are two idioventricular pacemakers. Pacemaker A has a rate of 35, and pacemaker B has a rate of 45. There is a fusion beat (FB) between complexes A and B.

7. How can you tell whether the idioventricular pacemaker is in the right ventricle (RV) or left ventricle (LV)?

ANS.: If it is in the LV, the QRS resembles right bundle branch block (RBBB). If it is in the RV, the QRS looks like left bundle branch block (LBBB). It is because in order to get to the opposite ventricle the conduction must go through retrograde pathways just as if the bundle branch on the opposite side were blocked.

*8. Where in the RV is the idioventricular pacemaker if there is an LBBB with (a) left axis deviation? (b) a normal axis? (c) right axis deviation?

ANS.: Picture the right side of the septum as if it were clear plastic, with the posterior division of the left bundle seen supplying the posterior apex and the anterior division seen supplying the upper anterior septum and anterior apex [8].

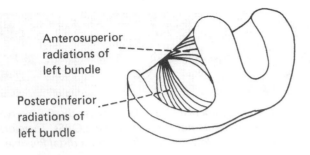

Anterosuperior radiations of left bundle

Posteroinferior radiations of left bundle

  a. If the impulse begins at the posterior apex, the posterior branch is reached first, and a left axis deviation is produced. It is an imitation of anterior divisional block.

  b. If the impulse begins in the middle of the septum, both branches are reached at the same time and a normal axis results.

  c. If the impulse begins in the outflow tract of the RV, the anterior branch is reached first, and a right axis deviation is produced. It is an imitation of posterior divisional block.

  Note: It is of interest to know the site of a ventricular pacemaker because today, with the implantation of artificial pacemakers, it can sometimes be useful to know where the pacemaker has been implanted or if it has shifted. There is also evidence that although frequent right ventricular ectopic beats are as serious as those from the LV, ectopic beats in a normal heart usually arise from the RV [125].

Atria in Complete AV Block

1. What are the atria doing during the usual complete AV block?

  ANS.: As in any AV dissociation, they may be doing anything.

*2. Why does complete AV block sometimes produce retrograde P waves?

  ANS.: One theory is that a P wave occurring after a QRS in complete AV block is really not due to retrograde conduction but merely to mechanical stimulation of an atrial pacemaker by the ventricle [83]. This questionable theory has been used by some authors to explain all so-called retrogradely produced P waves.

  Note: With bundle of His recordings and rapid ventricular pacing, retrograde conduction into or through the AV node can be found in more than 50 percent of subjects with complete anterograde AV block [67].

*3. What is meant by 'ventriculophasic' arrhythmia?

  ANS.: In complete AV block, the P waves, even though independent, are often seen to come closer together when there is a QRS between them. This pattern is called 'ventriculophasic arrhythmia' and is thought to be due to changes in coronary flow to the SA node caused by ventricular contraction. It suggests that ventricular contraction either shortens the phase 4 stage of the SA node action potentials or decreases the conduction time from the SA node to the atria. (See rhythm strips on pp. 484 and 486.)

  Note: Rarely, the P-P interval around a QRS is actually more prolonged than the other P-P intervals; i.e., it produces a negative chronotropic effect [37]. The probable cause is reflex vagal slowing after stimulation of the arterial pressor receptors by the pulse wave.

Complete AV Block with Acute Myocardial Infarction

1. What is the evidence that coronary disease is a relatively rare cause of chronic complete AV block?

ANS.: a. When due to posterior infarction, the AV block is almost always transient. When it is due to anterior infarction, the patient usually dies.

b. At necropsy, no significant coronary disease is usually found, and muscle adjacent to the damaged bundle branches is essentially intact [30].

Note: a. In complete AV block due to a posterior or inferior infarct, a proximal or His bundle pacemaker is expected because a posterior or inferior infarct is caused by a right coronary or circumflex occlusion, and these arteries supply the AV node but not much of the conduction tissue beyond the AV node.

b. In AV block due to an anterior infarction, the QRS complexes are usually wide because this block is usually due to a bilateral bundle branch block, and there must be a distal Purkinje pacemaker [124].

c. *Complete* or even *chronic complete* applied to AV block does not necessarily mean permanent block. Intermittent AV conduction is not uncommon even after years of AV block [127].

*2. In what type of infarction is complete AV block likely to be preceded by various degrees of AV block and then have narrow QRS complexes during the complete block? Why?

ANS.: In acute posterior or inferior myocardial infarction, which is usually caused by a right coronary occlusion [111]. The right coronary artery gives rise to the artery to the AV node in 90 percent of subjects. If the AV node is damaged, a His pacemaker usually takes over, and so the QRS is likely to be narrow.

Note: a. About one-half of the patients in whom second-degree AV block develops secondary to infarction go on to complete AV block. Complete AV block due to posterior myocardial infarction rarely lasts longer than a week [110].

b. The AV node is usually supplied by a branch of the right coronary artery, the ramus septi fibrosi, which is given off at the crux of the heart. (The crux is the point where the posterior intraventricular groove, or sulcus, meets the AV sulcus.) The ramus septi fibrosi penetrates the posterior portion of the AV node but leaves only a tiny branch to supply the distal AV node as well as the bundle of His. Anastomoses to this small branch from the anterior descending septal arteries are so poor that if the right coronary artery is suddenly blocked the perfusion to the AV node may be preserved only by anastomoses from the anterior descending artery. The distal end of the AV node and the bundle of His (which is not more than 2 mm long) only occasionally suffers enough hypoxia from a right coronary occlusion to produce a permanent AV block [146].

c. A common precursor of complete AV block in anterior myocardial infarction is the sudden appearance of RBBB. There is usually no progression from first-degree and second-degree to complete AV block, as in posterior infarction [142]. Complete AV block can occur within minutes after RBBB in anterior infarcts. Characteristic of the ECG picture of the RBBB that is followed by complete AV block within 24 hours is the presence of a Q in V1, because an anteroseptal infarction is usually present as the cause of RBBB [142].

    d. In about 30 to 50 percent of patients with acute infarction who have RBBB and anterior divisional block, complete AV block will develop [122]. In patients with *chronic* RBBB and anterior divisional block, complete AV block can be expected to develop in only about 10 percent [73].

3. If chronic complete AV block is not caused by infarction, what are the five most likely causes besides congenital maldevelopments?

    ANS.: a. Lev's disease (fibrous degeneration of the left side of the cardiac skeleton). This process is accelerated by hypertension [77]. It also refers to invasion of the conduction system from without by calcium spreading from the mitral ring or the aortic valve.

       b. Lenegre's disease (fibrosis of the proximal conduction tissue, i.e., bundle of His and bundle branches).

       c. Cardiomyopathies or myocarditis [58].

       d. Infiltrates such as sarcoid, amyloid, metastatic tumors, hemochromatosis, transfusion siderosis [13], or leukemic cells [86]. (Hemochromatosis has presented as complete AV block [140].)

       e. Inflammatory involvement of the bundle of His, as in collagen disease, ankylosing spondylitis [81, 136, 156], or uropolyarthritis [11].

    Note: a. Among rare causes of AV block are both thyrotoxicosis and myxedema (reversible with thyroxine) [45, 74, 139]. Chest trauma has also caused complete AV block [137].

       b. About half the patients with complete chronic AV block have Lenegre's or Lev's disease [17, 58].

       c. Progressive AV block to complete AV block may occur in families. It may be a form of Lenegre's disease [85, 128].

       d. In one study, two-thirds of children with congenital complete AV block were born to mothers with evidence of connective tissue disease, primarily disseminated lupus erythematosus [94].

Supernormal Conduction

1. What is meant by the term *supernormal conduction?*

    ANS.: It is the ability of conduction tissue to allow unexpectedly the passage of an impulse through the AV node or bundle branches that was blocked under usual conditions. Conduction is not actually supernormal but only temporarily improved in an area of depressed conduction.

    Note: a. Supernormal conduction occurs from 0 to 650 msec (0.65 sec) after the end of the T wave. It may coincide with the U wave of the ECG.

Supernormal
period of
conductivity

Supernormal
period of
excitability

b. The supernormal phase of conductivity must be distinguished from the supernormal phase of excitability. The latter enhances the generation of an impulse to permit an early or unexpected QRS to be generated. The supernormal phase of excitability occurs at the end of the downslope of the T wave.

2. When is supernormal conduction usually used to account for unexpected AV conduction?

ANS.: In otherwise complete AV block a P wave that occurs in the critical period of the junctional area (supernormal period) may be conducted to the ventricles. Any P wave that occurs earlier or later is blocked.

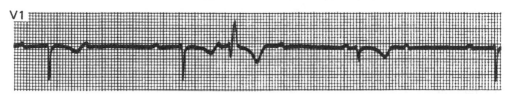

V1

This ECG is from the same patient with the arrhythmia described in question 9, p. 484. The RBBB QRS is not a PVC. We recorded from this 60-year-old woman many dozens of such early RBBB beats, and they followed all the P waves that came earliest on the previous T waves. Therefore it is probably a manifestation of supernormality in the AV node. The right bundle had not had time to recover, causing the appearance of RBBB. This temporary delay down a part of the conduction system is known as aberrant conduction. Note that the next two P waves are blocked and are followed by a slightly aberrant junctional beat.

*3. How can supernormality account for disappearance of a bundle branch block?

ANS.: Supernormal conduction can probably occur in the bundle branches so that a bundle branch block can disappear if, in sinus rhythm, a premature atrial beat (or in atrial fibrillation, an early QRS) occurs at just the right moment [70, 99].

Note: Electronic pacemakers, when failing, have often produced a QRS only if the pacemaker fired during the supernormal phase of excitability.

4. What is meant by the absolute refractory period of the cycle?

ANS.: It refers to that phase of the cycle during which the heart is unable to respond to a stimulus regardless of the stimulus strength. As reported in the literature, this period varies from the beginning of the QRS to

a. The end of the QRS [22].

    b. About halfway along the upstroke of the T [51].

    c. Near the end of the T [60]. A reason for these differences may be that the absolute refractory period is shortened by fast heart rates.

5. What is meant by the relative refractory period?

    ANS.: It is the period between the absolute refractory period and the supernormal period. During the relative refractory period a stronger-than-normal stimulus is required to evoke a response, and the resultant response is below normal; nevertheless, a response can be elicited.

ESCAPE BEATS

1. What protects against death when the sinus pacemaker fails?

    ANS.: Another pacemaker site takes over.

2. What term is used to describe another pacemaker that 'takes over' due to depression of the sinus pacemaker?

    ANS.: *Escape pacemaker.* It might also be called an auxiliary, subsidiary, emergency, or natural demand pacemaker. It does, however, imply that other automatic cells are always trying to reach threshold but are prematurely extinguished by the faster pacemaker's depolarization wave; i.e., the slower automatic cells 'escape' *from the dominance of the faster automatic cells* in the sinus node when the latter is depressed.

3. Which pacemaker site usually takes over when the sinus pacemaker site is depressed?

    ANS.: The one with the automatic cells that have the next fastest rate of rise when compared with the SA node, i.e., the junctional area. (See the arrhythmia below.)

    Note: The farther a pacemaker cell is from the SA node, the slower is its firing rate.

4. Can merely a slow sinus rate cause a junctional escape pacemaker to take over?

    ANS.: Yes, any long pause that delays depolarization of the AV node can cause a junctional pacemaker to escape. Thus in a young person or athlete with a marked sinus arrhythmia a junctional pacemaker may take over every time he or she breathes out (see the ECG strip that follows).

    Note: When the sinus node is depressed, the first few escape cycles may be longer than subsequent ones until a stable cycle length is reached. This 'warming-up' process has been called the 'Treppe phenomenon' or hysteresis [131].

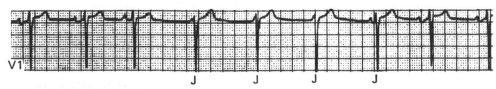

This ECG is from an 18-year-old girl with mitral disease and sinus arrhythmia. When she breathed out, the sinus rate suddenly slowed and a junctional pacemaker (J) escaped. The initial part of the P waves is barely visible in front of the junctional beats.

*5. What interval is long enough to allow a junctional escape beat to occur?

ANS.: The automatic cells in the junctional area would fire at a rate of 40 to 60 times per minute if they were allowed to. If we assume the slowest firing rate of 40, a pause of at least 1 second (seven large divisions on ECG paper) would be necessary to allow a junctional escape beat to manifest (see rhythm strip below).

Note: A series of consecutive escape beats constitutes an escape rhythm.

6. How can you recognize an escape beat?

ANS.: A long pause followed by a QRS that is preceded either by no P wave at all or by a P-R interval that is shorter than usual (see arrhythmia below).

7. Why are junctional escape beats often slightly different in appearance (aberrant) from the sinus beats?

ANS.: a. They may actually be arising in a bundle branch or one of its divisions and so must take a roundabout pathway to reach the other fascicles [91]. It may even occur in the bundle of His, with aberrancy caused by longitudinal dissociation at the distal end of the cable of fibers within the bundle [109].

b. If they occur after a P wave, they may even be ventricular escape beats that are not very wide because they are fusion beats (partly from above and partly from below) [91].

*c. They may travel down a Mahaim fiber, which passes from the bundle of His directly to muscle [153].

*d. They may be junctional with aberrancy due to phase 4 block.

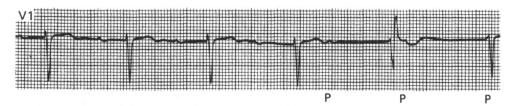

Type 1 second-degree AV block with two escape beats. The dropped beat causes a pause long enough to allow an RBBB escape beat, probably from one of the left bundle divisions. The next long pause (due to another blocked P wave) is followed by an escape beat from above the bifurcation of the bundles.

*8. What is meant by phase 4 block?

ANS.: If the depolarization of the ventricle's conduction system occurs after a long pause, the threshold potential may rise in some of the conduction system fibers. The next phase 0 of the action potential will be of lower amplitude in those conduction fibers, which may slow conduction enough to produce aberrancy.

Note: a. Phase 4 block usually implies damaged conduction tissue [117].

b. The mechanical equivalent of an escape pacemaker is a demand pacemaker implanted by a surgeon, i.e., a mechanical pacemaker that fires after a preset long pause. It fires on demand, as do nature's own 'escape' pacemakers.

*9. How can the ECG in hyperkalemia imitate that of a junctional escape rhythm secondary to sinus arrest?

ANS.: Hyperkalemia suppresses conduction through the atrial muscle much more than over the specialized conduction system of the atria. (There are three conduction pathways between the SA and AV nodes.) The impulses from the SA node have been shown to continue to travel to the AV node by the three potassium-resistant pathways without depolarizing atrial muscle [31]. This regular QRS rhythm with no visible P waves has been called sinoventricular rhythm.

Escape Pacemakers with Myocardial Infarction

*1. When can a junctional arrhythmia warn that a rupture of the left ventricular free wall has occurred in a patient with acute infarction?

ANS.: When there is sinus slowing, then junctional rhythm, then a return to sinus rhythm followed by a slower junctional rhythm. Such a sequence, each rhythm lasting for seconds or minutes, if followed by a state of shock, requires immediate pericardial aspiration [98].

2. What are some of the names given to a ventricular ectopic rhythm at a rate of 60 to 100 beats per minute that occurs primarily in acute myocardial infarction?

ANS.: a. Accelerated idioventricular rhythm.
b. Idioventricular rhythm.
c. Slow ventricular tachycardia.
d. Idioventricular tachycardia.
e. Nonparoxysmal ventricular tachycardia.

3. Why is the term *accelerated idioventricular rhythm* a satisfactory one?

ANS.: a. It tells you that the pacemaker is in the ventricle.
b. It tells you that the pacemaker is independent (*idio* means 'one's own'); i.e., it is not due to reentry.
c. It tells you that the pacemaker is enhanced in some way, so that it fires more rapidly than at the usual idioventricular rate of 20 to 40 beats per minute.
d. It avoids the word *tachycardia*, which is out of place with a rate of 60 to 100. By convention, tachycardia usually means a rate of more than 100.

4. Why is this ectopic rhythm not considered to be due to a junctional pacemaker?

ANS.: a. It very often begins and ends with fusion-like beats.
b. The QRS complexes are always wider than the patient's normal supraventricular complexes.
c. Ventricular parasystole from a similar focus has occurred on occasion [112].

*Note: a. Bundle of His recordings in six such patients showed that the accelerated pacemaker was in one of the bundle branches or at least below the bundle of His [53, 91].
b. These ventricular pacemakers may produce almost normal QRS widths, although on close analysis their QRSs are slightly wider than their supraventricular complexes. The reason is that the focus may be in a division of the left bundle branch.
c. An accelerated idioventricular rhythm that occurs during infarction is much more likely to occur during sinus arrhythmia than during sinus bradycardia [112], but it can start with
(1) A premature beat from the idioventricular focus.
(2) An escape beat after a long pause due to a premature contraction.
(3) A gradual process through several fusion beats.

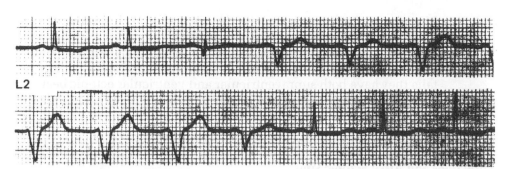

L2

An accelerated idioventricular rhythm in a patient with acute myocardial infarction. Fusion complexes begin and end the paroxysm. (There are seven idioventricular complexes in the 15-beat paroxysms that are not shown here.) The complexes that occur after complete P waves are slightly narrower than those without full P waves and are therefore fusion complexes. The idioventricular rate is slightly faster than the sinus rate.

5. Does accelerated idioventricular rhythm turn into ventricular tachycardia or ventricular fibrillation?

    ANS.: It has occasionally been the only prodrome to ventricular fibrillation [84]. In one study the rate occasionally suddenly doubled to more than 125 per minute [42]. As many as 85 percent of patients with accelerated idioventricular rhythm have developed ventricular tachycardia during acute infarction [32], especially if the idioventricular rate was more than 75 [143].

*6. What is the commonest cause of an accelerated idioventricular rhythm in the absence of myocardial infarction?

    ANS.: Digitalis overdose, especially with hypokalemia.

    Note: This rhythm has also been reported with rheumatic heart disease, primary myocardial disease, and patients with no evidence of heart disease [110].

    Note: a. With constant monitoring during the acute myocardial infarction, about 50 percent of subjects show this rhythm and nearly always within 24 hours [112].

    b. An accelerated idioventricular rhythm can remain active for a long time if it retrogradely activates the atrium (rare).

ATRIAL ECTOPIC BEATS AND PACEMAKERS

Physiology of Automatic Cells

1. Which areas of the atrium other than the SA node and bundle of His area can become a pacemaker?

    ANS.: Wherever Purkinje-like fibers are found.

    Note: These fibers act as special conduction pathways and contain automatic cells. An automatic cell is one with a phase 4 rise toward threshold potential.

2. How do hypokalemia and hyperkalemia affect phase 4 of automatic cells?

    ANS.: Hypokalemia increases their rate of rise; hyperkalemia does the opposite.

Note: a. Many antiarrhythmic drugs have the same effect as hyperkalemia; i.e., they decrease the rate of rise in phase 4.
  b. That hypokalemia stimulates automatic cells is suggested by the finding that even if hypokalemic patients are not receiving digitalis they have both supraventricular and ventricular ectopic beats 2.5 to 3.0 times more frequently than in a control hospital population [29].

P Wave Directions and Atrial Ectopic Sites

1. What is the direction of the P wave when the SA node is the pacemaker? Why?
   ANS.: 0° to + 90° is the range, but it is usually about + 60° because the SA node is high and to the right of the mean atrial mass that must be depolarized.
2. What is the expected direction of the P wave if the pacemaker is low in the atrium?
   ANS.: Superior and leftward or rightward.

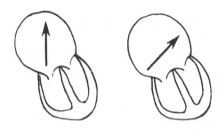

3. What is an ectopically produced P wave called?
   ANS.: P prime (P′).
*4. Why can you not tell by the spatial direction of the P′ wave exactly where in the left or right atrium the pacemaker is; i.e., if the P′ is ◤ why does it *not necessarily* mean that it is coming from high in the left atrium?
   ANS.: Because activation of the atria can be by the specialized conduction pathways. Thus a pacemaker even near the AV node may conduct rapidly to the left atrium first by way of special conduction tissue; then after depolarizing the left atrium the impulse may come back down to reach the right atrium last. However, a left atrial pacemaker rarely, if ever, produces an upright P in lead 1, i.e., right-to-left conduction [7].
     Note: a. In one study an electrode catheter stimulating various places in the right atrium always produced a P vector directed toward a point on the opposite end of the two atria, as if the atria were a sphere being concentrically depolarized [76].
       b. The P may point to the right and anteriorly and so appear to come from the left atrium. It can, however, be caused by retrograde P waves from junctional or ventricular pacemakers that were shown in one study to often point to the right at about − 110° and either posteriorly or anteriorly [41].
       c. If the P′ wave is negative in aVL and positive in V1, the focus is in the left atrium [143A].
*5. What is the only certain sign of a left atrial pacemaker?
   ANS.: The dome and dart P wave in V1, which is rare [100].

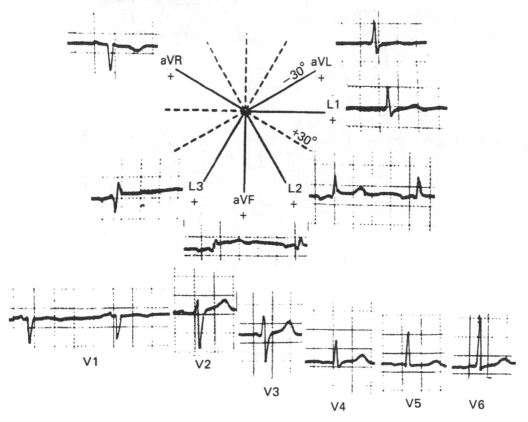

The dome is produced by the left atrium, which is activated first if there is a left atrial pacemaker. The dart represents late activation of the right atrium.

The P is equiphasic in L1, making an axis of − 90°. V1 has the dome and dart configuration of a left atrial pacemaker in this 40-year-old woman with a normal heart. Others have also found a left atrial type of P wave in subjects with apparently normal hearts [49].

Note: If dextrocardia is present, an ectopic pacemaker from the right-sided left atrium causes the P wave to be upright in lead 1. The dome and dart P in V1 tells you that it is due to a left atrial pacemaker [102].

*6. What is meant by coronary sinus rhythm?

ANS.: A rhythm with left axis deviation of the P wave and a P-R interval of 120 msec (0.12 sec) or more, thought to originate from the coronary sinus area or from the junctional area, but with markedly delayed conduction to the ventricles.

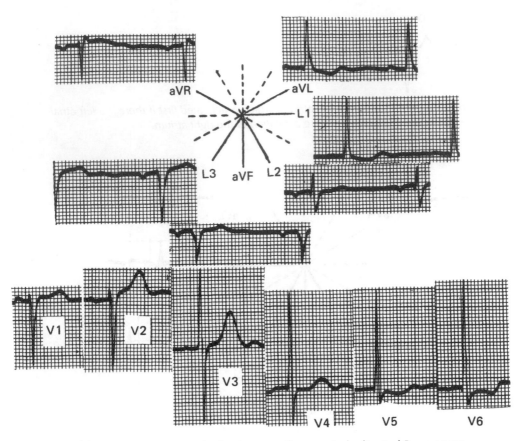

This ECG qualifies as coronary sinus rhythm because the superiorly directed P waves are associated with a P-R interval of 200 msec (0.20 sec). It is from a 69-year-old hypertensive man with cardiomegaly and angina.

> *Note:* a. The term *coronary sinus rhythm* may be incorrect because the same P direction and P-R interval can be produced experimentally by a pacemaker in the posterior left atrium or the lower lateral surface of the right atrium [152].
>
> b. 'Coronary sinus rhythm' is always a transient phenomenon [141].
>
> c. A leftward P, i.e., between 0 and + 30°, has been found in one series of ASDs to correlate with the presence of a sinus venosus defect or a persistent left superior vena cava [57]. (Some low atrial pacemakers produce only a leftward P, i.e., between 0° and 30° [57].) When a leftward or left axis of the P wave occurs in a patient with any congenital heart defect, there is a high likelihood of a persistent left superior cava draining into the coronary sinus [105].

*7. How can a low atrial pacemaker produce an inferiorly directed P wave?

ANS.: Activation is thought to occur rapidly up the atrial septum probably by way of the anterior internodal pathway to Bachmann's bundle, from which it spreads downward in a manner similar to that occurring during sinus rhythm [151]. This is further confirmed by the fact that artificial atrial stimulation at points a few millimeters apart can result in significant changes in P direction [152].

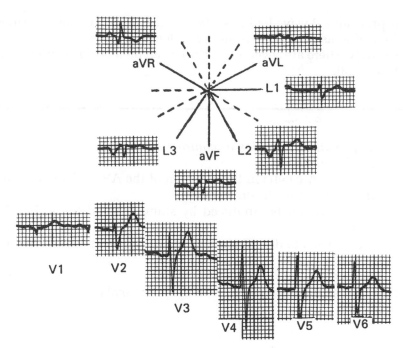

Low atrial or junctional pacemaker. The almost equiphasic P in L1 and negative P in L2 indicate a superior P vector of about − 90°. Because the P-R interval is only 100 msec (0.10 sec), it does not qualify as a coronary sinus rhythm.

*8. How can an ectopic atrial rhythm produce the appearance of left atrial overload?
  ANS.: If the pacemaker is in a high anterior location in the right atrium, its direction has been shown to be not only inferior and to the left, as in any sinus pacemaker, but also posterior to as much as − 60° in the horizontal plane, thus suggesting a left atrial overload. This pattern can usually be distinguished from that of left atrial overload if the ectopic P happens to produce negativity as far as V4 [101]. Left atrial overload rarely produces P negativity beyond V2 or V3.

Premature Atrial Contractions

1. What are the other terms used for premature atrial contractions (PACs)?
  ANS.: a. Atrial premature beats (APBs).
  b. Atrial extrasystoles.
  c. Premature atrial depolarizations. (See p. 515 for defense of the term *premature ventricular contractions*. The same defense may be used for PACs.)
2. How can you recognize an uncomplicated PAC?
  ANS.: a. You may see a premature ectopic P wave. (An ectopic P wave is called a P prime, or P′.)
  b. The QRS may look like all the other supraventricular QRS complexes. (A supraventricular QRS is one caused by conduction through the bundle of His.)
  c. The P should not look like that subject's sinus P wave.

Note: If the premature P wave looks exactly like the sinus P waves, consider the possibility of sinus premature beats; i.e., a focus in the SA node may be firing prematurely. There are several reports of such premature beats even in normal subjects [38].

P′ in Junctional and Low Atrial Pacemakers

1. Why is the term *nodal premature complex* or *contraction* a poor one for P′ waves that are retrogradely conducted?
   ANS.: a. There are no automatic cells in the N region of the AV node, where the main slowing work of the atrium is done.
   b. Retrograde P waves can be produced by stimulation of the atrium in non-nodal areas.
2. What term may be correctly used to describe premature pacemakers around the AV node?
   ANS.: Junctional pacemakers.
3. Diagram a premature contraction from very low in the junctional area.
   ANS.:

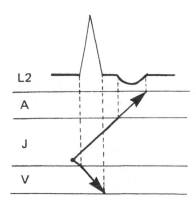

4. How can a low junctional ectopic pacemaker be imitated by a mid-junctional pacemaker?
   ANS.: If the mid-junctional pacemaker had a retrograde first-degree block, retrograde conduction (conduction upward or backward) through the AV node would be longer than anterograde conduction (forward or downward) conduction through the AV node. Thus it would look as if it were low junctional because the retrograde, delayed P wave would come after the QRS. Most junctional pacemakers are probably bundle of His pacemakers [27].

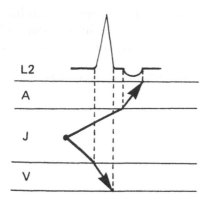

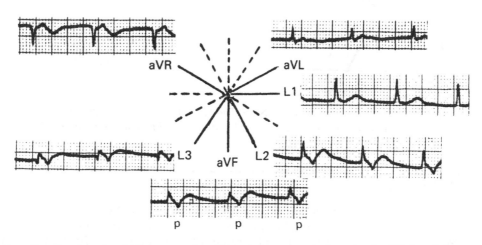

Junctional or bundle of His pacemaker. There is a retrograde P wave of − 90° (equiphasic in L1 and negative in L2) following each QRS.

5. Diagram a premature contraction from the middle of the junctional area with equal rates of anterograde and retrograde conduction.
   ANS.:

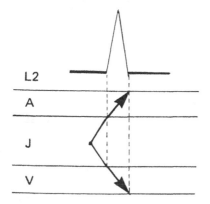

6. Where is the P' wave seen in relation to the QRS if a junctional pacemaker conducts in both directions at such a rate it reaches the atrium and ventricle simultaneously?
   ANS.: The P' is not seen, because it is hidden by the simultaneously occurring QRS.
7. Diagram a premature contraction from low in the atrium or very high in the junctional area.
   ANS.:

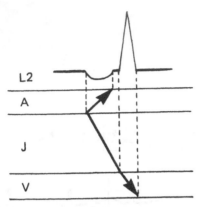

Here the P'' wave precedes the QRS. Note: *The high junctional pacemaker can be imitated by a mid-junctional pacemaker with anterograde block in the bundle of His.*

___

P'-R and P'-P Intervals

1. How is the P'-R interval affected by the early ectopic P wave? Why?
   ANS.: The P'-R is often prolonged, because the earlier that the AV node is depolarized, the more difficulty there is in transmitting the impulse through the AV node.
   Note: The function of the AV node is to block early impulses, and the earlier the impulse the more it is blocked.

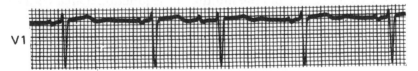

The relatively long P'-R interval in this PAC may have been exaggerated by the small amount of digitalis taken by this 78-year-old man with angina.

2. Why is a P'-R interval occasionally shorter than expected?
   ANS.: The ectopic atrial focus may be in one of the internodal pathways that partially or totally bypass the AV node. (See p. 197 for a discussion of atrio-His preexcitation.)
3. If the P' is very early, the AV node may be completely refractory, and conduction may not pass from the atrium to the ventricle. What is this condition called?
   ANS.: If you wish to refer only to the P' wave, you can call it a 'blocked premature atrial contraction' (blocked PAC). If you wish to refer to the missing QRS, you can call it a 'dropped beat' caused by a blocked PAC (see p. 503).

4. What commonly follows the pause caused by a blocked PAC?
   ANS.: A junctional escape beat; i.e., an automatic cell in the bundle of His area reaches threshold and produces a QRS.

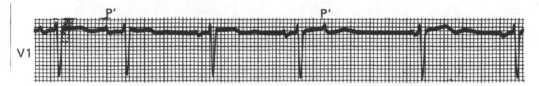

The first PAC is conducted with a relatively long P'-R interval. The second PAC is blocked and is followed by a junctional escape beat. The sudden short P-R indicates that that P wave is not producing the next QRS.

5. Can the SA node be depolarized by an ectopic atrial pacemaker?
   ANS.: Yes, it usually is.
   > *Note:* It follows the rule that if one cell of the conduction system is depolarized, all the cells are depolarized unless there is a pathologic or physiologic block.

6. When should the next P wave occur if the SA node was depolarized by a premature atrial focus?
   ANS.: The next P wave should occur when the SA node fires again at its usual firing rate; i.e., if the P-P interval was 1 second, the next P should occur 1 second after the ectopic P'.

7. What is meant by a P'-P interval?
   ANS.: The P' is the ectopic early P, and the P'-P is therefore the interval between the ectopic P and the next normal P.

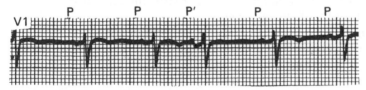

The P'-P interval following this premature atrial contraction is almost equal to the regular P-P interval; i.e., the ectopic premature atrial depolarization has reset the SA node firing interval. Careful measurement, however, shows that the P'-P interval is slightly longer than the regular P-P interval.

8. What usually happens to the P'-P interval following an atrial ectopic beat? Why?
   ANS.: It is usually prolonged. If the SA node is depolarized unusually early, an SA block is often produced. Therefore the next or postectopic P wave is delayed because of some SA block.
   > *Note:* If a P' occurs very late in diastole, it may reach the SA node after the latter has already fired and crossed the surrounding transitional cells into the atrium; i.e., the SA node may not be depolarized and no SA block occurs. Therefore a perfect compensatory pause occurs so that the P-P interval surrounding the PAC is exactly equal to two regular P-P intervals [19].

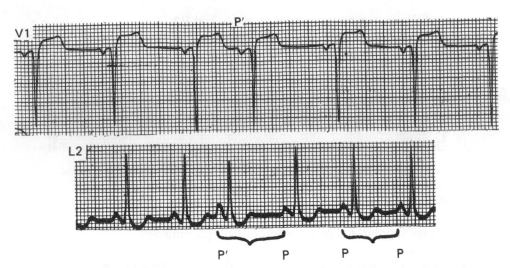

Two patients with PACs causing SA block. Note that the P'-P intervals in both strips are longer than any of the normal P-P intervals because of temporary SA block caused by the premature depolarization of the SA node.

Hidden Ectopic P Wave Diagnosis

1. What is the general term used to refer to all ectopic beats coming from above the bundle of His?

    ANS.: *Supraventricular.* Actually, this term applies to beats initiated from above the bifurcation of the bundle branches; i.e., it really means 'suprabifurcational,' or from the bundle of His or above.

2. What may make P' waves invisible even if they are not superimposed on a QRS?

    ANS.: a. They are often superimposed on a T wave.

         b. They are often low in voltage.

3. How can you tell by the appearance of the QRS that a premature ectopic pacemaker is in the atrium even if the P' wave is invisible?

    ANS.: If the ectopic pacemaker is supraventricular (above the bifurcation of right and left bundle branches), the normal pathways through the ventricles are ordinarily used. Thus the QRS complex of the early atrial beat usually appears like all the other QRS complexes on that ECG; i.e., it is expected to look like the other supraventricular beats.

4. If a P' is superimposed on a T, how can you detect its presence?

    ANS.: Always look for a slight difference in the contour of the T wave preceding an early beat. For example, if the T is slightly more peaked than the other T waves of that lead, a P' wave is probably superimposed on it. This trick is the most important when differentiating an aberrant premature atrial beat from a premature ventricular ectopic beat. An atrial ectopic beat may assume a wide bundle branch block configuration due to temporary delay in conduction along a bundle branch or one of its divisions and thus look like a premature ventricular ectopic beat. It is also the best way to diagnose one of the commonest causes of a pause, because a premature atrial contraction is often blocked at the AV node and does not produce a QRS at all.

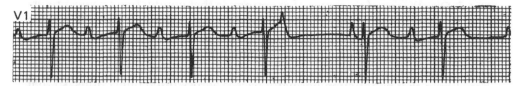

A nonconducted premature atrial P wave is seen peaking a T wave and explains the pause. The QRS ending the pause is probably junctional because it looks like all the other supraventricular QRS complexes and is preceded by a short P-R interval. Sudden shortening of a P-R interval nearly always implies that that QRS is ectopic (if the P wave looks like a sinus node P).

*5. What is unexpected about the sinus P wave following some PACs?

ANS.: It is often aberrantly conducted. Following about 60 percent of PACs in patients with myocardial disease [20], the next normal sinus P wave is aberrant. It can also occur after junctional or ventricular premature beats that retrogradely depolarize the atrium [21]. The aberrant conduction may be due to a change in atrial size produced by the long diastole [116].

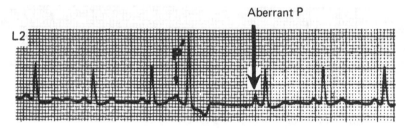

The P′ of the aberrant premature atrial beat distorts the previous T wave. The P following this premature beat is also aberrant in this elderly woman with coronary disease. (See also the aberrant P in the ECG of question 4.)

*6. What are the characteristics of an atrial escape rhythm?

ANS.: An atrial escape rhythm may occur when a sinus bradycardia or 2:1 SA block allows an atrial pacemaker to dominate. It is characterized by

a. An inherent rhythm at about the same rate as a junctional pacemaker.

b. Aberrant P′ deflections, but with anterograde conduction and often with varying degrees of aberrancy, so that the multiform P waves manifest what appears to be a 'wandering' atrial pacemaker.

Note: The basic disturbance leading to a 'wandering' atrial pacemaker is usually a sinus bradycardia with supraventricular escape beats. The term *wandering atrial pacemaker* is frequently incorrectly applied to multifocal PACs. A rapid rate of more than 100 due to multifocal PACs is called multifocal atrial tachycardia [134] (see p. 560).

Aberrant Conduction with Premature Atrial Contractions

1. Why can a PAC imitate a premature ventricular contraction (PVC)?

ANS.: Because a PAC can depolarize the ventricle with slow conduction through one of the bundles and thus look wide and bizarre like a bundle branch or divisional block. It is called *aberrant conduction*.

Note: One theory of the cause of aberrancy is that conduction travels preferentially down one of the bundle branches or divisions of the left bundle while they are still in the bundle of His. This theory is based on the concept of longitudinal dissociation of conduction fibers in the bundle of His. Each conduction strand in the bundle of His is like an isolated cable. One study has shown that conduction normally passes across interconnections, so that aberrancy may occur if these interconnections are damaged [6].

2. What is the specific meaning of 'aberrant' conduction?

ANS.: It is used to describe an *unexpected* temporary bundle branch or divisional block despite the fact that conduction proceeded from above the bifurcation of the bundle of His. That is, the stimulation was supraventricular but temporarily found one of the bundle branches or their divisions partially refractory, usually due to a change in previous cycle length.

If a pacemaker is in a ventricle, as in a PVC, aberrancy is bound to occur and is therefore expected. If a pacemaker is supraventricular, aberrancy is unexpected. It is the unexpected temporary aberrancy that is meant by the term *aberrant conduction.*

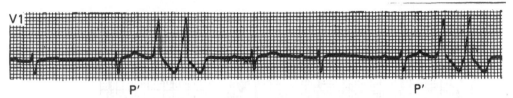

PACs in pairs with aberrant conduction. Note how a P' causes a slightly different T wave in front of each pair of bizarre RBBB-looking beats that would otherwise be passed off as premature ventricular complexes coming from the LV.

3. Which part of the bundle branch system is most commonly refractory when aberrancy is seen?

ANS.: The right bundle. In about 20 percent of instances of aberrancy, LBBB is seen. Although this finding suggests some damage to the left bundle branch system, it is occasionally seen with apparently normal hearts.

Note: a. At longer cycle lengths the relative refractory period of the right bundle branch is greater than that of the left bundle branch thus accounting for the appearance of either RBBB or LBBB aberrancy in a PAC depending on how early it occurs [19A].

*b. The three divisions of the left bundle have shorter action potential durations and functional refractory periods than the right bundle. Therefore they usually recover faster than the right bundle after an early impulse [64].

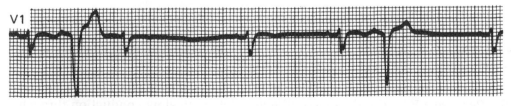

PACs with LBBB aberrancy in a 24-year-old man with an otherwise normal heart. Note the P' hidden in the preceding T wave and the various degrees of aberrancy. The third QRS is also a PAC with the P' hidden on the T of the aberrant beat.

*4. How does aberrancy relate to the U wave?

ANS.: One study has shown that aberrancy occurs with a PAC only when the premature QRS complex precedes the apex of the U wave. Because aberrancy probably results when conduction occurs early enough to take place during the relatively refractory period of the conduction system, and this period occurs during phase 3 of depolarization, the U wave may represent phase 3 depolarization of the conduction system.

Note: The presence of RBBB aberrancy is thought to be due to a longer action potential duration in the right than in the left bundle branch. If true, it may be postulated that the initial part of the U wave is produced by the left bundle branch and the terminal part by the right bundle branch. This situation is suggested by the observation that LBBB aberrancy occurs when the premature QRS takes place at least 50 msec before the apex of the U wave, and RBBB aberrancy occurs when the early QRS takes place less than 50 msec before the U wave apex [155].

*5. How can a PAC cause normal conduction in a patient with bundle branch block?

ANS.: Automatic cells exhibit a greater amplitude and rate of rise in phase 0 if they are depolarized just at the beginning of phase 4 than at any other time in diastole because at that time their resting potential has the greatest voltage, i.e., is farthest from the threshold potential. Therefore the slow bundle conduction that caused the bundle branch block is now changed to a normal rate of conduction, and no bundle branch block is seen [138].

*6. Why is a premature junctional beat more likely to be aberrant than a PAC?

ANS.: A PAC can cause slow AV node conduction, which allows time for the bundle branches to recover fully [104].

7. How does the length of a preceding cycle cause an early beat to be aberrant?

ANS.: If the early beat follows a QRS that is preceded by a long diastole, that early beat may be aberrantly conducted. It is known as the Ashman phenomenon.

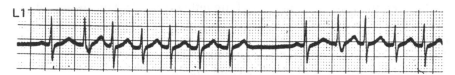

Two runs of atrial or junctional tachycardia. Note that the first early beat of each run is aberrant (wide S suggesting RBBB aberrancy). It is because they each follow a QRS that is preceded by a long diastole.

8. What is there about a long diastole that can cause the QRS that ends a short cycle after the long cycle to be aberrant?

ANS.: A long diastole causes the beat that ends the long diastole to have an action potential that is longer than usual. A longer action potential requires a longer recovery period. The length of the refractory period of branches of the conduction system is directly related to the length of the preceding cycle; a longer preceding cycle results in a longer refractory period than does a shorter cycle.

Note: The faster the heart rate, the shorter the refactory period of the bundle branches and the shorter must be the coupling interval to cause aberrancy [48A].

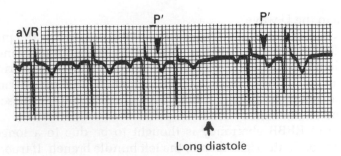

Long diastole

Two PACs, one with aberrant conduction. The tiny shoulder on the T waves (arrows) represents hidden P' waves. The second PAC is aberrant, with RBBB type of conduction, because it is the second QRS after a long diastole.

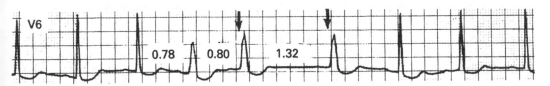

Tachycardia- and bradycardia-dependent bundle branch block in a 70-year-old woman with aortic stenosis and marked sinus arrhythmia. The short cycles of 0.78 and 0.80 second end with LBBB aberrancy. The long cycle of 1.32 seconds also ends with LBBB aberrancy owing to phase 4 aberrancy. (See p. 541 for explanation of phase 4 aberrancy.)

*RIGHT AND LEFT ATRIAL DISSOCIATION

*1. How has atrial dissociation been produced experimentally?

ANS.: By ligating the interatrial branch of the left coronary artery, following which the right atrium remained in sinus rhythm while the left atrium fibrillated [23].

*Note: There are reports of simultaneous

a. Atrial fibrillation and sinus rhythm [35].

b. Atrial fibrillation and atrial flutter [52].

c. P waves from two sources bearing no relation to one another, but each perfectly regular [90]. (Usually the right atrium is controlled by the sinus node [23].)

d. Atrial flutter and sinus rhythm [108, 132].

e. Bradycardia in one atrium and sinus tachycardia in the other (in the pressence of acute atrial infarction) [17].

f. Respiratory artifacts rather than true dissociation. These artifacts were thought to be due to use of accessory muscles of respiration in those reports in which dyspnea or pulmonary disease was present [59].

L1

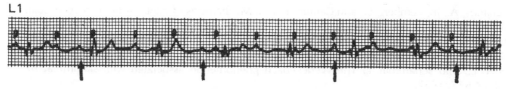

Pseudoatrial dissociation. The sinus rate is 115 per minute, and there is AV dissociation with a junctional rate of 70. The small P-like waves (at a rate of about 38/minute) marked off by pointers (two superimposed on P waves) are probably due to accessory muscles of respiration. The rate of this artifact was the patient's respiratory rate when the tracing was recorded.

*2. What are the usual clinical conditions in the presence of atrial dissociation?

ANS.: Such patients usually are in heart failure and taking digitalis or having an acute infarction [133]. One patient had infarction involving the atrial septum, and the ectopic left atrial focus controlled the ventricles despite sinus rhythm in the right atrium.

Note: Atrial dissociation has persisted for as long as 3 years [63].

REFERENCES

1. Abarquez, R. F., and LaDue, J. S. Atrial dissociation. *Am. J. Cardiol.* 8:448, 1961.
2. Alimurung, M. M., and Massell, B. F. The normal P-R interval in infants and children. *Circulation* 13:257, 1956.
3. Anderson, K. R., Yen Ho, S., and Anderson, R. H. Location and vascular supply of sinus node in human heart. *Br. Heart J.* 41:28, 1979.
4. Anderson, P. A. W., et al. Atrioventricular conduction in secundum atrial septal defects. *Circulation* 48:27, 1973.
5. Arguss, N. S., et al. Significance of chronic sinus bradycardia in elderly people. *Circulation* 46:924, 1972.
6. Bailey, J. C., Spear, J. F., and Moore, E. N. Functional significance of transverse conducting pathways within the canine bundle of His. *Am. J. Cardiol.* 34:790, 1974.
6A. Barold, S. S. Lingering misconceptions about type 1 second-degree atrioventricular block. *Am. J. Cardiol.* 88:1018–1020, 2001.
7. Beder, S. D., et al. Clinical confirmation of electrocardiographic criteria for left atrial rhythm. *Am. Heart J.* 103:848, 1982.
8. Bishop, L. F., and McGinn, F. X. Recurrent paroxysmal atrial fibrillation occurring in the absence of heart disease. *Vasc. Dis.* 5:31, 1968.
9. Bizarro, R. O., et al. Familial atrial septal defect with prolonged atrioventricular conduction. *Circulation* 41:677, 1970.
9A. Bond, R. C., Englem T. R., and Schaal, S. F. The effect of digitalis on sinoatrial conduction in man. *Am. J. Cardiol.* 33 (Abstracts): 128, 1974.
10. Bonke, F. I. M., et al. The effect of digitalis on the isolated sinus node of the rabbit heart as studied with microelectrodes. *Circ. Abstr.* (Suppl. 111) 55–56:135, 1977.
11. Bottiger, L. E., and Edhag, O. Heart block in ankylosing spondylitis and uropolyarthritis. *Br. Heart J.* 34:487, 1972.
12. Bower, P. J. Sick sinus syndrome. *Arch. Intern. Med.* 138:133, 1978.
13. Buckberg, G. D., and Fowler, N. O. Complete atrioventricular block due to cardiac metastasis of bronchogenic carcinoma. *Circulation* 24:657, 1961.
14. Caralis, G. D., and Varghese, P .J. Familial sinoatrial node dysfunction increased vagal tone: A possible aetiology. *Br. Heart J.* 38:951, 1976.
15. Carleton, R. A., Miller, P. H., and Graettinger, J. S. Effects of ouabain and atropine on A-V nodal conduction in man. *Circulation* 20:283, 1967.

16. Castellanos, A., Jr., Lemberg, L., and Centurion, M.J. Mechanisms of digitalis-induced ventricular fibrillation. *Dis. Chest* 54:221, 1968.

17. Chatterjee, K., et al. The electrocardiogram in chronic heart block. A histological correlation with ECG changes in 42 patients. *Am. Heart J.* 80:47, 1970.

18. Chesler, E., and Schamroth, L. The Wenckebach phenomenon associated with sialorrhea. *Br. Heart J.* 4:577, 1957.

19. Childers, R. W., et al. Sinus nodal echoes. Clinical case report and canine studies. *Am. J. Cardiol.* 31:220, 1973.

19A. Chilson, D. A., Zipes, D. P., Heger, J. J., Browne, K.F., Prystowsky, E.N. Functional bundle branch block: discordant response of right and left bundle branches to changes in heart rate. *Am. J. Cardiol.* 54:313–316, 1984.

20. Chung, E. K. Aberrant atrial conduction – unrecognized electrocardiographic entity. *Am. J. Cardiol.* 26:628, 1970.

21. Chung, E. K. Aberrant atrial conduction – unrecognized electrocardiographic entity. *Br. Heart J.* 34:341, 1972.

22. Chung, E. K. *Principles of Cardiac Arrhythmias.* Baltimore: Williams & Wilkins, 1971. P. 26.

23. Chung, K. Y., Walsh, T. J., and Massie, E. A review of atrial dissociation with illustrative cases in critical discussion. *Am. J. Med. Sci.* 250:106, 1965.

24. Clarke, M., and Keith, J. D. Atrioventricular conduction in acute rheumatic fever. *Br. Heart J.* 34:472, 1972.

25. Cohen, H. C., Ali, M., and D'Cruz, I. A. Electrocardiography and electrophysiology – 11. *Am. J. Cardiol.* 41:383, 1978.

26. Cranefield, P. F., Wit, A. L., and Hoffman, B. F. Genesis of cardiac arrhythmias. *Circulation* 47:24, 1973.

27. Damato, A. N., et al. His bundle rhythms. *Circ. Abstr.* [Suppl. 111] 39–40:65, 1969.

28. Das, G., Talmers, F. N., and Weissler, A. M. New observations on the effects of atropine on the SA and AV nodes. *Am. J. Cardiol.* 36:281, 1975.

29. Davidson, S., and Surawicz, B. Ectopic beats and atrioventricular conduction disturbances. *Arch. Intern. Med.* 120:280, 1967.

30. Davies, M., and Harris, A. Pathological basis of primary heart block. *Br. Heart J.* 31:219, 1969.

31. Davis, L., and Hoffman, B. E. Evidence for specialized pathways (abstract). *Fed. Proc.* 22:246, 1963.

32. DeSoyza, N., Bissett, J., and Doherty, J. E. Association of accelerated idioventricular rhythm and VT. *Am. J. Cardiol.* 34:667, 1974.

33. Dhingra, R. C. His bundle recording in acquired conduction disease. *Arch. Intern. Med.* 135:397, 1975.

34. Dhingra, R. C., Rosen, K. M., and Rahimtoola, S. Normal conduction intervals using His bundle recordings. *Chest* 64:55, 1973.

35. Dietz, G. W., III, et al. Atrial dissociation and uniatrial fibrillation. *Circulation* 15:883, 1957.

36. Dighton, D. H. Sinus bradycardia-autonomic influences and clinical assessment. *Br. Heart J.* 36:791, 1974.

37. Donoso, E., et al. Congenital heart block. *Am. J. Med.* 60:869, 1956.

38. Dorkin, J. R. Sinus premature systoles. *Am. J. Cardiol.* 9:804, 1962.

39. Dreifus, L. A. Myocardial infarction and heart block. *J.A.M.A.* 202:172, 1967.

40. Eliasen, P., and Andersen, M. Sinoatrial block during lithium treatment. *Eur. J. Cardiol.* 3:97, 1975.

41. El-Sherif, N. A-V junctional versus left atrial rhythm. *Br. Heart J.* 33:358, 1971.

42. El-Sherif, N., et al. Accelerated ventricular rhythms in acute myocardial infarction and differential effect of lidocaine. *Circ. Abstr.* [Suppl. 111] 55–56:66, 1977.

43. Emanuel, R., et al. Association of secundum atrial septal defect with abnormalities of atrio-ventricular conduction or left axis deviation: A new syndrome. *Br. Heart J.* 38:536, 1976.

44. Engle, T. R., Meister, S. G., and Frankl, W. S. Absence of Wedensky effect in man. *Am. Heart J.* 94:435, 1977.

45. Eraker, S. A., Wickamasekaran, R., and Goldman, S. Complete heart block with hyperthyroidism. *J.A.M.A.* 239:1644, 1978.

46. Eraut, D., and Shaw, D. B. Sinus bradycardia. *Br. Heart J.* 33:742, 1971.
47. Erikssen, J., et al. P-R interval in middle aged men with overt and latent coronary disease. *Clin. Cardiol.* 5:353, 1982.
48. Ferrer, M. E. The sick sinus syndrome. *Circulation* 47:635, 1973.
48A. Fisch, C. Aberration: 75 years after Sir Thomas Lewis. *Br. Heart J.* 50:297, 1983.
48B. Fleg, J. L. et al. Aging and the ECG. *J. Gerontol.* 45:M95, 1990.
49. Frankl, W. S., and Soloff, L. A. Left atrial rhythm. Analysis by intra-atrial electrocardiogram and the vectorcardiogram. *Am. J. Cardiol.* 22:645, 1968.
50. Friedberg, H. D. Mechanism of Wedensky phenomena in the left bundle branch. *Am. J. Cardiol.* 27:698, 1971.
51. Friedman, H. H. *Diagnostic Electrocardiography and Vectorcardiography.* New York: McGraw-Hill, 1971. P. 336.
52. Friedman, P. L., et al. Inter-and intra-atrial dissociation during spontaneous atrial flutter. *Am. J. Cardiol.* 50:756, 1982.
53. Gallagher, J. J., Damato, A. N., and Lau, S. H. Electrophysiologic studies during accelerated idio-ventricular rhythms. *Circulation* 54:671, 1971.
54. Gimbel, K. S. The reentry phenomenon. *Chest* 63:1, 1973.
55. Ginks, W., Siddons, H., and Leatham, A. Coronary artery disease as a cause of atrioventricular block or sinoatrial disease. In *VIII World Congress of Cardiology Abstracts*, 1978. P. 446.
56. Gochberg, S. H. Congenital heart block. *Am. J. Obstet. Gynecol.* 88:238, 1964.
57. Hancock, E. W. Coronary sinus rhythm in sinus venosus defect and persistent left superior vena cava. *Am. J. Cardiol.* 14:608, 1964.
58. Harris, A., et al. Aetiology of chronic heart block. A clinico-pathological correlation in 65 cases. *Br. Heart J.* 31:206, 1959.
59. Higgins, T. G., Phillips, J. H., and Sumner, R. G. Atrial dissociation. *Am. J. Cardiol.* 18:132, 1966.
60. Hoffman, B. F., and Cranefield, P. F. *Electrophysiology of the Heart.* New York: McGraw-Hill, 1960. P. 254.
61. Hoffman, B. F., and Cranefield, P. F. The physiological basis of cardiac arrhythmias. *Am. J. Med.* 37:670, 1964.
62. Hoffman, J. I. E. Heart block in congenital heart disease. *Bull. N.Y. Acad. Med.* 47:885, 1971.
63. Igarashi, M., Katayama, F., and Hinohara, S. Two cases of atrial dissociation. *Am. J. Cardiol.* 11:267, 1963.
64. Iwamura, N., et al. Functional properties of the left septal Purkinje network in premature activation of the ventricular conduction system. *Am. Heart J.* 95:60, 1978.
65. James, T. N., and Marshall, T. K. Multifocal stenoses due to fibromuscular dysplasia of the sinus node artery. *Circulation* 53:736, 1976.
66. Kahler, R. L., et al. Familial congenital heart disease. *Am. J. Med.* 40:384, 1966.
67. Khalilullah, M., et al. Unidirectional complete heart block. *Am. Heart J.* 97:608, 1979.
68. Kibler, L. E., and Gazes, P. C. Effect of clondine on atrioventricular conduction. *J.A.M.A.* 238:1930, 1977.
69. Klein, H. O., et al. Effect of extrasystoles on idioventricular rhythm. *Circulation* 47:758, 1973.
70. Klein, H. O., et al. The supernormal phase of intraventricular conduction. Normalization of premature beats. *J. Electrocardiol.* 15:89, 1982.
71. Kugler, J. D., Garson, A., Jr., and Gillette, P. C. Electrophysiologic effect of digitalis on sinoatrial nodal function in children. *Am. J. Cardiol.* 44:1344, 1979.
71A. Lange, H. W., Ameisen, O., Mack, R., Moses, J. W., Kligfield, P. Prevalence and clinical correlates of non-Wenckebach, narrow-complex second-degree atrioventricular block detected by ambulatory ECG. *Am. Heart J.* 115:114–120, 1988.
72. Langendorf, R. Terminology and classification of disturbances of A-V conduction. *Bull. N.Y. Acad. Med.* 47:877, 1971.
73. Lasser, R. P., Haft, J. I., and Friedberg, C. K. Relationship of right bundle branch block and marked left axis deviation (with left parietal or periinfarction block) to complete heart block and syncope. *Circulation* 37:429, 1968.

74. Lee, J. K., and Lewis, J. A. Myxoedema with complete A-V block and Adams-Stokes disease abolished with thyroid medication. *Br. Heart J.* 24:253, 1962.
75. Lee, Y. C. Ventricular fusion beats. *J.A.M.A.* 201:156, 1967.
76. Leon, D. F., et al. Right atrial ectopic rhythms: experimental production in man. *Am. J. Cardiol.* 25:6, 1970.
77. Lev, M. The normal anatomy of the conduction system in man and its pathology in atrioventricular block. *Ann. N.Y. Acad. Sci.* 111:817, 1964.
78. Lev, M., et al. Lack of connection between the atria and the more peripheral conduction system in congenital atrioventricular block. *Am. J. Cardiol.* 27:481, 1971.
79. Lightfoot, P. R., et al. His bundle electrograms in healthy adolescents with persistent second degree A-V block. *Chest* 63:358, 1973.
80. Lister, J. W., et al. Atrioventricular conduction in man. *Am. J. Cardiol.* 16:516, 1965.
81. Liu, S. M., and Alexander, C. S. Complete heart block and aortic insufficiency in rheumatoid spondylitis. *Am. J. Cardiol.* 25:623, 1970.
82. Lloyd-Mostyn, R. H., Kidner, P. H., and Oram, S. Sinoatrial disorder including the bradytachycardia syndrome. A review with addition of 11 cases. *Q.J. Med.* 42:41, 1973.
83. Louvros, N., and Costeas, E. Retrograde activation of atria in auriculoventricular block. *Arch. Intern. Med.* 116:778, 1965.
84. Lown, B., Temte, J. V., and Arter, W. J. Ventricular tachyarrhythmias: Clinical aspects. *Circulation* 47:1364, 1973.
85. Lynch, H. T., et al. Hereditary progressive A-V conduction defect. *J.A.M.A.* 225:1465, 1973.
86. Maguire, L. C., et al. Reversible heart block in acute leukemia. *J.A.M.A.* 240:668, 1978.
87. Mandel, W. J., et al. Assessment of sinus node function in patients with the sick sinus syndrome. *Circulation* 46:761, 1972.
88. Mandel, W. J., Laks, M. M., and Obayashi, K. Sinus node function. Evaluation in patients with and without sinus node disease. *Arch. Intern. Med.* 135:388, 1975.
89. Mangiola, S. Intermittent left anterior hemiblock with Wenckebach phenomenon. *Am. J. Cardiol.* 30:892, 1972.
90. Marquis, M. G. Atrial dissociation. *Br. Heart J.* 20:335, 1958.
91. Massumi, R. A., Ertem, G. E., and Vera, Z. Aberrancy of junctional escape beats. *Am. J. Cardiol.* 29:351, 1972.
92. Maytin, O., Castillo, C., and Castellanos, A., Jr. Marked sinus tachycardia and overdrive suppression. *Chest* 58:528, 1970.
93. McCammon, R. W. Preliminary report on the developmental aspects of the P-R interval in the electrocardiograms of healthy children. *Pediatrics* 18:873, 1955.
94. McCue, C. M., et al. Congenital heart block in newborns of mothers with connective tissue disease. *Circulation* 55:82, 1977.
95. McHenry, M. M. Factors influencing longevity in adults with congenital complete heart block. *Am. J. Cardiol.* 29:416, 1972.
96. Merideth, J., and Pruitt, R. D. Disturbances in cardiac conduction and their management. *Circulation* 47:1098, 1973.
97. Merideth, J., and Titus, J. L. The anatomic atrial connections between sinus and A-V node. *Circulation* 37:566, 1968.
98. Meurs, A. A. H., et al. Electrocardiogram during cardiac rupture by myocardial infarction. *Br. Heart J.* 32:232, 1970.
99. Mihalick, M. J., and Fisch, C. Electrocardiographic findings in the aged. *Am. Heart J.* 87:117, 1974.
100. Mirowski, M. Left atrial rhythm. *Am. J. Cardiol.* 17:203, 1966.
101. Mirowski, M., et al. Ectopic right atrial rhythms. Experimental and clinical data. *Am. Heart J.* 81:666, 1971.
102. Mirowski, M., Neill, C. A., and Taussig, H.G. Left atrial ectopic rhythm in mirror-image dextrocardia and in normally placed malformed hearts. Report of twelve cases with 'dome and dart' P waves. *Circulation* 27:864, 1963.
103. Mobitz, W. Über die unvollstandige Storung der Erregungsuberleitung zwischen Vorhof und Kammer des menschlichen Herzens. *Z. Ges. Exp. Med.* 41:180, 1924.

104. Moe, G. K., Mendez, C., and Han, J. Aberrant A-V impulse propagation in the dog heart: A study of functional bundle-branch block. *Circ. Res.* 16:261, 1965.

105. Momma, K., and Linde, L. M. Abnormal rhythms associated with persistent left superior vena cava. *Pediatr. Res.* 3:210, 1969.

106. Munoz-Armas, S., et al. Single atrium. Embryologic, anatomic, electrocardiographic and other diagnostic features. *Am. J. Cardiol.* 21:639, 1968.

107. Murray, A., et al. RR interval variations in young male diabetics. *Br. Heart J.* 37:882, 1975.

108. Mussafia, A., and Jacovella, G. Paroxysmal partial auricular flutter with sinus rhythm. *Cardiologia* 31:173, 1957.

109. Narula, O. S., and Linhart, J. W. Demonstration of longitudinal dissociation in the His bundle. *Am. J. Cardiol.* 39:326, 1977.

110. Norris, R. M. Heart block in posterior and anterior myocardial infarction. *Br. Heart J.* 31:352, 1969.

111. Norris, R. M., and Croxson, M. D. Bundle branch block in acute myocardial infarction. *Am. Heart J.* 79:728, 1970.

112. Norris, R. M., and Mercer, C. J. Significance of idioventricular rhythms in acute myocardial infarction. *Prog. Cardiovasc. Dis.* 16:455, 1974.

113. O'Rourke, G. W., and Greene, N. M. Autonomic blockade and the resting heart rate in man. *Am. Heart J.* 80:469, 1970.

114. Pease, W. E., Nordenberg, A., and Ladda, R. L. Familial atrial septal defect with prolonged atrioventricular conduction. *Circulation* 53:759, 1976.

115. Perlman, W. V., et al. An epidemiologic study of first degree atrioventricular block in Tecumseh, Michigan. *Chest* 59:40, 1971.

116. Probst, P., et al. Investigation of atrial aberration as a cause of altered P wave contour. *Am. Heart J.* 88:516, 1973.

117. Przybylski, J., et al. The occurrence of phase-4 block in the anomalous bundle of patients with Wolff-Parkinson-White syndrome. *Eur. J. Cardiol.* 3/4:267, 1975.

118. Reicheck, N., et al. Advanced congenital first degree atrioventricular block. *Arch. Intern. Med.* 130:765, 1972.

119. Reiffel, J. A., Bigger, J. T., and Cramer, M. Effects of digoxin after vagal blockade in sinus node dysfunction. *Am. J. Cardiol.* 43:983, 1979.

120. Reiffel, J. A., et al. The human sinus node electrogram: A transvenous catheter technique. *Circulation* 62:1324, 1980.

121. Roberts, N., and Olley, P. His bundle electrogram in children. Statistical correlation of the atrioventricular conduction times in children with their age and heart rate. *Br. Heart J.* 34:1099, 1972.

122. Roos, J. C., and Dunning, A. J. Right bundle branch block and left axis deviation in acute myocardial infarction. *Br. Heart J.* 32:847, 1970.

123. Rosen, K. M., et al. Mobitz type II block without bundle-branch block. *Circulation* 44:1111, 1971.

124. Rosen, K. M., Loeb, H. S., and Rahimtoola, S. H. Mobitz type II block with narrow QRS complex and Stokes-Adams attacks. *Arch. Intern. Med.* 132:595, 1973.

125. Rosenbaum, M. B. Classification of ventricular extrasystoles according to form. *J. Electrocardiol.* 2:289, 1969.

126. Rosenbaum, M. D., et al. Wenckebach periods in the bundle branches. *Circulation* 40:79, 1969.

127. Rytand, D. A., Stinson, E., and Kelly, J. J., Jr. Remission and recovery from chronic, established, complete heart block. *Am. Heart J.* 91:645, 1976.

128. Sarachek, N. S., and Leonard, J. J. Familial heart block and sinus bradycardia. *Am. J. Cardiol.* 29:451, 1972.

129. Saraf, K. R., Klein, D. F., and Gittelman-Klein, R. Effect of imipramine treatment in children. *J. Am. Acad. Child Psychiatry* 17:60, 1978.

130. Scarpa, W. J. The sick sinus syndrome. *Am. Heart J.* 92:648, 1976.

131. Schamroth, L. *The Disorders of Cardiac Rhythm.* Oxford: Blackwell, 1971. P. 116.

131A. Scherf, D. The priority is Wenckebach's chest. *Chest* 62:239, 1972.

132. Schwartz, E. L. Atrial dissociation. *N.Y. State J. Med.* 69:3042, 1969.

133. Scott, M. E., and Finnegan, O. C. Atrial dissociation. *Br. Heart J.* 47:539, 1975.
134. Shine, K. I., Kastor, J. A., and Yurchak, P. M. Multifocal atrial tachycardia. *N. Engl. J. Med.* 279:344, 1968.
134A. Shoung, H. W., Lee, G. S., and Toh, C. C. S. The sick sinus syndrome. A study of 15 cases. *Br. Heart J.* 34:942, 1972.
135. Silvertssen, E., and Jorgensen, L. Atrial dissociation. *Am. Heart J.* 85:103, 1973.
136. Simonson, E., et al. Sex differences in the electrocardiogram. *Circulation* 22:598, 1960.
137. Sims, B. A., and Geddes, J. S. Traumatic heart block. *Br. Heart J.* 31:140, 1969.
138. Singer, D. H., and TenEick, R. E. Aberrancy: Electrophysiologic aspects. *Am. J. Cardiol.* 28:381, 1971.
139. Singh, J. B., et al. Reversible atrioventricular block in myxedema. *Chest* 63:582, 1973.
140. Slama, R. Atrioventricular heart block and hemochromatosis. *Presse Med.* 79:747, 1971.
141. Spodick, D. H., and Colman, R. Observations on coronary sinus rhythm and its mechanism. *Am. J. Cardiol.* 7:198, 1961.
142. Stock, R. J., and Macken, D. L. Observations on heart block during continuous electrocardiographic monitoring in myocardial infarction. *Circulation* 38:993, 1968.
143. Talbot, S., and Greaves, M. Association of ventricular extrasystoles and ventricular tachycardia with idioventricular rhythm. *Br. Heart J.* 38:457, 1976.
143A. Tang, C. W., Scheinman,, M. M. Van Hare G. F., Epstein, L. M., et al. P wave morphology during automatic atrial tachycardia in man. *J.A.C.C. (Abstr.)* iA–484A, 1994.
144. Thery, C., et al. Pathology of sinoatrial node. Correlations with electrocardiographic findings in 111 patients. *Am. Heart J.* 93:735, 1977.
145. Urthaler, F., et al. Mathematical relationship between automaticity of the sinus node and the AV junction. *Am. Heart J.* 86:189, 1973.
146. Van der Hauwaert, L. G., Stroobandt, R., and Verhaeghe, L. Arterial blood supply of the atrioventricular node and main bundle. *Br. Heart J.* 34:1045, 1972.
147. Vitasalo, M. T., Kala, R., and Eisalo, A. Ambulatory electrocardiographic recording in endurance athletes. *Br. Heart J.* 47:213, 1982.
148. Vohra, J., et al. The effect of toxic and therapeutic doses of tricyclic antidepressant drugs on intracardiac conduction. *Eur. J. Cardiol.* 3/3:219, 1975.
149. Waldo, A. L., et al. Effects on the canine P wave of discrete lesions in the specialized atrial tracts. *Circ. Res.* 29:452, 1971.
150. Waldo, A. L., et al. Etiology of prolongation of the P-R interval in patients with an endocardial cushion defect. *Circulation* 58:19, 1973.
151. Waldo, A. L., et al. Sequence of retrograde atrial activation of the human heart. Correlation with P wave polarity. *Br. Heart J.* 39:634, 1977.
152. Waldo, A. L., et al. The P wave and P-R interval. *Circulation* 42:653, 1970.
153. Walsh, T. J. Ventricular aberration of A-V nodal escape beats. Comments concerning the mechanism of aberration. *Am. J. Cardiol.* 10:217, 1962.
154. Wan, S., Lee, G. S., and Toh, C. The sick sinus syndrome. A study of 15 cases. *Br. Heart J.* 34:942, 1972.
155. Watanabe, Y., and Toda, H. The U wave and intraventricular conduction: Further evidence for the Purkinje repolarization theory on genesis of the U wave. *Am. J. Cardiol.* 41:23, 1978.
156. Weed, C. L., et al. Heart block in ankylosing spondylitis. *Arch. Intern. Med.* 117:800, 1966.
157. Wit, A. L., and Rosen, M. R. Cellular electrophysiology of cardiac arrhythmia. *Mod. Concepts Cardiovasc. Dis.* 50:1, 1981.
158. Yabek, S. M. Evaluation of sinus node automaticity and sinoatrial conduction in children with normal and abnormal sinus node function. *Clin. Cardiol.* 1:136, 1978.
159. Young, E., et al. Wenckebach atrioventricular block (Mobitz type 1) in children and adolescents. *Am. J. Cardiol.* 40:393, 1977.
160. Zakauddin, V., et al. Effect of digoxin on sinus node recovery time and resting and postexercise heart rates in patients with sick sinus syndrome. *Am. J. Cardiol.* 39:264, 1977.
161. Zema, M. J., Restivo, B., Pizzarello, R. A. Persistent atrial quiescence in adult rheumatic heart disease. *J. Electrocardiol.* 15(1):85–88, 1982.

28. Arrhythmia Diagnosis: Part 2. Premature Ventricular Contractions, Alternans, and Ectopic Tachycardias

PREMATURE VENTRICULAR CONTRACTIONS

What other terms are used for premature ventricular contractions (PVCs)?
ANS.: a. Ventricular premature beats (VPBs).
       b. Ventricular extrasystoles.
       c. Premature ventricular depolarizations (PVDs).

Note: There are no strong arguments for any of these terms. Against the use of VPB and PVC is the inability to see a 'beat' or a 'contraction' on an electrocardiogram (ECG). Against the use of ventricular extrasystole is the fact that most premature ectopic ventricular depolarizations prevent the regular QRS from occurring and so are not 'extra,' as well as the fact that systole cannot be seen on an ECG. Against the use of PVD is mainly its newness.

The only defense of PVC is that it has long usage and that the letter C can be translated into 'complex,' so that the purist may interpret the expression as 'premature ventricular complex.'

In atrial fibrillation the word *premature* may be out of place because some of the supraventricular complexes may come even earlier than the ectopic impulse. Here the term *ectopic ventricular complex* is more correct, even though the abbreviation EVC has not yet been used.

Site of Origin of PVCs

1. Where is the ectopic origin for a PVC?
    ANS.: Usually it is anywhere in the conduction system of either ventricle.
         Note: It is conceivable that under extremely abnormal metabolic conditions a PVC may originate in nonautomatic tissue.
2. What is the characteristic configuration of a PVC?
    ANS.: PVCs characteristically display an abnormal, wide QRS, imitating a bundle branch block. The appearance is often called bizarre.
         Note: If they occur high in the septum, they may be only slightly widened.
3. When does the shape of a PVC look like right bundle branch block (RBBB)? Why?
    ANS.: When the PVC originates in the left ventricle (LV). In this case the LV is depolarized first. The right ventricle (RV) can be reached only through a circuitous pathway and is depolarized last, as if RBBB were present.
4. When does a PVC look like left bundle branch block (LBBB)?
    ANS.: When it comes from either the RV, the LV, or the septum. How a PVC from the LV can produce a LBBB pattern is unknown.

Note: a. Because both RBBB and LBBB PVCs can come from the LV, it is not surprising that in patients with chest pain there is no correlation between the configuration of a PVC and either the presence or the severity of coronary disease [11].

b. In an apparently normal heart, about 75 percent of PVCs come from the RV and have marked anterior initial forces and a rightward QRS; i.e., the anterior division of the left bundle is probably reached first [103]. In an abnormal heart, at least 90 percent of PVCs come from the LV [72]. Acute injury to the anteroseptal region can result in arrhythmias from either ventricle [55].

*5. How can you tell whether a PVC is coming from the posterior or anterior wall of the LV?

ANS.: If the posterior wall is activated first, the PVC gives the same QRS direction as an anterior divisional block. Conversely, a PVC with an RBBB with *right axis deviation* tells you that it probably arises from the *anterior wall* of the LV [80].

6. What is the best term for PVCs that have different shapes in the same lead?

ANS.: *Multiform PVCs.*

Note: The term *multifocal PVCs* is commonly used but is misleading because the different shapes may be due to varying degrees of aberrancy, i.e., to varying degrees of refractoriness of portions of the ventricles rather than to initiation from different foci. The preferred term is *multiform.*

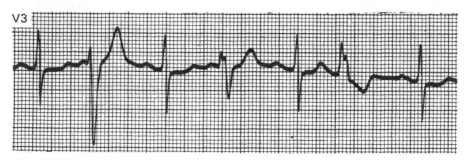

Multiform PVCs in bigeminy. It is bigeminy because every other complex is a PVC. The first PVC is near the peak of the P wave (end-diastolic), the second is on the downslope of the P, and the third is at the end of the T. Therefore the different shapes of PVC are probably due to different degrees of refractoriness of conduction tissue and are not necessarily multifocal.

Timing of PVCs in the Cycle

1. Where does a PVC usually occur in the cycle?

ANS.: Usually between the T and the next P.

---

* Material marked with an asterisk is included for reference and for advanced students in cardiology.

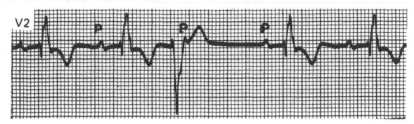

PVC probably from the RV (LBBB) pattern in a 59-year-old man with an atrial septal defect. There is RBBB and first-degree AV block (P-R interval 220 msec). The PVC occurs between the T and the next P.

2. When can a PVC occur during a P-R interval, i.e., at the end of diastole? Why?

    ANS.: It may occur after a P wave if diastole is short owing to rapid rates. This is because the P waves then come just at the end of every T wave, especially if the P-R interval is prolonged. If a sinus P comes very early, any PVC must occur after it unless the PVC occurs unusually early.

    Note: A PVC after a P wave is called an end-diastolic PVC.

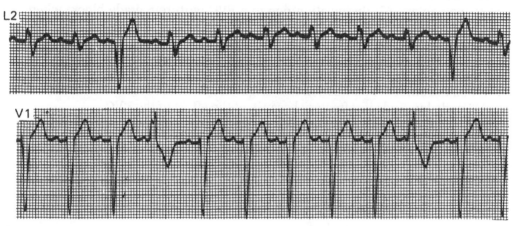

These strips are from different patients. Note that the two abnormal beats in each strip occur after P waves. Because the P waves preceding each wide QRS are not premature, these QRSs are not due to premature atrial complexes but are end-diastolic PVCs. If the rate is fast and the coupling interval is long, there is a good chance that the PVCs will be end-diastolic.

*3. With what can an end-diastolic PVC be confused? Why?

    ANS.: An atrioventricular (AV) preexcitation complex, because the P-R is short and the QRS of the PVC is wide.

4. What is the earliest that a PVC can occur in relation to the previous T wave? What is the significance of an early PVC?

    ANS.: It can occur near the peak of the previous T wave. This type is dangerous and may signify the imminent onset of a repetitive phenomenon, e.g., ventricular tachycardia or fibrillation. (See p. 566 for a discussion of the vulnerable zone of a T wave.)

Post-PVC Perfect Compensatory Pause

1. What happens to the sinus pacemaker when the PVC is producing its QRS and T?
   ANS.: It remains undisturbed, unless the PVC propagates backward through the AV node to depolarize the atrium and sinoatrial (SA) node.
2. What is upward or backward conduction through the AV node called?
   ANS.: Retrograde conduction. It is also called ventriculoatrial (VA) conduction.
      Note: Blockage of backward conduction through the AV node is called retrograde block.
3. If there is retrograde block following a PVC, what happens to the regular P-P interval during and around the PVC?
   ANS.: Nothing. The SA node is not disturbed and continues firing independently. The sinus P wave may be hidden in the QRS-T of the PVC, but if it is visible you will find the P-P interval undisturbed. (See the discussion of ventriculophasic arrhythmia, p. 488, for an explanation of one of the exceptions to this answer.)
4. What may we call a lack of connection between a ventricular depolarization and atrial depolarization, as when a PVC has retrograde block?
   ANS.: AV dissociation.
5. If there is momentary AV dissociation due to a PVC with retrograde block, when does the next regular QRS occur after the PVC?
   ANS.: When the next P wave can produce one. (See the upper rhythm strip, p. 517.)
6. When does a PVC not allow the sinus P wave (which may be hidden in the PVC) to produce a QRS?
   ANS.: When the atrial depolarization that originated from the SA node reaches the AV node but finds it refractory because of the effect of the PVC.
      Note: A PVC can retrogradely depolarize the AV node and make it refractory to the downcoming sinus P wave.

Hidden P would be here

The dropped QRS would have
occurred here

A sinus P was produced but is hidden by the abnormal QRS-T of the PVC. A QRS was not produced because the AV node was refractory, owing to the retrograde depolarization of the AV node by the premature beat.

7. If the PVC replaces the next expected regular QRS by making the AV node refractory to the downcoming P wave, when does the next QRS occur?
   ANS.: After the next P wave that comes down to a recovered AV node.
8. What is the pause called that results from a PVC replacing a regular QRS but with the postpause QRS coming at its usual time?
   ANS.: A perfect, complete, or fully compensatory pause. Sometimes it is simply called a compensatory pause.
      Note: A PVC occurring in the presence of complete AV block does not necessarily have the postextrasystolic QRS at the usual R-R interval. If the

PVC occurs early, the next QRS may come slightly early. If the PVC occurs late, the next QRS may come slightly late.

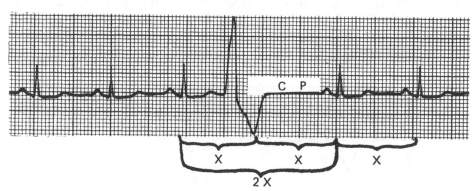

A complete compensatory pause is said to exist when the R-R interval containing the PVC is two times the R-R interval of the basic rhythm. If X = the basic R-R interval, bcause the R-R interval containing the PVC is 2X there is a complete compensatory pause (CP).

9. If retrograde conduction into the atria occurs from a PVC, what is the usual P wave vector direction?

   ANS.: Superior; i.e., there are usually negative P waves in the inferior leads.

   Note: Because the retrograde P is also directed anteriorly, it is typically positive in V1.

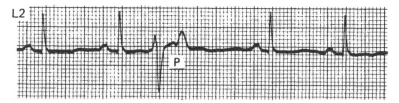

PVC with retrograde atrial conduction. The negative P on the upstroke of the T wave represents retrograde atrial conduction.

*10. If retrograde atrial conduction occurs from a PVC, when, after the P wave, does the next sinus P wave occur? Why?

   ANS.: The next P wave generally occurs at an interval slightly longer than the usual sinus cycle. See p. 502 for explanation.

*11. How can you sometimes differentiate a PVC with a retrograde atrial P' wave from a junctional premature complex with aberrant QRS conduction and a retrograde P'?

   ANS.: If the R-P' interval is less than 120 msec (0.12 sec), it is highly unlikely to be due to a PVC.

Interpolated PVCs

1. When does a PVC not replace a regular QRS? Why?

   ANS.: When there is retrograde VA block and the sinus rate is slow. A slow rate or a relatively early PVC allows the sinus P wave to occur late enough after the

PVC for the partially depolarized AV node to have recovered enough to allow the anterograde atrial depolarization to pass through the AV node.

2. What is a PVC called that does not interfere with the next QRS, i.e., does not prevent a regular QRS from occurring from the P wave that may be hidden in the PVCs' QRS-T?

    ANS.: An interpolated PVC.

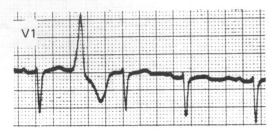

Interpolated PVC. The PVC did not prevent the regular P wave, buried in the T of the PVC, from getting through the AV node and producing its QRS.

3. How can a PVC conduct retrogradely through the AV node and not depolarize the atrium?

    ANS.: For some unexplained reason, especially when the ventricular rate is relatively slow, a PVC may only partially penetrate the AV node retrogradely and may merely make it relatively refractory for the downcoming impulse.

    Note: If conduction is not strong enough to traverse a length of tissue completely and ends in a gradual manner because of progressive weakening of the impulse, it is known as 'decremental conduction.'

4. How can one tell if a PVC has produced retrograde decremental conduction through the AV node if it never reaches the atrial muscle and so no retrograde P wave is produced by it?

    ANS.: The next P-R interval is prolonged because the AV node is now partly refractory if there was retrograde conduction through it from the PVC.

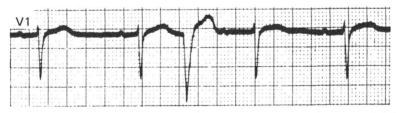

The PVC must have at least partially depolarized the AV node retrogradely because the next P-R interval is markedly prolonged (delaying the next QRS).

5. If the next P-R interval after a PVC is prolonged, and you infer that there was retrograde conduction through the AV node produced by the PVC, what is this inferred retrograde conduction called?

    ANS.: Retrograde *concealed conduction.*

    Note: Concealed conduction in the AV junction refers to penetration of this part of the conduction tissue by either an atrial or a ventricular impulse. The effects of the penetration, however, are seen only by the effect on the subsequent beat. The retrograde depolarization produced by the impulse may either delay conduction through the AV junction or delay the formation of a junctional beat.

6. If concealed VA conduction from an interpolated PVC prolongs the subsequent P-R interval, what does it do to the R-R interval of the sinus beats surrounding the PVC; i.e., what happens to the distance between the R waves preceding and following the PVC?

    ANS.: The sinus R-R interval with the interpolated beat in between is prolonged.

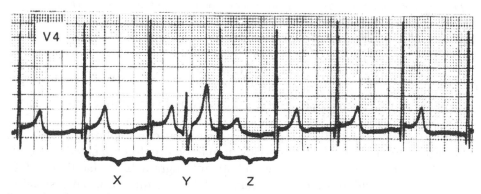

Interpolated PVC. The PVC allowed the regular P wave, buried in the T of the PVC, to get through the AV node and produce its QRS. Note that the R-R around the PVC (the interval Y) is longer than the regular R-R interval (X), and the subsequent R-R interval (Z) is shorter than the regular R-R interval.

7. If the QRS following an interpolated PVC is delayed because of prolongation of the P-R interval, what happens to the R-R interval of the two sinus beats after the interpolated PVC?

    ANS.: It is shortened. Now you have the pattern of an interpolated PVC with concealed conduction. There is a PVC between an R-R interval that is slightly longer than usual, followed by a slightly shorter-than-usual R-R interval. (See the diagram and rhythm strip that follow.)

    Note: A late train serves as an analogy for the short R-R interval following an interpolated PVC. If one train is late and the next train comes on time, the time interval between the two trains is shortened.

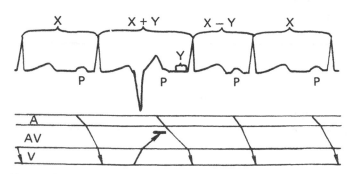

X = regular R-R interval; Y = degree of prolongation of P-R interval caused by the concealed retrograde VA conduction.

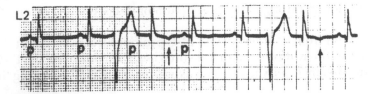

Interpolated PVCs. Note that the QRS following each PVC is not prevented from occurring, although it appears late owing to a prolonged P-R interval. The cause of the prolonged P-R interval is the retrograde conduction through the AV node. The late postinterpolated QRS causes the pattern of a long R-R around the PVC, followed by a shorter R-R than expected. Note the postextrasystolic T change (arrows) due to a change in previous cycle length.

*8. What is the significance of an interpolated PVC?
   ANS.: On auscultation it may imitate a three-beat run of ventricular or atrial tachycardia.
   Note: An interpolated junctional depolarization can explain an ECG with intermittent prolonged P-R intervals. It may be due to concealed firing of a junctional or ventricular focus with both anterograde block (so that no QRS is produced) and retrograde decremental VA conduction. This situation might produce either a pseudo AV block (Mobitz type 2) or, if the background rate is slow enough, only a sudden prolongation of the next P-R interval (concealed VA conduction) [102, 113].

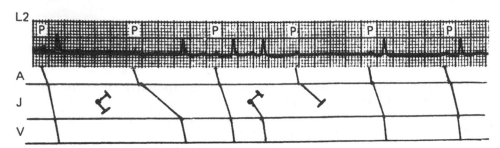

The second P wave finds the AV node partially refractory owing to a probable concealed premature junctional impulse that is blocked in both directions. The premature impulse partially depolarizes the AV node and therefore is followed by a long P-R interval. The second junctional premature impulse is blocked only retrogradely, but it depolarized the AV node enough to block the sinus impulse completely and produce a pause.

Group Beating[1]

1. What is meant by the term *bigeminy*?
   ANS.: A rhythm in which the beats occur in groups of two.
2. What can cause bigeminal rhythm?
   ANS.: There are many causes, the commonest being a PVC or PAC every other beat.

---

[1] A regularly recurrent pattern of irregularity is termed an *allorhythmia*.

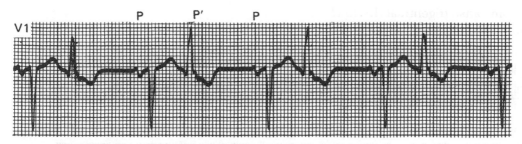

Bigeminy due to PVCs. Note that the P' waves are seen near the end of each ectopic QRS. Every PVC of this tracing conducts retrogradely into the atrium.

3. How can a bigeminal rhythm be produced by a conduction system block?
   ANS.: If every third beat is dropped owing to complete SA or AV block at every third beat, bigeminy is produced.

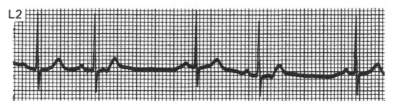

Bigeminy due to blocked PACs. The negative notch at the bottom of every second S-T segment is a P'. If there were no PACs, the diagnosis would be 3:2 type 1 second-degree AV block at the SA node, i.e., a sinus Wenckebach.

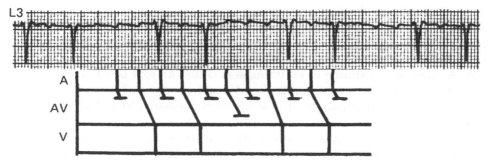

Bigeminy due to dropped beats. Sawtoothed atrial flutter waves at a rate of 230 are visible. Every other flutter wave is always blocked. Every nonblocked flutter wave gets through the AV node with a progressively longer F-R interval, resulting in a dropped beat with every third AV conducted beat (Wenckebach periods or type 1 second-degree AV block).

4. Is the word *coupling* synonymous with bigeminy?
   ANS.: No. Coupling merely refers to the interval between a normal beat and a subsequent ectopic premature beat. Thus we use the terms *fixed* or *variable* coupling to describe their relation.
   Note: To call two PVCs in a row 'coupled' is redundant, as all PVCs are coupled. They may be called 'couplets' or, better still, 'PVCs in pairs' or 'paired PVCs.'

5. What can cause trigeminal rhythm?
   ANS.: The causes are the same as for bigeminal rhythm.

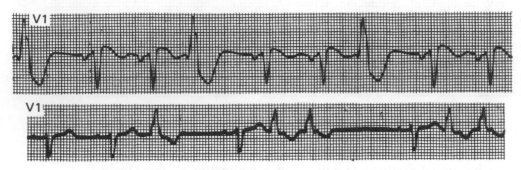

PVCs in trigeminy in two patients. Retrograde P waves follow the paired PVCs in the lower tracing. A long P'-P interval follows the retrograde P' waves, caused by SA block. (See p. 503 for SA block due to premature P waves.)

6. What is meant by the 'rule of bigeminy'?
   ANS.: Long cycles favor the appearance of PVCs. The compensatory pause follow-ing a PVC constitutes a long R-R interval, and it in turn favors precipitation of a further PVC. Bigeminal rhythm therefore tends to perpetuate itself.
7. What is the commonest cause of group beating with a repeat pattern making groups of 2, 3, or 4 other than PVCs or PACs?
   ANS.: Type 1 second-degree block.

---

*Concealed Extrasystoles

*1. What is meant by a concealed extrasystole?
   ANS.: It refers to a series of PVCs appearing at apparently random intervals but which are actually in trigeminy or bigeminy and blocked near their source, so that they often never enter the ventricles at all.
   Note: A block at the source of an impulse is called an exit block; i.e., it is failure of an impulse to exit from its site of origin.
*2. How can you recognize the presence of a series of concealed PVCs that are (a) bigeminal or (b) trigeminal?
   ANS.: a. The interectopic intervals always contain an odd number of sinus beats, e.g., 3, 5, 7, 9 [110, 112].

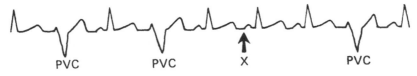

At X, a concealed PVC leaves three sinus beats.

   b. The interectopic intervals always contain two sinus beats plus a multiple of 3, e.g., 5, 8, 11.
   Note: Concealed extrasystoles are usually missed because long strips are not obtained when random PVCs with occasional bigeminy or trigeminy are seen.

Possible Causes of PVCs

Reentry Theory

1. Why is the term *irritable heart* a poor one for the heart of a patient with PVCs?

    ANS.: One of the theories that explains the cause of PVCs depends on the presence of a *depressed* area in conduction tissue.

2. What is the theory of PVCs produced by reentry into and from a depressed area of myocardium called?

    ANS.: Reentry theory.

3. Describe the two types of reentry.

    ANS.: a. For the 'tail-catching' type of reentry

    (1) Assume that somewhere in a ventricle a normal impulse traveling along a conducting fiber comes to a bifurcation because of the presence of a side branch. The impulse must divide and travel along both the main fiber and the side branch.

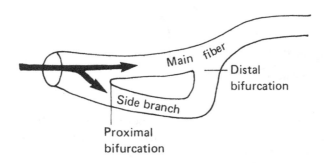

    (2) Now suppose that, because of an incomplete forward block along the side branch, only very slow conduction can occur along the side branch. This slowed impulse traveling along a side branch never reaches the main fiber because when conduction along the main fiber reaches the distal end of the side branch, where there is another bifurcation, it must again divide and travel retrogradely along the side branch. This sequence extinguishes the slow anterograde conduction in the side branch.

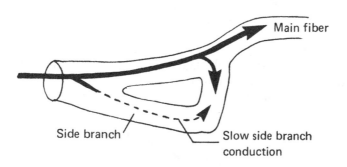

    (3) Now assume that this retrograde pathway is *blocked.* The very slow forward conduction in the side branch now may reach the normal pathway so late that it finds the normal fiber recovered from its refractoriness and ready for another impulse.

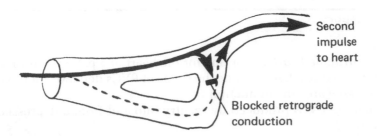

Second
impulse
to heart

Blocked retrograde
conduction

b. For the circular type of reentry
   (1) Assume that an impulse down a Purkinje fiber must divide at the proximal bifurcation of a side branch, and that the side branch has a complete block to forward conduction.

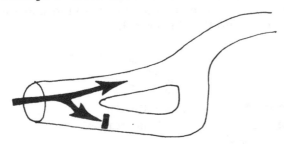

   (2) When the impulse along the main fiber reaches the distal end of the side branch, there is another bifurcation, and again the impulse must divide. Therefore it travels retrogradely down the side branch as well as forward along the main fiber; i.e., there is only unidirectional block.

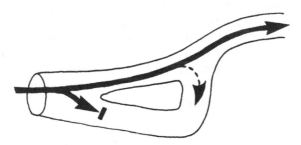

   (3) Finally, assume that very *slow* retrograde conduction occurs along the side branch that is blocked anterogradely. If it is slow enough, it finds the main fiber recovered enough to send another impulse to the rest of the heart.

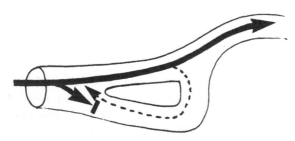

4. Why is the reentry theory useful?

ANS.: a. It helps to explain why PVCs seem to depend on the preceding sinus beat.
   b. It can explain repetitive tachycardias.
   c. It helps to explain 'fixed coupling,' i.e., why PVCs tend to occur at a nearly constant, or fixed, interval after the previous normal beat.

   *Note: a. Unidirectional block has been produced experimentally in depressed sections of Purkinje fibers [25]. If these depressed fibers are fired by an early beat such as an ectopic focus, the unidirectional block is exaggerated, and reentry could then occur, producing a second early beat.
   b. It has been shown that depressed conduction can be slow enough to allow sufficient time for the normal area of the reentry pathway to recover from its refractoriness which may require as long as 300 msec (0.3 sec). Depressed segments may conduct at 1/100 of normal velocity.
   c. The usual conduction fiber has an action potential with a rapid phase 0 and a resting potential of about – 85 mv. The depolarization of these fibers is due to rapid sodium influx. These fibers are called fast cardiac fibers. If damage such as acute ischemia alters the resting membrane potential to between – 60 and – 40 mv, the fast fibers are no longer depolarized by the sodium influx. Depolarization of the fast fibers becomes slow because of calcium influx through a slow membrane channel. This influx is called the slow response. The slow rate of depolarization and low amplitude of action potential results in slow conduction, a necessary condition for reentry [147].
   d. When the AV node, bundle of His, and bundle branches are involved in a reentry circuit, it is known as macroreentry. When reentry occurs in the peripheral Purkinje system, it is microreentry. Microreentry has been demonstrated in a variety of experimental preparations [41A].

*5. What can exaggerate the asynchrony of conduction between a slowly conducting, depressed Purkinje fiber and an adjacent normally conducting branch, so that the slow retrograde conduction is more likely to find the normal fiber ready for reentry?

ANS.: a. Early depolarization, i.e., a short preceding diastole [3].
   b. Vagotonia (by shortening refractory periods nonuniformly). This occurs primarily in the atria.
   c. Bradycardia. (It accounts for the observation that slow rates are likely to lead to PACs or PVCs.)
   d. Many antiarrhythmic drugs. (Further slowing of the already slow conduction may convert delayed conduction into complete block.)

   *Note: a. Digitalis toxicity can also cause PVCs by complex effects on the Purkinje fibers. In canine experiments, digitalis affects the left Purkinje fibers earlier than those on the right and may account for the observation that the left ventricle is often the site of origin of digitalis-induced arrhythmias [99].
   b. Exercise can also bring out PVCs. If treadmill exercise brings out PVCs, it has no meaning in a healthy subject. In patients with

known or suspected cardiac disease, however, exercise-induced PVCs increase the incidence of future coronary events, but not significantly more than with ischemic S-T changes alone, i.e., about 10 percent per year [132].

c. Subjects with thick and longitudinal false tendons are 30 times more likely to have PVCs than those without such false tendons. It is well known that most false tendons contain Purkinje fibers which when stretched may be arrhythmogenic [127A].

Multiform Versus Multifocal PVCs

1. What can cause PVCs to change configuration? What are different forms of PVCs called?

ANS.: PVCs can change configuration owing to

   a. Aberrant conduction caused by different degrees of slowing along the partially blocked reentry pathway, so that the reentrant impulse finds the main conduction system at different stages of recovery. They should therefore be called multiform, not multifocal.

   *Note: Stimulation of the ventricular endocardium at one site can produce multiform complexes if the stimulus is induced during the relative refractory period of the previous cycle [13].

   b. The occurrence of PVCs after P waves (end-diastolic PVCs). This situation can cause fusion of different degrees between the initial depolarization of the ventricle from the ectopic ventricular focus and final depolarization of the ventricle from the sinus node.

   *Note: Aberrant conduction may imitate a pair of multiform PVCs because if a PVC is conducted retrogradely through the AV node and enters an AV bypass or return pathway, the returning impulse may occur so early that it is aberrantly conducted. (See section on reciprocal beats, p. 534.)

*2. When does a PVC cause a QRS that is narrower than the supraventricular QRS?

ANS.: If the patient's supraventricular QRS has a bundle branch block and the focus for the PVC is in the blocked bundle, beyond the area of block.

   Note: a. Multiform PVCs are listed under the heading 'complex PVCs,' because they are more likely than uniform PVCs to be associated with myocardial disease and the development of fatal arrhythmias [4]. Also included under this heading are frequent PVCs, runs of two or more in a row, and those encroaching on a preceding T wave (R on T phenomenon). Frequent PVCs and the R on T phenomenon, however, are probably dangerous only in the presence of acute ischemia or a prolonged Q-T interval.

   b. Myocardial abnormalities can also manifest through PVCs if they are wider than 120 msec (0.12 sec), have an S-T segment with an initial isoelectric shelf, or have a T wave in the same direction as the QRS.

*3. If PVCs vary between RBBB and LBBB patterns, are they multifocal?

ANS.: It has been shown that a single focus in the LV can produce ectopic beats that change intermittently between LBBB and RBBB patterns. This situation is especially likely if an aneurysm is the source of the PVCs [53].

Ectopic Focus Theory

1. How can a premature ventricular depolarization occur without reentry but still be dependent on a previous depolarization and so produce fixed coupling?

   ANS.: Action potential studies have shown that under some abnormal metabolic conditions spontaneous depolarization can occur as soon as phase 3 drops to about − 40 mv [133].

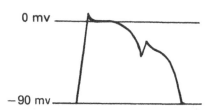

2. What is an oscillatory after-potential and how may it cause a PVC?

   ANS.: Under abnormal metabolic conditions an action potential may undershoot the resting potential (hyperpolarization) and then rebound toward threshold to produce an after-potential. If the rebound is high enough, it may reach threshold itself or allow a subthreshold stimulus to reach threshold and produce one or a series of early depolarizations [35].

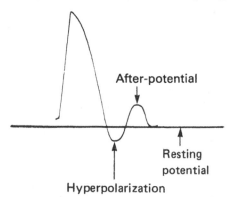

This abnormal premature depolarization may have such a high-amplitude after-potential that it reaches threshold and causes another premature complex.

3. What abnormal conditions have been shown to produce oscillatory after-potentials experimentally?

   ANS.: Digitalis excess, especially with low potassium, excess calcium, beta-adrenergic stimulation, and rapid stimulation [36, 130].

PVCs Versus Parasystole

Parasystole Defined

1. Because every part of the ventricle that contains Purkinje fibers can become a pacemaker, why do these automatic cells not fire and produce a QRS whenever the ventricle is not refractory?

   ANS.: The SA node's automatic cells have a faster (steeper) phase 4 rise and reach threshold sooner than do any other automatic cells in the conduction system. This faster phase 4 causes depolarization that spreads throughout the heart and extinguishes all the slower automatic cells before they can reach firing threshold.

2. What do we call an automatic cell that is not extinguished by the faster depolarization generated by the SA node?

    ANS.: Such a pacemaker focus is called a parasystolic focus. It is said to be 'protected' by an entrance block.

3. If an unextinguishable parasystolic focus is present, when does it produce a depolarization complex in the ECG?

    ANS.: Whenever the myocardium is not refractory.

4. What are a series of parasystolic beats called?

    ANS.: Parasystole.

5. What is the surgical equivalent of a parasystolic focus in the ventricle?

    ANS.: A fixed-rate electronic ventricular pacemaker competing with the patient's basic rhythm.

    Note: A fixed-rate pacemaker may fire during the vulnerable period of a previous QRS if the patient resumes his or her own sinus rhythm. (See p. 566 for an explanation of the vulnerable period.) It can produce ventricular tachycardia or fibrillation (usually only if the patient has an episode of transient ischemia or electrolyte imbalance). Therefore it is surprising that parasystolic ectopic beats in the early or late postinfarction period are less likely to cause sudden coronary death than are other types of PVCs [5, 66]. The fact that parasystole is often found in normal hearts may explain some of these results [88].

Parasystole and Coupling

1. Does a parasystolic QRS have a fixed relation to the previous QRS?

    ANS.: No. On the contrary, the hallmark of the ECG diagnosis of parasystole is the absence of fixed coupling.

2. What is the variable relation of a parasystolic QRS to the previous QRS called?

    ANS.: Variable coupling.

3. When should you always suspect ventricular parasystole?

    ANS.: Any time you see what appear to be PVCs but with variable coupling.

    Remember: Marked variable coupling always suggests parasystole.

    Note: a. Some degree of a variable coupling is seen, even with ordinary PVCs [77]. As much variation as 140 msec (0.14 sec) has been seen in the absence of parasystole. Any greater variation is considered a sign of parasystole.

    *b. Because a relatively long R-R interval is followed by a relatively long refractory period, there may be some delay in the exit of an ectopic impulse from its circuit, thereby increasing the coupling interval. Therefore you may observe longer coupling intervals after longer cycle lengths, even in cases of reentry. If the reverse occurs, suspect parasystole.

    *c. When a parasystolic rhythm is intermittent, each 'run' is usually initiated by an ordinary PVC. Also, a parasystolic rhythm can change for a few seconds into a bigeminal rhythm with PVCs from the same focus as the parasystolic rhythm.

    *d. It is common to have 'couplets' or PVCs in pairs if there is variable coupling of more than 0.11 second [127].

Parasystolic Entrance and Exit Blocks

1. What protects a slow parasystolic focus from being depolarized by the faster sinus beats, as are all other automatic cells with a slower phase 4?

   ANS.: It must be protected by what is called an 'entrance block,' the nature of which is unknown. This unidirectional insulation is the essential difference between a parasystolic focus and all other automatic cells.

   Note: a. One well-defended theory suggests that the parasystolic focus is actually firing at a rapid rate with varying degrees of exit block. The rapid firing keeps the adjacent tissue refractory to any impulses coming into it, because if a center fires rapidly enough the absolute refractory period occupies the whole of the ectopic cycle [113].

   b. A parasystolic ectopic focus does not always occur when expected, even when the ventricle is not refractory. It is because there may be first-, second-, or third-degree exit blocks from the parasystolic focus [60]. Entrance blocks can also be intermittent. When a sinus beat occurs within a certain critical period after the ectopic beat, the entrance block may be ineffective and the ectopic focus can be discharged [21].

   c. When two parasystolic beats occur consecutively, thus representing the shortest ectopic cycle length, the cycle length may be slightly longer than that calculated from longer interectopic intervals. The reason is unknown [109]. One study showed that if a nonparasystolic beat falls either during the first or last half of the ectopic cycle, there is often about a 10 percent shortening of the parasystolic cycle length [16].

*2. Why is it important to realize that a parasystolic focus may have variable degrees of exit blocks?

   ANS.: It accounts for

   a. The occasional nonappearance of a parasystolic beat when it should have occurred at a time when the ventricle was no longer refractory.

   b. The occasional occurrence of parasystolic ventricular tachycardia at an exact multiple (twice or more) of the parasystolic rate when the exit block suddenly disappears.

*3. Other than the degree of exit block, what controls how often a parasystolic QRS shows itself in a continuous tracing?

   ANS.: The sinus rate. If the sinus rate QRS complexes are frequent, the ventricle is refractory for most of the parasystolic ectopic beats. If the sinus rate is slow, many of the ectopic beats find the ventricles recovered, and so more of them show.

   Note: a. Occasionally, the parasystolic rate increases if the sinus rate increases perhaps because the parasystolic pacemaker cells are under influences similar to those that modulate the sinus rate.

   b. A ventricular focus that was previously entered by each sinus impulse may intermittently acquire a protective entrance block and change into an autonomous parasystolic form of discharge. Intermittent parasystole is usually initiated by a typical PVC with fixed coupling [111].

Parasystole and Fusion Beats

1. What happens if a ventricular ectopic focus fires just after a P wave, so that the normal supraventricular depolarization through the AV node is able to proceed through some of the ventricle?
   ANS.: The ventricle is partly depolarized from above and partly from the ectopic ventricular focus.
2. What is the beat called that is produced by depolarization that is partly from a PVC and partly from above through the usual conduction system?
   ANS.: A fusion beat.
3. How can you recognize a fusion beat?
   ANS.: a. It shows a QRS that looks intermediate between the patient's normal sinus beat and the QRS of the ventricular ectopic focus.
   b. It will follow a P wave with a P-R interval shorter than usual for that subject.

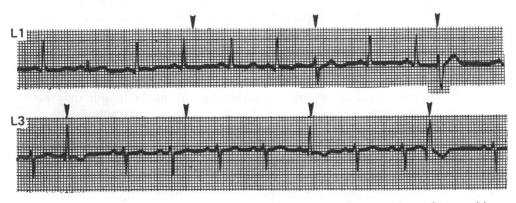

Ventricular parasystole in a 58-year-old woman with a severe cardiomyopathy and intractable failure. Note the markedly variable coupling. The arrows march out the shortest apparent interectopic interval. The arrows without an ectopic beat beneath them represent the time when the parasystolic focus fires but finds the ventricle refractory. Note the fusion beats when the focus fires just after a P wave.

Note: a. Because retrograde conduction from the peripheral Purkinje system to the bundle of His is probably not more than 60 msec (unless an electronic pacemaker has produced the ventricular beat [73]), the P-R of a fusion beat should never be shortened by more than 60 msec [79].
   b. A fusion beat may be narrower than the supraventricular beat in the presence of a bundle branch block because a premature beat from *beyond* the blocked area may allow almost simultaneous conduction along both bundle branches; i.e., the supraventricular impulse depolarizes the unblocked branch while the ectopic premature focus depolarizes the blocked branch almost simultaneously.
4. When are fusion beats commonly seen other than in parasystole?
   ANS.: Any time a premature ventricular focus fires during a P-R interval (in the absence of complete AV block, e.g., if there is an end-diastolic PVC or AV dissociation).

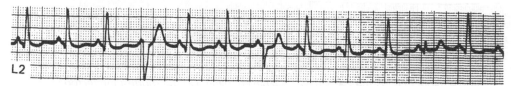

Two fusion complexes due to PVCs and a sinus arrhythmia. The fourth complex shows no fusion because it came earlier in relation to the P wave than did the second and third ectopic complexes. Thus the sinus P could not contribute to this complex. There may also be a 10-msec increase in the coupling interval in the last PVC. This pattern is not parasystole because the coupling is almost fixed.

Parasystole Recognition

1. What are three major characteristics of ventricular parasystole?

    ANS.: a. Variable coupling.
    b. Fusion beats.
    c. R-R intervals of the widely separated ectopic beats are some multiple of the shortest interectopic intervals.

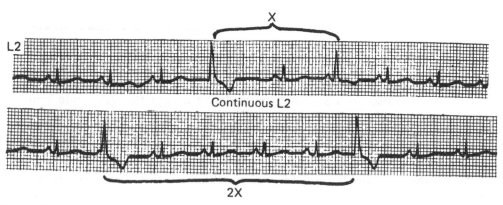

Ventricular parasystole. Note the varying coupling, the long interectopic interval (2X), exactly twice the short one (X), and the ectopic QRS that comes after a P wave, causing fusion (halfway in contour between the normal QRS and the ectopic QRS).

2. How can you prove the presence of parasystole?

    ANS.: When you see variable coupling, measure the distance between the ectopic beats with the shortest interectopic interval. Let your calipers mark this shortest interectopic interval along to see if all the ectopic beats occur at distances from one another that are multiples of the shortest interectopic intervals. The only time a parasystolic impulse should not be expected is when the ventricle is obviously refractory owing to the presence of the sinus-produced QRS.

    Note: a. Atrial parasystole is much rarer than ventricular parasystole [23].

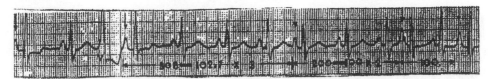

Atrial parasystole. Note that (1) the PACs have variable coupling, (2) the shortest interectopic interval (labelled 100 [msec]) is approximately one-half or one-third the other interectopic intervals.

*b. It is a curious fact that the P′ waves in many of the reported cases of atrial parasystole resemble one another in that the initial upstroke in lead 2 tends to be tall and peaked [109].

*c. When an ectopic rhythm depolarizes the atrium but not the SA node owing to a protection block, sinus parasystole may occur [108].

*d. Because the sinus node may be constantly reset by the atrial parasystolic depolarization, there may be a constant P′-P interval. It is termed *reversed coupling* or parasystolic bigeminy.

RECIPROCAL BEATS

1. How can VA retrograde conduction through the AV node also produce forward conduction through the AV node?
    ANS.: When the impulse goes slowly retrogradely through the AV node and reaches the middle or top of the AV node, it can divide into two forces: one depolarizing the atrium retrogradely and the other coming back down again (by way of a separate AV pathway in the AV node and bundle of His) to stimulate the ventricles and produce another (early) QRS.

2. What do we call the early beats caused by back-and-forth conduction through the AV node?
    ANS.: Reciprocal or echo beats. The pair of beats is called a reciprocal couplet.

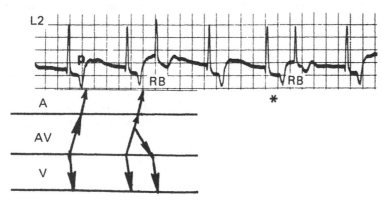

The negative P following the QRS signifies a junctional pacemaker. The premature beats are reciprocal beats (RB). Because it requires slow retrograde conduction through the AV node area to allow the forward AV pathway to recover conduction properties, the R-P′ interval is often slightly prolonged if it produces a reciprocal beat (*), usually to at least 200 msec (0.20 sec). Note that the reciprocal beat is slightly aberrant (no q wave).

*3. How is a reciprocal beat recognized at a glance?

ANS.: It is an early beat with these characteristics: a PVC or junctional pacemaker QRS is followed by a retrograde P wave with a prolonged R-P′ interval, which in turn is followed by a QRS that usually looks like the ordinary QRS for that patient (if there is no aberrancy).

Note: If a ventricular focus acts as the initiating stimulus it may

a. reach the top of the AV node or even the atrium and then come back down by a different pathway in the AV node and bundle of His.

b. travel part way up the bundle of His or AV node and then back by a different pathway in the AV node and bundle of His.

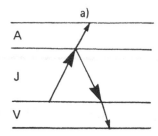
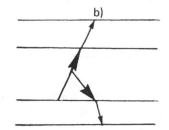

c. Reciprocal beating can even occur in the presence of AV block if the AV block is high in the node and the stimulating source is a ventricular ectopic beat [107].

*4. What is a reversed reciprocal or echo atrial depolarization?

ANS.: It is a retrograde P′ wave preceded by a QRS that is generated from the atrium. It is difficult to distinguish from a blocked premature atrial contraction (PAC). One explanation is that an anomalous pathway (with slight anterograde block) bypassing the AV node carries the impulse retrogradely [81]. An early PAC with a long enough P-R interval (long refractory period of the anterograde AV conduction pathway) can allow time for the accessory pathway to recover from refractoriness and so favor a retrograde reentry [115].

*5. What is the effect of digitalis on reciprocal beating from junctional pacemakers?

ANS.: It may encourage it by slowing retrograde VA conduction, allowing the forward pathway to recover [39].

Note: Retrograde conduction through the AV node is normally more difficult (slower) than anterograde conduction [26]. (The R-P′ interval is usually longer than the P-R interval.)

*6. What does a reciprocal beat following a PVC most imitate?

ANS.: It mimics an interpolated PVC at first glance. However, the long R-R, short R-R pattern of interpolation is missing (see p. 521).

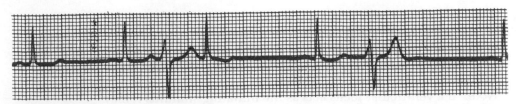

An imitation of an interpolated PVC. The pattern of interpolation is missing; i.e., the R-R of the normal beats surrounding the PVC is not longer than the basic R-R interval, and the cycle length after the postextrasystolic beat is not shorter than the basic R-R interval. This pattern, then, is probably a PVC followed by a reciprocal or echo beat. The second PVC in the strip came after a long diastole that probably lengthened the refractory period of the His-Purkinje fibers, so that retrograde conduction and a reciprocal beat could not occur.

ECTOPIC TACHYCARDIAS

What is the 'rule of hundreds' for tachycardias?

ANS.: The rule refers to atrial rates: 400 ± 50 beats per minute = atrial fibrillation
300 ± 50 beats per minute = atrial flutter
200 ± 50 beats per minute = atrial tachycardia

Note: a. Ventricular tachycardia also has about the same range as atrial tachycardia, i.e., 200 ± 50, but it is more likely to have a rate on the slower side.

b. These ranges are, of course, not absolute but apply to about 90 percent of all the various tachycardias.

Atrial Fibrillation

Atrial and Ventricular Rates

1. Does the atrium actually contract at 400 ± 50 times per minute in atrial fibrillation (AF)?
   ANS.: Yes, even though most of the contractions are weak or incomplete.
2. What is the usual range of the rate of ventricular response in untreated AF?
   ANS.: 120 to 180.
3. Why is the ventricular response so much less than the rate of atrial contractions in AF?
   ANS.: a. Although the atria contract at 400 ± 50 per minute, each contraction has a different strength and many depolarization waves may never penetrate the AV node.
   b. The AV node is usually refractory to more than 200 impulses per minute.
   c. Those impulses that are too weak to travel entirely through the AV node make the AV node partially refractory for the next impulse, which might otherwise have been strong enough to get through.
4. Why is the ventricular response grossly irregular in AF?
   ANS.: Probably because atrial depolarization waves of different strengths reach the AV node in haphazard order.
5. What are the undulations at 400 ± 50 per minute in the ECG called?
   ANS.: They are called f waves.

Characteristics of f Waves
1. In which leads are f waves best seen? Why?
   ANS.: In V1. Probably because V1 is closest to the atria and the direction of f waves is usually anterior and to the right (suggesting that they usually start in the left atrium).
2. List four characteristics of the f waves of AF.
   ANS.: They are
   a. Usually best seen in V1 [125].
   b. Irregularly spaced.
   c. Irregular in height.
   d. The waves closest together are separated by a distance that would make a rate of about 400 ± 50.
3. What is the significance of coarse fibrillation f waves, i.e., f waves 1 mm or more high?
   ANS.: Coarse f waves suggest the presence of atrial overload, either right or left (more likely due to volume than merely to a thick wall). All patients in one study with coarse fibrillation had left atrial enlargement on x-ray film [125, 129].
4. What is the significance of a fast f wave rate?
   ANS.: The faster the rate, the more likely is the probability that atherosclerotic heart disease is present. It may be because the atria are not damaged as much as in rheumatic valvular disease. The f rate in coronary heart disease tends to be more than 500 per minute, but in valvular disease it is usually less.
   Note: The configuration in coronary disease tends to have rounded apexes, whereas in valvular disease the apexes are sharper and more uniform; i.e., the f waves tend to look more alike [1, 100].
5. How can you quickly count the rate of f wave undulations?
   ANS.: Count the number of small divisions between undulations and divide into 1500.
*6. What is the significance of a slow, irregular ventricular rate with AF in the absence of drugs that block AV conduction, e.g., digitalis and propranolol?
   ANS.: It signifies that AV node disease is present. Because patients with AV node disease often have SA node disease as well, there is little hope of achieving or maintaining sinus rhythm with electroversion.

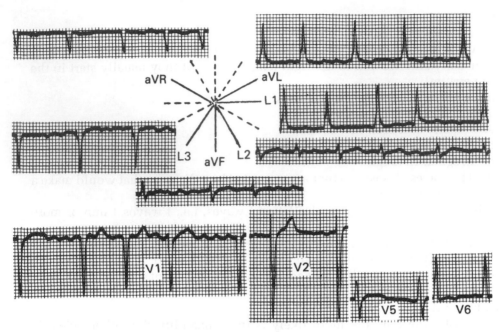

AF in a 58-year-old man with a cardiomyopathy probably due to coronary disease. The irregular baseline undulations of f waves are best seen in V1. They are small in amplitude, and the shortest f-f intervals are three small divisions apart; i.e., they would give a rate of 500 per minute.

7. Is there such a rhythm as 'flutter-fibrillation'?
   ANS.: Probably. Occasionally, the f waves have some of the characteristics of both fibrillation and flutter. It may be due to atrial dissociation, with one atrium fluttering and the other fibrillating [136]. The usual flutter-fibrillation, however, is a misreading of coarse fibrillation f waves. The differentiation from flutter is described on p. 550.

Causes of AF

1. What are the usual causes of AF?
   ANS.: a. Atherosclerotic coronary disease, chronic or with acute myocardial infarction.
         Note: AF develops in about 8 percent of patients with acute infarction but lasts less than 24 hours in 90 percent of cases [63].
      b. Left atrial enlargement, as in rheumatic mitral disease.
      c. Idiopathic cardiomyopathies (including 'lone' fibrillation [91]).
      d. Right atrial enlargement, as in atrial septal defects (usually after age 30).
      e. Thoracotomy, especially when done for cancer of the lung [6].
      f. Toxic effect of drugs such as alcohol.
      g. Thyrotoxicosis.
      Note: Digitalis can cause AF, but this cause is extremely rare.

2. What percentage of patients with AF have been found clinically to have no heart disease?
   ANS.: Five to ten percent [10]. Transient AF can be precipitated in normal subjects by some event that causes vagotonia, e.g., coughing or vomiting [91]. Excess alcohol ingestion occasionally results in a bout of AF, especially on the 'morning after' [69].

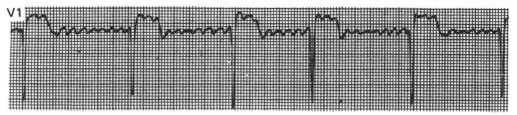

This pattern was called atrial flutter-fibrillation by several readers. Against flutter, however, is the fact that not only is the QRS rhythm irregular but also the f waves are of varying shapes, heights, and distances apart. There are f wave rates of 500 (three small divisions apart), and the f waves were smaller in L2, L3, and aVF (not shown). All these are typical of AF. Therefore this ECG should be called AF with coarse f waves.

3. Which arrhythmias usually initiate AF from sinus rhythm?
    ANS.: a. An accelerating short run of atrial tachycardia (fewer than six beats) [58].
    b. A single PAC.
    Note: Characteristic of the PAC that initiates AF is the short coupling interval from the previous sinus beat. In one study a coupling interval (P-P′ interval) that was 50 percent or less of the sinus cycle length (P-P interval) generally led to AF [58].

AF and Digitalis

1. Why can digitalis cause different rates of junctional pacemakers to occur in patients with AF?
    ANS.: a. Too much digitalis can cause AV block, and so the next fastest automatic cells take over, or 'escape.' These cells are usually in the AV junctional area. (Digitalis excess rarely allows a takeover by a ventricular pace-maker.) It results in a slow junctional pacemaker of between 40 and 60. It is a *passive* junctional rhythm, or junctional escape rhythm.

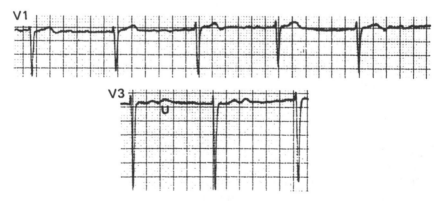

The regular rhythm at a rate of 60 in the presence of AF indicates that junctional escape rhythm is present. The relatively high U waves in V3 tell us that hypokalemia has probably exaggerated the toxic effect of digitalis on the AV node and caused the complete AV block.

b. Digitalis excess can cause increased automaticity (a steeper slope of phase 4) in automatic cells near the AV node, resulting in a shorter diastole and thus causing junctional rates as rapid as 70 to 150. It has been called an *active* junctional rhythm in general, but specifically it has been referred to by the confusing term *nonparoxysmal AV junctional tachycardia* when it accelerates and then ends gradually. The word *tachycardia* was applied because even a rate of 70 is faster than normal for the junctional area [57]. It has also been termed an *accelerated junctional rhythm*, which is the expression that is used here, as *nonparoxysmal* does not seem to apply and *tachycardia* is better used for rates of more than 100 (see ECG below).

Note: Whether the phase 4 slope of either the NH or His bundle automatic cells increases with digitalis is in doubt. A study has shown that NH or His bundle rhythms (induced in dogs by destroying the SA or AV node) are slowed with increasing doses of digitalis [114]. If true, either the rapid pacemakers induced by digitalis are in the Purkinje-like cells of the internodal tracts near the AV node or the addition of other abnormalities such as hypokalemia is required for digitalis to induce rapid pacemakers in the His bundle.

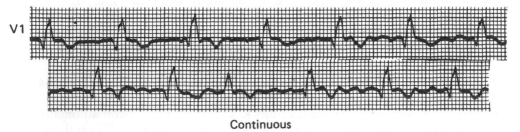

Continuous

Digitalis excess in a cyanotic woman with congestive failure due to an atrial septal defect with severe pulmonary hypertension and reversed shunt. Note the regular QRS rhythm in the top row despite AF. Because the QRS rate is about 80 and the configuration is the same as when the rhythm is irregular, this pattern represents an accelerated junctional pacemaker.

2. In a subject with AF, what should make you suspect that digitalis has produced an active or passive pacemaker?

ANS.: The appearance of a regular rhythm, either slow or fast, whether persistent or for only a few beats.

*3. In a subject with AF, how can digitalis cause an increase in ventricular rate but with the rhythm still irregular?

ANS.: It can cause a rapid junctional pacemaker, but at the same time it can cause type 1 second-degree block in the bundle of His, thus producing an irregular ventricular response [49, 94]. It may be called 'junctional tachycardia with type 1 second-degree exit block.' It can be recognized by seeing a type 1 second-degree block R-R pattern (see p. 541).

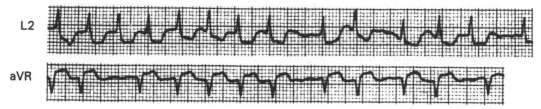

L2

aVR

This ECG is from a 55-year-old woman with AF due to rheumatic heart disease. Despite digitalis and diuretics, she was showing increasing symptoms of heart failure. Lead 2 shows a run of junctional tachycardia at a rate of 160. The groups of two suggest type 1 second-degree block. The groups of three in lead 2 and five in aVR show a type 1 block pattern, i.e., a decreasing R-R interval for at least two cycles and pauses that are less than twice the shortest R-R. Therefore digitalis toxicity is producing not only a junctional tachycardia but a type 1 second-degree exit block from the junctional pacemaker.

AF with Aberrant Conduction

1. How can both a very short and a very long cycle in AF cause aberrancy (see pp. 505–508)?

   ANS.: a. If diastole is extremely short, one of the bundle branches or their divisions may still be partly refractory when the QRS begins again.

   b. A very long diastole may allow the threshold potential to rise so that the phase 4 of some action potentials rise closer to zero potential by the time they reach threshold [32]. This could slow conduction—more in some fibers than in others, thus producing aberrancy. This situation is known as phase 4 aberrancy, which can occur only if the AV junctional cells are sufficiently depressed that they cannot reach threshold first and capture the ventricles. Phase 4 aberrancy also explains why when the AV junctional cells capture the ventricles with a slow escape rhythm they often show aberrant conduction.

2. What circumstances cause the same short cycle length to produce aberrancy only intermittently? Why?

   ANS.: Only when the short cycle is preceded by a long one may aberrancy be produced at the end of the short cycle. It is known as the Ashman phenomenon.

   Note: a. After excitation, the myocardial cell passes through a period of nonresponsiveness known as the absolute refractory period. The refractory period of the right bundle branch is longer than that of the left bundle branch, and the anterior division has a longer Q-T (longer refractory period) than the posterior division. Therefore the right bundle and anterior division of the left bundle are more susceptible to conduction delays when depolarization is early.

   b. The Ashman phenomenon can change the T wave even in the absence of QRS aberration [1B].

3. If a wide, abnormal QRS occurs in the presence of AF, what are the two major possible causes?

   ANS.: a. An ectopic beat (generated below the bundle of His) may have occurred.

   b. Aberrant conduction has occurred.

   Note: It has been argued that a ventricular ectopic beat, contraction, or complex should not be called a PVC in a patient with AF because it may be no more 'premature' than many of the other early complexes in this irregular rhythm.

4. How can you tell that a single abnormal-looking beat in a run of fast beats in AF is aberrant rather than ectopic?

ANS.: A wide second QRS in a run of fast beats is probably aberrancy because that second QRS is the only beat of the group that follows a short cycle preceded by a long cycle (see p. 507 and ECG for question 8).

5. Which is more likely to have fixed coupling, an aberrant beat or a PVC?

ANS.: A PVC. (Beware of the fortuitous fixed coupling occasionally seen in aberrant beats.)

6. Why does a PVC often cause a postextrasystolic pause in AF?

ANS.: Because a PVC may partially depolarize the AV node retrogradely and make it refractory for a longer period than usual. This pause is therefore due to concealed VA conduction (see p. 520, question 5).

Note: The pause after a bizarre-looking complex should be considered due to a PVC with retrograde conduction if it is longer than the average cycle length of 10 normally conducted beats [45].

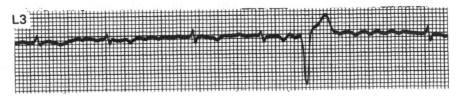

AF with a post-PVC pause due to concealed retrograde conduction.

7. Because both aberrant conduction and a left ventricular ectopic QRS are likely to resemble RBBB, how can you tell the difference by contour alone?

ANS.: An ectopic complex from the LV is more likely to have

a. A notched or slurred R or qR in V1, with the initial peak taller than the second, rather than an RSR′ (triphasic complex) of the usual RBBB [34, 45, 128].

b. A deep S in V6 (QS or rS), rather than the shallow, wide S of the usual RBBB [45]. The deep S of a PVC in V6 probably reflects the marked left axis deviation often seen in PVCs. If, however, an anterior divisional block is already present, even an aberrant QRS may show a deep S in V6.

c. An axis either in the right upper quadrant or markedly anterior.

d. An initial vector that is different from the patient's usual vector. (This also occurs in about 50 percent of aberrantly conducted beats.)

Note: It is so unusual for an RBBB type of ventricular ectopic complex to have the same initial forces as the patient's usual QRS that a similar initial force is strong evidence against ectopy [106].

e. An excessively wide QRS, i.e., 140 msec (0.14 sec) or more.

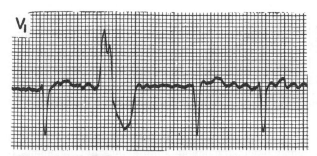

PVC from the left ventricle in V1. The initial peak is taller than the second peak.

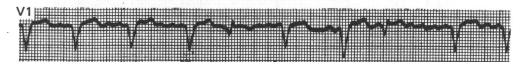

AF in a 68-year-old man with a severe idiopathic cardiomyopathy and failure. The wide QRS is due to LBBB. The two early beats are probably PVCs because they have fixed coupling, there is an extra-long diastole following the second one (concealed retrograde VA conduction), and they have a QR configuration.

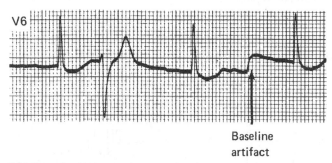

Baseline
artifact

PVC from the LV in V6 showing the deep S and the change in initial vector.

*8. How can you tell the difference between a right ventricular ectopic complex and the occasional aberrant conduction that looks like LBBB?

ANS.: Aberrancy is the most probable cause of an occasionally abnormal QRS if

    a. The coupling interval is variable but not due to parasystole.

    b. The abnormal QRS ends a short cycle that is preceded by a long cycle (Ashman phenomenon). See p. 524 for the rule of bigeminy, which competes with the Ashman phenomenon and makes it less useful.

    c. The abnormal QRS looks like RBBB, especially if the V1 has a triphasic complex with a small septal r (an rSR' or rSr'), and it has a shallow, wide S in V6, with the initial QRS contour the same as the usual one for that subject.

    d. There are varying degrees of RBBB in many abnormal beats.

    e. There is no long pause following the abnormal QRS.

    Note: a. See Chap. 30, p. 605, for a definitive differentiation by bundle of His recordings.

          b. The only really useful ECG criterion for differentiation is the presence of fixed coupling, which tells you that the wide QRS is very likely *not* due to aberrancy.

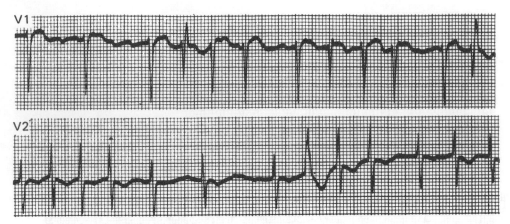

AF with aberrant conduction. The widened QRS complexes are probably not PVCs because not only do they follow the long R-R, short R-R sequence, but also there is slightly variable coupling, their initial vectors have not changed, their pattern is that of RBBB (with an rSr' in V1), and there is no long pause after them. The eighth QRS in V1 is only partially aberrant. The slight variations in amplitude in V1 are probably due to respiration. Equiphasic leads often show respiratory voltage changes. Although a monophasic complex as in V2 here is unusual with aberrancy, it can occur, especially if posterior myocardial infarction is present.

9. What is the value of differentiating aberrant conduction from PVCs in AF?
   ANS.: PVCs may mean digitalis toxicity; with aberrant conduction the patient may have more digitalis to slow the rate.

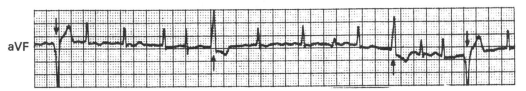

A 35-year-old woman had mitral stenosis and intractable heart failure despite daily administration of 0.5 mg of digoxin. Multiform PVCs (arrows) in the presence of AF are usually a sign of digitalis toxicity. Stopping digitalis eliminated the PVCs.

10. Can an ectopic premature atrial depolarization with a P' occur in AF?
    ANS.: No. Any complete depolarization of the atrium very likely causes conversion to sinus rhythm, even if only for one beat.

*11. Why is it dangerous when AF develops in a patient with atrioventricular pre-excitation, i.e., with the Wolff-Parkinson-White syndrome?
    ANS.: An accessory bundle does not have the built-in delay that is found in the AV node. Therefore the ventricle receives the irregular impulses at a very fast rate and may fail to maintain a normal cardiac output.

Note: a. In AF the ventricular response depends on the conduction properties of the accessory pathway. The ventricular rate may be as slow
as 210 per minute in some patients to 310 in others [17]. Digitalis
and verapamil may speed up the ventricular response because
they may shorten the refractory period of the accessory pathway.
Lidocaine or beta blockers usually have no significant effect on
the accessory bundle [4]. However, lidocaine has abolished atrial
tachycardia in the WPW syndrome [29].

b. If a patient with WPW syndrome shows only intermittent accessory AV bundle conduction during sinus rhythm, the refractory
period of the accessory bundle is usually long enough to prevent a
very rapid ventricular response if AF develops. Therefore sudden
death is probably not a hazard in such patients.

c. About 20 percent of patients with the WPW syndrome (i.e., with
tachycardias) have episodes of AF. About 90 percent of those who
have AF episodes have type A delta waves [17, 130].

d. If submaximal treadmill exercise or procainamide 10 mg per
kilogram intravenously does not block the accessory bundle, the
bundle's refractory period is probably short enough to suggest a
high risk of sudden death [142] if AF occurs [71, 142].

e. With age, the accessory pathway may become blocked to various
degrees so that high ventricular rates with AF diminish with
increasing age [140].

Atrial Flutter

Atrial Flutter F Wave Characteristics
1. What is the usual rate of atrial flutter F waves?
   ANS.: It is usually 300 ± 50 waves per minute.
2. What are the two theories used to explain the origin of atrial flutter?
   ANS.: a. The rapid atrial rate results from the rapid firing of an ectopic focus in
   the atrium, similar to atrial tachycardia but faster.

   b. A rapid wave of excitation encircles the roots of the superior and inferior
   venae cavae. 'Daughter waves' of excitation then spread from the circular
   pathway to the remainder of the atria. It is known as the *circus movement*
   theory.

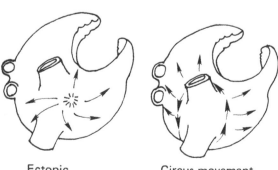

Ectopic   Circus movement
atrial focus

3. What is characteristic of flutter waves? Why?
    ANS.: In the leads with the largest and most characteristic F waves, flutter waves
        tend to be sawtoothed in shape, and there are no isoelectric periods between
        waves. As an atrial pacemaker rate increases, the Ta wave becomes larger
        and the isoelectric periods shorter [97].

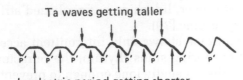

As the rate of the ectopic P′ waves increases, the Ta amplitude increases and the
isoelectric period shortens. When the rate is fast enough, the isoelectric shelf finally
disappears, to leave fully developed flutter waves.

4. In which leads are sawtooth-shaped flutter waves usually best seen?
    ANS.: In the inferior leads, i.e., leads 2, 3, and aVF.
        Note: In the commonest type of flutter the F waves are really retrograde P′
        waves because they are negative in the inferior leads 2, 3, and aVF. The
        ectopic focus seems to be low in the atrial septum. There is a rare type,
        however, in which the focus is high in the right atrium [41].
5. Are flutter waves regular in timing, size, and shape?
    ANS.: Yes, invariably.

F Wave–QRS Relations
1. What is the usual ratio between an atrial flutter rate and its ventricular rate?
    ANS.: The ratio is usually 2:1, i.e., one ventricular response to every two flutter
        waves. For example, if the flutter rate is 300, the ventricular rate is usually
        150. This relation is so common that whenever you see a patient with a
        regular tachycardia at a rate of approximately 150 per minute, you are
        correct most of the time if you predict that the patient has atrial flutter with
        a 2:1 AV block.

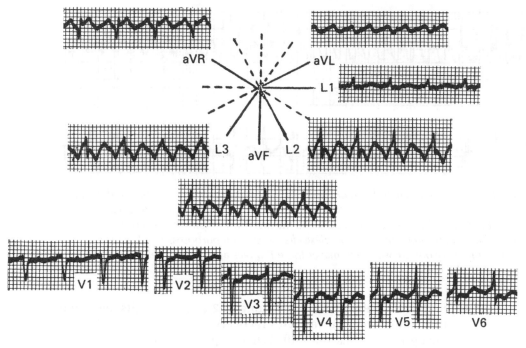

Atrial flutter. Because this 68-year-old man has chronic obstructive pulmonary disease and heart failure, his QRS voltage is low and the F waves are exaggerated. Note that the F waves are best seen in the inferior limb leads (L2, L3, and aVF), and that in V1 they are only barely visible. The flutter rate is 300, and the ventricular rate is 150; i.e., there is the usual 2:1 block.

Note: *a. High AV conduction ratios can occur. When the AV block is regular, the high conduction ratios are usually even-numbered, i.e., 4:1, 6:1, or 8:1.

b. It used to be thought that quinidine, simply because of its vagolytic effect, was capable of causing a 1:1 response with flutter. It is now believed that it also produces 1:1 AV conduction by slowing the flutter rate and thereby reducing the rate at which impulses enter the AV node thus decreasing the amount of physiologic AV block. Digitalis usually, but not always, prevents this [105]. Large doses of quinidine can, however, depress AV nodal conduction.

*c. If 1:1 conduction occurs in an adult with atrial flutter in the absence of a drug such as quinidine, suspect an AV nodal bypass pathway such as an atrio-His accessory bundle [16]. In infants with atrial flutter, 1:1 conduction may occur in the absence of drugs or accessory bundles.

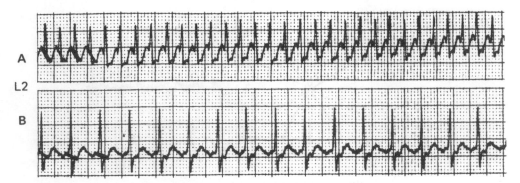

These two strips are from a 6-month-old boy with an atrial septal defect. The atria are fluttering at a rate of about 332. A. There is an unusual phenomenon of 1:1 conduction. B. Taken a few hours later, the usual 2:1 conduction can be seen. The first few complexes of each strip have the F waves drawn in through the QRS complexes for orientation purposes. The T wave is superimposed on every other F wave and makes these F waves appear taller than the ones superimposed on the QRSs.

> *d. Ventricular rates of 300 for as long as 2 days in adults and 5 days in infants have occurred with recovery, despite a shock-like state during the tachycardia [30]. When it persisted for 5 days in one young patient with an otherwise normal heart, it resulted in death from congestive failure [37].

2. If the AV block is irregular, what happens to the ventricular rhythm?
   ANS.: It is irregular.

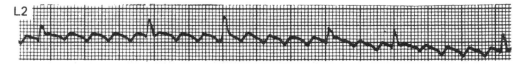

Atrial flutter at rate of 250, with variable AV block, probably secondary to digitalis effect.

3. When does the irregularity have an easily recognizable pattern in atrial flutter?
   ANS.: If the F-R intervals follow a type 1 second-degree AV block (Wenckebach) pattern.

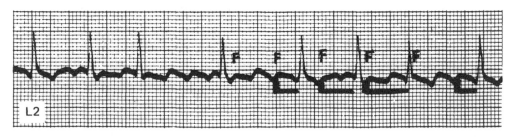

Every other F wave is always blocked while the unblocked ones (marked F) are conducting with a type 1 second-degree AV block (Wenckebach periods).

4. How can you recognize or bring out F waves in atrial flutter if the QRS and T are superimposed on them?

ANS.: a. If you try to picture what the baseline would look like without the QRSs, a pattern of sawtoothed F waves are usually visualized in leads 2, 3, and aVF.

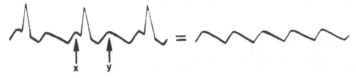

The F wave at x did not produce the QRS perched on it because the F-R interval is too short. The F wave at y probably conducted to the next QRS. The F waves on the right are exactly the same as the ones on the left but without QRS complexes to obscure the pattern. Note that the classic F wave pattern has a short initial rising limb and a longer downward limb.

b. Try vagal stimulation, e.g., carotid sinus pressure which often produces a temporary AV block and uncovers the F waves, because there then are fewer QRSs.

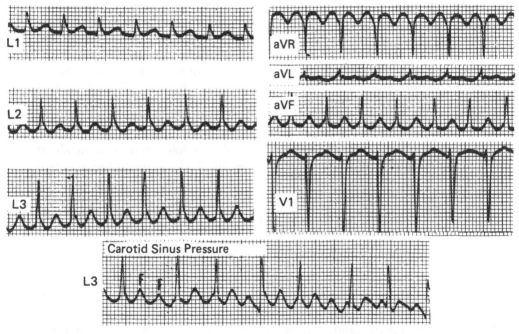

Atrial flutter with F waves hidden by QRS complexes. In the bottom strip, from lead 3, the vagal stimulation of carotid sinus pressure has uncovered large F waves by producing intermittent AV block.

5. If no F waves are apparent (F waves can be very small) and the AV block is chaotically irregular, so that an irregular response of the ventricle occurs, what may flutter mimic?

ANS.: AF.

6. Describe three major differences, already discussed, between AF and atrial flutter.
   ANS.: a. In timing, shape, and size, atrial flutter waves are regular and AF waves are irregular.

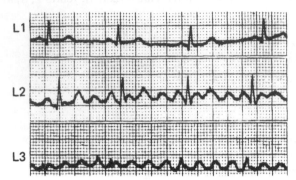

A 75-year-old man had a parkinsonian tremor. Lead 1 shows that the rhythm is really sinus, but leads 2 and aVF give a false first impression of atrial flutter due to the hand tremor. Note that the false F waves are more like giant AF f waves because they tend to have different heights and widths.

   b. Atrial flutter F waves are best seen in leads 2, 3, and aVF. The f waves of AF are best seen in V1 or V2. (On rare occasions the reverse is true; i.e., the f waves of AF are best seen in leads 2, 3, and aVF, and the F waves of flutter are best seen in V1.)
   c. The distance between the F waves in atrial flutter would make a rate of 300 ± 50, whereas in AF the shortest interval between f waves would make a rate of about 400 ± 50 (see the arrhythmia on p. 538).
      Note: *a. Type II flutter is an unusually rapid atrial flutter that can be as fast as 400 per minute and may be transitional between classic flutter and AF. This type of flutter has been seen in about one-third of patients in whom flutter develops following open heart surgery [143].
         b. The faster ventricular and atrial rates of AF, flutter, and tachycardia are expected in infants and children because the refractory periods of their conduction tissue, including the AV node, are shorter than in adults [28].
         c. The larger the atria, the slower the flutter rate.
7. Why does atrial flutter sometimes imitate atrial tachycardia?
   ANS.: In both atrial flutter and atrial tachycardia, V1 often shows an isoelectric shelf or space between F waves.
      Note: In the common caudocranial type, with typical F waves in L2, L3, and aVF, V1 may look like a series of P′ waves with an isoelectric shelf between F waves. It is postulated that it is because the circular (circus movement) loop of atrial excitation is probably an ellipsoid, mostly in the sagittal plane, with the largest diameter in the Y (inferosuperior) axis.

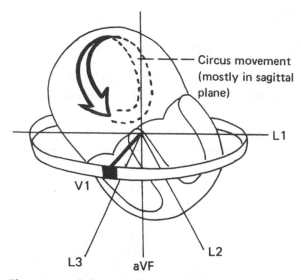

There is very little vector force parallel to the X axis (L1 axis) or Z axis (V1 axis). The major forces are parallel to L2, L3, and aVF.

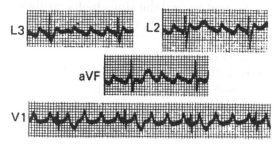

Note that even though the F waves of atrial flutter are typical in L2, L3, and aVF, V1 has a nearly isoelectric line between F waves. Thus in V1 it looks more like an atrial tachycardia.

*8. What is the effect of digitalis on the rate of atrial flutter waves?

ANS.: It is variable, depending on whether a vagal or a direct effect predominates; a vagal effect speeds up the rate by shortening the atrial refractory period, and a direct effect slows it up by some unknown mechanism.

Note: Speeding up the flutter rate with digitalis may convert the flutter to AF. Stopping the digitalis lengthens the refractory period and may convert the fibrillation to sinus rhythm.

Causes of Atrial Flutter

1. Which atrial arrhythmias tend to come from a damaged or enlarged (a) right atrium? (b) left atrium?

ANS.: a. Right atrial damage produces all the atrial arrhythmias, i.e., fibrillation, flutter, and tachycardia.

b. Left atrial damage tends to produce only AF.

2. Can digitalis toxicity cause atrial flutter?

ANS.: There are rare reports of this happening [22, 48].

Note: Atrial flutter, as well as AF, has been induced by vagal stimulation (carotid sinus stimulation) [31]. When experimental AF is required in dogs, bilateral vagal stimulation is used plus electrical stimulation of the atrium.

3. About what percentage of subjectswith atrial flutter have pulmonary disease?

ANS.: About 50 percent [24].

Note: Although pulmonary embolism rarely causes atrial flutter, when flutter suddenly occurs in an adult for no apparent reason, a pulmonary embolism should be suspected.

Atrial Tachycardia

1. How is the P-R interval affected by atrial tachycardia (AT)? Why?

ANS.: It tends to become prolonged because the earlier an impulse reaches the AV node, the more it is blocked.

Note: If the atrium is paced at faster and faster rates by an electronic pacemaker, the P-R becomes longer and longer due to the effect of early beats on the cells in the N region of the AV node (see p. 471, question 1).

2. How is the P-R interval affected by sinus tachycardia? Why?

ANS.: The P-R interval tends to remain normal even at rates similar to that of AT because the sympathetic stimulation that caused the sinus tachycardia tends also to shorten the P-R interval. Sympathetic stimulation accelerates conduction through the AV node.

3. When is it difficult to tell an AT from a sinus tachycardia?

ANS.: a. When the P vector of the AT is normal in amplitude and direction, the rate is below 180, and the P-R interval is not prolonged.

   b. When a sinus tachycardia is more than 150.

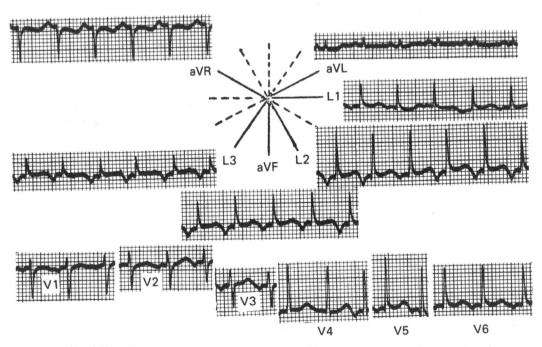

AT at a rate of about 150. The − 90° P vector makes the diagnosis of a low atrial or junctional pacemaker obvious.

4. Because sinus tachycardia can have about the same rate as AT, i.e., about 150, how can you tell the difference between them on an ECG if the P vector directions are normal?

    ANS.: a. In sinus tachycardia the P waves are more likely to be tall (the faster the sinus rate, the taller the P waves); in AT the P' waves are likely to be small.

           b. In sinus tachycardia the P-R interval is more likely to be normal; in AT the P-R is more likely to be long.

           c. Carotid sinus pressure can often slow a sinus tachycardia significantly [87]. With vagal stimulation an AT either remains unaffected, is slowed slightly, or suddenly breaks into sinus rhythm.

           d. SA node reentry type of supraventricular tachycardia is a type of atrial tachycardia that uses the SA node as part of its pathway. This should be suspected if the rate is about 125 (too slow for the usual atrial tachycardia) and they run in paroxysms rather than gradual increases and decreases as in sinus tachycardia.

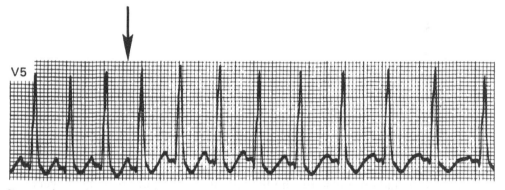

Sinus tachycardia at a rate of 150 per minute. Carotid sinus pressure (at the arrow) induced a gradual slowing to 115 per minute. With release of pressure, you should also expect gradual acceleration to the original rate.

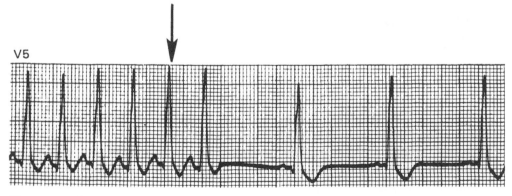

AT at a rate of 155 per minute. Carotid sinus pressure (at the arrow) induced an abrupt change to sinus rhythm at a rate of about 60 per minute.

    Note: a. The incidence of AT in acute infarction is about 5 percent [52, 133].

           b. It was extremely rare to find ATs in acute infarction before 1966 because before the days of continuous monitoring, many transient

episodes must have been missed and many ATs have aberrant conduction and thus may have been mistakenly called ventricular
tachycardias.

Reciprocal Beat Theory for ATs
*1. Show how a reciprocal beat can follow a surpaventricular beat.
     ANS.: a. Assume that the downcoming impulse divides to travel down two
     pathways (alpha and beta) through the AV node.

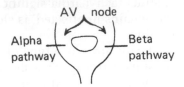

b. Then assume that one pathway, e.g., the beta one, is blocked to
anterograde conduction but not to retrograde conduction.

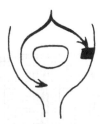

c. Assume next that the impulse divides at the distal end of the normally
conducting alpha pathway into a forward impulse that produces a QRS
and a retrograde impulse up the beta pathway, which, however, is very
slow.

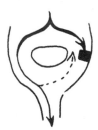

d. Now assume that this slow retrograde unblocked impulse divides high in
the node, one branch producing a retrograde P wave and the other reen-
tering the alpha pathway. The retrograde conduction must be so slow
that the alpha pathway has had time to recover from its refractoriness.

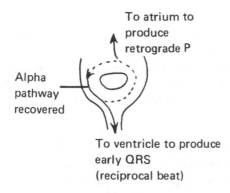

To atrium to
produce
retrograde P

Alpha
pathway
recovered

To ventricle to produce
early QRS
(reciprocal beat)

Note: a. This path is the circular type of reentry as described for Purkinje fibers on p. 526.

    b. If the retrograde beta pathway has recovered enough to conduct each impulse from the alpha pathway, a 'reciprocating tachycardia' can result [42]. It is also known as 'reentrant tachycardia.'

   *c. An earlier premature atrial beat causes a more delayed reciprocal beat because both alpha and beta pathways are more refractory after an earlier impulse. That this actually happens is demonstrated by the fact that atrial tachycardias have shown an inverse relation between the earliness of the first ectopic beat and the lateness of the second beat of the paroxysm [9].

   *d. Digitalis encourages reciprocal beating, presumably by depressing retrograde conduction in the junctional area via vagal stimulation, giving time for anterograde junctional conduction to recover and to produce another QRS. A report of AT induced by swallowing suggests that vagal stimulation can cause reentrant tachycardias [84].

    e. The QRS of reciprocal beats often shows aberrant conduction.

*2. What are the necessary conditions before an artificial PAC produced by a stimulating electrode in the right atrium can initiate an episode of AT?

  ANS.: The stimulation must produce a long P-R interval because a certain degree of AV block is necessary to cause enough slowing through the retrograde beta pathway for the alpha pathway to recover from its refractoriness [42].

  Note: Artificial stimulation does not produce a supraventricular tachycardia in normal subjects. Therefore this technique can be used to document the occurrence of AT if the arrhythmias have been too rare or fleeting for ECG evidence to be obtained [42].

*3. What is the 'unitary' theory of AT and atrial flutter? How does it affect terminology?

  ANS.: Some investigators believe that both atrial flutter and AT are due to an ectopic pacemaker that fires more rapidly for flutter than for AT [98]. They prefer the term *atrial tachysystoles* to describe them [51].

  Note: ATs may be due to reentry or to an ectopic atrial focus. The latter is rare in adults but common in children. The diagnosis of an ectopic focus is strongly suspected if

    a. The first P wave of the tachycardia has an anterograde direction.

    b. The P-R intervals are normal.

    c. The P waves are clearly visible [40]. Unfortunately, sinus node reentry tachycardias may have the same characteristics, except that the P-R intervals are usually prolonged [148].

AT in the WPW and Lown-Ganong-Levine Syndromes

1. How has the reentry theory been invoked to account for the supraventricular tachycardias seen in patients with an accessory AV bundle?

   ANS.: Assume that a premature atrial depolarization is blocked only anterogradely at the accessory bypass pathway but not at the AV node. The AV node pathway depolarizes the ventricle to reenter the anomalous pathway retrogradely and slowly. This action could establish a circular reentry tachycardia.

   Note: His bundle recordings and atrial and ventricular mapping studies have shown that the circus pathway usually uses anterograde AV conduction and retrograde Kent bundle conduction. It is known as orthodromic type of circus movement. 'Ortho' means 'right, correct, or straight.' It is usually easier to go down an AV node than retrogradely. However, occasionally the circus movement is down the accessory bundle and up the AV node (antidromic reentry) [68].

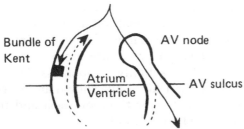

2. What other type of preexcitation syndrome probably uses bypass fibers as part of a circular pathway to produce supraventricular tachycardias?

   ANS.: With atrio-His preexcitation fibers, reentrant tachycardias can also occur and this is known as the Lown-Ganong-Levine (LGL) syndrome [76].

3. What usually is necessary before an AT is initiated by a PAC in a patient with an accessory bundle?

   ANS.: The impulse from a PAC must be early enough to conduct slowly through the AV node. By the time it reaches the bundle of His or ventricle, the accessory bundle has recovered and may now conduct the impulse retrogradely to excite the atrium and start a reentrant tachycardia [12].

   Note: AV node reentrant tachycardia is a misnomer because the two limbs of the reentrant circuit are outside the compact portion of the AV node. The accessory pathway (which may not function and does not produce a delta wave with sinus rhythm) will usually be the slow retrograde pathway and produce a late retrograde wave very close to the end of the QRS. Thus it may produce a pseudo R′ in V1 and a pseudo S in inferior leads [54A, 151A].

4. What is the difference between AV reentrant tachycardia and AV nodal reentrant tachycardia?

   ANS.: In AV reentrant tachycardia the reentry is through a slowly conducting accessory pathway outside the AV node. Therefore the P′ will come after the QRS. The R-P′ is always over 70 msec. The long R-P can cause the P to come just in front of the next QRS and be confused with sinus tachycardia and atrial tachycardia.

   Note: An AV nodal reentrant tachycardia uses the node for reentry and the classic ECG shows a short R-P′ interval.

AT with Block
1. What is meant by AT with block?
   ANS.: It means that with the AT there is a second-degree AV block. (A first-degree AV block alone is expected with atrial tachycardias and is therefore not referred to as AT with block.)
   Note: Because almost all ATs are paroxysmal (i.e., not permanent), the term paroxysmal atrial tachycardia (PAT) seems redundant. Even if it is chronic and persistent, as it is in the occasional patient, when reading an ECG it is impossible to know if it is one of those rare sustained types that can go on for years [85].

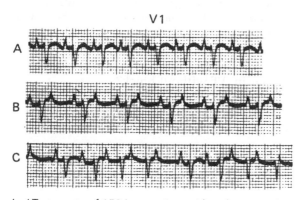

A. AT at a rate of 150 in a patient with pulmonary disease and digitalis toxicity. The tall, peaked P waves are due to the right atrial overload. B. AT with 2:1 block has developed. C. AT with type 1 second-degree AV block (Wenckebach periods) has occurred a minute later. Therefore B and C are two types of atrial tachycardia with block.

2. What are the clinical differences between AT with block and AT without block?
   ANS.: a. In AT without block, because they are due to reentry:
      (1) Vagal stimulation (as with carotid pressure) either does nothing or completely suppresses the reentry and allows sinus rhythm to take over.
      (2) The rhythm is regular unless it occurs in a short burst or is multifocal.
      (3) The cause is unknown. It is only occasionally caused by digitalis [89].
   b. In AT with block because they are due to an ectopic focus:
      (1) Carotid pressure or other vagal stimulation simply increases the degree of AV block without suppressing the ectopic pacemaker; i.e., the arrhythmia responds as if it were atrial flutter.
      (2) The rhythm is often irregular owing to variable degrees of AV block.
      (3) There is digitalis excess in about half the patients, often with hypokalemia.
   Note: a. If only patients with valvular or congenital heart disease with AT and block are analyzed, digitalis toxicity is rare [124].
      b. AT with block has been precipitated by anxiety and hyperventilation in one subject with a normal heart [144].

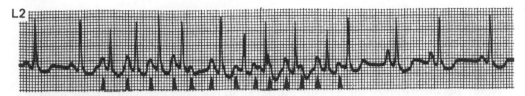

This ECG is from a 59-year-old man with runs of AT every few beats. It began 2 days after gallbladder surgery, although there was no abnormal cardiovascular history. Note the irregularity of the P′ waves in this short burst. Because only the fifth, ninth, and eleventh beats are blocked (i.e., there is only occasional second-degree AV block), it is not the usual AT with block. The P′ waves probably all look different because they fall on different places on the S-T, T waves. The tall P falling after the paroxysm is due to the aberrant atrial conduction after PACs in hearts with myocardial damage [19]. Note also the sagging S-Ts due to digitalis.

3. When is the ventricular rhythm irregular in AT without block?
   ANS.: a. When a short burst occurs.
         b. When there is multifocal or chaotic atrial tachycardia.
4. How does AT with block due to digitalis toxicity differ from that not due to digitalis?
   ANS.: a. Carotid sinus pressure probably does not stop AT due to digitalis. If AT is not due to digitalis, it occasionally reverts to sinus rhythm with this maneuver.
         b. In AT due to digitalis, atropine does not speed the atrial rate, and carotid pressure does not slow it [89]. If the AT is not due to digitalis, the atrial rate may quicken with atropine and slow with carotid pressure.

Junctional Tachycardias
1. Can you always tell the difference between a junctional tachycardia and AT?
   ANS.: No. When no P′, fibrillation, or flutter waves are seen with a supraventricular tachycardia, it is presumed to be either an AT with the P′ waves superimposed on the T or a junctional tachycardia with retrograde P waves superimposed on the QRS. However, there are occasional atrial tachycardias with P′ waves so small they are invisible to the naked eye despite the fact that they are not superimposed on QRS complexes [151].

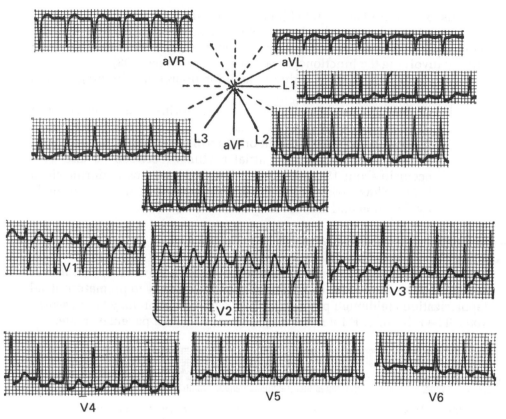

Atrial or junctional tachycardia at a rate of 185 in a 25-year-old man with tonsillitis and no cardiac abnormality. Because no P waves are visible and the QRS is not wide, it may be either a junctional tachycardia with the P waves superimposed on the QRS, or an AT with the P waves too small to be seen. Because it is not atrial flutter or fibrillation or a sinus tachycardia, the usual expression, 'supraventricular tachycardia,' is inappropriate because it does not stress that there are only two possibilities. Note the electrical alternans in V2 to V5.

2. What is meant by an accelerated junctional rhythm?

    ANS.: Because the normal junctional escape rate is between 40 and 60 beats per minute, a junctional rate above 60 (but not more than 100) is an accelerated junctional rhythm. (If, however, it begins and ends by acceleration and deceleration, it has been called by the confusing term nonparoxysmal junctional tachycardia [93].)

    Note: A junctional rate of more than 100 should be called simply a junctional tachycardia.

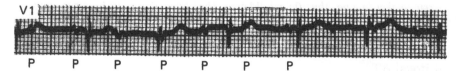

An accelerated junctional pacemaker with AV dissociation. The junctional rate is 85. The faster atrial rate of 135 should have controlled the ventricles. Because it did not, there must be marked AV block. This patient had acute inferior infarction, a common cause of transient AV block.

*3. What are the usual causes of accelerated junctional rhythms?
ANS.: Most are caused by digitalis, but accelerated junctional rhythms are also found in about 10 percent of patients with acute myocardial infarction [65]. Surgery involving the junctional area can also cause them [93].
Note: a. When this rhythm is due to anterior infarction, the prognosis is grave [65].
b. Ambulatory and intensive care monitoring can disclose brief episodes of relatively slow asymptomatic atrial tachycardias (below rates of 150) in about one-fourth of cardiac patients. Accelerated junctional or slow atrial rhythms (between 80 and 100) occur in about 15 percent of cardiac patients, mostly during sleep [122]. Slow atrial rhythms may be associated with sinus node dysfunction and sick sinus syndrome [35].

Wandering and Shifting Atrial Pacemakers

1. What is meant by a wandering atrial pacemaker?
ANS.: Haphazard changes in P wave configuration due to a pacemaker that moves from one site to another in the atrium but not due entirely to premature atrial depolarizations (although premature atrial depolarization may be present).
Note: The P-R and R-R intervals may change with each pacemaker site.

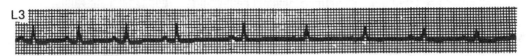

The varying shape of P waves and varying R-R intervals here are not respiration-dependent. This pattern therefore represents a wandering atrial pacemaker. Some believe that it is merely wandering within the sinus node.

2. What is another name for an atrial pacemaker that shifts between only two sites?
ANS.: A shifting atrial pacemaker.
3. What are two of the usual sites of origin of shifting atrial pacemakers?
ANS.: Pacemaking commonly shifts back and forth between the sinus node and one junctional or low atrial area.
Note: When a P wave begins at nearly the same time from the two separate sites, a fusion P wave results.

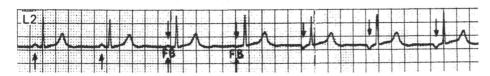

Shifting atrial pacemaker in a healthy 20-year-old man. The pacemaker shifts between sinus and low atrial or junctional areas. The intermediate-looking P waves (FB) are due to fusion.

Note: A shifting atrial pacemaker rhythm only rarely evolves into a multifocal AT.

Multifocal or Chaotic AT

1. Above what rate should a wandering pacemaker be considered to be a multifocal AT?

ANS.: Above 100. Multifocal AT rates range from 100 to 250 per minute [118, 120].

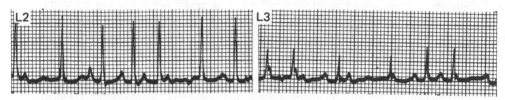

Multifocal or chaotic AT in a 70-year-old woman with chronic obstructive pulmonary disease (COPD), pulmonary fibrosis, and pneumonia. The irregularly spaced P waves, at a rate of about 160, vary in direction and amplitude.

2. In what type of patient is multifocal AT usually found? Is it due to digitalis?

   ANS.: Elderly patients who are very ill with COPD and are usually taking bronchodilators [120]. They are also commonly diabetic. It is not related to digitalis excess [74].

   Note: The hospital mortality in these patients is about 55 percent and is not related to the arrhythmia [8]. However, there is a rare benign variety of multifocal atrial tachycardia in young persons with otherwise normal hearts and a good long-term prognosis [27].

3. Which arrhythmia most commonly precedes multifocal AT?

   ANS.: Multifocal premature atrial beats [74].

4. Which other arrhythmia can multifocal AT most imitate?

   ANS.: It often looks like AF when the P waves are small.

   Note: Multifocal AT commonly develops into AF [74]. (It does not become AT with block.)

*5. What is meant by a 'chaotic atrial mechanism'?

   ANS.: A slow multifocal atrial pacemaker, i.e., a slow wandering atrial pacemaker [2]. This arrhythmia occasionally becomes a multifocal AT but usually remains slow [92].

   Note: Excessive accumulation of fat in the interatrial septum, termed *lipomatous hypertrophy of the interatrial septum*, is an uncommon atrial abnormality found in some elderly obese patients with multifocal or unifocal atrial tachycardias, wandering atrial pacemakers, or atrial fibrillation [47]. A 'dome and dip' configuration of the P wave in L2, L3, and aVF with a prolonged duration is found in about half of these patients [50]. Others simply have a low atrial pacemaker with purely negative P wave in L2, L3, and aVF [33].

I-II-III   **aVR-aVL-aVF**   **V₁-V₂-V₃**

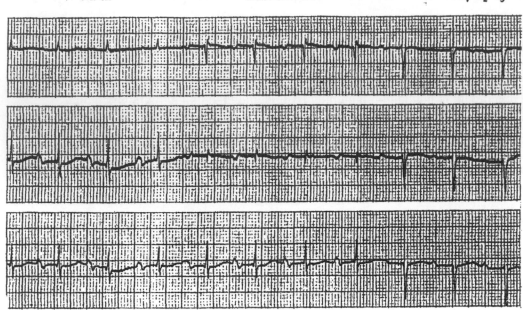

This is from a patient whose echocardiogram showed lipomatous hypertrophy of the atrial septum.

Isorhythmic Dissociation

1. What is meant by 'isorhythmic dissociation'?
   ANS.: Because *iso* means 'same,' it is easy to remember that the term refers to two pacemakers, one in the atrium and one below the atrium, each firing at almost the same time. It therefore refers to some attempt at synchronization of two pacemakers.
2. What are the two types of isorhythmic dissociation patterns seen?
   ANS.: a. The P oscillates rhythmically back and forth across the QRS.

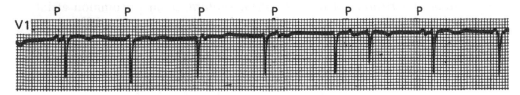

Isorhythmic dissociation due to independent atrial and junctional pacemakers. The conducted early beat (capture beat) suggests that AV conduction is intact.

     b. The P remains relatively fixed with respect to the QRS, being either inside or just after the QRS [70].

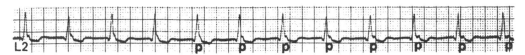

Isorhythmic dissociation. The notch on the downstroke of each QRS is a P wave.

3. How can the second type of isorhythmic dissociation just described be accounted for other than by AV dissociation?

   ANS.: It may not be AV dissociation at all but the effect of a junctional pacemaker with retrograde conduction [70]. An inferiorly directed P vector has been thought to be possible with a junctional pacemaker [83, 134] (see p. 496).

*4. What is the word sometimes used to describe a short burst of isorhythmic dissociation?

   ANS.: *Accrochage*, which is the French word for 'grappling.'

   Note: a. The term was coined when it was shown that if two fragments of isolated frog heart muscle are placed close together without touching one another they tend to discharge impulses at the same rate because of a 'pulling in' effect of the faster-moving fragment [117]. For it to occur, the rates of the two fragments must not differ by more than 25 percent. Whether the influence is mechanical or electrical is uncertain.

   b. Accrochage can occur even in complete AV block [78].

ELECTRICAL ALTERNANS

1. What is meant by electrical alternans?

   ANS.: Alternating amplitudes or configurations of P, QRS, or T complexes (or any combination) in which all the complexes originate from one pacemaker.

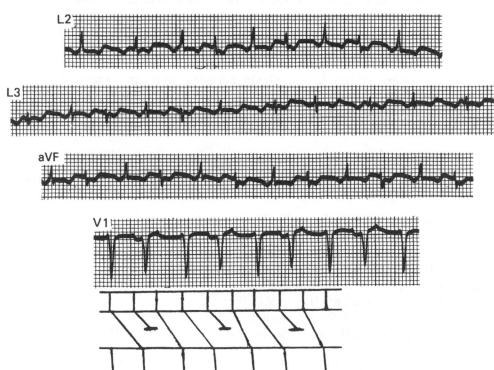

Electrical alternans in a man with malignant pericardial effusion. The atria are fluttering, and the F-R intervals are varying in Wenckebach periods. These leads were the only ones of the entire ECG that showed the intermittent runs of alternans.

2. What is the commonest type of alternans?
   ANS.: One in which only the QRS changes in alternate beats.
3. What is meant by total alternans? What is its significance?
   ANS.: Alternans in which the P, QRS, and T are all different in alternate beats.
   Tamponade with pericardial thickening is almost always present clinically
   with total alternans [20]. Rarely, however, pericardial disease is not present,
   but severe four-chamber enlargement is present instead.
   Note: The commonest causes of the effusion that can produce total alternans
   are malignant tumors, tuberculosis, or disseminated lupus erythematosus.
4. What are the three common causes of the usual QRS alternans?
   ANS.: Marked tachycardia, pericardial effusion, and severe myocardial damage
   (especially during a cardiac operation on a damaged myocardium).
   Note: a. Rates of more than 100 are usually necessary before even pericardial effusion or tamponade can produce electrical alternans [121].
   b. The removal of as little as 50 ml of pericardial fluid can abolish
   the electrical alternans [121].
*5. What is the most likely cause of electrical alternans in tamponade?
   ANS.: Anatomic oscillations or alternation of cardiac position.
*6. What rare type of alternans has been seen other than 2:1, i.e., for every two beats
   there is one alternation?
   ANS.: There is a 3:1 type but with transition complexes between the recurrent
   third complexes [121]. These patients often have no pericardial disease [20].
   Note: T wave alternans alone is seen clinically in severe myocardial disease
   [38], severe hyperkalemia due to uremia, acute myocardial ischemia especially during vasospastic angina, and in the post-tachycardia state if there is
   coexistent myocardial damage [137].
*7. Is electrical alternans an arrhythmia?
   ANS.: It is called an arrhythmia in many texts, but because it can occur with regular rhythms it is a misuse of the term. It is really an alternating aberrancy.
   Note: Electrical alternans in the absence of tamponade is highly indicative
   of a reentrant arrhythmia using a retrograde accessory pathway [43].

VENTRICULAR TACHYCARDIA

1. What is meant by ventricular tachycardia (VT)?
   ANS.: A rapid succession of at least three ventricular ectopic complexes.
   Note: A group of two abnormal-looking complexes may be due to a PVC
   followed by a reciprocal beat with aberrant conduction and so give the false
   appearance of a pair of multiform PVCs.
2. What do the QRS complexes look like in VT? Why?
   ANS.: They are wide and different from the normal QRS. It is because each
   complex originates in the ventricle, below the bifurcation of the His bundle.
3. What is the rate of a VT?
   ANS.: Its range is roughly the same as the slower ATs; i.e., instead of the AT range
   of 200 ± 50, it is between 150 and 200.
   Note: If the rate of a series of wide QRS complexes is more than 200, there is
   no time for an isoelectric space between them, which is one of the characteristics of ventricular flutter.

4. Is VT irregular?

ANS.: It may be grossly irregular only if it occurs in a short burst or paroxysm. (A short burst from any ectopic pacemaker in the atrium or ventricle can be grossly irregular.)

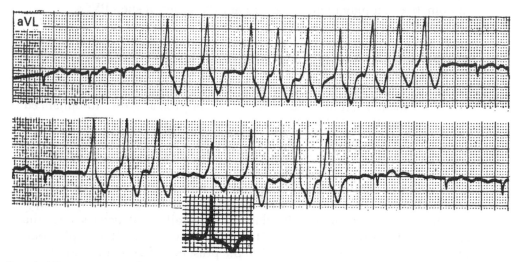

Pseudo VT in a 30-year-old woman with rheumatic mitral disease and AF. This strip is continuous. The first three complexes are the patient's regular QRSs. Then follows a series of very wide QRSs due to complete use of an AV bundle of Kent. Above the inset is a more classic fusion beat between AV accessory bundle and AV conduction. The inset shows a similar aVL complex in a previous ECG when a classic AV accessory bundle conduction was seen while the patient was in sinus rhythm.

The wide QRS complexes can easily be mistaken for a run of VT. Such ECGs have led to the mistaken belief that VT is grossly irregular. The intermittent Kent bundle conduction is probably due to the vagal effects of respiration; i.e., when the patient breathed out, the increased vagal tone blocked the AV node sufficiently to allow accessory bundle conduction.

Note: A slight irregularity may occur with slower rates of VT when a sinus P wave or an AF f wave occasionally manages to get through the AV node and partially captures the ventricles. Also, bidirectional VT may be slightly irregular (see p. 583).

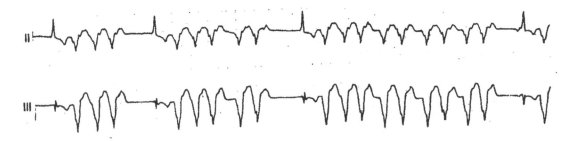

This is from a patient with heart failure due to dilated cardiomyopathy. The short bursts of repetitive VT show marked irregularity which is not a feature of sustained VT. Junctional escape beats interrupt the paroxysms of VT.

Mechanisms and Causes of VT

*1. What are the possible sources of the ectopic depolarization of a VT?
ANS.: a. The same source as for a PVC; i.e., it may be initiated by a preceding normal beat through some mechanism such as reentry or increased automaticity. It may in effect be a repetitive series of such PVCs.
b. A sudden loss of 'exit block' by a rapidly firing parasystolic focus, so that instead of manifesting a slow rate due to a variable degree of exit block, it reaches the ventricles at double or triple its blocked rate. (See p. 529 for an explanation of parasystole.)
Note: a. In acute myocardial infarction, early arrhythmias are usually due to reentry. After about 6 hours VT is probably due to enhanced automaticity [138, 147].
b. A VT that is initiated by a PVC falling late in diastole, outside the relative refractory period of the ventricles, is likely to be due to focal automaticity [138, 147].

2. When is a PVC likely to precipitate a VT?
ANS.: When the PVC occurs before the end of the previous T wave, it may precipitate either VT or ventricular fibrillation, especially if it occurs near the beginning of the downstroke of the T [14]. It is known as the R on T phenomenon and is probably dangerous only in the presence of acute infarction or if the Q-T interval is prolonged.
Note: Most episodes of VT, however, are initiated by late PVCs and not by R on T phenomena [18, 61, 146].

3. What is meant by the 'vulnerable zone' of the T wave?
ANS.: There are two meanings:
a. An area on the upstroke and peak of the T wave where a depolarization impulse can precipitate VT or ventricular fibrillation. Because it is in the absolute refractory period of the ventricle, it requires either a defibrillation shock (the way it was originally discovered in dogs) or severe myocardial damage as in acute infarction.
b. Anywhere on the downstroke of the T wave during the relative refractory period if there is ischemia, electrolyte imbalance, or a prolonged Q-T.

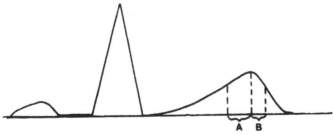

A depolarization stimulus at A often produces ventricular fibrillation. Because it occurs during the absolute refractory period, depolarization can occur here only with electroshock from a defibrillator or if the patient has an acute myocardial infarction. At B, or anywhere on the downstroke of the T, there can be a vulnerable zone in the presence of acute ischemia or other metabolic abnormalities.

Note: A PVC anywhere in the cycle can precipitate a VT if there are two in a row, because the second one can occur in the vulnerable zone of the PVC's T wave.

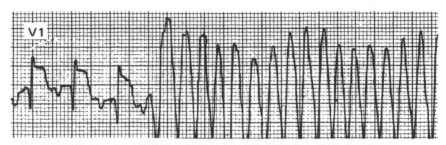

A run of VT and ventricular flutter beginning at the end of diastole. The S-T elevation is due to acute anterior myocardial infarction. Although the run of VT and flutter occur long after the previous T wave, this run is probably due to the second PVC occurring near the peak of the first premature beat's T wave.

4. Which heart rates tend to favor VT? Why?

    ANS.: Bradycardias, in the absence of acute ischemia. In animal studies progressive reductions in pulse rates cause increasing degrees of nonhomogeneous recovery of excitability, and so bradycardias lend themselves to reentry [46] (see ECG strip on p. 572). In the presence of acute ischemia, however, tachycardias tend to trigger VT.

*5. What kind of acute viral infection has been associated with VT?

    ANS.: A myocarditis caused by an echovirus. (AT has also been seen with it.)

    Note: A VT that is refractory to almost all medical treatment has been caused by a ruptured congenital aneurysm of the basilar artery with subarachnoid hemorrhage [44].

*6. What is meant by *torsade de pointes*?

    ANS.: A literal translation is 'twisted coil of points.' It refers to a paroxysm of multiform VT in which the QRS axis undulates over every 5 to 20 beats owing to changes in QRS axes. (It sometimes looks more like ventricular flutter or fibrillation.) It usually starts with a relatively late premature QRS in a patient with a bradycardia and a long Q-T interval [67]. It has been caused by low potassium, low magnesium, and anything that prolongs the Q-T interval, e.g., quinidine. It has been incriminated as the cause of syncope and death in a woman on a liquid protein weight reduction diet [119]. It has also occurred as a fatal arrhythmia in the presence of mitral valve prolapse [7].

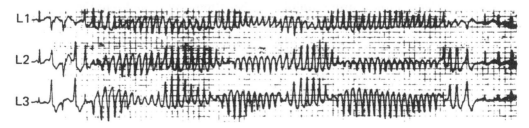

Simultaneous leads from a patient with hypokalemia showing the torsade de pointes type of VT. The last three sinus beats show an underlying sinus tachycardia of about 140 beats per minute. The run of VT with a gradually rotating axis begins with a bidirectional VT. (Adapted from D. M. Krickler and P. V. L. Curry, Br. Heart J. 38:117, 1976.)

    Note: a. In one study, in which it was called 'polymorphous VT,' shortening the Q-T by isoproterenol prevented recurrences [116]. Another report, in which it was called VT 'with reversal of points,' also found that acceleration of the heart rate by either drugs or a pacemaker eliminated the VT [64].

b. A drug-induced polymorphic ventricular tachycardia. It usually begins after a pause produced by a PVC. Over one-half begin a few days after the drug has started but if it occurs later, it is probably because a new drug such as a thiazide or digitalis was added.

c. Q-T prolongation which is common during sinus rhythm in patients with torsade favors the possibility of a premature stimulus occurring at the height of the vulnerable period, i.e., near the peak of the T wave [4A]. The torsade of patients who have a long Q-T (usually females) is usually preceded by a pause. The torsade caused by quinidine is pause dependent [133A]. Early afterdepolarizations are exacerbated by long cycles and suppressed by short cycles such as by rapid pacing.

d. Active ischemia and hypokalemia are predisposing factors so that any short enough coupling interval can produce torsade even without Q-T prolongation [87A].

e. If the Q-T is normal, then class 1 antiarrhythmic agents may be beneficial. If the Q-T is prolonged, such drugs are contraindicated and rapid pacing or magnesium is advised [43A].

---

*Chronic VT

*1. What is unexpected about the frequency and prognosis of repeated short paroxysms of VT in the absence of any other cardiac abnormality?

ANS.: a. The paroxysms may be more frequent than sinus rhythm [90].

b. The paroxysms usually disappear within a few years if there is no underlying cardiac disease. The prognosis is good, and it often requires no treatment [99].

Note: a. These repeated paroxysms are called 'repetitive VT.' The same paroxysmal phenomena can occur with atrial and junctional tachycardia, with the same prognosis. Although they are often eliminated by 'overriding' with the rapid rates produced by exercise or drugs, propranolol can also often eliminate them [56].

b. In the presence of underlying heart disease, sudden death is not uncommon with repetitive VT [123].

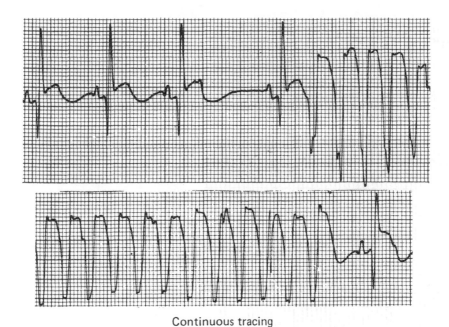

Continuous tracing

A paroxysm of VT at a rate of 230 in a man with acute myocardial infarction. The blocked PAC (note the P' on the third T wave) caused a long diastole that probably caused inhomogeneous repolarization, which in turn caused a reentry PVC to occur. This PVC, which occurred on the downstroke of a T wave, caused a run of VT. Note that the P-P interval between the end of the paroxysm and the first sinus beat is not longer than the basic sinus rate. Therefore the SA node has probably been firing independently.

*2. What is probably the longest recorded duration of a VT?

ANS.: It is 62 days [59]. Most patients with VT go into a shock-like state within a few minutes or hours because the asynchronous contraction that occurs when an impulse originates in an odd place in the ventricle can seriously impair cardiac function.

Arrhythmogenic Right Ventricular Dysplasia (ARVD)

What is ARVD?

ANS.: It is an idiopathic familial RV cardiomyopathy with fibrofatty replacement of myocytes surrounding islands of visible myocytes. They have recurrent VT originating from the RV. The RV is hypokinetic with localized areas of dyskinesis. The T waves are typically inverted from V1 to V3 and very small baseline wiggles (late potentials) occur on the S-T segment of V1 to V3 which are known as epsilon waves [46A, 104A].

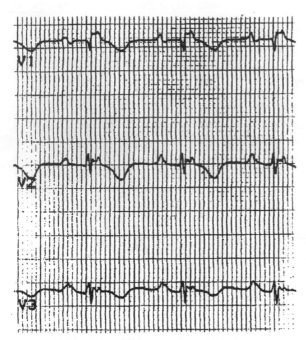

Intraventricular conduction delay due to slow conduction in the RV free wall makes a secondary spike resulting in an epsilon wave.

The Brugada Syndrome

What are the ECG findings characteristic for the Brugada syndrome?

ANS.: a. Incomplete RBBB.

b. S-T elevation in R precordial leads which are saddle-shaped or coved.

c. No S wave in V5 and 6.

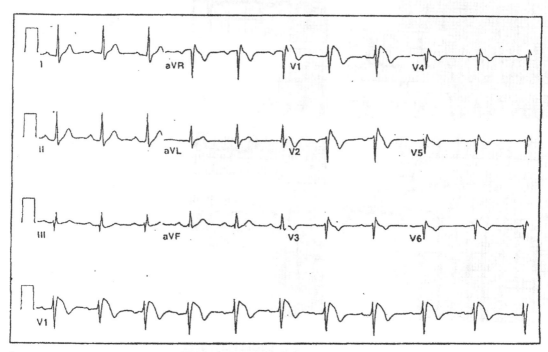

From an asymptomatic 35-year-old man with a normal heart and BP on history and physical examination. His S-Ts are coved and elevated as in the Brugada syndrome.

Differentiation of VT from Supraventricular Tachycardias

1. When are supraventricular tachycardias with QRS complexes abnormally wide and may therefore mimic VT?

    ANS.: a. If there was a bundle branch block before the tachycardia occurred (see ECG strips on p. 576, question 5c).

    b. If there is a rate-dependent bundle branch block (aberrant conduction) due to the rapid rate.

    c. If there is anterograde conduction over an AV bypass tract.

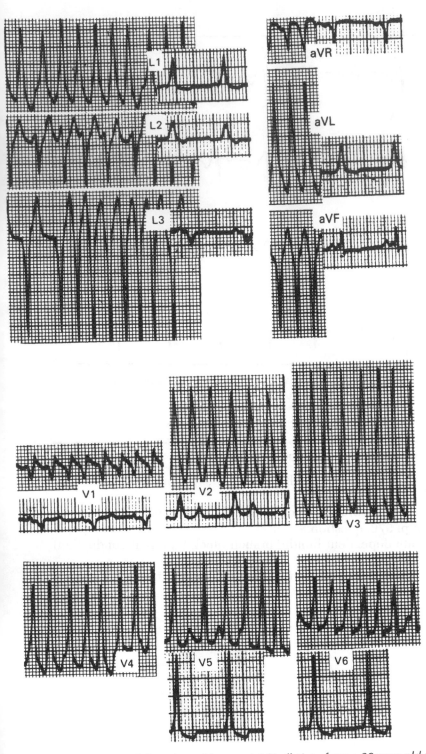

Two ECGs, one with and the other without atrial fibrillation, from a 29-year-old man with WPW syndrome and a normal heart except for episodes of palpitations due to rapid AF. The tachycardia with the wide complexes at a rate of 280 would have the appearance of a VT if it were not for the gross irregularity and the suggestion of a delta wave. After electrical cardioversion, the patient's normal sinus complexes (mounted beside the preconversion ECG) are seen to have AV preexcitation. The delta wave is best seen in V6. It was this kind of imitation of VT that led early ECG readers to believe that VT can be grossly irregular. There is a left axis deviation only during the tachycardia.

2. What is meant by a rate-dependent bundle branch block?

ANS.:   It is a bundle branch block that occurs only with rapid rates or short diastoles, so that one of the branches, either right or left, has had insufficient time to recover from its refractory period. A more complex explanation is given in the answers to questions 3 and 4.

Note: A much rarer bradycardia-dependent bundle branch block also occurs, and its mechanism is explained by understanding phase 4 block (see p. 493). According to the phase 4 block theory, bradycardia can produce bundle branch block or divisional block only if there are abnormal junctional cells, thereby explaining the absence of an escape beat. An escape beat would prevent bradycardia-dependent blocks.

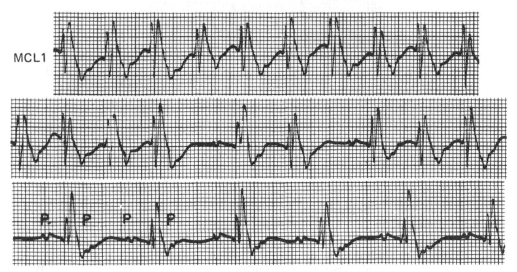

These strips were obtained a few seconds apart.

AT temporarily imitating a VT on a monitor MCL1 lead from a patient in a coronary care unit. The pattern is that of an RBBB (MCL1 is much like V1). The upper strips look like a VT at a rate of about 135. The distortion at the end of each QRS suggests a hidden P wave, but these areas could have been wrongly interpreted as retrograde P waves from each ventricular ectopic QRS. The middle strip a few seconds later shows a sudden halving of the rate with a P wave and long P-R interval in front of two complexes. The third strip shows an atrial rate of about 135, with a 2:1 AV block.

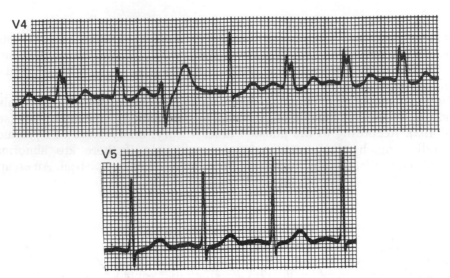

The LBBB in V4 was interrupted by a PVC that caused a long pause. This pause allowed recovery of left bundle conduction and produced a normal QRS. By the time V5 was being recorded, the rate had slowed from 100 to about 80 per minute, and normal conduction occurred.

*3. How can retrograde invasion into a bundle branch perpetuate a functional bundle branch block during tachycardia?

ANS.: If the first early beat of the tachycardia finds one of the bundles refractory, the impulse travels down the recovered bundle and invades the refractory bundle retrogradely. Thus the last structure to be depolarized is the bundle branch that was refractory. This bundle, which is activated later, is likely to be refractory enough for the next downcoming impulse to go down a recovered bundle again and up the bundle that had been refractory thereby causing a self-perpetuating bundle branch block [139]. This phenomenon may even be the cause of all rate-dependent bundle branch blocks.

*4. How can the R-R interval after a run of tachycardia differentiate VT from AT with aberrant conduction?

ANS.: The R-R interval is longest following the first normal sinus beat terminating a paroxysm of AT. Its length is due to a prolonged SA node recovery time. The subsequent R-R intervals often become progressively shorter. Termination of the tachycardia with a fixed R-R interval for the first sinus beat indicates that the SA node was not depressed and that a ventricular (or junctional) tachycardia with retrograde block must have been present.

5. How can inspecting another ECG when the tachycardia is absent help to decide whether a tachycardia with bizarre QRSs is due to aberrant conduction or to VT?

ANS.: a. If another ECG shows exactly the same type of complex in a PVC, that of course would make the tachycardia a VT.

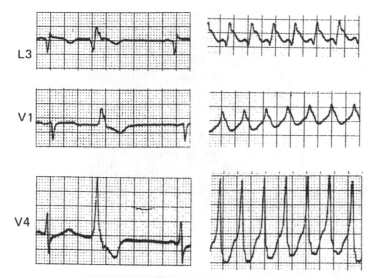

This ECG is from a 50-year-old man with an acute inferior infarction. The tachycardia on the right (rate about 185) was electrically cardioverted, and occasional PVCs (as on the left) were then seen. The contours of the PVCs are similar to the tachycardia complexes. Therefore the tachycardia is probably a VT. (Note the QR in the PVC of lead 3, indicating an inferior infarct.)

b. If another ECG shows exactly the same type of complex in a PAC with aberrancy, it would make the tachycardia an atrial or junctional tachycardia with aberrant conduction.

c. If another ECG shows a fixed bundle branch block pattern that is exactly repeated in the tachycardia, the tachycardia is an AT or junctional tachycardia in a patient with bundle branch block. See the following ECGs A and B.

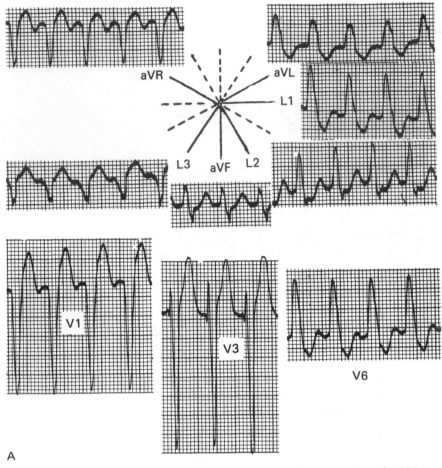

A

This fast rate could be due either to an atrial or junctional tachycardia with LBBB or to a ventricular tachycardia. This ECG is from a 70-year-old hypertensive diabetic woman with acute pulmonary edema (see ECG B, p. 577).

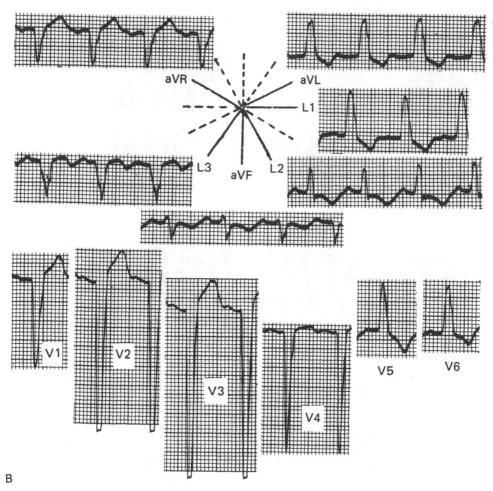

B

ECG from the same woman as in ECG A (p. 576), taken a few minutes later. It can be seen that in sinus rhythm she also has an LBBB with exactly the same QRS configuration as during the tachycardia. Thus an atrial or junctional tachycardia would have been the correct interpretation of A.

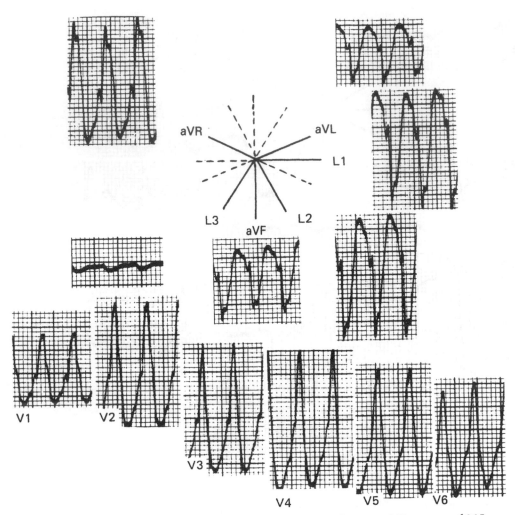

ECG from a 56-year-old man with an acute anterior infarction. That it is a VT at a rate of 215 per minute is indicated by the following: (1) The QRS is markedly anterior (upright in all precordial leads), and (2) the frontal QRS is markedly rightward and superior at about − 150°. This VT was converted to sinus rhythm with 100 mg of lidocaine.

AV Dissociation

1. What are the atria doing during VT?
   ANS.: Almost anything; i.e., there may be
   a. Sinus rhythm, AF, atrial flutter, or AT.
   b. Sinus arrest and no atrial activation (rare). Persistent atrial standstill has been described in patients with muscular dystrophy, amyloidosis, and idiopathic cardiomyopathy.

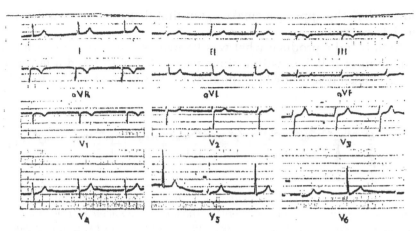

Atrial standstill in a patient with an idiopathic dilated cardiomyopathy. No A waves were present in the right atrial pressure tracings. No premature beats could be induced by stimulation of the right atrium and an intracardiac electrocardiogram did not show P or fibrillary waves.

    c. Retrogradely produced P waves from all or some of the ectopic ventricular beats. If all the ectopic beats retrogradely fire the atria, the atria and ventricles beat at the same rate. This pattern occurs in about two-thirds of VTs [62].

2. What term is used to describe a situation in which the atria and ventricles have independent pacemakers?

    ANS.: *AV dissociation.*

*3. Is there any specific meaning for the term *AV dissociation?*

    ANS.: It used to have a specific meaning, i.e., an independent atrial and junctional pacemaker *without* complete AV block. It used to be called 'interference dissociation' because the lower pacemaker was usually so fast that the upper pacemaker always found the ventricles refractory when it tried to get through to them. Therefore the lower pacemaker *interfered* with the upper pacemaker's ability to produce a QRS, and the occasional beats that got through the AV node from above *interfered* with the regular rhythm of the lower pacemaker. It is no longer correct to use the term *AV dissociation* to mean a specific arrhythmia.

        Therefore *AV dissociation* is no longer a diagnosis but a general term that must be identified in detail. You must say what the rhythm is at both pacemaker sites. Even a complete AV block is a kind of AV dissociation due to independent atrial and ventricular pacemakers.

4. What is necessary before there can be independent atrial and ventricular pacemakers without complete AV block?

    ANS.: The lower pacemaker must prevent the supraventricular pacemaker from producing most of the QRS complexes.

5. When does a lower pacemaker prevent the supraventricular pacemaker from controlling the ventricle?

    ANS.: If the lower pacemaker is

        a. Able to produce retrograde conduction into the atrium.

        b. Faster than the upper pacemaker.

    c. Slower than the upper pacemakers, but first-degree or second-degree AV block is present.
Note: Both b and c produce what was known as interference dissociation. The commonest is b, i.e., with a sinus pacemaker above and a faster junctional pacemaker below blocking the slower sinus beats at the AV node [82].

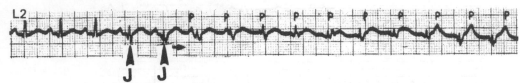

A double tachycardia due to the sudden onset of junctional tachycardia with aberrant conduction. The J-J intervals are slightly shorter than the P-P intervals. The junctional pacemaker of 115 is therefore slightly faster than the sinus rate of 108, which prevents any of the sinus beats from penetrating the AV node. This pattern used to be called interference dissociation.

6. When does a lower pacemaker not result in retrograde depolarization of the upper pacemaker?
    ANS.: If there is retrograde (VA) block.
        Note: Both junctional and ventricular pacemakers can have retrograde block and therefore can result in AV dissociation.

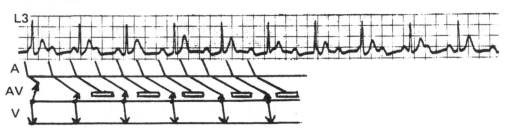

AV dissociation with the sinus or atrial pacemaker of 150 faster than the junctional pacemaker. The only reason that the faster pacemaker does not capture the ventricles is that there is at least a 2:1 AV block.

7. How is AV dissociation detected on an ECG when P waves are visible?
    ANS.: AV dissociation is present
        a. If the P-R intervals gradually shorten or are intermittently short.
        b. If the P-R interval gradually lengthens, but the R-R intervals are constant except for occasional early (capture) beats.

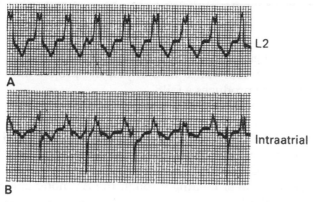

A

L2

B

Intraatrial

Ventricular tachycardia at a rate of 140 with AV dissociation proved by a simultaneous lead 2 and an intraatrial lead. In the intraatrial lead the P wave deflections are of greater amplitude than the QRS. In lead 2 the fourth QRS has a P wave in front of it, and the fifth has a P wave on its S-T segment. That these are P waves is proved by the simultaneous P deflections in the intraatrial lead. The last P wave seems to get through the AV node to produce a fusion beat (narrower QRS).

Note: a. During VT it is often possible to see disturbances of the S-T, T by the independent P waves going at their own rate.

b. The easiest way to detect AV dissociation is by physical examination. Listen to the first heart sound. It varies in loudness from beat to beat because changing P-R intervals produce changing S1 loudness. A varying systolic blood pressure also occurs because of the changing Starling effects [145]. Intermittent jugular cannon waves may be seen.

8. What can imitate exactly the ECG picture of VT with AV dissociation?

ANS.: A junctional tachycardia with aberrant conduction or bundle branch block and AV dissociation.

Note: It is often said that a good way to diagnose VT is to look for signs of AV dissociation. In practice, however, you must rule out a junctional tachycardia with AV dissociation. Furthermore, VT produces retrograde conduction into the atrium even more often than with single PVCs, so that AV dissociation is commonly *not* present [96]. On the other hand, AV dissociation with junctional tachycardia is so rare that finding dissociation in the presence of a tachycardia with abnormal QRS morphology is strong presumptive evidence of a VT.

9. How can the ECG prove that independent supraventricular and ventricular pacemakers are present if no P waves are seen?

ANS.: If the pacemaker from above the ventricle occasionally gets through the AV node and assists in the depolarization of the ventricles, it causes capture or fusion beats.

Capture and Fusion Beats

1. What is a 'capture' beat?
   ANS.: It is the occasional early beat seen in AV dissociation *with no AV block*, when the higher pacemaker sometimes fires at just the proper time to get through the AV node and so produces a QRS.
2. In the presence of a VT, how can you tell that a supraventricular pacemaker has succeeded in getting through the AV node to assist in producing part of the wide QRS?
   ANS.: By seeing an occasional QRS looking halfway between a normal QRS and a very wide QRS; i.e., when an occasional QRS looks *slightly narrower* than the usual lower pacemaker QRS.
3. Why does a supraventricular pacemaker coming through the AV node change the width of the lower pacemaker's QRS?
   ANS.: If the initial part of the QRS is produced by a ventricular pacemaker and the terminal part is finished by the upper pacemaker, or vice versa, the QRS can be narrower than expected for a ventricular pacemaker.
4. What do we call a beat that is slightly narrower because it is composed of both a supraventricular and a ventricular QRS?
   ANS.: A fusion beat. (It is occasionally called a Dressler beat.) *It is the most reliable sign of VT.*

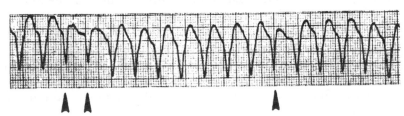

VT at a rate of 165. The arrows point to QRS complexes that are slightly narrower than the others. They are therefore fusion beats.

5. When is there never a fusion beat in VT despite the absence of complete AV block?
   ANS.: a. When the supraventricular pacemaker cannot get through the junctional area because the ventricular pacemaker is too fast (interference dissociation).
   b. When there is retrograde depolarization of the atrium, so that every lower pacemaker beat produces its own P wave.
6. How can the width of the QRS suggest that a tachycardia is VT rather than aberrant conduction?
   ANS.: Aberrancy is not likely to prolong a QRS beyond 140 msec (0.14 sec). VT can prolong a QRS beyond 140 msec.
7. How can the rate suggest that a tachycardia is due to a VT rather than to an AT with aberrancy?
   ANS.: A rate of more than 170 favors aberrant conduction.
   Note: Although VT rates have a range of 200 ± 50 beats per minute, the vast majority are slower than 200 [146].
8. How can the frontal plane axis help to distinguish aberrancy from VT?
   ANS.: Supraventricular tachycardias with aberrancy do not usually show an anterior divisional block (left axis deviation) unless the divisional block was present before the tachycardia [145].

Distinguishing VT from Its Commonest Mimic, a Regular Supraventricular Tachycardia with Aberrancy: Summary

1. *Presumptive evidence for VT is present if there is*
   a. An anterior divisional block and you know there was none before the tachycardia [145], especially if the axis is − 90° or more.
   b. A QRS > 140 msec with RBBB and > 160 msec with LBBB [1A].
   c. An RBBB complex in V1 in which the complexes are either
      (1) Monophasic
      (2) Biphasic, *or*
      (3) The initial positivity is higher than the second positivity if there is a notch or S wave present.
   d. An LBBB pattern with
      (1) QR or QS complex in V6 [141].
      (2) Entirely upright or entirely inverted complexes across the precordium.
      (3) An R of 30 msec or more in V1 or V2 (more common with inferior infarction).
      (4) R to nadir of S in V1 or V2 of 80 msec or more.
      (5) Notching on the downslope of the S wave in V1 or V2 (uncommon with anterior infarction) [59A].
   e. AV dissociation.
2. *Absolute evidence for VT is present if*
   a. Fusion or capture beats are seen.
   b. The same complexes as in the tachycardia are seen in PVCs in a pretachycardia or post-tachycardia ECG.
   c. In a lead with an R and S measure from the beginning of the R to the nadir of the S. If it is over 100 msec, it is highly specific for ventricular tachycardia [13A].
3. If there is a short paroxysm with wide QRS complexes, look for a P′ distorting the T wave preceding the tachycardia. Then look for a lack of post-tachycardia P-P lengthening that tells you that the sinus pacemaker has not been depressed by a succession of rapid P′ waves—a strong sign of a VT.
   Note: Entirely upright or inverted complexes in the precordium is called concordance.

Bidirectional Tachycardia

1. What is meant by bidirectional tachycardia?
   ANS.: A tachycardia with alternating directions of wide QRS complexes.
2. What characteristics have been found in almost all ECGs with bidirectional tachycardia?
   ANS.: a. The precordial leads always show an RBBB picture in all complexes [104].
   b. The frontal QRS directions for alternate beats are about − 60° and 120° [104].
   c. The rhythm is regular.

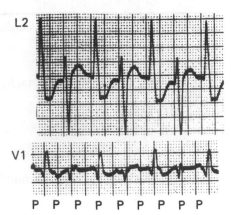

L2

V1

P P P P P P P P P

Bidirectional tachycardia at a rate of 150 one-half hour after intravenous digitalis was given. The P waves are independent at a rate of about 210. Therefore this ECG signals a double tachycardia. Bidirectional tachycardias and double tachycardias are both accepted signs of digitalis toxicity. Rarely a double tachycardia can be induced by exercise without digitalis and without apparent heart abnormalities [30A].

3. How can this alternating conduction be explained?
   ANS.: One beat has RBBB with anterior divisional block, and the other has RBBB with posterior divisional block; i.e., it is either a supraventricular tachycardia with fixed RBBB and alternate anterior and posterior divisional blocks, or a VT with a focus in the main left bundle branch with alternating anterior and posterior divisional block [86, 104].
4. What is almost always present as a cause when a biventricular tachycardia is present?
   ANS.: Myocardial damage and excess digitalis.
   Note: a. If a patient has VT with an RBBB at one time and an LBBB at another, it does not necessarily mean a left and right ventricular focus. Both foci have been shown to arise usually from the same ventricle and most likely from within an aneurysm [53].
   b. Patients with chronic recurrent tachycardias that appear to come from the left ventricle (RBBB configuration) have more overt heart disease, more abnormal left ventricular and coronary angiograms, and a higher yearly mortality than patients with 'right ventricular' tachycardias [95].

VENTRICULAR FLUTTER AND FIBRILLATION

1. What is meant by ventricular flutter?
   ANS.: Regular waves without an isoelectric baseline between them, usually a precursor to fibrillation.

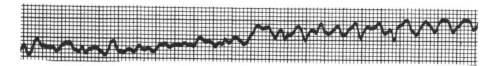

Ventricular flutter at a rate of about 210. The rate range is the same as for VT, i.e., about 200 ± 50.

2. What does ventricular fibrillation (VF) look like on an ECG?
   ANS.: Chaotic undulations of the baseline.

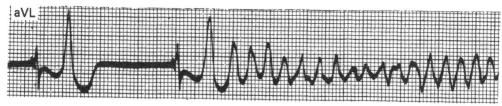

3. How do episodes of VF begin other than from a PVC in the vulnerable zone of a T? (See p. 566 for an explanation of the vulnerable zone.)
   ANS.: a. Some begin as part of the progress of a sustained VT, often through a stage of ventricular flutter.

Junctional pacemaker with bigeminy due to PVCs near the peak of a negative T wave, the second of which initiates a run of VF.

   b. Some are precipitated by a PVC that occurs after a P wave. During acute infarction, there is a greater incidence of VF with a PVC after a P than on a T [131].

4. List the most important conditions facilitating VF.
   ANS.: The VF threshold can be lowered by anything that produces inhomogeneity of recovery or shortens the refractory period of the ventricles. Thus an early depolarization due to a PVC shortens the refractory period and increases inhomogeneity of recovery [54]. These conditions are exaggerated by myocardial ischemia, prolongation of the Q-T, electrolyte imbalance, drugs that can increase automaticity, and hypothermia [126].
   Note: a. Digitalis toxicity can produce any kind of onset of VF, with the additional features that a preceding ventricular tachycardia is likely to be bidirectional or to develop gradually widening QRS complexes, and the tachycardia resists cardioversion [14].
          b. The VF that occurs after prolonged alcoholic bouts may be due to magnesium deficiency, which in turn may allow loss of intracellular potassium [75].

SYSTEMATIC APPROACH TO INTERPRETATION OF AN ARRHYTHMIA

If the following questions are answered in the order given, most arrhythmias are well on the way to being understood.

1. Is the QRS rhythm regular or irregular?
2. If the QRS rhythm is irregular, is there a pattern to it (especially a repeat pattern), or is it chaotic? A repeat pattern should make you very suspicious of a second-degree SA or AV block.
3. Is there a P wave in front of or after every QRS?
4. Are the P waves that are in front of or after the QRSs related to those QRSs, or are they independent?
5. If the P waves are related to the QRSs, is there a fixed relation between the P waves and their QRSs?
6. If there are QRSs without P waves, are the P waves hidden, or are the QRS complexes ectopic?
7. If the QRSs are ectopic, where is the focus?
8. If there are no P waves, is the atrial rhythm fibrillation or flutter, or are the P waves hidden in the QRS (retrograde P waves)?
9. Can you account for any temporary anomalous, bizarre, different-appearing QRS or P contours by utilizing concepts of aberrancy, ectopy, or fusion?
10. Can you account for any pauses or early QRSs?

REFERENCES

1. Aberg, H. Atrial fibrillation. A study of the fibrillatory waves using a new technique. *Acta Soc. Med. Upsal.* 74:17, 1969.
1A. Akhtar, M., Shenasa, M., Jazayeri, M., Caceres, J., Tchou, P. J. Wide QRS complex tachycardia. *Ann. Int. Med.* 109; 905–912, 1988.
1B. Akiyama, T., et al. Ashman phenomenon of the T wave. *Am. J. Cardiol.* 63:886, 1989
2. Akre, P. R. Multifocal premature contractions. *Aerospace Med.* 38:197, 1967.
3. Anderson, G. J., Greenspan, K., and Bandura, J. Asynchrony of conduction and reentry. *Am. J. Cardiol.* 26:623, 1970.
4. Barrett, P. A., et al. The electrocardiographic effects of lidocaine in the Wolff-Parkinson-White syndrome. *Am. Heart J.* 100:23, 1980.
4A. Bashour, T. T., Lehrman, K., Edgett, J. Torsade de pointes: a maximal vulnerability arrhythmia. *Am. Heart J.* 109:167–9, 1985.
5. Baxter, R. H., and McGuinness, J. B. Comparison of ventricular parasystolic with other dysrhythmias after acute infarction. *Am. Heart J.* 88:443, 1974.
6. Beck-Nielsen, J., Sorensen, H. R., and Alstrup, P. Arrhythmia more likely when thoracotomy done for cancer of the lung. *Acta Med. Scand.* 133:425, 1973.
7. Bennett, K. R. Torsade de pointes and mitral valve prolapse. *Am. J. Cardiol.* 45:715, 1980.
8. Berlinerblau, R., and Feder, W. Chaotic atrial rhythm. *J. Electrocardiol.* 5:135, 1972.
9. Bigger, J. T., Jr., and Goldreyer, B. N. The mechanism of supraventricular tachycardia. *Circulation* 30:330, 1968.
10. Bishop, L. F., and McGinn, F. X. Recurrent paroxysmal atrial fibrillation occurring in the absence of heart disease. *Vasc. Dis.* 5:31, 1968.
11. Bodenheimer, M. M., Banka, V. S., and Helfant, R. H. Relation between the site of origin of ventricular premature complexes and the presence and severity of coronary artery disease. *Am. J. Cardiol.* 40:865, 1977.

12. Boineau, J. P., et al. Epicardial mapping in Wolff-Parkinson-White syndrome. *Arch. Intern. Med.* 125:422, 1975.

13. Booth, D. C., Popio, K. A., and Gettes, L. S. Multiformity of induced unifocal ventricular premature beats. *Am. J. Cardiol.* 49:1643, 1982.

13A. Brugada, P., et al. A new approach to the differential diagnosis of a wide QRS tachycardia. *Circulation* 83:1649, 1991.

14. Castellanos, A., Jr., Lemberg, L., and Centurion, M. J. Mechanisms of digitalis-induced ventricular fibrillation. *Dis. Chest* 54:221, 1968.

15. Castellanos, A., Jr., et al. Modulation of ventricular parasystole by extraneous depolarizations. *J. Electrocardiol.* 17:195, 1984.

16. Castellanos, A., Jr., et al. Syndrome of short P-R, narrow QRS: the possible occurrence of R on T. *Eur. J. Cardiol.* 2:337, 1975.

17. Castellanos, A., Jr., et al. Factors regulating ventricular rates during atrial flutter and fibrillation in pre-excitation (Wolff-Parkinson-White) syndrome. *Br. Heart J.* 35:811, 1973.

18. Chou, T.-C., and Wenzke, F. The importance of R on T phenomenon. *Am. Heart J.* 96:191, 1978.

19. Chung, E. K. Aberrant atrial conduction – unrecognized electrocardiographic entity. *Am. J. Cardiol.* 26:628, 1970.

20. Chung, K.-Y., Walsh, T. J., and Massie, E. Electrical alternans: A report of twelve cases. *Am. J. Med. Sci.* 248:110, 1964.

21. Cohen, H., Langendorf, R., and Pick, A. Intermittent parasystole – mechanism of protection. *Circulation* 48:761, 1973.

22. Cole, S. L. Digitalis intoxication chronic effects manifested by diarrhea and auricular flutter. *Am. Heart J.* 39:900, 1950.

23. Collado, A., Mower, M. M., and Tabatznik, B. Left atrial parasystole. *Chest* 59:214, 1971.

24. Cosby, R. S., and Herman, L. M. Atrial flutter and pulmonary disease. *Geriatrics* 21:140, 1966.

25. Cranefield, P. F., Klein, H. O., and Hoffman, B. F. Delay, block and one-way block in depressed Purkinje fibers. *Circulation* 28:199, 1971.

26. Damato, A. N., Lau, S. H., and Bobb, G. A. Studies on ventriculo-atrial conduction and the reentry phenomenon. *Circulation* 41:423, 1970.

27. D'Cruz, I. A., et al. Benign repetitive multifocal ectopic atrial tachycardia. *Am. Heart J.* 88:671, 1974.

28. DuBrow, I. W., et al. Comparison of cardiac refractory periods in children and adults. *Circulation* 51:485, 1975.

29. Dye, C. L. Atrial tachycardia in Wolff-Parkinson-White syndrome. *Am. J. Cardiol.* 24:265, 1969.

30. Edeiken, J. Extreme tachycardia with report of nonfatal paroxysms following myocardial infarction. *Am. J. Med. Sci.* 205:52, 1943.

30A. Eldar, M., Belhassen, B., Hod, H., Schuger, C. D., Scheinman, M. M. Exercise-induced double (atrial and ventricular) tachycardia: a report of three cases. *J.A.C.C.* 14:1376–1381, 1989.

31. El-Sherif, N. Paroxysmal atrial flutter and fibrillation. Induction by carotid sinus compression and prevention by atropine. *Br. Heart J.* 34:1024, 1972.

32. El-Sherif, N. Tachycardia- and bradycardia-dependent bundle branch block. *Br. Heart J.* 36:291, 1974.

33. Erhardt, L. R. Abnormal atrial activity in lipomatous hypertrophy of the interatrial septum. *Am. Heart J.* 87, 571, 1974.

34. Fellstrom, B., and Nordgren, L. Initial vector rates in differentiation between aberration and extrasystoles. *J. Electrocardiol.* 12:49, 1979.

35. Ferrer, M. I. Significance of slow atrial rhythm. *Am. J. Cardiol.* 46:176, 1980.

36. Ferrier, G. R. Digitalis arrhythmias: Role of oscillatory afterpotentials. *Prog. Cardiovasc. Dis.* 19:459, 1977.

37. Finkelstein, D., Gold, H., and Bellet, S. Atrial flutter with 1:1 A-V conduction. *Am. J. Med.* 20:65, 1956.

38. Fisch, C., Edmands, R. E., and Greenspan, K. T. wave alternans: An association with abrupt rate change. *Am. Heart J.* 81:817, 1971.

39. Fletcher, E., and Stevenson, M. The effect of digitalis on nodal rhythm with reciprocal beats. *Br. Heart J.* 18:557, 1956.
40. Gillette, P. C., and Garson, A., Jr. Electrophysiologic and pharmacologic characteristics of automatic ectopic atrial tachycardia. *Circulation* 56:571, 1977.
41. Girard, G., Latour, H., and Puesch, P. Flutter in man: A study of auricular activation by esophageal and cavitary leads. *Arch. Mal Coeur* 58:819, 1955.
41A. Gimbel, K. S. The reentry phenomenon. *Chest* 63:1, 1973.
42. Goldreyer, B. N., and Damato, A. N. The essential role of atrioventricular conduction delay in the initiation of paroxysmal supraventricular tachycardia. *Circulation* 43:679, 1971.
42A. Gomez, J. A., et al. Sustained sinus node reentrant tachycardia. *J. Am. Coll. Cardiol.* 5:45, 1985.
43. Green, M., et al. Value of QRS alternation in determining the site of origin of narrow QRS tachycardia. *Circulation* 68:386, 1983.
43A. Griffin, J., and Most, A. S. True and false torsade. *Am. Heart J.* 109:404, 1985.
44. Grossman, M. A. Cardiac arrhythmias in acute central nervous system disease. *Arch. Intern. Med.* 136:203, 1976.
45. Gulamhusein, S., et al. Electrocardiographic criteria for differentiating aberrancy and ventricular extrasystole in atrial fibrillation. *J. Electrocardiol.* 18:41, 1985.
46. Han, J., et al. Temporal dispersion of recovery of excitability in atrium and ventricle as a function of heart rates. *Am. Heart J.* 71:481, 1966.
46A. Hurst, J. W. Naming of the waves in the ECG, with a brief account of their genesis. *Circulation* 98:1937–1942, 1998.
47. Hutter, A. M., Jr., and Page, D. L. Atrial arrhythmias and lipomatous hypertrophy of the cardiac interatrial septum. *Am. Heart J.* 82:16, 1971.
48. Igarashi, M. Electrocardiogram in potassium depletion. *Jpn. Circ. J.* 27:476, 1963.
49. Irons, G. V., and Orgain, E. S. Digitalis-induced arrhythmias and their management. *Prog. Cardiovasc. Dis.* 8:539, 1966.
50. Isner, J. M., et al. Lipomatous hypertrophy of the interatrial septum. *Circulation* 66:470, 1982.
51. Janvier, R. P., Narula, O. S., and Samet, P. Atrial tachysystole (flutter) with apparent exit block. *Circulation* 40:179, 1969.
52. Jewitt, D. E., et al. Incidence and management of supraventricular arrhythmias after acute myocardial infarction. *Lancet* 2:734, 1967.
53. Josephson, M. E., et al. Recurrent sustained ventricular tachycardia. *Circulation* 59:459, 1978.
54. Josephson, M. E., et al. Mechanism of ventricular fibrillation in man: Observations based on electrode catheter recordings. *Am. J. Cardiol.* 44:623, 1979.
54A. Kalbfleisch, B., et al. Diagnosis of supraventricular tachycardia. *J.A.C.C.* 21:85–89, 1993.
55. Kaplinsky, E., et al. Origin of so-called right and left ventricular arrhythmias in acute myocardial ischemia. *Am. J. Cardiol.* 42:774, 1978.
56. Kariv, I., Kreisler, B., and Behar, S. Repetitive tachycardia: Effects of exercise tests and amyl nitrite. *Br. Heart J.* 33:115, 1971.
57. Kastor, J. A., and Yurchak, P. M. Recognition of digitalis intoxication in the presence of atrial fibrillation. *Ann. Intern. Med.* 67:1045, 1967.
58. Killip, T., and Gault, J. H. Mode of onset of atrial fibrillation in man. *Am. Heart J.* 70:172, 1965.
59. Kilpatrick, T. R., Moore, C. B., and Maza, E. S. Drug-resistant ventricular tachycardia of 62 days' duration. *J.A.M.A.* 197:108, 1966.
59A. Kindwall, E., Brown, J., Josephson, M. E. Electrocardiographic criteria for ventricular tachycardia in wide complex left bundle branch block morphology tachycardias. *Am. J. Cardiol.* 61: 1279–1283, 1988.
60. Kinoshita, S. Mechanisms of intermittent ventricular parasystole due to type II second degree entrance block. *J. Electrocardiol.* 16:7, 1983.
61. Kinoshita, S., et al. Ventricular tachycardia initiated by late-coupled extrasystoles, due to longitudinal dissociation. *Am. Heart J.* 103:1090, 1982.
62. Kistin, A. D. Problems in differentiation of ventricular arrhythmia from supraventricular arrhythmia with abnormal QRS. *Prog. Cardiovasc. Dis.* 9:1, 1966.

63. Klass, M., and Haywood, L. J. Atrial fibrillation associated with acute myocardial infarction. A study of thirty-four cases. *Am. Heart J.* 79:752, 1970.

64. Klauser, H. Ventricular tachycardia 'with reversal of points' and electrolyte disorders. *J.A.M.A.* 239:453, 1978.

65. Konecke, L. L., and Knoebel, S. B. Nonparoxysmal junctional tachycardia complicating acute myocardial infarction. *Circulation* 45:367, 1972.

66. Kotler, M. N., et al. Prognostic significance of ventricular ectopic beats with respect to sudden death in the late postinfarction period. *Circulation* 47:959, 1973.

67. Krickler, D. M., and Curry, P. V. L. Torsade de pointes, an atypical VT. *Br. Heart J.* 38:117, 1976.

68. Kuck, K. H., Brugada, P., and Wellens, H. J. J. Observations on the antidromic type of circus movement tachycardia in the Wolff-Parkinson-White syndrome. *J. Am. Coll. Cardiol.* 2:1003, 1983.

69. Lamb, L. E., and Pollard, L. W. Atrial fibrillation in flying personnel: Report of 60 cases. *Circulation* 29:694, 1964.

70. Levy, M. N., and Edelstein, J. The mechanism of synchronization in isorhythmic A-V dissociation. *Circulation* 42:689, 1970.

71. Levy, S. Exercise testing in the Wolff-Parkinson-White syndrome. *Am. J. Cardiol.* 48:976, 1981.

72. Lewis, S., et al. Significance of site of origin of premature ventricular contractions. *Am. Heart J.* 97:159, 1979.

73. Linenthal, A. J., and Zoll, P. M. Ventricular fusion beats during electrical stimulation in man. *Circulation* 31:651, 1965.

74. Lipson, M. J., and Naimi, S. Multifocal atrial tachycardia (chaotic atrial tachycardia). *Circulation* 42:397, 1970.

75. Loeb, H. S., et al. Paroxysmal ventricular fibrillation in two patients with hypomagnesemia. Treatment by transvenous pacing. *Circulation* 37:210, 1968.

76. Lown, B., Ganong, W. F., and Levine, S. A. The syndrome of short P-R interval, normal QRS complex and paroxysmal rapid heart action. *Circulation* 5:693, 1952.

77. MacDonald, G. Ventricular ectopic beats. *Am. J. Cardiol.* 13:198, 1964.

78. Marriott, H. J. L. Atrioventricular synchronization and accrochage. *Circulation* 14:38, 1956.

79. Marriott, H. J. L., Schwartz, N. L., and Bix, H. H. Ventricular fusion beats. *Circulation* 28:880, 1962.

80. Mautner, B., and Girotti, A. L. Premature ventricular contractions. Experimental study. *Am. Heart J.* 85:389, 1973.

81. Mehta, M. C., and Singh, S. V. Reversed reciproacting paroxysmal tachycardia. *Dis. Chest* 56:352, 1969.

82. Miller, R., and Sharrett, R. H. Interference dissociation. *Circulation* 16:803, 1957.

83. Mirowski, M., and Tabatznik, B. The spatial characteristics of atrial activation in ventriculoatrial excitation. *Chest* 57:9, 1970.

84. Mirvis, D. M., Bandura, J. P., and Brody, D. A. Symptomatic swallowing-induced paroxysmal supraventricular tachycardia. *Am. J. Cardiol.* 39:741, 1977.

85. Morgan, C. L., and Nadas, A. S. Chronic ectopic tachycardia in infancy and childhood. *Am. Heart J.* 67:617, 1964.

86. Morris, S. N., and Zipes, D. P. His bundle electrocardiography during bidirectional tachycardia. *Circulation* 48:32, 1973.

87. Moss, A. J., and Aledort, L. M. Use of endrophonium (Tensilon) in the evaluation of supraventricular tachycardia. *Am. J. Cardiol.* 17:58, 1966.

87A. Motte, G., Siami, R. True and false torsade de pointes. *Am. Heart J.*, 111:1404, 1985.

88. Myburgh, D. P., and Lewis, B. S. Ventricular parasystole in healthy hearts. *Am. Heart J.* 82:307, 1971.

89. Oram, S., Resnekov, L., and Davies, P. Digitalis as a cause of paroxysmal atrial-tachycardia with atrioventricular block. *Br. Med. J.* 2:1402, 1960.

90. Parkinson, J., and Papp, C. Repetitive paroxysmal tachycardia. *Br. Heart J.* 9:241, 1947.

91. Peter, R. H., Gracey, J. G., and Beach, T. B. Clinical profile of idiopathic atrial fibrillation. *Ann. Intern. Med.* 68:1288, 1968.

92. Phillips, J., Spano, J., and Burch, G. Chaotic atrial mechanism. *Am. Heart J.* 78:171, 1969.

93. Pick, A., and Dominguez, P. Nonparoxysmal A-V node tachycardia. *Circulation* 16:1022, 1957.

94. Pick, A., Langendorf, R., and Katz, L. N. A-V nodal tachycardia with block. *Circulation* 24:112, 1961.

95. Pietras, R. J., et al. Chronic recurrent right and left ventricular tachycardia: Comparison of clinical, hemodynamic and angiographic findings. *Am. J. Cardiol.* 40:32, 1977.

96. Pooya, M., et al. Incidence and patterns of retrograde ventriculoatrial conduction (VAC) in man. *Circulation* (Suppl. III) 38–40:163, 1969.

97. Prinzmetal, M., et al. *The Auricular Arrhythmias*. Springfield. IL: Charles C. Thomas, 1952, P. 145.

98. Prinzmetal, M., et al. Auricular flutter. *Am. J. Med.* 11:410, 1951.

99. Rahilly, G. T., Prystowsky, E. N., and Zipes, D. P. Clinical and electrophysiologic findings in repetitive monomorphic ventricular tachycardia and normal electrocardiogram. *Am. J. Cardiol.* 50:459, 1982.

100. Rizzon, P., and Bacca, F. The clinical significance of some patterns of auricular fibrillation. *Cuore Circ.* 49:847, 1970.

101. Roos, J. C., and Dunning, A. J. Right bundle branch block and left axis deviation in acute myocardial infarction. *Br. Heart J.* 32:847, 1970.

102. Rosen, K. M., Rahimtoola, S. H., and Gunnar, R. M. Pseudo A-V block secondary to premature nonpropagated His bundle depolarization. *Circulation* 42:367, 1970.

103. Rosenbaum, M. B. Classification of ventricular extrasystoles according to form. *J. Electrocardiol.* 2:289, 1969.

104. Rosenbaum, M. B., Elizari, M. V., and Lasari, J. O. The mechanism of bidirectional tachycardia. *Am. Heart J.* 78:4, 1969.

104A. Rossi, P., Massumi, A., Gillette, P., Hall, R. J. Arrhythmogenic right ventricular dysplasia: clinical features, diagnostic teahniques, and current management. *Am. Heart J.* 103:415–420, 1982.

105. Rubeiz, G. A., and Bey, S. K. Atrial flutter with 1:1 A-V conduction. *Am. J. Cardiol.* 7:753, 1961.

106. Sandler, A., and Marriott, H. J. L. The differential morphology of anomalous ventricular complexes of RBBB-type in lead V1. Ventricular ectopy versus aberration. *Circulation* 31:551, 1965.

107. Schamroth, L. Reciprocal rhythm of ventricular origin during atrial fibrillation with complete A-V block. *Br. Heart J.* 32:564, 1970.

108. Schamroth, L. Sinus parasystole. *Am. J. Cardiol.* 3:434, 1967.

109. Schamroth, L. *The Disorders of Cardiac Rhythm*. Oxford: Blackwell, 1971, P. 4.

110. Schamroth, L., and Marriott, H. J. L. Concealed ventricular extrasystoles. *Circulation* 27:1043, 1963.

111. Schamroth, L., and Marriott, H. J. L. Intermittent ventricular parasystole. *Am. J. Cardiol.* 7:799, 1961.

112. Schamroth, L., and Surawicz, B. Concealed interpolated A-V junctional extrasystoles and A-V junctional parasystole. *Am. J. Cardiol.* 27:703, 1971.

113. Scherf, D., and Bornemann, C. Parasystole with a rapid ventricular center. *Am. Heart J.* 62:320, 1961.

114. Scherlag, B. J., et al. The differential effects of ouabain on sinus, A-V nodal, His bundle, and idioventricular rhythms. *Am. Heart J.* 81:227, 1971.

115. Schuilenburg, R. M., and Durrer, D. Atrial echo beats in the human heart elicited by induced atrial premature beats. *Circulation* 37:680, 1968.

116. Sclarovsky, S., et al. Polymorphous ventricular tachycardia: Clinical features and treatment. *Am. J. Cardiol.* 44:339, 1979.

117. Segers, M., Lequime, J., and Denolin, H. Synchronization of auricular and ventricular beats during complete heart block. *Am. Heart J.* 33:685, 1947.

118. Shine, K. I., Kastor, J. A., and Yurchak, P. M. Multifocal atrial tachycardia. *N. Engl. J. Med.* 279:344, 1968.

119. Singh, B. N., et al. Liquid protein diets and torsade de pointes. *J.A.M.A.* 240:115, 1978.

120. Spano, P. J., and Burch, G. Chaotic atrial mechanism. *Am. Heart J.* 78:171, 1969.

121. Spodick, D. H. Electric alternation of the heart. *Am. J. Cardiol.* 10:155, 1962.

122. Stemple, D. R., Fitzgerald, J. W., and Winkle, R. A. Benign slow paroxysmal atrial tachycardia. *Ann. Intern. Med.* 87:44, 1977.

123. Stock, J. P. P. Repetitive paroxysmal ventricular tachycardia. *Br. Heart J.* 24:297, 1962.

124. Storstein, P., and Rasmussen, K. Digitalis and atrial tachycardia with block. *Br. Heart J.* 36:171, 1974.

125. Strasburger, K. H., and Klepsiz, H. The significance of coarse and fine atrial fibrillation. *Z. Kreislaufforsch.* 51:871, 1962.

126. Surawicz, B. Ventricular fibrillation. *Am. J. Cardiol.* 28:268, 1971.

127. Surawicz, B., and Kuo, C.-S. Association of ventricular couplets with variable coupling interval and ventricular parasystole. *Circulation* (Suppl. III) 55–56:243, 1977.

127A. Suwa, M., Hirota, Y., Kaku, K., Yoneda Y., Nakayama, A., et al. Prevalence of the coexistence of left ventricular false tendons and premature ventricular complexes in apparently healthy subjects: A prospective study in the general population. *J. Am. Coll. Cardiol.* 12:910–914, 1988.

128. Swanick, E. J., LaCamera, F., Jr., and Marriott, H. J. L. Morphologic features of right ventricular ectopic beats. *Am. J. Cardiol.* 30:888, 1972.

129. Thurmann, M., and Janney, J. G., Jr. The diagnostic importance of fibrillatory wave size. *Circulation* 25:991, 1962.

130. Trautwein, W. Mechanisms of tachyarrhythmias and extrasystoles. In *Symposium on Cardiac Arrhythmias*. Sodertalje, Sweden: Astra, 1970, P. 56.

131. Tye, H.-H., et al. R on T or R on P phenomenon? Relation to the genesis of ventricular tachycardia. *Am. J. Cardiol.* 44:632, 1979.

132. Udall, J. A., and Ellestad, M. H. Predictive implications of ventricular premature contractions associated with treadmill stress testing. *Circulation* 56:988, 1977.

133. Vazifder, J. P., and Levine, S. A. Rarity of atrial tachycardia in acute myocardial infarction and in thyrotoxicosis. *Arch. Intern. Med.* 118:41, 1966.

133A. Viskin, S. Long QT syndromes and torsade de pointes. *Lancet* 354:1625–1632, 1999.

134. Waldo, A. L., et al. The mechanism of synchronization in isorhythmic A-V dissociation. *Circulation* 38:880, 1968.

135. Waldo, A. L., et al. The P wave and P-R interval. *Circulation* 42:653, 1970.

136. Wallach, J., et al. Auricular fibrillation and mitral stenosis in bacterial endocarditis. *Circulation* 9:908, 1954.

137. Wellens, H. J. J. Isolated electrical alternans of the T wave. *Chest* 62:319, 1972.

138. Wellens, H. J. J. Pathophysiology of ventricular tachycardia in man. *Arch. Intern. Med.* 135:473, 1975.

139. Wellens, H. J. J., and Durrer, D. Supraventricular tachycardia with left aberrant conduction due to retrograde invasion into the left bundle branch. *Circulation* 38:474, 1968.

140. Wellens, H. J. J., and Durrer, D. Wolff-Parkinson-White syndrome in atrial fibrillation. *Am. J. Cardiol.* 34:777, 1974.

141. Wellens, H. J. J., Bar, F. W. H. M., and Lie, K. I. The value of the electrocardiogram in the differential diagnosis of a tachycardia with a widened QRS complex. *Am. J. Med.* 64:27, 1978.

142. Wellens, H. J. J., et al. Procainamide in Wolff-Parkinson-White syndrome to disclose a short refractory period. *Am. J. Cardiol.* 50:1087, 1982.

143. Wells, J. L., Jr., et al. Characterization of atrial flutter: Studies in man after open heart surgery using fixed atrial electrodes. *Circulation* 60:665, 1979.

144. Wildenthal, K., Fuller, D. S., and Shapiro, W. Paroxysmal atrial arrhythmias induced by hyperventilation. *Am. J. Cardiol.* 21:436, 1968.

145. Wilson, W. S., Judge, R. D., and Siegel, J. H. A simple diagnostic sign in ventricular tachycardia. *N. Engl. J. Med.* 270:446, 1964.

146. Winkle, R. A., Derrington, D. C., and Schroeder, J. S. Characteristics of ventricular tachycardia in ambulatory patients. *Am. J. Cardiol.* 39:487, 1977.

147. Wit, A. L., and Friedman, P. L. Basis for ventricular arrhythmias accompanying myocardial infarction. *Arch. Intern. Med.* 135:459, 1975.

148. Wu, D., and Denes, P. Mechanisms of paroxysmal supraventricular tachycardia. *Arch. Intern. Med.* 135:437, 1975.

149. Yoneda, S., Murata, M., and Akaike, A. Persistent atrial standstill developed in a patient with rheumatic heart disease: Electrophysiological and histological study. *Clin. Cardiol.* 1:43, 1978.

150. Young, D., et al. Wenckebach atrioventricular block (Mobitz type 1) in children and adolescents. *Am. J. Cardiol.* 40:393, 1977.

151. Zipes, D. P., et al. Atrial tachycardia without P waves masquerading as an A-V junctional tachycardia. *Circulation* 55:253, 1977.

151A. Zivin, A. Evaluation and management of supraventricular tachycardia in adults. *Curr. Pract. Med.* 2:2133, 1999.

9. Electronic Pacemakers

1. How can you recognize immediately on an electrocardiogram (ECG) that an electronic pacemaker is present?
   ANS.: Several of the ECG leads show vertical spikes repeatedly at the same place in the cycle.
2. List the common types of pacemakers by their triggering arrangement.
   ANS.: a. Fixed-rate ventricular.
   b. Demand, of which there are two types: a ventricular-inhibited type and a ventricular-synchronous type.
   c. Atrial and P wave-triggered.
   d. Atrioventricular (AV) sequential.
3. What is meant by (a) a bipolar system and (b) a unipolar system?
   ANS.: a. In a bipolar system the two pacing electrodes (anode and cathode) are both in the heart at the end of the wire.
   b. In a unipolar system one pacing electrode (cathode) is in the heart and the other (anode) is at some distant site under the skin (usually incorporated into the pacemaker casing).
   Note: Bipolar pacing produces small spikes, which do not distort the QRS complexes that follow. On the other hand, because unipolar spikes are generally of great amplitude and biphasic, they can markedly distort the subsequent QRS.

FIXED-RATE PACEMAKERS

1. How can a fixed-rate ventricular pacemaker be recognized?
   ANS.: A vertical pacemaker spike occurs at regular intervals despite the kind of arrhythmia. If the pacemaker is working well, the spike is followed by a QRS whenever the ventricle is not refractory. This kind of pacemaker is rare today.

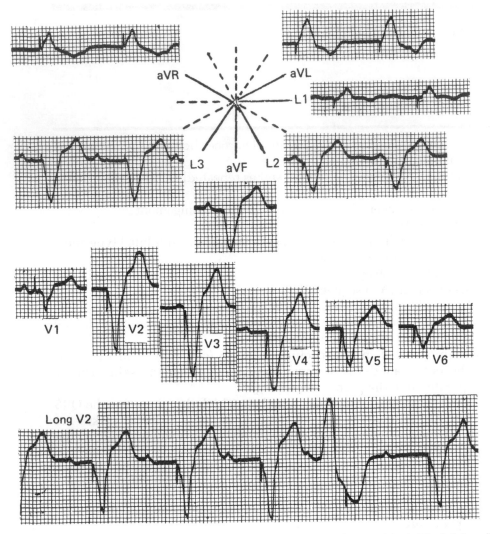

Fixed-rate pacemaker in a 75-year-old man with acquired complete AV block. The left bundle branch block configuration indicates that the pacemaker is implanted in the right ventricle. Because the premature ventricular contraction (PVC) in the long strip has an uninterrupted pacemaker spike (on the S-T segment), it is a fixed rate pacemaker. A demand pacemaker would have been inhibited by the PVC. Note that the pacemaker has fired on the vulnerable zone of the T of the PVC.

2. What risk is posed by a fixed-rate pacemaker?
   ANS.: a. If the patient can conduct through the AV node (because he or she either regains AV conduction or never had AV block), the pacemaker spikes are in 'competition' for the ventricle. The spikes can then occur in the vulnerable zone of a sinus beat's T wave and produce ventricular tachycardia (VT) or fibrillation if the patient has ischemia or electrolyte imbalance or is under the influence of cardiac drug excess.

*b. Even in the presence of complete AV block, it can also fire on the vulnerable zone of a T wave produced by an early QRS, e.g., PVC or reciprocal beat [2]. (See p. 534 for an explanation of reciprocal beats.)

L2

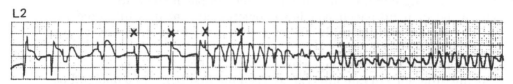

A patient with acute inferior infarction. A fixed-rate pacemaker is set at 90 in an attempt at overdrive pacing to prevent refractory VT. A pacemaker spike on the peak of a T wave produces ventricular fibrillation.

3. What protects most patients from the dangerous effects of a pacemaker spike's falling in the vulnerable zone of a T wave?
   ANS.: A pacemaker spike has too little strength to produce dangerous arrhythmias in the absence of ischemia, electrolyte abnormalities, or cardiac drugs.

DEMAND PACEMAKERS

1. What is a demand pacemaker?
   ANS.: It is a ventricular pacemaker that is set to fire after a pause whose duration is preset by the physician. The common type is inhibited by an early R wave and is usually known as an R wave or ventricular-inhibited pacemaker. A sensing mechanism can detect all R waves occurring earlier than the preset pacing interval. These sensed R waves will inhibit the pacemaker.

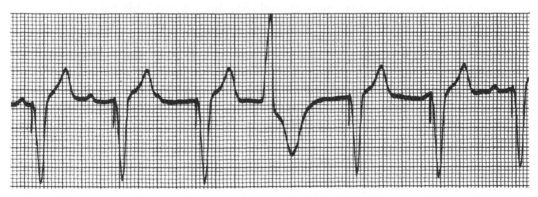

R wave-inhibited demand pacemaker. Note that an early QRS inhibits the pacemaker, so that no spike is seen when the PVC occurs and the pacemaker is reset.

* Material marked with an asterisk is included for reference and for advanced students in cardiology.

2. Why is a demand pacemaker preferable to a fixed-rate pacemaker?

   ANS.: A demand pacemaker fires only when a long pause occurs. Therefore it never fires near the peak of the T wave if there are premature beats or if the patient produces his or her own QRS-Ts in competition with the pacemaker.

3. What controls the length of the pause before a demand pacemaker fires?

   ANS.: The usual demand pacemaker is so constructed that it is inhibited by an early R wave, and it fires only after a preset pause. (It must 'sense' an R wave before it can be inhibited.)

*4. What is meant by pacemaker hysteresis?

   ANS.: It is the difference in rate interval between the first firing of a demand pacemaker and its subsequent firing rate, which is usually faster. For example, a pacemaker may be set to fire when the patient's own rate drops to below 50 per minute, but if it continues to fire it usually fires at a rate faster than 60. Hysteresis allows the patient's own intrinsic rate to fall to as low as possible before the electronic pacemaker fires, so that both sinus rhythm and battery life are preserved as much as possible. However, once the pacemaker has to take over, its successive firing rate is fast enough to give the patient a good cardiac output.

5. How can you recognize an R wave-inhibited type of demand pacemaker on an ECG?

   ANS.: When there are no pacemaker spikes except after long R-R intervals and a pacemaker induced a series of QRSs are reset by a PVC or a premature atrial contraction (PAC).

6. What is an R wave-triggered, or ventricular-triggered, demand pacemaker?

   ANS.: It is a pacemaker that always fires in response to the patient's own QRS; i.e., it is triggered by an R wave. This pacemaker produces fusion beats and is rarely used today.

7. When are atrial stimulating pacemakers used?

   ANS.: When there is no AV block but the sinus mechanism is so slow that it gives rise to cerebral symptoms, heart failure symptoms, or symptomatic ventricular arrhythmias. (This complex is known as the sick sinus syndrome.) An atrial demand pacemaker is inhibited when a P wave is sensed. An AV sequential pacemaker is a type of dual chamber pacing. This pacemaker both paces and senses in the ventricle but only paces in the atrium. The atrial and ventricular stimuli are separated by an appropriate AV delay simulating an AV node. A premature QRS will inhibit the ventricular pacemaker.

8. What are the two types of dual-chamber modes?

   ANS.: Those in which the ventricles are paced following a patient's own P waves (VDD, DDD) or those in which there is sequential atrial and ventricular pacing (DV1, DD1, and DDD).

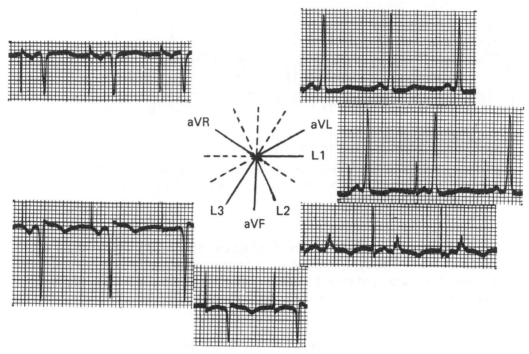

A 69-year-old man had severe coronary cardiomyopathy with episodes of ventricular tachycardia that could not be prevented by overdriving with a fixed-rate pacemaker. They could be prevented only by the improved cardiac function resulting from the atrial 'kick' provided by a demand atrial pacemaker plus a rate faster than 70.

9. What is the purpose of P wave-triggered ventricular pacing? How does it work?

    ANS.: Its purpose is to allow the patient's sinoatrial (SA) node to control a ventricular pacemaker rate and to have an atrial contraction preceding every ventricular contraction, thereby increasing stroke volume. The P wave is sensed by a sensing electrode in or on an atrial surface. This atrial sensing electrode is connected to a pacing electrode in or on a ventricle so that an AV sequential system is used. A delay of about 240 msec (0.24 sec) is built in between the atrial sensing and the ventricular pacing electrode (an electronic AV node).

10. How can you recognize P wave-triggered pacing on an ECG?

    ANS.: At the end of each P-R interval there is a pacemaker spike, followed immediately by a wide QRS.

11. What built-in safeguards are there in P wave-triggered ventricular pacemakers against the effects of atrial arrhythmias such as tachycardias or fibrillation?

    ANS.: Atrial tachycardia causes a 2:1 or 3:1 AV block in the pacemaker mechanism. Atrial fibrillation causes the pacemaker to convert to a fixed-rate mode, and it then paces independently of the atrium.

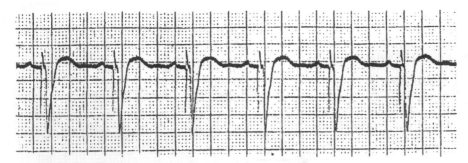

Atrial triggered pacing. An electrode in the R atrium picks up the P wave which is fed into a pacemaker which paces the ventricle after a predetermined P-R interval. The heart rate can respond to exercise and emotion.

12. How can you tell that the AV node is normal when considering putting in an atrial pacemaker in a patient with symptomatic sinus node dysfunction?

ANS.: If rapid atrial pacing of over 130 does not produce any more than a type 1 second-degree AV block or if carotid sinus pressure does not produce an AV block.

Note: Dual-chamber pacing is necessary:
a. If the atrial 'kick' must be preserved as in patients with stiff ventricles.
b. In those with pacemaker syndromes.
c. If the sinus node is unable to respond to metabolic needs so that a single chamber atrial pacemaker is not indicated.

Since a pacemaker QRS hides the patient's pre-pacemaker QRS, you can find out if the patient has any QRS abnormalities using an external pulse generator. One terminal of the generator is placed over the pacemaker pocket on the patient's chest and the other terminal is placed near the apex beat. The external pulse generator rate is set at a rate faster than the implanted pacemaker rate, and the voltage is gradually increased until the implanted pacemaker is completely inhibited. The rhythm will then be the patient's slow sinus rhythm, junctional, or ventricular escape rhythm. Or the patient may show a ventricular arrest. But as soon as the external pacemaker is turned off, the implanted pacemaker will resume pacing.

THREE-LETTER PACEMAKER CODE

1. Which letters are used to describe pacemakers and their functions?

ANS.: A = atrium
V = ventricle

D = dual (atrium and ventricle)
I = inhibited
T = triggered
O = no inhibition or triggering

2. In the three-letter code what does each letter signify?
   ANS.: The letters are placed in positions 1, 2, and 3. The first letter signifies the chamber paced, i.e., A, V, or D. The second signifies the chamber sensed, i.e., A, V, or D. The third signifies what is done with what it senses; i.e., it is either inhibited or triggered by what complex is seen in the chamber that the second letter shows.

3. Give the three-letter code for a demand or R wave-inhibited pacemaker.
   ANS.: VVI; i.e., it is pacing the ventricle (the first V), it is sensing the QRS in the ventricle (the second V), and it is inhibited by that QRS (the I).

4. What are the most advanced pacemakers called?
   ANS.: DDD; i.e., they can be programmed to pace and sense either atrium or ventricle, as well as be triggered or inhibited by either atrium or ventricle.

*5. What is the rarely used five-letter pacemaker code?
   ANS.: The fourth position refers to programmable functions:
   P = programmable (rate and/or output)
   M = multiprogrammable
   C = communicating
   O = none
   The fifth position refers to special antitachyarrhythmia functions:
   B = bursts
   N = normal rate competition
   S = scanning
   E = external

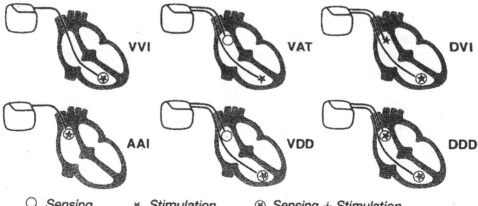

○ *Sensing*   ✳ *Stimulation*   ⊛ *Sensing + Stimulation*

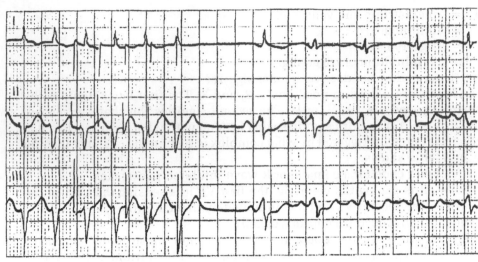

Burst pacing for 1 sec at 214/min to end atrial tachycardia in WPW syndrome. The antitachycardia pacemaker electrode was in the coronary sinus.

PACEMAKER FAILURE

1. What is the most sensitive way of detecting incipient pacemaker battery failure?
   ANS.: The firing rate slows down, and the height of the pacemaker spike decreases. A slowing of as little as 1 beat per minute is significant for suggesting battery failure.

   Note: An ordinary ECG machine cannot pick up a change of 1 beat per minute. Paper speed can vary by as much as 2 beats per minute. Therefore most centers require a change of 5 beats per minute before a pacemaker is replaced.

2. If it takes more than the usual amperage from a pacemaker to stimulate the myocardium, what is said to be happening?
   ANS.: The myocardial threshold for stimulation has risen and may continue to rise until it does not capture the ventricle at all.

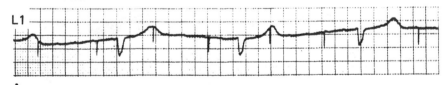

A

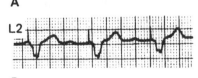

B

A 60-year-old man had a pacemaker implanted 3 months before and was re-admitted because of recurrent Stokes-Adams attacks. He was taking no medication. A. The pacemaker spikes are firing at its present rate of 70, but the pacemaker does not capture the ventricles which are controlled by an idioventricular pacemaker. B. After the pacemaker electrode was repositioned, each spike captured the ventricle.

*3. What factors other than fibrosis or other causes of poor electrode contact with the myocardium can raise the stimulation threshold?

ANS.: Hypoxia, myocardial depressant drugs such as quinidine, and electrolyte problems such as hypokalemia or marked hyperkalemia [4].

Note: If the stimulation threshold is high, the pacemaker may still be able to stimulate the myocardium near the terminal portion of the T wave, i.e., during the supernormal period (see p. 490).

*4. How can you prove that low voltage is the cause of malsensing?

ANS.: By showing that the sensing mechanism itself is actually intact. You can demonstrate it if you apply chest wall stimulation with an external pacemaker. By gradually increasing the spike amplitude of an external pacemaker, an amperage is reached that turns off the internal pacemaker, provided the sensing mechanism is intact.

5. What is meant by the 'pacemaker syndrome'? What is the treatment?

ANS.: Symptoms of weakness and orthostatic dizziness due to retrograde conduction into the atrium. This results from atrial contraction during ventricular systole, i.e., while the AV valves are closed. The pacemaker should be removed and a single chamber atrial pacemaker (if AV conduction is intact) or dual-chamber pacing can be substituted.

RECOGNITION OF IMPLANTATION SITE

1. If a pacemaker is in the right or left ventricle, what kind of bundle branch block is seen?

ANS.: A pacemaker in the right ventricle produces a left bundle branch block (LBBB), and one in the left ventricle produces a right bundle branch block (RBBB).

2. How can a pacemaker in the right ventricle produce a right bundle branch block pattern in V1 and a left bundle branch block pattern in the limb leads? How is this confusion resolved?

ANS.: If the pacemaker is at the apex of the right ventricle, it can produce an anterior divisional block so that the terminal force is superior and slightly anterior. If the V1 electrode is placed one interspace lower, the QS of the left bundle block will be seen [2A].

*3. What can cause the sudden appearance of RBBB morphology in a patient with a right ventricular pacemaker?

ANS.: a. The tip of the catheter may have perforated the myocardium or the septum and may be stimulating the left ventricle.

b. The tip may have entered the coronary sinus.

c. The pacemaker may be stimulating small branches of the left bundle that extend to the right side of the septum [1].

Note: The terminal force in V1 is a more reliable sign of which ventricle contains the pacemaker than are the limb leads. The slightest terminal negativity in V1 should suggest a left bundle branch block pattern and therefore a right ventricular pacemaker.

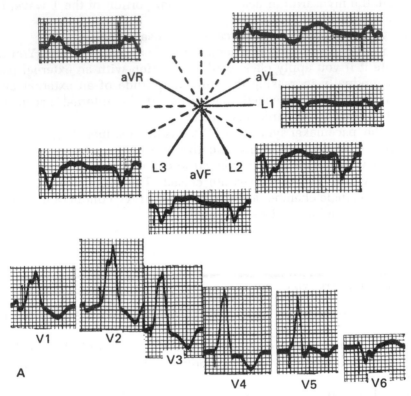

A

ECG obtained after a transvenous demand pacemaker was supposed to have been placed in the right ventricle of a 73-year-old man. Although it was pacing well, the RBBB configuration with left axis deviation suggested that the electrodes were stimulating the left ventricle. It was discovered that the electrode had been accidentally placed in the coronary sinus.

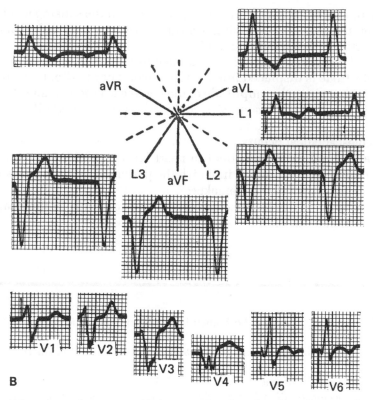

B

When the catheter was withdrawn and replaced in the right ventricle, this ECG was obtained and showed an LBBB.

*4. What is meant by a programmable pacemaker?
    ANS.: The application of a magnet externally can change the rate of firing, voltage output, spike, firing threshold, sensing threshold, or refractory period.

PACEMAKER ARRHYTHMIAS

*1. What can cause a type 1 second-degree pacemaker-to-QRS block?
    ANS.: High doses of procainamide plus hyperkalemia, or lidocaine plus metabolic acidosis [3].
*2. How can a demand pacemaker that is controlling each QRS have an occasional unexpectedly delayed spike?
    ANS.: A demand pacemaker is occasionally inhibited by a T wave if the sensing device is oversensitive.
        *Note: a. A persistently T-sensing (T-inhibited) demand pacemaker never produces asystole. It can only result in a bradycardia that has a cycle that is never longer than the escape rate of the pacemaker plus the Q-to-peak-of-T interval. It usually leads to a rate of 40 to 50 per minute.

b. A method of testing for oversensing is to turn off the sensing mechanism altogether by applying a magnet over the pacemaker and converting it to a fixed-rate mode.

*3. What causes unexpected P wave sensing? How is it diagnosed by ECG?

ANS.: If the sensing electrode is displaced into the right atrium or proximal portion of the coronary sinus, since the amplitude of the P wave is much greater than that of the QRS, the pacemaker 'senses' each P wave and is turned off. If the patient has complete AV block the ECG then shows a series of P waves with no QRS until an escape beat occurs.

4. What gives a better cardiac output for a patient in heart failure, an AV sequential pacemaker or a P wave triggered pacemaker in which the patient's own P waves are sensed in order to drive the ventricular pacemaker?

ANS.: A P synchronous pacemaker, because the pacemaker responds to the heart rate needs of emotion or exertion.

REFERENCES

1. Abernathy, W. S., and Crevey, B. J. Right bundle branch block during transvenous ventricular pacing. *Am. Heart J.* 90:774, 1975.
2. Barold, S. S., Linhart, J. W., and Samet, P. Reciprocal beating induced by ventricular pacing. *Circulation* 38:330, 1968.
2A. Klein, H. O. Unusual QRS associated with pacemakers. *Chest* 87:517, 1985.
3. Mehta, J., and Khan, A. J. Pacemaker Wenckebach phenomenon due to antiarrhythmic drug toxicity. *Cardiology* 61:189, 1976.
4. O'Reilly, M. V., Murnaghan, D. P., and Williams, M. B. Transvenous pacemaker failure induced by hyperkalemia. *J.A.M.A.* 228:336, 1974.

0.*Bundle of His Recordings

*TECHNIQUE

*1. How is a clinical recording made of the bundle of His?

    ANS.: A cardiac catheter is passed from the inferior vena cava into the right atrium, then through the tricuspid valve into the right ventricle. At the end of the catheter are two or more tiny electrodes, 5 to 10 mm apart. The proximal ends of the catheter leads are connected to an ECG amplifier for intracardiac recording of a bipolar electrogram, i.e., for recording the result of current flowing between any two of the tiny electrodes at the distal end of the catheter. As the catheter is pulled back slowly through the tricuspid valve, the electrodes pass over the region of the bundle of His when the catheter lies across it. When the catheter tip is in the ideal position against the septal leaflet of the tricuspid valve, a sharp, tiny biphasic or triphasic spike is recorded [13].

*2. How can you tell that a recorded spike is from the bundle of His?

    ANS.: The His bundle spike (H) occurs between the P wave and the QRS of the simultaneously recorded external ECG. It also occurs between the atrial depolarization spikes (A) and QRS depolarization spikes (V) on the bipolar electrogram (His bundle electrogram).

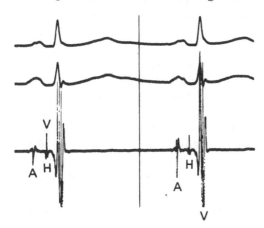

Normal bundle of His recording. The A-H interval is 110 msec. The H-V interval is 35 msec.

    Note: a. Two groups of vibrations other than the bundle of His spike are seen on His bundle electrograms. One represents atrial electrical activity close to the atrioventricular (AV) node (A in the preceding electrogram); the other represents ventricular depolarization activity (V in the preceding electrogram).

* Material marked with an asterisk is included for reference and for advanced students in cardiology.

   b. His bundle spikes can be best recorded by using the highest frequency on the ECG amplifier, preferably as high as 500 Hz.
*3. Can AV nodal or bundle branch activity be recorded by the preceding catheter technique?
   ANS.: Yes. The N or AV nodal potential is a slow wave with a notched upstroke and downstroke between the atrial ECG and the His bundle spike. A right bundle potential can often be seen as a spike following the His spike.
   Note: No recordings have so far been made from the anterior or posterior divisions of the left bundle branch in humans.

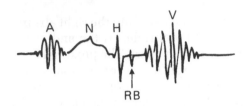

*INTERVALS FROM THE HIS BUNDLE ELECTROGRAM

*1. What is the interval between the beginning of the P to the His bundle spike called?
   ANS.: The P-H interval.
*2. What is the ventricular and atrial electrical activity in a His bundle electrogram called?
   ANS.: Ventricular depolarization is called the V deflection, or the ventricular electrogram. The local atrial activity close to the AV node that is recorded from the His bundle electrode catheter is called the A deflection, or atrial electrogram.
   Note: The P-A interval measures intraatrial conduction and is 45 ± 15 msec. The A-H interval represents AV nodal conduction time and is about 90 ± 30 msec; i.e., AV nodal conduction takes about twice as long as intraatrial conduction [12].
*3. What does the P-H interval represent, and what is its normal duration?
   ANS.: It measures intraatrial plus AV nodal conduction times and is about 120 ± 30 msec.
   Note: Because the timing of the A deflections depends on catheter position, which may change slightly from moment to moment, the A deflection is usually ignored; i.e., changes in AV nodal conduction are usually measured by P-H intervals.
*4. What is the interval between the His bundle potential (H) and the QRS called, and what is its duration?
   ANS.: It has been called the H-V interval (His to ventricular activation), as well as the H-Q or H-R interval. It is about 40 ± 15 msec.
   Note: a. The P-H interval is about three times the H-V interval.
       b. The interval between the onset of H to the onset of QRS represents conduction time through the bundle of His and bundle branches to the beginning of muscle activation.

*SUMMARY OF WHAT HAS BEEN LEARNED OR CONFIRMED ABOUT THE CONDUCTION SYSTEM BY HIS BUNDLE ELECTROGRAMS

*AV Blocks

*1. Atrial pacing (with a pacing catheter in the right atrium) prolongs the P-R interval by prolonging only the A-H interval [5]. A sufficiently early paced beat can also prolong the H-V time and produce differential blocks along the right and left bundles and their divisions, but probably only in subjects with latent conduction problems [7].

*2. First-degree AV block may be due to
    a. Intraatrial delay alone (P-A time prolonged).
    b. AV nodal delay alone (A-H time prolonged).
    c. Bundle branch delay (H-Q time prolonged) [10].
    d. Intra-His block, i.e., either a wide His electrogram or a split H electrogram (H,H').
    e. Combinations of the above [4].
    Note: Congenital first-degree AV block is usually due to a prolonged A-H interval (AV nodal delay) [4].

*3. Although the vast majority of type 1 second-degree AV blocks (Wenckebach periods) are due to blocks proximal to the bundle of His, some are due to intra-His blocks with gradually increasing H to H' intervals [9].

*4. Although the vast majority of type 2 second-degree AV blocks are due to blocks beyond the bundle of His, they are occasionally due to blocks proximal to the bundle of His [9]. A sudden block between a split H and H' has also been recorded. A sudden 'dropped beat' may even be caused by a nonpropagated His bundle premature depolarization with both proximal and distal blocks.

*5. All complete, acquired AV blocks with wide QRSs that have been studied have been found to have a pacemaker below the bundle of His. If the QRS is narrow, however, the pacemakers are usually just proximal to the bundle of His [9, 10]. Idioventricular beats are often preceded by a right or left bundle branch deflection; i.e., they often originate in the main bundle branches.
    Note: In acute inferior or posterior wall infarction, a delay or block in conduction is usually proximal to the His bundle; AV block following anteroseptal myocardial infarction is usually related to a delay or a block distal to the His bundle.

*Effect of Drugs

*1. Isoproterenol, phenytoin sodium (diphenylhydantoin), and atropine shorten only the P-H interval while digitalis and propranolol lengthen the A-H interval [4].

2. Lidocaine has very little effect on either A-H or H-V times, but intravenous procainamide can increase both [4]. In ischemic hearts, lidocaine can prolong conduction in the His bundle and the right bundle branch [6].

*Bundle Branch Block and Aberrant Conduction

*1. In right bundle branch block (RBBB), fixed or intermittent, the H-V interval is usually normal, indicating normal conduction through the left bundle branch [1, 11].

*2. In left bundle branch block (LBBB), fixed or intermittent, even with normal R-R intervals, H-V time is often prolonged (more than 50 msec), suggesting that patients with LBBB often have conduction delays in the right bundle as well. Therefore trifascicular disease is probably often present with LBBB [12].

Note: In alternating bundle branch block with a changing P-R interval, the latter is related to changing conduction along the bundle branches rather than through the AV node (as shown by the changing H-V intervals) [11].

Preexcitation

Atrioventricular (AV) preexcitation complexes have been shown to be due to fusion between normal AV and accessory pathway conduction [3].

---

*Ectopic Pacemakers

Junctional beats with slight aberrancy have sometimes been shown actually to be due to a pacemaker in the left or right bundle.

REFERENCES

1. Berkowitz, W. D., et al. The use of His bundle recordings in the analysis of unilateral and bilateral bundle branch block. *Am. Heart J.* 81:340, 1971.
2. Castellanos, A., Jr., et al. His bundle electrograms in patients with short P-R intervals, narrow QRS complexes, and paroxysmal tachycardias. *Circulation* 43:667, 1971.
3. Castellanos, A., Jr., et al. His bundle electrograms in two cases of Wolff-Parkinson-White (preexcitation) syndrome. *Circulation* 41:399, 1970.
4. Damato, A. N., and Lau, S. H. Clinical value of the electrogram of the conducting system. *Prog. Cardiovasc. Dis.* 13:119, 1970.
5. Damato, A. N., et al. A study of atrioventricular conduction in man using premature atrial stimulation and His bundle recordings. *Circulation* 40:61, 1969.
6. Gerstenblith, G., et al. Effect of lidocaine on conduction in the ischemic His-Purkinje system of dogs. *Am. J. Cardiol.* 42:587, 1978.
7. Haft, J. E., et al. Assessment of atrioventricular conduction in left and right bundle branch block using His bundle electrograms and atrial pacing. *Am. J. Cardiol.* 27:474, 1971.
8. Lau, S. H., et al. A study of atrioventricular conduction in atrial fibrillation and flutter in man using His bundle recordings. *Circulation* 40:71, 1969.
9. Narula, O. S., et al. Significance of His and left bundle recordings from the left heart in man. *Circulation* 42:385, 1970.
10. Narula, O. S., et al. Atrioventricular block localization and classification by His bundle recordings. *Am. J. Med.* 50:146, 1971.
11. Ranganathan, N., et al. His bundle electrogram in bundle branch block. *Circulation* 45:282, 1972.
12. Rosen, K. M., et al. Bundle branch and ventricular activation in man. *Circulation* 43:193, 1971.
13. Scherlag, B. J., et al. Catheter technique for recording His bundle activity in man. *Circulation* 39:13, 1969.

1. Systematic Approach to Reading an Electrocardiogram

On the left side of the reporting sheet, make a note of the heart rate, P-R interval, QRS width, and then of all abnormalities. On the right side, note your impressions, i.e., the conclusions reached as a result of finding the abnormalities.

1. To read the heart rate use one of the many rate rules available, or count large divisions between R waves and divide into 300. Take the heart rate to the nearest 5 or 10. Do not read a rate as 74; it is not only easier to remember 75, but a heart rate usually changes at least slightly from minute to minute. Read a sinus rate of 55 or less as sinus bradycardia and a sinus rate of more than 100 as sinus tachycardia. If the patient is in atrial fibrillation, count the number of R waves in 6 seconds (it is 3 seconds between two vertical lines in the margin of many ECG paper rolls) and multiply by 10. Do not give a range. It is more important to know the average rate per minute. If no vertical 3-second marks are present, count the number of R waves in 30 large divisions (30 × 0.2 second = 6 seconds) and multiply by 10.

2. To measure the P-R interval count the small divisions between the beginning of the P and the beginning of the QRS. Multiply this figure by 4, and then put in the decimal point, e.g., four divisions = 16 = 0.16 second (160 msec). Read any P-R of more than 200 msec (0.2 sec) as first-degree atrioventricular (AV) block; even a P-R of 200 msec should be read as first-degree AV block if there is a sinus tachycardia or the patient is a young child. Read any P-R of less than 120 msec (0.12 sec) as some sort of preexcitation unless the P vector is abnormal (e.g., negative in leads 1, 2, or aVF), in which case report it as an ectopic atrial pacemaker.

3. To measure the QRS duration measure the duration of white space between the initial and terminal direction of the QRS. Use the lead with the widest QRS in the entire ECG, but be careful to avoid using QRSs with slurred or rounded endings, which make the QRS appear to be artifactually wide. If you report a QRS duration as short as 40 msec (0.04 sec), you are probably making an error (unless you are reading pediatric ECGs). Read a QRS of more than 90 msec (0.09 sec) as some sort of conduction defect, which usually is some degree of bundle branch or divisional block but occasionally is a periinfarction block or AV accessory bundle conduction. If it is not any of these, call it a 'nonspecific intraventricular conduction defect.'

4. Look for QRS negativity in the 'critical leads,' leads 1, 2, and aVF. If negativity is found, an axis abnormality is present and should usually be read as follows: right axis deviation if more than + 90°; left axis deviation if between 0° and − 30°; and marked left axis deviation if more than − 30°. The latter is recognized by predominant negativity in lead 2. All left axes are anterior divisional blocks if there is a terminal positivity in aVR and no S in lead 1.

5. Look for left ventricular hypertrophy (LVH) voltage criteria in the limb leads (index of Lewis: RL1 + SL3 = 17 after subtracting opposites). Then look at the chest leads for LVH voltage criteria, especially SV1 + RV5 or SV2 + RV6 = 35 mm. (Do not subtract opposites.) However, do not report LVH unless some other sign of it is seen

in the ECG, e.g., S-T, T abnormalities, left atrial overload, or incomplete left bundle branch block pattern. If no other changes are present, report it as a 'nonspecific voltage increase' in limb or chest leads unless the patient is under 30, in which case simply report it as a normal ECG. If an LVH strain pattern is present and no voltage criteria for LVH are present, report 'LVH without voltage criteria suggested.'

Note: A diagnosis of hypertension, aortic stenosis, or some other cause of LVH should be considered as a secondary criterion for LVH, to use if voltage criteria are present.

6. Look for T negativity in critical and left precordial leads. If they are probably secondary to LVH or bundle branch block, nothing need be written about them. If the T is more deeply negative than expected for LVH alone, e.g., 5 mm or more, report it as 'myocardial ischemia' or 'fibrosis.' Ischemia, however, implies that the changes are acute. A notched T alone is read as a 'nonspecific minor T abnormality.'

7. Look for progression of the R/S ratio across the precordium. If it does not progress, look for signs of infarction or early right ventricular hypertrophy (RVH). If the initial or terminal forces are disturbed by a conduction abnormality such as right bundle branch block or anterior divisional block, a poor R/S progression does not mean infarction or early RVH.

8. Look for the septal vector and be sure it is normal. Mention a q in the limb leads only if it is more than 30 msec (0.03 sec) wide or is relatively deep in aVF, i.e., at least one-third of the R height in aVF or 50 percent of the R in aVL (provided there is no S wave). Do not mention a relatively deep Q in lead 3 as a sign of infarction. It represents LVH, not infarction.

   In the chest leads, the tiniest q in the wrong place (i.e., if it is not a septal q) suggests an infarct. A normal septal q in the precordium is seen only in the left ventricular leads and perhaps in the transitional lead. With incomplete left bundle branch block (LBBB) patterns (i.e., without a left precordial Q), do not read a Q only in V1, V2, or only in V1, V2, and V3 as an infarct. Only a Q from V1 to V4 indicates definite infarction (in the absence of complete LBBB), even if the q in V4 is minute. Because a Q in V1, V1 and V2, or V1 to V3 *may* be an infarct, you could mention 'anterolateral infarction *may* be present or it may be an incomplete LBBB pattern.'

9. Read infarcts as 'old' if only abnormal q waves and no S-T, T changes are seen. If an injury current is present, read an acute infarct. If the T is going in the same direction as the S-T, call it hyperacute. If nonspecific T changes are present, report the infarct as 'age indeterminate.' If an injury current is present in a patient not suspected of having an acute infarct, report it as 'acute infarction or old aneurysm.'

10. If the requisition says 'no digitalis' or fails to say whether digitalis has been administered, yet obviously sagging S-Ts with relatively high U waves, low T amplitude, and short Q-Ts are present, report 'digitalis effect suggested.' The patient may have been taking digitalis recently. Do not describe T waves as 'flat' when you mean 'low.' Only S-Ts should be described as flat. Because T waves never really have flat tops, such an artifactual appearance means a notched T.

11. Look for relatively high U waves. Do not mention U waves at all unless the T waves are low. Record them as 'hypokalemia suggested,' but only in the absence of LVH, digitalis effect, or notched T waves, unless the U is markedly exaggerated. (All notched T waves have relatively high U waves. The abnormality here is the notched T, not the U.)

12. Read tall P waves (more than 2.5 mm) as right atrial overload. Do not read a wide, notched P as left atrial overload. Record it as an intraatrial block. If in V1 there are

negative terminal P forces one small division in area, read it as left atrial overload. Remember that it is a minor sign of LVH (in the absence of mitral stenosis).

A NOTE ON DESCRIBING PREMATURE BEATS OR COMPLEXES

1. Interpret arrhythmias separately, either before or after the foregoing steps are taken. If more than one premature complex is seen, report 'frequent PVCs or PACs'; otherwise, report 'occasional PVCs or PACs.' If every other complex is premature, add the word *bigeminy* to the description, e.g., 'premature ventricular complexes in bigeminy.' Trigeminy or quadrigeminy should be used for other appropriate groupings.
2. Describe where a premature complex occurs in the cycle if it is unusual, e.g., 'end-diastolic or interpolated PVCs.'
3. If the premature atrial complex has a QRS that looks different from the usual ones, report aberrancy.
4. If marked variable coupling is seen between the premature complex and the preceding complex, look for parasystole (see p. 529). See p. 586 on steps to take when reading a complicated arrhythmia.

A NOTE ON DIASTOLIC PREMATURE BEATS OR COMPLEXES

Index

Printed and bound by CPI Group (UK) Ltd, Croydon, CR0 4YY

23/10/2024

01778245-0015